Advances in Cancer Multimodal Approach: Biomarkers, Mechanisms, Surgical Procedures and Oncological Therapies

Advances in Cancer Multimodal Approach: Biomarkers, Mechanisms, Surgical Procedures and Oncological Therapies

Editors

Valentin Titus Grigorean
Daniel Alin Cristian

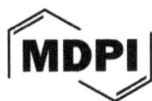

Basel • Beijing • Wuhan • Barcelona • Belgrade • Novi Sad • Cluj • Manchester

Editors
Valentin Titus Grigorean
"Carol Davila" University of
Medicine and Pharmacy
Bucharest
Romania

Daniel Alin Cristian
"Carol Davila" University of
Medicine and Pharmacy
Bucharest
Romania

Editorial Office
MDPI AG
Grosspeteranlage 5
4052 Basel, Switzerland

This is a reprint of articles from the Special Issue published online in the open access journal *Medicina* (ISSN 1648-9144) (available at: https://www.mdpi.com/journal/medicina/special_issues/0WZ3R01AI4).

For citation purposes, cite each article independently as indicated on the article page online and as indicated below:

Lastname, A.A.; Lastname, B.B. Article Title. *Journal Name* **Year**, *Volume Number*, Page Range.

ISBN 978-3-7258-1843-3 (Hbk)
ISBN 978-3-7258-1844-0 (PDF)
doi.org/10.3390/books978-3-7258-1844-0

© 2024 by the authors. Articles in this book are Open Access and distributed under the Creative Commons Attribution (CC BY) license. The book as a whole is distributed by MDPI under the terms and conditions of the Creative Commons Attribution-NonCommercial-NoDerivs (CC BY-NC-ND) license.

Contents

Valentin Titus Grigorean and Daniel Alin Cristian
Cancer—Yesterday, Today, Tomorrow
Reprinted from: *Medicina* **2023**, *59*, 98, doi:10.3390/medicina59010098 1

Irinel-Gabriel Dicu-Andreescu, Marian-Augustin Marincaș, Anca-Angela Simionescu, Ioana Dicu-Andreescu, Sînziana-Octavia Ionescu, Virgiliu-Mihail Prunoiu, et al.
The Role of Lymph Node Downstaging Following Neoadjuvant Treatment in a Group of Patients with Advanced Stage Cervical Cancer
Reprinted from: *Medicina* **2024**, *60*, 871, doi:10.3390/medicina60060871 3

Suji Lee, Jee Yeon Kim, So Jeong Lee, Chung Su Hwang, Hyun Jung Lee, Kyung Bin Kim, et al.
Impact of Neoadjuvant Chemotherapy (NAC) on Biomarker Expression in Breast Cancer
Reprinted from: *Medicina* **2024**, *60*, 737, doi:10.3390/medicina60050737 19

Ola Abu Al Karsaneh, Arwa Al Anber, Sahar AlMustafa, Hussien AlMa'aitah, Batool AlQadri, Abir Igbaria, et al.
Human Papillomavirus Is Rare and Does Not Correlate with $p16^{INK4A}$ Expression in Non-Small-Cell Lung Cancer in a Jordanian Subpopulation
Reprinted from: *Medicina* **2024**, *60*, 660, doi:10.3390/medicina60040660 33

Lucian Dragoș Bratu, Michael Schenker, Puiu Olivian Stovicek, Ramona Adriana Schenker, Alina Maria Mehedințeanu, Tradian Ciprian Berisha, et al.
Retrospective Evaluation of the Efficacy of Total Neoadjuvant Therapy and Chemoradiotherapy Neoadjuvant Treatment in Relation to Surgery in Patients with Rectal Cancer
Reprinted from: *Medicina* **2024**, *60*, 646, doi:10.3390/medicina60040656 48

Seunghak Lee, Sunmin Park, Chai Hong Rim, Young Hen Lee, Soon Young Kwon, Kyung Ho Oh and Won Sup Yoon
A Potential Radiomics–Clinical Model for Predicting Failure of Lymph Node Control after Definite Radiotherapy in Locally Advanced Head and Neck Cancer
Reprinted from: *Medicina* **2024**, *60*, 92, doi:10.3390/medicina60010092 63

Tomas Januskevicius, Ieva Vaicekauskaite, Rasa Sabaliauskaite, Augustinas Matulevicius, Alvydas Vezelis, Albertas Ulys, et al.
Germline DNA Damage Response Gene Mutations in Localized Prostate Cancer
Reprinted from: *Medicina* **2024**, *60*, 73, doi:10.3390/medicina60010073 74

Wee Liam Ong, Sorinel Lunca, Stefan Morarasu, Ana-Maria Musina, Alina Puscasu, Stefan Iacob, et al.
Evaluation of Changes in Circulating Cell-Free DNA as an Early Predictor of Response to Chemoradiation in Rectal Cancer—A Pilot Study
Reprinted from: *Medicina* **2023**, *59*, 1742, doi:10.3390/medicina59101742 83

Yeshong Park, Jai Young Cho, Ho-Seong Han, Yoo-Seok Yoon, Hae Won Lee, Boram Lee, et al.
Comparison of Open versus Laparoscopic Approaches in Salvage Hepatectomy for Recurrent Hepatocellular Carcinoma after Radiofrequency Ablation
Reprinted from: *Medicina* **2023**, *59*, 1243, doi:10.3390/medicina59071243 95

Horia-Dan Liscu, Bogdan-Radu Liscu, Ruxandra Mitre, Ioana-Valentina Anghel, Ionut-Lucian Antone-Iordache, Andrei Balan, et al.
The Conditioning of Adjuvant Chemotherapy for Stage II and III Rectal Cancer Determined by Postoperative Pathological Characteristics in Romania
Reprinted from: *Medicina* **2023**, *59*, 1224, doi:10.3390/medicina59071224 105

Petru Radu, Dragos Garofil, Anca Tigora, Mihai Zurzu, Vlad Paic, Mircea Bratucu, et al.
Parathyroid Cancer—A Rare Finding during Parathyroidectomy in High Volume Surgery Centre
Reprinted from: *Medicina* 2023, 59, 448, doi:10.3390/medicina59030448 122

Mahsa Naghashpour, Dian Dayer, Hadi Karami, Mahshid Naghashpour, Mahin Taheri Moghadam, Seyed Mohammad Jafar Haeri and Katsuhiko Suzuki
Evaluating the Magnolol Anticancer Potential in MKN-45 Gastric Cancer Cells
Reprinted from: *Medicina* 2023, 59, 286, doi:10.3390/medicina59020286 135

Oana Gabriela Trifanescu, Radu Iulian Mitrica, Laurentia Nicoleta Gales, Serban Andrei Marinescu, Natalia Motas, Raluca Alexandra Trifanescu, et al.
Validation of a New Prognostic Score in Patients with Ovarian Adenocarcinoma
Reprinted from: *Medicina* 2023, 59, 229, doi:10.3390/medicina59020229 147

Suk Hun Ha, Moonho Kim, Hyojin Kim, Boram No, Ara Go, Miso Choi, et al.
Cancer-Oriented Comprehensive Nursing Services in Republic of Korea: Lessons from an Oncologist's Perspective
Reprinted from: *Medicina* 2023, 59, 144, doi:10.3390/medicina59010144 159

Laura Lopez-Gonzalez, Alicia Sanchez Cendra, Cristina Sanchez Cendra, Eduardo David Roberts Cervantes, Javier Cassinello Espinosa, Tatiana Pekarek, et al.
Exploring Biomarkers in Breast Cancer: Hallmarks of Diagnosis, Treatment, and Follow-Up in Clinical Practice
Reprinted from: *Medicina* 2024, 60, 168, doi:10.3390/medicina60010168 170

Valentina-Fineta Chiriac, Daniel Ciurescu and Daniela-Viorica Moșoiu
Cancer Pain and Non-Invasive Brain Stimulation—A Narrative Review
Reprinted from: *Medicina* 2023, 59, 1957, doi:10.3390/medicina59111957 197

Petru Radu, Mihai Zurzu, Vlad Paic, Mircea Bratucu, Dragos Garofil, Anca Tigora, et al.
CD34—Structure, Functions and Relationship with Cancer Stem Cells
Reprinted from: *Medicina* 2023, 59, 938, doi:10.3390/medicina59050938 219

Melanie Schubert, Dirk Olaf Bauerschlag, Mustafa Zelal Muallem, Nicolai Maass and Ibrahim Alkatout
Challenges in the Diagnosis and Individualized Treatment of Cervical Cancer
Reprinted from: *Medicina* 2023, 59, 925, doi:10.3390/medicina59050925 233

Valentin Titus Grigorean, Anwar Erchid, Ionuț Simion Coman and Mircea Lițescu
Colorectal Cancer—The "Parent" of Low Bowel Obstruction
Reprinted from: *Medicina* 2023, 59, 875, doi:10.3390/medicina59050875 252

Marco Agostini, Pietro Traldi and Mahmoud Hamdan
Mass Spectrometry Contribution to Pediatric Cancers Research
Reprinted from: *Medicina* 2023, 59, 612, doi:10.3390/medicina59030612 263

Petru Radu, Mihai Zurzu, Vlad Paic, Mircea Bratucu, Dragos Garofil, Anca Tigora, et al.
Interstitial Cells of Cajal—Origin, Distribution and Relationship with Gastrointestinal Tumors
Reprinted from: *Medicina* 2023, 59, 63, doi:10.3390/medicina59010063 285

Donatella Coradduzza, Serenella Medici, Carla Chessa, Angelo Zinellu, Massimo Madonia, Andrea Angius, et al.
Assessing the Predictive Power of the Hemoglobin/Red Cell Distribution Width Ratio in Cancer: A Systematic Review and Future Directions
Reprinted from: *Medicina* 2023, 59, 2124, doi:10.3390/medicina59122124 292

Valentin Titus Grigorean, Radu Serescu, Andrei Anica, Violeta Elena Coman, Ştefan Iulian Bedereag, Roxana Corina Sfetea, et al.
Spindle Cell Rhabdomyosarcoma of the Inguinal Region Mimicking a Complicated Hernia in the Adult—An Unexpected Finding
Reprinted from: *Medicina* 2023, *59*, 1515, doi:10.3390/medicina59091515 306

Elena-Cristina Marinescu, Horia Bumbea, Iuliana Iordan, Ion Dumitru, Dan Soare, Cristina Ciufu and Mihaela Gaman
The Philadelphia Chromosome, from Negative to Positive: A Case Report of Relapsed Acute Lymphoblastic Leukemia Following Allogeneic Stem Cell Transplantation
Reprinted from: *Medicina* 2023, *59*, 671, doi:10.3390/medicina59040671 318

Veronica Aran, Vinicius Mansur Zogbi, Renan Lyra Miranda, Felipe Andreiuolo, Nathalie Henriques Silva Canedo, Carolina Victor Nazaré, et al.
The Use of Liquid Biopsy in the Molecular Analysis of Plasma Compared to the Tumour Tissue from a Patient with Brain Metastasis: A Case Report
Reprinted from: *Medicina* 2023, *59*, 459, doi:10.3390/medicina59030459 325

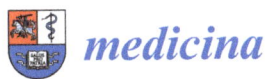

Editorial

Cancer—Yesterday, Today, Tomorrow

Valentin Titus Grigorean [1,2,*] and Daniel Alin Cristian [2,3]

1 "Bagdasar-Arseni" Clinical Emergency Hospital, 041915 Bucharest, Romania
2 "Carol Davila" University of Medicine and Pharmacy, 050474 Bucharest, Romania
3 "Colțea" Clinical Hospital, 030167 Bucharest, Romania
* Correspondence: grigorean.valentin@yahoo.com; Tel.:+40-213-343-025 (ext. 1301)

Citation: Grigorean, V.T.; Cristian, D.A. Cancer—Yesterday, Today, Tomorrow. *Medicina* **2023**, *59*, 98. https://doi.org/10.3390/medicina59010098

Received: 24 November 2022
Revised: 19 December 2022
Accepted: 21 December 2022
Published: 31 December 2022

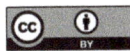

Copyright: © 2022 by the authors. Licensee MDPI, Basel, Switzerland. This article is an open access article distributed under the terms and conditions of the Creative Commons Attribution (CC BY) license (https://creativecommons.org/licenses/by/4.0/).

The COVID-19 pandemic has brought infectious and contagious diseases back to the forefront of medical concerns worldwide [1]. Prior to this period, the global mosaic of pathologies was dominated by cardiovascular diseases and cancers, as a cumulative result of the risk factors of our civilization [2,3].

Oncological pathology, unfortunately, has permanently occupied an undesirable leading position, even if, in previous decades, it was underdiagnosed. The more consistent application of screening methods and the improvement of diagnostic tools have given us an understanding that is closer to the true dimension of the phenomenon [4].

Genetic, molecular, histopathological, immunohistochemical, clinical and statistical studies have highlighted new facets of the neoplastic disease and found certain mutations suffered due to it (appearance at younger and younger ages, atypical evolutions, accompanying bizarre paraneoplastic phenomena, resistance to established therapeutic means, more frequent and more aggressive recurrence, etc.) [5,6].

The increase in average life expectancy has also induced an increase in the incidence of neoplasms in older people, with the appearance of new histological or evolutive types and the association of several concurrent or successive neoplasms in the same person [7,8].

Given that almost any component structure of the human body can develop multicellular malignant degeneration, with the possibility that the biology and "own strategy" of development and manifestation are different for each; that confirmed histological forms evolve (in the sense of worsening) from one stage to another; and that there is a loss of efficiency of some therapeutic means used (increasing resistance to chemotherapy, drug tachyphylaxis, radioresistance, etc.), we have a more complete picture of this puzzle [9,10].

The therapeutic means, in turn, have been developed and improved considerably, but must be permanently aligned with the dynamics of the development and manifestation of the neoplastic disease. Oncological surgery is often the pivot in cancer treatment as a practice of radical interventions on the primary tumor and resectable metastases. Unfortunately, it is possible to reach a capping of the surgical performance, considering that multivisceral resection (in locoregionally advanced forms) is not always applicable, and sometimes, its consequences are incompatible with survival or generate unacceptable suffering or sequelae. Often, oncological cases are completely inoperable and only palliative interventions can be practiced [11,12].

Transplantation surgery in oncology has obtained encouraging results, but currently, it is only applicable in a limited number of cancers that are in an early evolutive stage [13].

From this perspective emerges the idea that superior results in the fight against this disease can be obtained through a better understanding of predisposing genetic factors, of the particular neoplastic biology of each individual variant, of risk factors (environment, food, toxins, etc.) and of the development of nonsurgical therapeutic methods.

The COVID-19 pandemic has also produced profound changes regarding the issue of oncological pathology. It is worth noting, on the one hand, the reluctance of patients to access medical services during that period, and on the other hand, the overcrowding of medical units with the prioritization of medico-surgical emergencies.

Certainly, the effect of the SARS-CoV-2 infection on the patient's oncological background could potentiate immunosuppression, along with other systemic effects, but, thus far, this has been insufficiently studied. Medical researchers are also called to clarify the general biological, disimmunity, vascular and individual reactivity mutations produced by the virus in the body of oncological patients [14].

Despite the significant progress made in the area of diagnosis and treatment of neoplastic disease, there remains a huge field to explore, considering the current unknowns and the alert dynamics under which cancer evolves. Oncology is the medical field that requires the mobilization of most medical specialties in order to outline the particular profile of each individual patient and optimize the necessary treatment [15].

The results of research from the various fields that deal with oncological issues must be capitalized and "assembled" into a unitary whole in order for them to have scientific and practical value.

This is the direction in which this Special Issue of the *Medicina* journal is headed, and is an invitation for all specialists working in the oncological field to present their experience and research results.

Conflicts of Interest: The authors declare no conflict of interest.

References

1. Aimrane, A.; Laaradia, M.A.; Sereno, D.; Perrin, P.; Draoui, A.; Bougadir, B.; Hadach, M.; Zahir, M.; Fdil, N.; El Hiba, O.; et al. Insight into COVID-19's epidemiology, pathology, and treatment. *Heliyon* **2022**, *8*, e08799. [CrossRef] [PubMed]
2. Roth, G.A.; Mensah, G.A.; Johnson, C.O.; Addolorato, G.; Ammirati, E.; Baddour, L.M.; Barengo, N.C.; Beaton, A.Z.; Benjamin, E.J.; Benziger, C.P.; et al. Global Burden of Cardiovascular Diseases and Risk Factors, 1990–2019: Update From the GBD 2019 Study. *J. Am. Coll. Cardiol.* **2020**, *76*, 2982–3021. [CrossRef] [PubMed]
3. Santucci, C.; Carioli, G.; Bertuccio, P.; Malvezzi, M.; Pastorino, U.; Boffetta, P.; Negri, E.; Bosetti, C.; La Vecchia, C. Progress in cancer mortality, incidence, and survival: A global overview. *Eur. J. Cancer Prev.* **2020**, *29*, 367–381. [CrossRef] [PubMed]
4. Okoli, G.N.; Lam, O.L.T.; Reddy, V.K.; Copstein, L.; Askin, N.; Prashad, A.; Stiff, J.; Khare, S.R.; Leonard, R.; Zarin, W.; et al. Interventions to improve early cancer diagnosis of symptomatic individuals: A scoping review. *BMJ Open* **2021**, *11*, e055488. [CrossRef] [PubMed]
5. Vasan, N.; Baselga, J.; Hyman, D.M. A view on drug resistance in cancer. *Nature* **2019**, *575*, 299–309. [CrossRef] [PubMed]
6. Kang, T.W.; Lim, H.K.; Cha, D.I. Aggressive tumor recurrence after radiofrequency ablation for hepatocellular carcinoma. *Clin. Mol. Hepatol.* **2017**, *23*, 95. [CrossRef] [PubMed]
7. Estape, T. Cancer in the Elderly: Challenges and Barriers. *Asia Pac. J. Oncol. Nurs.* **2018**, *5*, 40. [CrossRef] [PubMed]
8. Bittorf, B.; Kessler, H.; Merkel, S.; Brückl, W.; Wein, A.; Ballhausen, W.; Hohenberger, W.; Günther, K. Multiple primary malignancies: An epidemiological and pedigree analysis of 57 patients with at least three tumours. *Eur. J. Surg. Oncol.* **2001**, *27*, 302–313. [CrossRef] [PubMed]
9. Mansoori, B.; Mohammadi, A.; Davudian, S.; Shirjang, S.; Baradaran, B. The Different Mechanisms of Cancer Drug Resistance: A Brief Review. *Adv. Pharm. Bull.* **2017**, *7*, 339. [CrossRef] [PubMed]
10. Lin, X.; Kong, D.; Chen, Z.S. Editorial: Chemo-Radiation-Resistance in Cancer Therapy. *Front. Pharmacol.* **2022**, *13*, 904063. [CrossRef] [PubMed]
11. de Nes, L.C.F.; van der Heijden, J.A.G.; Verstegen, M.G.; Drager, L.; Tanis, P.J.; Verhoeven, R.H.A.; de Wilt, J.H.W. Predictors of undergoing multivisceral resection, margin status and survival in Dutch patients with locally advanced colorectal cancer. *Eur. J. Surg. Oncol.* **2022**, *48*, 1144–1152. [CrossRef] [PubMed]
12. Lilley, E.J.; Cooper, Z.; Schwarze, M.L.; Mosenthal, A.C. Palliative Care in Surgery: Defining the Research Priorities. *Ann. Surg.* **2018**, *267*, 66–72. [CrossRef] [PubMed]
13. Abdelrahim, M.; Esmail, A.; Abudayyeh, A.; Murakami, N.; Saharia, A.; McMillan, R.; Victor, D.; Kodali, S.; Shetty, A.; Fong, J.V.N.; et al. Transplant Oncology: An Evolving Field in Cancer Care. *Cancers* **2021**, *13*, 4911. [CrossRef] [PubMed]
14. Geisslinger, F.; Vollmar, A.M.; Bartel, K. Cancer patients have a higher risk regarding COVID-19—And vice versa? *Pharmaceuticals* **2020**, *13*, 143. [CrossRef] [PubMed]
15. Schilsky, R.L.; Nass, S.; le Beau, M.M.; Benz, E.J. Progress in Cancer Research, Prevention, and Care. *N. Engl. J. Med.* **2020**, *383*, 897–900. [CrossRef] [PubMed]

Disclaimer/Publisher's Note: The statements, opinions and data contained in all publications are solely those of the individual author(s) and contributor(s) and not of MDPI and/or the editor(s). MDPI and/or the editor(s) disclaim responsibility for any injury to people or property resulting from any ideas, methods, instructions or products referred to in the content.

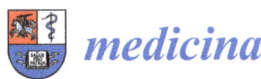

Article

The Role of Lymph Node Downstaging Following Neoadjuvant Treatment in a Group of Patients with Advanced Stage Cervical Cancer

Irinel-Gabriel Dicu-Andreescu [1,2], Marian-Augustin Marincaș [1,2,*], Anca-Angela Simionescu [1,3,*], Ioana Dicu-Andreescu [1], Sînziana-Octavia Ionescu [1,2], Virgiliu-Mihail Prunoiu [1,2], Eugen Brătucu [1,2] and Laurențiu Simion [1,2]

[1] Clinical Department No 10, General Surgery, University of Medicine and Pharmacy "Carol Davila", 050474 Bucharest, Romania; andreescugabriel43@gmail.com (I.-G.D.-A.)
[2] Department of Oncological Surgery, Oncological Institute "Prof. Dr. Alexandru Trestioreanu", 022328 Bucharest, Romania
[3] Department of Obstetrics and Gynecology, Filantropia Clinical Hospital, 011171 Bucharest, Romania
* Correspondence: augustin.marincas@gmail.com (M.-A.M.); anca.simionescu@umfcd.ro (A.-A.S.)

Citation: Dicu-Andreescu, I.-G.; Marincaș, M.-A.; Simionescu, A.-A.; Dicu-Andreescu, I.; Ionescu, S.-O.; Prunoiu, V.-M.; Brătucu, E.; Simion, L. The Role of Lymph Node Downstaging Following Neoadjuvant Treatment in a Group of Patients with Advanced Stage Cervical Cancer. *Medicina* **2024**, *60*, 871. https://doi.org/10.3390/medicina60060871

Academic Editor: Konstantinos Dimas

Received: 29 March 2024
Revised: 13 May 2024
Accepted: 24 May 2024
Published: 26 May 2024

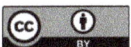

Copyright: © 2024 by the authors. Licensee MDPI, Basel, Switzerland. This article is an open access article distributed under the terms and conditions of the Creative Commons Attribution (CC BY) license (https://creativecommons.org/licenses/by/4.0/).

Abstract: *Background and Objectives*: Cervical cancer is the fourth most frequent type of neoplasia in women. It is most commonly caused by the persistent infection with high-risk strands of human papillomavirus (hrHPV). Its incidence increases rapidly from age 25 when routine HPV screening starts and then decreases at the age of 45. This reflects both the diagnosis of prevalent cases at first-time screening and the likely peak of HPV exposure in early adulthood. For early stages, the treatment offers the possibility of fertility preservation.. However, in more advanced stages, the treatment is restricted to concomitant chemo-radiotherapy, combined, in very selected cases with surgical intervention. After the neoadjuvant treatment, an imagistic re-evaluation of the patients is carried out to analyze if the stage of the disease remained the same or suffered a downstaging. Lymph node downstaging following neoadjuvant treatment is regarded as an indubitable prognostic factor for predicting disease recurrence and survival in patients with advanced cervical cancer. This study aims to ascertain the important survival role of radiotherapy in the downstaging of the disease and of lymphadenectomy in the control of lymph node invasion for patients with advanced-stage cervical cancer. *Material and Methods*: We describe the outcome of patients with cervical cancer in stage IIIC1 FIGO treated at Bucharest Oncological Institute. All patients received radiotherapy and two-thirds received concomitant chemotherapy. A surgical intervention consisting of type C radical hysterectomy with radical pelvic lymphadenectomy was performed six to eight weeks after the end of the neoadjuvant treatment. *Results*: The McNemar test demonstrated the regression of lymphadenopathies after neoadjuvant treatment—*p*: <0.001. However, the persistence of adenopathies was not related to the dose of irradiation (*p*: 0.61), the number of sessions of radiotherapy (*p*: 0.80), or the chemotherapy (*p*: 0.44). Also, there were no significant differences between the adenopathies reported by imagistic methods and those identified during surgical intervention—*p*: 0.62. The overall survival evaluated using Kaplan-Meier curves is dependent on the post-radiotherapy FIGO stage—*p*: 0.002 and on the lymph node status evaluated during surgical intervention—*p*: 0.04. The risk factors associated with an increased risk of death were represented by a low preoperative hemoglobin level (*p*: 0.003) and by the advanced FIGO stage determined during surgical intervention (*p*-value: 0.006 for stage IIIA and 0.01 for stage IIIC1). In the multivariate Cox model, the independent predictor of survival was the preoperative hemoglobin level (*p*: 0.004, HR 0.535, CI: 0.347 to 0.823). Out of a total of 33 patients with neoadjuvant treatment, 22 survived until the end of the study, all 33 responded to the treatment in varying degrees, but in 3 of them, tumor cells were found in the lymph nodes during the intraoperative histopathological examination. *Conclusions*: For advanced cervical cancer patients, radical surgery after neoadjuvant treatment may be associated with a better survival rate. Further research is needed to identify all the causes that lead to the persistence of adenopathies in certain patients, to decrease the FIGO stage after surgical intervention, and, therefore, to lower the risk of death. Also, it is mandatory to correctly evaluate and treat the anemia, as it seems to be an independent predictor factor for mortality.

Keywords: cervical cancer; lymph node; downstaging; neoadjuvant treatment; adenopathy

1. Introduction

With more than 604,000 new cases reported in 2020, cervical cancer is the fourth most frequent cancer in women worldwide, according to GLOBOCAN [1]. It is most commonly caused by the the persistent infection with high-risk strands of human papillomavirus (hrHPV), especially HPV 16, 18, 31, and 45, and favored by some additional risk factors [2,3]. These risk factors are represented by a weakened immune system caused by co-infection with HIV/AIDS [4], age [5], obesity [6], smoking [7], multiple sexual partners and multiparity [8], or a diet low in fruits and vegetables [9]. It is important to highlight that, of these factors, the co-infection HIV-HPV is a significant one, as women who are HIV positive have a six-fold increased risk of developing cervical cancer compared to the non-exposed population. Moreover, it is believed that the two viral infections are linked to 5% of all cases of cervical cancer [10]. Regular follow-up through Pap smear-based testing, detection and typing of HPV, and using HPV vaccination has remarkably reduced cervical cancer incidence worldwide [11]. Also, high-risk HPV is an important biomarker of prognosis in cervical cancer [12]. When routine screening begins at age 25, the incidence rises quickly and then starts to decline at age 45. This reflects both the diagnosis of prevalent cases at first-time screening and the likely peak of HPV exposure in early adulthood [13].

About 90% of deaths reported to be due to cervical cancer in 2020 (342,000 deaths) occurred in low- and middle-income countries [4]. The level of income is correlated with the screening measures and programs that allow the identification of pre-cancerous lesions and, consequently, an earlier therapeutic approach. In low- and middle-income countries, there is limited access to these measures, and consequently, cervical cancer is often identified in advanced stages [14]. Furthermore, access to treatment, for example, surgical interventions, radiotherapy, and chemotherapy, may be also limited, leading to a higher death rate.

After establishing an accurate diagnosis and stage confirmed by the post-biopsy histopathological result and by imagistic exploration, the treatment plan is elaborated according to The European Society of Gynaecological Oncology (ESGO), the European Society for Radiotherapy and Oncology (ESTRO), the European Society of Pathology (ESP) and National Comprehensive Cancer Network (NCCN) [15–17]. This treatment plan takes into account the age of the patient, the stage of the tumor, and other tumor-related factors, and comorbidities [18].

Figure 1 briefly presents a summary of ESGO/ESTRO/ESP guidelines for treatment of cervical cancer [19].

The options vary according to the International Federation of Gynecology and Obstetrics (FIGO) staging of the disease so that in the early stages (IA1, IA2) patient can opt for fertility-preserving methods such as cervical conization or radical trachelectomy [20], or non-fertility-sparing surgery such as extrafascial hysterectomy (Type A Querleu-Morrow classification [21] for stage IA1) or modified radical hysterectomy (Type B for Stage IA2) [13]. For stages IB1, IB2, and IIA1 in which the tumor does not exceed 4 cm in diameter and is limited to the cervix, the recommended intervention is Type C radical hysterectomy with pelvic lymphadenectomy [22].

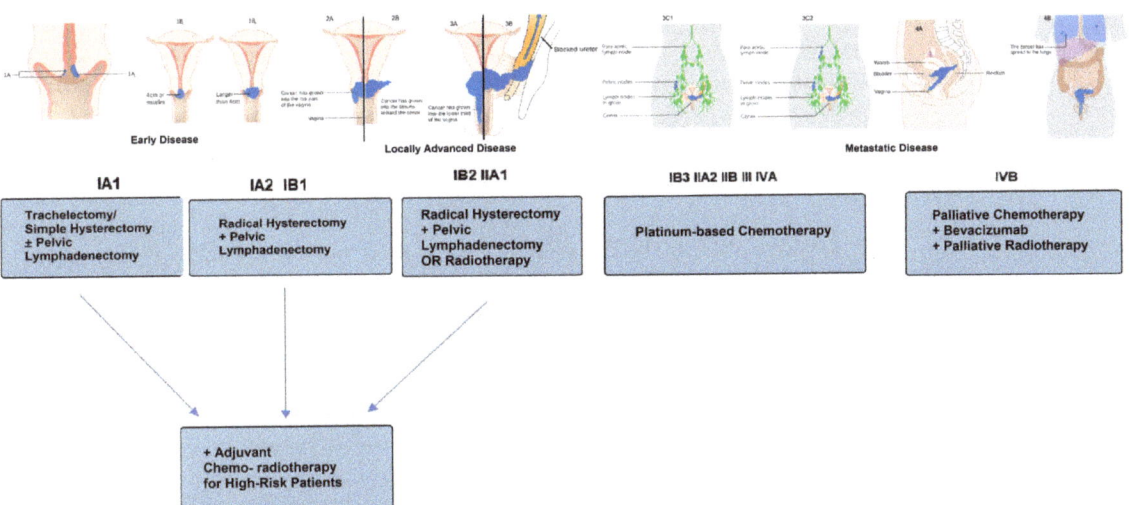

Figure 1. Summary of ESGO/ESTRO/ESP guidelines for neoadjuvant treatment in cervical cancer. Cervical cancer stage images modified from Wikimedia Commons.

In 2008, the Querleu-Morrow Classification was adopted to simplify and accurately establish the lateral resection limits in radical hysterectomy [23]. Thus, in Type A radical hysterectomy the main goal is to ensure the removal of the cervix in its entirety down to the vaginal fornix, together with a paracervical margin. Type B hysterectomy consists of resection of the paracervix at the ureter level and includes two subtypes: B1 and B2. Type B1 is the classical "modified" radical hysterectomy. The ureter is unroofed and mobilized laterally, allowing the transection of the paracervix at the level of the ureteral tunnel. For a type B2 resection, a paracervical lymphadenectomy can be added to increase the radicality of node dissection. Combined with pelvic lymphadenectomy, type B2 surgeries aim to remove the pelvic nodes as completely as possible. In Type C hysterectomy the transection of the paracervix is performed at its junction with the internal iliac vascular system. This operation corresponds to the classical radical hysterectomy. Transection of the rectovaginal and rectouterine ligaments is performed at the rectum. Transection of the ventral parametrium ligament is performed at the bladder. The vesico-uterine and vesicovaginal ligaments are resected and the ureter is completely mobilized and lateralized. The length of the vaginal cuff is then adjusted to the vaginal extent of the tumor. The last type of radical hysterectomy is type D which is a less common intervention with additional ultra-radical procedures, in which structures lateral to the paracervix are resected. It has two subtypes: D1 with resection of the entire paracervix at the pelvic sidewall together with the hypogastric and obturator vessels, exposing the roots of the sciatic nerve. The resection plane is lateral to the internal iliac vessels, ligating branches of the gluteal superior, gluteal inferior, and pudendal vessels. This procedure corresponds to the Palfalvi–Ungar laterally extended parametrectomy [24]. And type D2 which is D1 plus resection of the adjacent fascial and muscular structures.

For stages IB3 and IIA2, external radiotherapy associated with concurrent platinum-based chemotherapy followed by intracavitary brachytherapy is recommended. Another alternative is external pelvic radiotherapy associated with concurrent chemotherapy and brachytherapy followed by complementary radical hysterectomy (type C) for certain selected cases. From stage IIB onwards, NCCN recommends concurrent chemoradiotherapy, with the possibility of additional external irradiation with 5–10 Gy, in the case of parametrial invasion, as well as irradiation of the paraaortic lymph nodes [15].

This study aims to ascertain the important role of downstaging of the adenopathies after radiotherapy or concomitant chemo-radiotherapy in advanced stages of cervical cancer. To do this, we evaluated the reduction in the size of ilio-obturator lymph node metastases after neoadjuvant treatment as well as the survival rate of patients in relation to disease stage, radiation dose, and necessity for concurrent chemotherapy. The findings could help determine or customize the optimal dosage of radiation to the pelvic lymph nodes, which may directly improve the survival rate of patients with cervical cancer.

2. Materials and Methods

The study group consists of 33 patients hospitalized between 1 January 2019 and 31 December 2019 in the Department of Oncologic Surgery of Bucharest Oncological Institute with the diagnosis of biopsy-confirmed cervical neoplasm and pelvic lymph node $\geq$10 mm in diameter, reported by imagistic techniques, like CT and MRI, that were considered metastatic, which meant stage IIIC1 FIGO and beyond.

All patients had an ECOG (Eastern Cooperative Oncology Group) Score between 0 and 2. Also, in our group, a higher ECOG score was due to other co-morbidities of the patients, not to the neoplastic disease. Patients who had distant metastases in other organs or those with an ECOG performance status $\geq$3 were excluded from the study

The local guideline of the Bucharest Oncological Institute including our Oncology department follows the ESGO/ESTRO/ESP treatment guidelines [17] but also provides an alternative option, in selected cases, for patients with stages considered loco-regionally advanced (Stages IIB, III, and IVA) but non-metastatic [25]. In such cases, our guideline recommends that after the concurrent radio-chemotherapy, if the patients show an important regression of the tumor and of the adenopathies, (which suggests a favorable response to the treatment), surgery is recommended after an interval of six to eight weeks.

It has to be mentioned that the downstaging term used by the multidisciplinary team consisting of surgeon, radiotherapist, and oncologist, is an unofficial term used to reevaluate the response to neoadjuvant treatment and the practical possibility of performing the surgical intervention and it has no counterpart in current clinical practice, the official cancer stage of the patients remaining the one established before radiochemotherapy.

The patients should receive 50 Gray (Gy) external-beam radiotherapy to the entire pelvic region divided into 17 to 25 sessions of 2 Gy/day, 5 days/week, over the five weeks of chemotherapy. After completion of external-beam radiotherapy with chemotherapy, patients undergo high-dose-rate brachytherapy. A brachytherapy dose of 7.5 Gy is delivered and divided into 5 sessions, to result in a cumulative dose of 80 to 87.5 Gy combining external-beam radiotherapy and brachytherapy.

The surgical approach consists of type C radical hysterectomy with bilateral pelvic lymphadenectomy for stage IIIC1, and para-aortic lymph node sampling or para-aortic lymphadenectomy for stage IIIC2 if, preoperatively, the multidisciplinary team considers that the tumor could be resected with margins free of disease [25]. Of note, cervical cancer is most often associated with pelvic lymph node metastases, up to 20% according to some studies when the tumor size is above 4 cm [26]. Postoperative low-dose-rate brachytherapy is mandated only if the surgical specimen revealed positive surgical margins and has to be administered within 4 weeks after surgery at a median dose of 30 Gy to the vaginal mucosa delivered to a depth of 0.5 cm.

In our cohort, the multidisciplinary team decided that the first step of treatment for our patients, included in stage IIIC1, should be concurrent chemo-radiotherapy. Patients were evaluated after four to six weeks by CT or MRI. In our institution, according to the internal guidelines, if no pelvic nodes with suspicion of metastasis are detected during the post-radiation imaging investigations, it is decided to perform the surgical intervention consisting of type C radical hysterectomy with radical pelvic lymphadenectomy six to eight weeks after the end of the neoadjuvant treatment, to avoid as much as possible the post-radiation fibro-inflammatory remodeling of tissues that could appear later.

The patients were closely monitored for three years postoperatively. The outcome was represented by the death of the patient, or by the end of the three years of follow-up, considered enough time for assessing the survival, by taking into consideration the advanced stage of the cancer in our cohort.

In summary, we included in the study all patients hospitalized in our clinic in 2019 diagnosed with cervical cancer who had pelvic nodes ≥ 10 mm in diameter at the imaging investigations (stage IIIC1), with an ECOG score between 0 and 2, and who underwent neoadjuvant treatment. Each of them was evaluated through imaging after the completion of the neoadjuvant treatment and if they showed a significant reduction of the primary tumor and adenopathies, after six weeks, the surgical intervention was performed (type C radical hysterectomy with bilateral pelvic lymphadenectomy).

We excluded the patients with cervical cancer without adenopathies, those with an ECOG score above 2, or those who refused surgery.

Statistical analysis was performed with the SPSS program. The p-value was considered significant at a value under 0.05. The null hypothesis is that there are no significant differences between the two sub-groups—those who remained alive at three years of follow-up and those who did not survive, regarding the response to neoadjuvant therapy, which was focused especially on the downstaging of the lymph nodes, the radiation dose and the use of concurrent chemo-radiotherapy.

The differences between the two subgroups were evaluated using the Mann-Whitney U test for continuous variables (only the age and the preoperative hemoglobin were normally distributed, and, therefore, could be assessed using the Student t-test) and Pearson chi-square and Fisher's exact test for the categorical ones. Also, we used the McNemar test to explore the evolution of the involvement of the lymph nodes after neoadjuvant treatment. We opted for this test because it is appropriate for the evaluation of how related categorical variables change according to an event, in our case the chemo-radiotherapy. We also used the univariate Cox model for identifying the risk factors for a worse survival, by analyzing each of the variables in relation to the end-point, and the multivariate one to identify the independent predictors of survival. Each significant variable from the univariate Cox model was added and analyzed to simultaneously evaluate the effect of several risk factors on survival time. Last, but not least, we built Kaplan-Meier curves to assess the survival related to categorical variables explored in this cohort.

3. Results

In one of the three wards of the Oncological Surgery Department in our Institute, 150 patients with cervical cancer were operated on in the year 2019. Of these, 33 patients presented stage IIIC1 FIGO cervical cancer, with apparent pelvic lymph node invasion on imaging investigations. According to our internal treatment guidelines, all 33 patients received tele-irradiation by a 3D-CRT linear accelerator, at the level of the pelvis, including in the irradiation field the area of the cervix and pelvic lymph node groups with a total irradiation dose of 50 Gy, administered in 17–25 sessions, depending on the clinical tolerance or acceptance of the patients. Also according to the irradiation protocol from the total of 33, 31 of them received five sessions of endocavitary high-dose-rate (HDR) brachytherapy with doses of 7.5 Gy per session– the remaining two patients developed radiation cystitis or vaginal pain after tele-irradiation and it was and it was considered better and it was considered better not to do brachytherapy. The total irradiation dose, received by patients, which is the cumulation of external irradiation and brachytherapy, was between 82.5 and 87.9 Gy and the total duration of treatment was 35 days. Throughout the tele-irradiation, five sessions of concurrent cisplatin-based chemotherapy (40 mg/m^2) were administered in 22 patients—the other 11 either did not tolerate it or refused it from the beginning. No cases of acute toxicity following irradiation were reported in any patient, but four of them presented radiation cystitis, one presented radiation colitis, 13 patients presented anemia after radio-chemotherapy and four patients developed moderate leukopenia.

Table 1 highlights the main characteristics of the patients included in the study before the start of the neoadjuvant treatment, divided into two groups, those who were alive at three years after neoadjuvant treatment and those who did not survive this follow-up period.

Table 1. Main characteristics of the patients.

	Total (33)	Alive at 3 Years (22)	Deceased at 3 Years (11)	p-Value
Age, years, median (SD)	55.3 (11.5)	56 (14)	54 (26)	0.895
Environment, n (%)	urban: 12 (36) rural: 21 (64)	urban: 8 (36) rural: 14 (64)	urban: 4 (36) rural: 7 (64)	0.801
Histological types of cancer, (biopsy) n (%)	1. Squamous cell carcinoma 30 (90) 2. Adenocarcinoma-2 (6) 3. Adenosquamous carcinoma-1 (3)	1. Squamous cell Carcinoma-20 (90) 2. Adenocarcinoma-1 (4) 3. Adenosquamous Carcinoma-1 (4)	1. Squamous cell carcinoma-10 (90) 2. Adenocarcinoma-1 (9)	0.687
Pre-RT FIGO stage, n (%)	III C1 33 (100)	IIIC1: 22 (100)	IIIC1: 11 (100)	1
Pre-RT Parametrial Invasion n (%)	19 (57)	11 (50)	8 (72)	0.210
Initial Tumor size (cm), median (IQR)	2 (1.6)	1.95 (0.9)	3 (2.5)	0.048
Pre-RT leukocyte count, median (IQR)	6200 (2000)	6350 (2100)	6050 (2700)	0.825
Pre-RT hemoglobin, mean (SD)	12.5 (1.4)	12.8 (1.1)	11.5 (1.3)	0.03

SD—standard deviation; n—number; IQR—inter-quartile range.

In Table 2 we present the main adverse reactions encountered after neoadjuvant treatment.

Table 2. The main adverse reactions encountered after neoadjuvant treatment.

Post-Neoadjuvant Treatment Adverse Reactions	Alive at 3 Years after Treatment	Dead at 3 Years after Treatment	p-Value
Radiation colitis	0	1	0.33
Radiation cystitis	0	4	0.008
Anemia	6	7	0.06
Leukopenia	1	3	0.09

From a total of 33 patients, at the end of the study, 22 patients were alive. We present below in the Figure 2 a summary diagram with the evolution of the patients enrolled in our study.

Table 3 highlights the details regarding adjuvant and neoadjuvant treatment. We note that we did not find any statistically significant differences between the two groups, concerning the administration of neoadjuvant treatment, since all patients followed the same treatment plan.

Table 4 highlights the post-radio-chemotherapy staging and also the intraoperative findings. It should be mentioned that we obtained a downstaging of the disease for 29 patients, and we also had 15 patients with complete disappearance of the tumor at the intraoperative anatomopathological examinations.

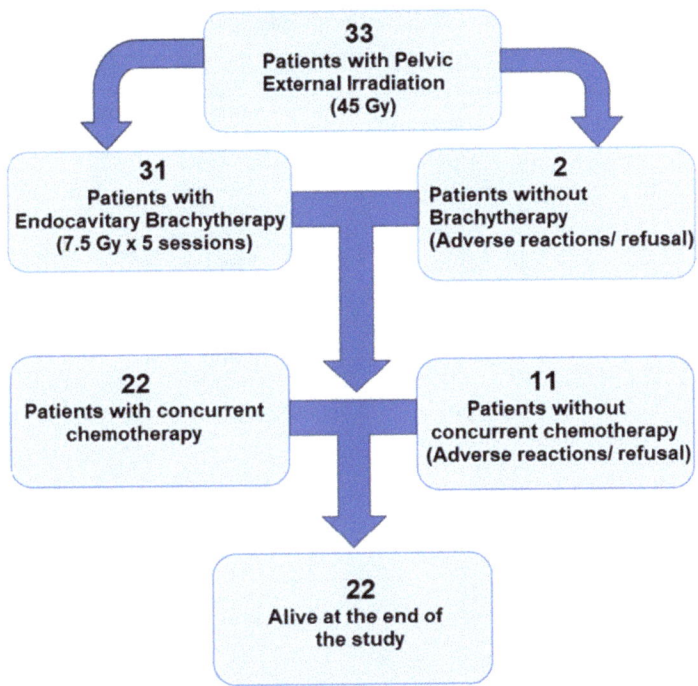

Figure 2. Evolution and outcome of patients under treatment.

Table 3. Details of adjuvant and neoadjuvant treatment.

	Total (33)	Alive at 3 Years (22)	Deceased at 3 Years (11)	*p*-Value
RT dose, median (IQR)	50 (0.2)	50 (0.4)	50 (0)	0.611
Nr. of RT sessions, median (IQR)	25 (1)	25 (1)	25 (1)	0.807
Sensitization chemotherapy, median (IQR)	5 (5)	5 (5)	3 (5)	0.440
Postoperatively chemotherapy, n (%)	10 (30)	5 (22)	5 (45)	0.181

The only significant difference identified in the two subgroups is the pre-RT as shown in Table 1 and post-RT hemoglobin (Table 4) which is much higher in those who survived—*p* values of 0.03 and 0.02.

To evaluate the downstaging of the lymph nodes we used the McNemar test, which demonstrated the regression of lymphadenopathies after neoadjuvant treatment—*p*-value: <0.001. To further investigate the correspondence between the adenopathies identified through imagistic methods after neoadjuvant treatment and those found intraoperative and confirmed by biopsy and histopathological examination, we performed again the McNemar test, but, this time, it was not significant—*p*-value: 0.62, which confirms the accuracy of the imagistic techniques. It has to be mentioned that for all patients the size of the pelvic lymph nodes decreased considerably, a fact that could represent an argument to consider it a complete therapeutic response. However, for five patients, subcentimetric lymph nodes were found intraoperatively on the same site as the old adenopathies, which, if they still contain malignant cells could potentially act, in the future, as reservoirs of tumoral cells.

Table 4. Post-radiochemotherapy staging and intraoperative findings.

	Total (33)	Alive at 3 Years (22)	Deceased at 3 Years (11)	p-Value
Post-RT FIGO stage, n (%)	Absence of tumor: 10 (30) IA1-2 (6) IA2-1 (3) IB1-10 (30) IB2-1 (3) IIA1-1 (3) IIA2-1 (3) IIB-1 (3) IIIA-1 (3) IIIC1-5 (15)	Absence of tumor: 10 (45) IA1-2 (9) IA2-0 (0) IB1-6 (27) IB2-0 (0) IIA1-1 (4) IIA2-0 (0) IIB-1 (5) IIIA-0 (0) IIIC1-2 (9)	Absence of tumor: 0 (0) IA1-0 (0) IA2-1 (9) IB1-4 (36) IB2-1 (9) IIA1-0 (0) IIA2-1 (9) IIB-0 (0) IIIA-1 (9) IIIC1-3 (27)	0.121
Post-RT lymphadenopathy, n (%)	5 (15)	2 (9)	3 (27)	0.304
Preoperative leukocyte count, median (IQR)	5600 (2100)	5630 (2070)	5600 (3500)	0.721
Preoperative hemoglobin, mean (SD)	11.9 (1.4)	12.3 (1.2)	11 (1.4)	0.02
Intraoperative FIGO stage, n (%)	Absence of tumor: 15 (45) IA1-2 (6) IA2-3 (9) IB1-3 (9) IB2-0 (0) IIA1-1 (3) IIA2-1 (3) IIB-1 (3) IIIA-1 (3) IIIC1-4 (12)	Absence of tumor: 13 (59) IA1-1 (4) IA2-2 (9) IB1-1 (4) IB2-0 (0) IIA1-1 (4) IIA2-0 (0) IIB-1 (4) IIIA-0 (0) IIIC1-1 (4)	Absence of tumor: 2 (18) IA1-1 (9) IA2-1 (9) IB1-2 (18) IB2-0 (0) IIA1-0 (0) IIA2-1 (9) IIB-0 (0) IIIA-1 (9) IIIC1-3 (27)	0.119
Intraoperative histological type of cancer n (%)	Absence of tumor: 15 (45) In situ carcinoma: 1 (3) Squamous cell carcinoma: 15 (45) 2. Adenocarcinoma: 1 (3) 3. Adenosquamous Carcinoma: 1 (3)	Absence of tumor: 13 (59) In situ carcinoma: 0 (0) Squamous cell carcinoma: 8 (36) 2. Adenocarcinoma: 0 (0) 3. Adenosquamous Carcinoma: 1 (4)	Absence of tumor: 2 (18) In situ carcinoma: 1 (9) Squamous cell Carcinoma: 7 (63) 2. Adenocarcinoma: 1 (9) 3. Adenosquamous Carcinoma: 0 (0)	
Intraoperative parametrial Invasion n (%)	2 (6)	1 (4)	1 (9)	0.601
Positive intraoperative lymph nodes, n (%)	3 (9)	1 (4)	2 (18)	0.252
Lymphovascular invasion, n (%)	7 (21)	3 (13)	4 (36)	0.186

n—number; FIGO—International Federation of Obstetrics and Gynecology.

A particularity of this study is that our guidelines allowed us to combine chemo-radiotherapy with surgical intervention and, therefore, to evaluate the real response to neoadjuvant treatment. This allowed us to confirm the role and the sensitivity of imagistic methods. A fact that is of great importance is that neither the dose of radiotherapy—p: 0.5, nor the number of sessions differed in those with persistent lymphadenopathies after neoadjuvant treatment versus those without—p: 0.5.

For evaluating the survival, we have built Kaplan-Meier curves, in which we explored the effect of each variable on the outcome.

According to Figure 3, the size of the initial tumor significantly influences survival, which is lower the larger the size of the tumor.

The FIGO stage post-radiotherapy based on imaging investigations had also a significant impact on survival (Figure 4). The best result was, as expected, in the case of a complete response to neoadjuvant treatment, meaning the complete disappearance of the tumor. Those patients had a better survival rate of at least 40% compared to those who presented post-RT tumors in different stages—p-value (Log Rank): 0.002.

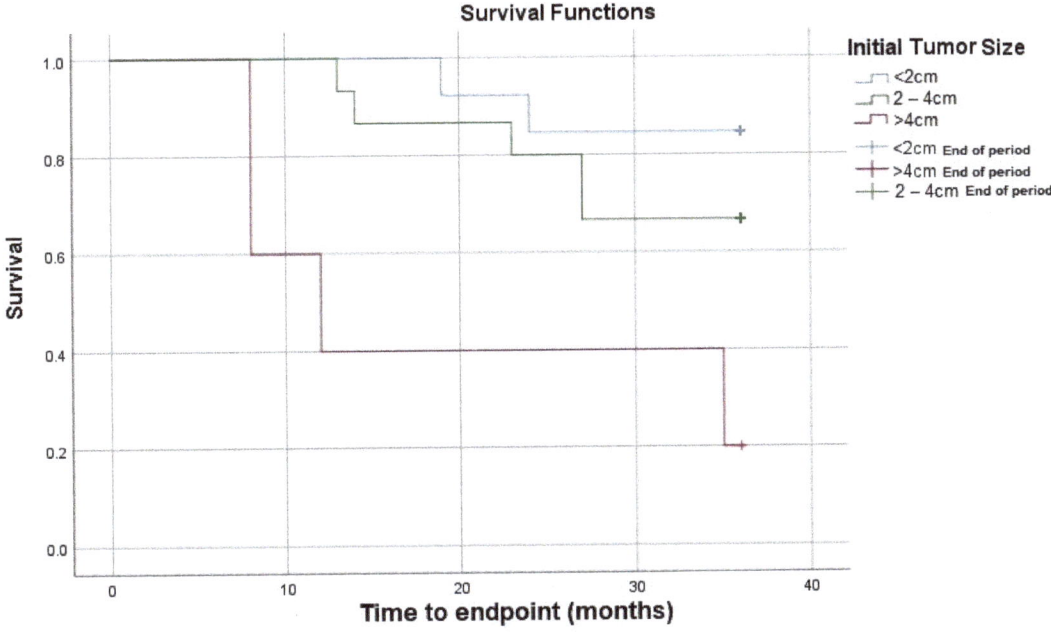

Figure 3. Survival rate according to initial tumor size.

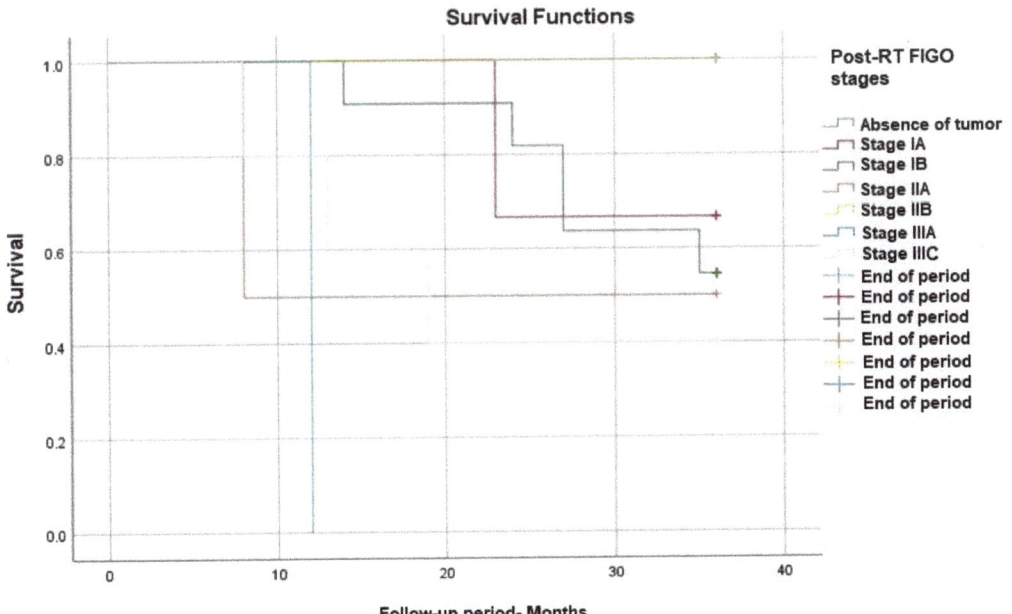

Figure 4. Survival rate according to post-RT FIGO stage.

We also evaluated with Kaplan-Meyer curves the influence of intraoperatively lymph node status on survival during the three years of follow-up. Again, we found that the survival rate in patients with nodal invasion is 40% lower than those without nodal invasion with a *p*-value (Log Rank) of 0.04 (Figure 5).

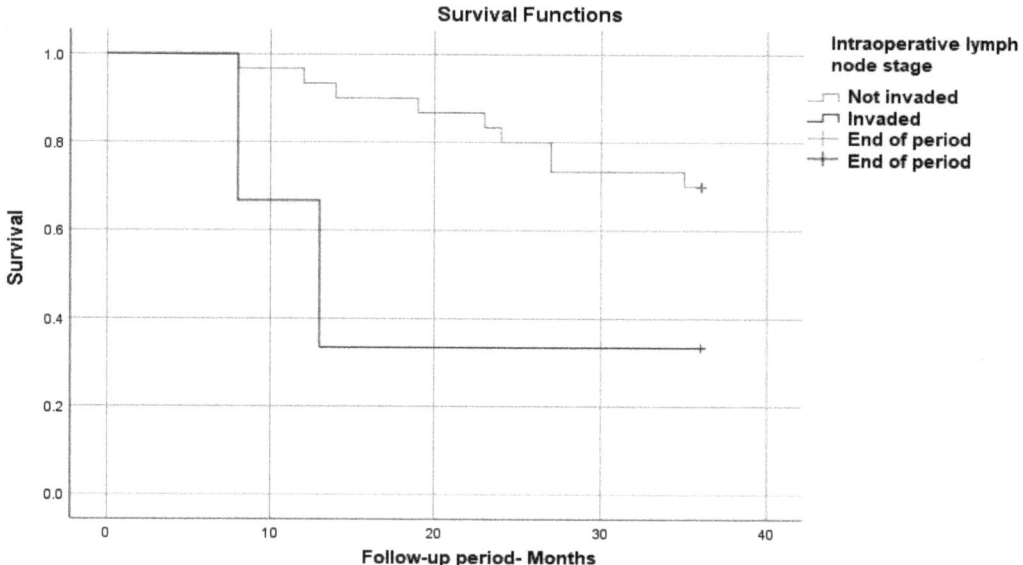

Figure 5. Survival rate according to Intraoperative lymph node stage.

To identify the risk factors associated with an increased risk of death in our cohort, we used a univariate Cox model which showed that only the hemoglobin level, both before and after neoadjuvant treatment, and the advanced intraoperative FIGO stage were statistically significant. The hemoglobin level has an inversely proportional relationship with the risk of death with a *p*-value—0.003, and intraoperative stage IIIC1 FIGO has a directly proportional one—*p*-value—0.006. The explanation is that the hemoglobin level is a parameter that can estimate the state of health, as a normal or near normal level is correlated with the absence of inflammatory states, blood loss, or infections, aspects that can have an independent effect on survival. Furthermore, the advanced stage of FIGO after the neoadjuvant treatment means a lack of response and, as it is expected, a lower rate of survival. Taking into consideration that all the patients received the same dose of irradiation and that both neo- and adjuvant chemotherapy did not differ in the two subgroups, a part of the patients responded completely, with the best chances of survival in the cohort, and other part remaining in stage IIIC1 FIGO, with persistent lymph node involvement, further research is needed to explore and identify the predictor factors associated with the response to neoadjuvant treatment. Interestingly, the lymphovascular invasion, despite being claimed in literature as a negative prognostic factor [27], did not differ significantly in the two subgroups—*p*: 0.18, and, at least in our cohort, did not represent a risk factor for a worse survival—*p*: 0.07.

Table 5 shows the results for the univariate Cox model in which the factors associated with increased risk of death were evaluated.

In the multivariate Cox model, the only independent predictor of survival was the preoperative hemoglobin level with a *p*-value: 0.004, hazard ratio of 0.535, and confidence interval between 0.347 to 0.823. Again, this aspect is very important both in clinical practice and for further research to better identify the patients with an optimal therapeutic response.

Table 5. Factors associated with increased risk of death.

Factors	HR	CI	p-Value
Age	0.987	0.935–1.041	0.621
Environment	1.001	0.292–3.423	0.999
Histological types of cancer, (biopsy)	1.241	0.159–9.706	0.979
Pre-RT hemoglobin	0.702	0.397–0.912	0.005
Initial Tumor size	1.746	1.248–2.441	0.001
Pre-RT parametrial invasion	2.445	0.647–9.227	0.187
RT dose	0.970	0.792–1.187	0.766
Nr. of RT sessions	0.971	0.689–1.368	0.867
Post-RT Lymphadenopathy	3.186	0.835–12.153	0.09
Post-RT FIGO	2.965	0.972–7.842	0.573
Sensitization chemotherapy	0.937	0.761–1.155	0.543
Pre-RT hemoglobin	0.702	0.397–0.912	0.005
Preoperative hemoglobin	0.506	0.325–0.789	0.003
Preoperative leukocyte count	1.153	0.895–1.486	0.271
Intraoperative FIGO	47.447 9.203	3.078–731.400 1.529–55.372	Stage IIIA: 0.006 Stage IIIC1: 0.01
Intraoperative parametrial invasion	2.162	0.275–16.970	0.600
Positive intraoperative lymph nodes	4.064	0.862–19.164	0.076
Postoperatively chemotherapy	2.617	0.795–8.610	0.113
Lymphovascular invasion	3.04	0.885–10.442	0.07

Clinical parameters that were statistically significant in our study are marked in red.

4. Discussion

Annually, around 1300 patients with cervical cancer are treated in our institute. Of these, in the three wards of the Department of Oncological Surgery, approximately 500 patients are operated on annually. So, the experience of the surgery clinic is vast. This experience led to the development of an internal protocol that takes into account international recommendations but offers treatment alternatives for selected cases, considered loco-regionally advanced.

Radiotherapy in combination with sensitizing chemotherapy is considered the standard method of treatment for patients with cervical cancer in locally advanced stages [15]. In our study, all the pelvic lymph nodes that showed dimensions greater than 10 mm on the short axis during CT or MRI imaging investigations were considered metastatic. The sensitivity and specificity of these imaging methods for highlighting nodal structures larger than 10 mm were evaluated at approximately 80% for CT and 85% for MRI, percentages consistent with data from the literature [28,29], and later confirmed during radical surgery. In the case of lymph nodes with dimensions over 15 mm, the specificity of CT and MRI increases, with a positive prediction rate between 75–100% [29].

Although standard regimens of adjuvant treatment are established by the institutional or European treatment protocols, the radiotherapy regimens for lymph node metastases leave room for nuances [30]; the treatment dose is ultimately determined by the radiation therapist. This can be another thing that should be reevaluated, as our results, despite being conducted on a small number of patients, revealed that the persistence of adenopathies is not related to the dose of irradiation, the number of sessions of radiotherapy, or the chemotherapy. One of the reasons could be represented by the histological type of the primary tumors. According to some studies response to chemoradiotherapy varies depending on the histologic subtype, patients with adenocarcinoma or adenosquamous carcinoma of the cervix having a worse therapeutic response [31–33]. Due to this aspect, current guidelines for cervical cancer may not be sufficient for all patients, hence the need for a tailored regimen.

To date, few studies have addressed the relationship between radiation doses to pelvic lymph node groups suggestive of metastases and their response to treatment [34]. Following pelvic radiotherapy combined with chemotherapy, pelvic lymph nodes considered metastatic were no longer visualized on imaging investigations (CT, MRI) in all 33 patients, but in three of them, pelvic nodes with cancer invasion were present during surgery. All three patients presented the histological type of adenosquamous carcinoma at the intraoperative anatomopathological examination. Two of them died due to the progression of the disease, and one survived until the end of the follow-up period.

In our study, the hemoglobin level before and after neoadjuvant treatment was a statistically significant factor for the survival rate, a better survival being observed in patients with a hemoglobin level above 12 g/dL. The relationship between mild or moderate anemia before and after neoadjuvant treatment and the evolution of patients with cervical cancer is controversial. Some studies have shown that changes in the level of hemoglobin before and after the administration of neoadjuvant treatment are correlated with a poorer prognosis [35]. Although an exact cause could not be established, the reasons may be changes in iron metabolism, suppression of erythroid progenitor cells by releasing tumor cytokines, impaired erythropoietin response on erythroid progenitor cells, and hemorrhage [36]. A hypothesis is also that tumor hypoxia resulting from decreased oxygen-carrying capacity of the blood in case of anemia leads to a relative tumor radio-resistance [37]. Other studies have shown that certain forms of cancer with aggressive biological behavior are often associated with anemia even in the early stages [38].

We consider that a strong point of our study is the possibility of evaluating the response to the neoadjuvant treatment by intraoperative verification and by the histopathological result of the resection pieces to see if there is any residual tumor. Another advantage is the fact that we can compare the survival of our patients in the advanced stages of cervical cancer with neoadjuvant treatment and radical surgery with the data from the literature of those who only received neoadjuvant treatment.

However, our study has a few important limitations. First of all, the small number of patients explained by the rarity of advanced cases do not allow us to draw strong conclusions regarding the variants of neoadjuvant treatment, doses, or regimens. The small study group is influenced by the relatively rare cases of patients with cervical cancer in an advanced stage but without invasion into adjacent organs or distant metastases and also who are strong enough to undergo surgical intervention [39]. Another disadvantage is that we do not have a comparative group in the same stage of cervical cancer in which only neoadjuvant treatment was performed, since the internal protocol applies to all patients, thus being limited to the comparison only with data from the literature.

In low and middle-income countries, the initial stage of cervical cancer presentation is usually an advanced one [40]. On the other hand, being a study made exclusively on patients with stage IIIC1 cervical cancer, the survival predictors identified can lead to a future direction for research, for example, the emphasis on targeted therapy [41,42]. We consider it crucial to identify the main therapeutic factors associated with a good therapeutic response [43] that can lead to an improved quality of life for the patients [44,45].

Unfortunately, it was not possible to collect data on the exact size and number of metastatic nodes of each patient, due to the incomplete descriptions of the CT and MRI examinations, often performed in other medical units, descriptions in which nodules larger than 10 mm or 15 mm are roughly mentioned. This could have helped us to observe also the variation in the number of lymph nodes, not just their sizes.

Last, but not least, in our study, neither the presence of residual adenopathies post neoadjuvant treatment nor the lymphovascular invasion did not seem to impact the survival, however, other studies have found that both nodal invasion and lymphovascular invasion represent strong negative predictive factors in survival [27,46,47]. Again, our results may be influenced by the small size of our group. On the other hand, the FIGO stage determined during surgical intervention was an independent predictor factor, which means that even though adenopathies alone do not seem to be risk factors for a lower survival rate when combined with the tumor size [48] and the presence or absence of metastases [49,50], which create the FIGO stage, can independently predict the survival [51].

Some studies take into account that for patients with early cervical cancer the sentinel lymph node biopsy is an alternative to pelvic lymphadenectomy to avoid the complications and risks of this intervention [52]. However, in the case of our patients, being in a stage considered advanced, in an attempt to increase the intraoperative control, both visual and palpatory, in all cases, an open pelvic lymphadenectomy was done.

According to the latest studies, the size of the primary tumor is a factor with a strong impact on survival [53,54]. In our study, this parameter did also appear to be statistically significant, despite the small number of patients. Also, according to recent studies, a favorable response to radio-chemotherapy, which means a decrease in tumor size, is an important parameter in predicting survival [55].

For all patients, the surgical intervention consisted of type C1 radical hysterectomy, which is the standard operation for bulky or high-risk tumors. During the procedure, we identified and preserved the lower hypogastric plexus and the bladder nerve branches. Preservation of these structures substantially decreases the rate of postoperative complications, including bladder or sexual dysfunctions [56]. A fact that is of crucial importance is that post-irradiation fibrous-inflammatory changes make the surgical intervention much more difficult, and also, with lower chances to obtain radicality, as a part of lymph nodes can be overlooked and metastasize in the future. The best moment for the surgical intervention is after six-to-eight weeks after the neoadjuvant treatment.

5. Conclusions

This study evaluates the lymph node status after neoadjuvant treatment and its correlation with the rate of mortality documented at three years of follow-up in a cohort of patients with advanced-stage cervical cancer. Because the local guidelines allow us to complete the neoadjuvant treatment with surgical intervention, we could also verify the real correspondence between the adenopathies identified through imagistic methods and those confirmed after surgical intervention by histopathological examination. After neoadjuvant treatment, the adenopathies regressed significantly, thus obtaining a lymph node downstaging but, intraoperatively findings revealed that the response was only 90%, 10% of the patients still presenting lymph node involvement. Interestingly, the lymph node response was not correlated with the dose of irradiation, the number of sessions of radiotherapy, or the concurrent chemotherapy, on the survival, which, at first view, can appear as a confirmation of the null hypothesis. However, when residual adenopathies are combined with the tumor size and the presence or absence of metastases, which create the FIGO stage, can independently predict the survival, those with the best response to neoadjuvant treatment having the highest chances of survival at three years, a fact that infirmed the null hypothesis. This aspect is of great importance, in treating patients with advanced-stage cervical cancer because it raises the need for a better exploration of the causes of resistance to treatment.

Moreover, a better understanding of this can improve the therapeutic approach and also limit unnecessary exposure to chemo-radiotherapy. Also, by adding the radical surgery, we could verify the real histological response to neoadjuvant treatment and, by revising the intraoperative FIGO stage, we found that it represents a major risk factor that can lead to a decreased survival rate.

Last, but not least, the presence of anemia evaluated both at the time of the first visit to the clinic and before the surgical intervention seems to play a very important role in the survival of the patients, as we found that it is an independent predictor factor. This fact is related, most probably, to a worse overall status of the patient, a frailty-related characteristic, that can decrease the chances of survival, and, therefore, a correct pre-therapeutic evaluation is very important. Further research is needed in order to complete these findings with the factors associated with a poor response to chemo-radiotherapy and to ensure an optimal therapeutic approach.

Author Contributions: Conceptualization: I.-G.D.-A., M.-A.M., A.-A.S., I.D.-A., S.-O.I., E.B. and L.S.; Data curation: I.-G.D.-A. and I.D.-A.; Formal analysis: I.-G.D.-A. and I.D.-A.; Investigation: I.-G.D.-A.; Methodology, I.-G.D.-A. and M.-A.M.; Project administration: M.-A.M., E.B. and L.S.; Resources: M.-A.M., E.B. and L.S.; Software: I.-G.D.-A. and I.D.-A.; Supervision: M.-A.M., A.-A.S., S.-O.I., V.-M.P., E.B. and L.S.; Validation: M.-A.M., A.-A.S., S.-O.I., V.-M.P., E.B. and L.S.; Visualization: I.-G.D.-A., M.-A.M., A.-A.S. and E.B.; Writing–original draft, I.-G.D.-A.; Writing—review & editing: I.-G.D.-A., A.-A.S., I.D.-A. and S.-O.I. All authors have read and agreed to the published version of the manuscript.

Funding: This research received no external funding.

Institutional Review Board Statement: The study was conducted in accordance with the Declaration of Helsinki, and approved by the Ethics Committee of the Bucharest Oncological Institute (protocol code 1A and date of approval 8 January 2024).

Informed Consent Statement: Informed consent was obtained from all subjects involved in the study.

Data Availability Statement: The patients' data were obtained from the medical documents of the Bucharest Oncological Institute and they cannot be publicly available, as they contain personal and confidential data of the patients, but any information about these documents can be obtained on request from the corresponding author.

Acknowledgments: Publication of this paper was supported by the University of Medicine and Pharmacy Carol Davila, through the institutional program Publish not Perish.

Conflicts of Interest: The authors declare no conflict of interest.

References

1. Sung, H.; Ferlay, J.; Siegel, R.L.; Laversanne, M.; Soerjomataram, I.; Jemal, A.; Bray, F. Global Cancer Statistics 2020: GLOBOCAN Estimates of Incidence and Mortality Worldwide for 36 Cancers in 185 Countries. *CA Cancer J. Clin.* **2021**, *71*, 209–249. [CrossRef]
2. Crosbie, E.J.; Einstein, M.H.; Franceschi, S.; Kitchener, H.C. Human Papillomavirus and Cervical Cancer. *Lancet* **2013**, *382*, 889–899. [CrossRef]
3. Everett, T.; Bryant, A.; Griffin, M.F.; Martin-Hirsch, P.P.; Forbes, C.A.; Jepson, R.G. Interventions Targeted at Women to Encourage the Uptake of Cervical Screening. *Cochrane Database Syst. Rev.* **2011**, *5*, CD002834. [CrossRef]
4. Gilles, C.; Konopnicki, D.; Rozenberg, S. The Recent Natural History of Human Papillomavirus Cervical Infection in Women Living with HIV: A Scoping Review of Meta-analyses and Systematic Reviews and the Construction of a Hypothetical Model. *HIV Med.* **2023**, *24*, 877–892. [CrossRef]
5. Olusola, P.; Banerjee, H.N.; Philley, J.V.; Dasgupta, S. Human Papilloma Virus-Associated Cervical Cancer and Health Disparities. *Cells* **2019**, *8*, 622. [CrossRef] [PubMed]
6. Wichmann, I.A.; Cuello, M.A. Obesity and Gynecological Cancers: A Toxic Relationship. *Int. J. Gynecol. Obstet.* **2021**, *155*, 123–134. [CrossRef] [PubMed]
7. Roura, E.; Castellsagué, X.; Pawlita, M.; Travier, N.; Waterboer, T.; Margall, N.; Bosch, F.X.; de Sanjosé, S.; Dillner, J.; Gram, I.T.; et al. Smoking as a Major Risk Factor for Cervical Cancer and Pre-Cancer: Results from the EPIC Cohort. *Int. J. Cancer* **2014**, *135*, 453–466. [CrossRef]
8. Tekalegn, Y.; Sahiledengle, B.; Woldeyohannes, D.; Atlaw, D.; Degno, S.; Desta, F.; Bekele, K.; Aseffa, T.; Gezahegn, H.; Kene, C. High Parity Is Associated with Increased Risk of Cervical Cancer: Systematic Review and Meta-Analysis of Case-Control Studies. *Womens Health* **2022**, *18*, 17455065221075904. [CrossRef] [PubMed]
9. Dicu-Andreescu, I.-G.; Marincaș, M.-A.; Prunoiu, V.-M.; Dicu-Andreescu, I.; Ionescu, S.-O.; Simionescu, A.-A.; Brătucu, E.; Simion, L. The Impact of Patient Characteristics, Risk Factors, and Surgical Intervention on Survival in a Cohort of Patients Undergoing Neoadjuvant Treatment for Cervical Cancer. *Medicina* **2023**, *59*, 2147. [CrossRef]

10. Ghebre, R.G.; Grover, S.; Xu, M.J.; Chuang, L.T.; Simonds, H. Cervical Cancer Control in HIV-Infected Women: Past, Present and Future. *Gynecol. Oncol. Rep.* **2017**, *21*, 101–108. [CrossRef]
11. Foran, C.; Brennan, A. Prevention and Early Detection of Cervical Cancer in the UK. *Br. J. Nurs.* **2015**, *24*, S22–S24, S26, S28–S29. [CrossRef]
12. Lei, J.; Arroyo-Mühr, L.S.; Lagheden, C.; Eklund, C.; Nordqvist Kleppe, S.; Elfström, M.; Andrae, B.; Sparén, P.; Dillner, J.; Sundström, K. Human Papillomavirus Infection Determines Prognosis in Cervical Cancer. *J. Clin. Oncol.* **2022**, *40*, 1522–1528. [CrossRef]
13. Cervical Cancer Statistics by Age. Available online: https://www.cancerresearchuk.org/health-professional/cancer-statistics/statistics-by-cancer-type/cervical-cancer/incidence#heading-One (accessed on 15 February 2024).
14. Hull, R.; Mbele, M.; Makhafola, T.; Hicks, C.; Wang, S.; Reis, R.; Mehrotra, R.; Mkhize-Kwitshana, Z.; Kibiki, G.; Bates, D.; et al. Cervical Cancer in Low and Middle-income Countries (Review). *Oncol. Lett.* **2020**, *20*, 2058–2074. [CrossRef]
15. NCCN Guidelines for Cervical Cancer. Available online: https://www.nccn.org/professionals/physician_gls/pdf/cervical.pdf (accessed on 18 June 2023).
16. Marth, C.; Landoni, F.; Mahner, S.; McCormack, M.; Gonzalez-Martin, A.; Colombo, N. Cervical Cancer: ESMO Clinical Practice Guidelines for Diagnosis, Treatment and Follow-Up. *Ann. Oncol.* **2017**, *28*, iv72–iv83. [CrossRef]
17. Cibula, D.; Raspollini, M.R.; Planchamp, F.; Centeno, C.; Chargari, C.; Felix, A.; Fischerová, D.; Jahnn-Kuch, D.; Joly, F.; Kohler, C.; et al. ESGO/ESTRO/ESP Guidelines for the Management of Patients with Cervical Cancer—Update 2023*. *Int. J. Gynecol. Cancer* **2023**, *33*, 649–666. [CrossRef]
18. Perelli, F.; Mattei, A.; Scambia, G.; Cavaliere, A.F. Editorial: Methods in Gynecological Oncology. *Front. Oncol.* **2023**, *13*, 1167088. [CrossRef]
19. Áyen, Á.; Jiménez Martínez, Y.; Boulaiz, H. Targeted Gene Delivery Therapies for Cervical Cancer. *Cancers* **2020**, *12*, 1301. [CrossRef]
20. Ramirez, P.T.; Pareja, R.; Rendón, G.J.; Millan, C.; Frumovitz, M.; Schmeler, K.M. Management of Low-Risk Early-Stage Cervical Cancer: Should Conization, Simple Trachelectomy, or Simple Hysterectomy Replace Radical Surgery as the New Standard of Care? *Gynecol. Oncol.* **2014**, *132*, 254–259. [CrossRef]
21. Querleu, D.; Cibula, D.; Abu-Rustum, N.R. 2017 Update on the Querleu-Morrow Classification of Radical Hysterectomy. *Ann. Surg. Oncol.* **2017**, *24*, 3406–3412. [CrossRef]
22. Dicu-Andreescu, I.-G.; Marincaș, A.-M.; Ungureanu, V.-G.; Ionescu, S.-O.; Prunoiu, V.-M.; Brătucu, E.; Simion, L. Current Therapeutic Approaches in Cervical Cancer Based on the Stage of the Disease: Is There Room for Improvement? *Medicina* **2023**, *59*, 1229. [CrossRef]
23. Querleu, D.; Morrow, C.P. Classification of Radical Hysterectomy. *Lancet Oncol.* **2008**, *9*, 297–303. [CrossRef]
24. Palfalvi, L.; Ungar, L. Laterally Extended Parametrectomy (LEP), the Technique for Radical Pelvic Side Wall Dissection: Feasibility, Technique and Results. *Int. J. Gynecol. Cancer* **2003**, *13*, 914–917. [CrossRef]
25. Nagy, V.; Rancea, A.; Coza, O.; Kacso, G.; Aldea, B. Alexandru Eniu Ghid MS Conduita Cancer Col Uterin. Available online: http://old.ms.ro/index.php?pag=181&pg=5 (accessed on 4 March 2024).
26. Cao, L.; Kong, W.; Li, J.; Song, D.; Jin, B.; Liu, T.; Han, C. Analysis of Lymph Node Metastasis and Risk Factors in 975 Patients with FIGO 2009 Stage IA–IIA Cervical Cancer. *Gynecol. Obstet. Investig.* **2023**, *88*, 30–36. [CrossRef]
27. Ronsini, C.; Anchora, L.P.; Restaino, S.; Fedele, C.; Arciuolo, D.; Teodorico, E.; Bizzarri, N.; Zannoni, G.F.; Ferrandina, G.; Scambia, G.; et al. The Role of Semiquantitative Evaluation of Lympho-Vascular Space Invasion in Early Stage Cervical Cancer Patients. *Gynecol. Oncol.* **2021**, *162*, 299–307. [CrossRef]
28. Luo, L.; Luo, Q.; Tang, L. Diagnostic Value and Clinical Significance of MRI and CT in Detecting Lymph Node Metastasis of Early Cervical Cancer. *Oncol. Lett.* **2020**, *19*, 700–706. [CrossRef]
29. Zhu, Y.; Shen, B.; Pei, X.; Liu, H.; Li, G. CT, MRI, and PET Imaging Features in Cervical Cancer Staging and Lymph Node Metastasis. *Am. J. Transl. Res.* **2021**, *13*, 10536–10544.
30. Kondo, E.; Yoshida, K.; Tabata, T.; Kobayashi, Y.; Yamagami, W.; Ebina, Y.; Kaneuchi, M.; Nagase, S.; Machida, H.; Mikami, M. Comparison of Treatment Outcomes of Surgery and Radiotherapy, Including Concurrent Chemoradiotherapy for Stage Ib2-IIb Cervical Adenocarcinoma Patients: A Retrospective Study. *J. Gynecol. Oncol.* **2022**, *33*, e14. [CrossRef]
31. Voinea, S.; Herghelegiu, C.; Sandru, A.; Ioan, R.; Bohîlțea, R.; Bacalbașa, N.; Chivu, L.; Furtunescu, F.; Stanica, D.; Neacșu, A. Impact of Histological Subtype on the Response to Chemoradiation in Locally Advanced Cervical Cancer and the Possible Role of Surgery. *Exp. Ther. Med.* **2020**, *21*, 93. [CrossRef]
32. Kaidar-Person, O.; Yosefia, S.; Abdah-Bortnyak, R. Response of Adenocarcinoma of the Uterine Cervix to Chemoradiotherapy. *Oncol. Lett.* **2015**, *9*, 2791–2794. [CrossRef]
33. Kang, J.-H.; Cho, W.K.; Yeo, H.J.; Jeong, S.Y.; Noh, J.J.; Shim, J.I.; Lee, Y.-Y.; Kim, T.-J.; Lee, J.-W.; Kim, B.-G.; et al. Prognostic Significance of Tumor Regression Rate during Concurrent Chemoradiotherapy in Locally Advanced Cervix Cancer: Analysis by Radiation Phase and Histologic Type. *J. Clin. Med.* **2020**, *9*, 3471. [CrossRef]
34. Wakatsuki, M.; Ohno, T.; Kato, S.; Ando, K.; Noda, S.-e.; Kiyohara, H.; Shibuya, K.; Karasawa, K.; Kamada, T.; Nakano, T. Impact of Boost Irradiation on Pelvic Lymph Node Control in Patients with Cervical Cancer. *J. Radiat. Res.* **2014**, *55*, 139–145. [CrossRef] [PubMed]

35. Serkies, K.; Badzio, A.; Jassem, J. Clinical Relevance of Hemoglobin Level in Cervical Cancer Patients Administered Definitive Radiotherapy. *Acta Oncol.* **2006**, *45*, 695–701. [CrossRef]
36. Mercadante, S.; Gebbia, V.; Marrazzo, A.; Filosto, S. Anaemia in Cancer: Pathophysiology and Treatment. *Cancer Treat. Rev.* **2000**, *26*, 303–311. [CrossRef]
37. Dunst, J.; Kuhnt, T.; Strauss, H.G.; Krause, U.; Pelz, T.; Koelbl, H.; Haensgen, G. Anemia in Cervical Cancers: Impact on Survival, Patterns of Relapse, and Association with Hypoxia and Angiogenesis. *Int. J. Radiat. Oncol. Biol. Phys.* **2003**, *56*, 778–787. [CrossRef] [PubMed]
38. Caro, J.J.; Salas, M.; Ward, A.; Goss, G. Anemia as an Independent Prognostic Factor for Survival in Patients with Cancer: A Systemic, Quantitative Review. *Cancer* **2001**, *91*, 2214–2221. [CrossRef] [PubMed]
39. Zhang, H.; Kong, W.; Chen, S.; Zhao, X.; Luo, D.; Xie, Y. Surgical Staging of Locally Advanced Cervical Cancer: Current Status and Research Progress. *Front. Oncol.* **2022**, *12*, 940807. [CrossRef] [PubMed]
40. Arbyn, M.; Weiderpass, E.; Bruni, L.; de Sanjosé, S.; Saraiya, M.; Ferlay, J.; Bray, F. Estimates of Incidence and Mortality of Cervical Cancer in 2018: A Worldwide Analysis. *Lancet Glob. Health* **2020**, *8*, e191–e203. [CrossRef] [PubMed]
41. Vora, C.; Gupta, S. Targeted Therapy in Cervical Cancer. *ESMO Open* **2018**, *3*, e000462. [CrossRef] [PubMed]
42. Watkins, D.E.; Craig, D.J.; Vellani, S.D.; Hegazi, A.; Fredrickson, K.J.; Walter, A.; Stanbery, L.; Nemunaitis, J. Advances in Targeted Therapy for the Treatment of Cervical Cancer. *J. Clin. Med.* **2023**, *12*, 5992. [CrossRef]
43. Qin, C.; Chen, X.; Bai, Q.; Davis, M.R.; Fang, Y. Factors Associated with Radiosensitivity of Cervical Cancer. *Anticancer Res.* **2014**, *34*, 4649–4656.
44. Singh, U.; Verma, M.L.; Rahman, Z.; Qureshi, S.; Srivastava, K. Factors Affecting Quality of Life of Cervical Cancer Patients: A Multivariate Analysis. *J. Cancer Res. Ther.* **2019**, *15*, 1338–1344. [CrossRef]
45. Osann, K.; Hsieh, S.; Nelson, E.L.; Monk, B.J.; Chase, D.; Cella, D.; Wenzel, L. Factors Associated with Poor Quality of Life among Cervical Cancer Survivors: Implications for Clinical Care and Clinical Trials. *Gynecol. Oncol.* **2014**, *135*, 266–272. [CrossRef]
46. Mereu, L.; Pecorino, B.; Ferrara, M.; Tomaselli, V.; Scibilia, G.; Scollo, P. Neoadjuvant Chemotherapy plus Radical Surgery in Locally Advanced Cervical Cancer: Retrospective Single-Center Study. *Cancers* **2023**, *15*, 5207. [CrossRef]
47. Cui, H.; Huang, Y.; Wen, W.; Li, X.; Xu, D.; Liu, L. Prognostic Value of Lymph Node Ratio in Cervical Cancer: A Meta-Analysis. *Medicine* **2022**, *101*, e30745. [CrossRef]
48. Sun, C.; Wang, S.; Ye, W.; Wang, R.; Tan, M.; Zhang, H.; Zhou, J.; Li, M.; Wei, L.; Xu, P.; et al. The Prognostic Value of Tumor Size, Volume and Tumor Volume Reduction Rate During Concurrent Chemoradiotherapy in Patients With Cervical Cancer. *Front. Oncol.* **2022**, *12*, 934110. [CrossRef] [PubMed]
49. Zhang, S.; Wang, X.; Li, Z.; Wang, W.; Wang, L. Score for the Overall Survival Probability of Patients With First-Diagnosed Distantly Metastatic Cervical Cancer: A Novel Nomogram-Based Risk Assessment System. *Front. Oncol.* **2019**, *9*, 1106. [CrossRef] [PubMed]
50. Berman, M.L.; Keys, H.; Creasman, W.; DiSaia, P.; Bundy, B.; Blessing, J. Survival and Patterns of Recurrence in Cervical Cancer Metastatic to Periaortic Lymph Nodes. *Gynecol. Oncol.* **1984**, *19*, 8–16. [CrossRef] [PubMed]
51. Mileshkin, L.R.; Moore, K.N.; Barnes, E.H.; Lee, Y.C.; Gebski, V.; Narayan, K.; Bradshaw, N.; Diamante, K.; Fyles, A.W.; Small, W.; et al. Staging Locally Advanced Cervical Cancer with FIGO 2018 versus FIGO 2008: Impact on Overall Survival and Progression-Free Survival in the OUTBACK Trial (ANZGOG 0902, RTOG 1174, NRG 0274). *J. Clin. Oncol.* **2022**, *40*, 5531. [CrossRef]
52. Ronsini, C.; De Franciscis, P.; Carotenuto, R.M.; Pasanisi, F.; Cobellis, L.; Colacurci, N. The Oncological Implication of Sentinel Lymph Node in Early Cervical Cancer: A Meta-Analysis of Oncological Outcomes and Type of Recurrences. *Medicina* **2022**, *58*, 1539. [CrossRef]
53. Ronsini, C.; Köhler, C.; De Franciscis, P.; La Verde, M.; Mosca, L.; Solazzo, M.C.; Colacurci, N. Laparo-Assisted Vaginal Radical Hysterectomy as a Safe Option for Minimal Invasive Surgery in Early Stage Cervical Cancer: A Systematic Review and Meta-Analysis. *Gynecol. Oncol.* **2022**, *166*, 188–195. [CrossRef]
54. Ronsini, C.; Solazzo, M.C.; Molitierno, R.; De Franciscis, P.; Pasanisi, F.; Cobellis, L.; Colacurci, N. Fertility-Sparing Treatment for Early-Stage Cervical Cancer ≥ 2 Cm: Can One Still Effectively Become a Mother? A Systematic Review of Fertility Outcomes. *Ann. Surg. Oncol.* **2023**, *30*, 5587–5596. [CrossRef] [PubMed]
55. Ronsini, C.; Solazzo, M.C.; Bizzarri, N.; Ambrosio, D.; La Verde, M.; Torella, M.; Carotenuto, R.M.; Cobellis, L.; Colacurci, N.; De Franciscis, P. Fertility-Sparing Treatment for Early-Stage Cervical Cancer ≥ 2 Cm: A Problem with a Thousand Nuances-A Systematic Review of Oncological Outcomes. *Ann. Surg. Oncol.* **2022**, *29*, 8346–8358. [CrossRef] [PubMed]
56. Scotti, R.J.; Bergman, A.; Bhatia, N.N.; Ostergard, D.R. Urodynamic Changes in Urethrovesical Function After Radical Hysterectomy. *Obstet. Gynecol.* **1986**, *68*, 111–120. [PubMed]

Disclaimer/Publisher's Note: The statements, opinions and data contained in all publications are solely those of the individual author(s) and contributor(s) and not of MDPI and/or the editor(s). MDPI and/or the editor(s) disclaim responsibility for any injury to people or property resulting from any ideas, methods, instructions or products referred to in the content.

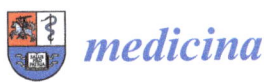

Article

Impact of Neoadjuvant Chemotherapy (NAC) on Biomarker Expression in Breast Cancer

Suji Lee [1,2], Jee Yeon Kim [2,3], So Jeong Lee [4], Chung Su Hwang [2,3], Hyun Jung Lee [2,3], Kyung Bin Kim [1,2], Jung Hee Lee [2,3], Dong Hoon Shin [2,3], Kyung Un Choi [1,2], Chang Hun Lee [1,2], Gi Yeong Huh [1,2] and Ahrong Kim [1,2,*]

1. Department of Pathology, Pusan National University Hospital, Biomedical Research Institution, 179 Gudeok-ro, Seo-gu, Busan 49241, Republic of Korea
2. Department of Pathology, School of Medicine, Pusan National University, Beomeori, Mulgeum-eop, Yangsan 50612, Republic of Korea
3. Department of Pathology, Yangsan Pusan National University Hospital, Medical Research Institute, Beomeori, Mulgeum-eop, Yangsan 50612, Republic of Korea
4. Department of Pathology, Seegene Medial Foundation Busan, Joongangdaero 297, Busan 48792, Republic of Korea
* Correspondence: ahrong2h@naver.com; Tel.: +82-240-7000

Abstract: *Background and Objectives*: This study aimed to explore biomarker change after NAC (neoadjuvant chemotherapy) and to investigate biomarker expression as a prognostic factor in patients with residual disease (RD) after NAC. *Materials and Methods*: We retrospectively evaluated 104 patients with invasive breast cancer, who underwent NAC and surgery at Pusan National University Hospital from 2015 to July 2022. The expression of the biomarker was assessed, and the overall survival (OS) and disease-free survival (DFS) were investigated. *Results*: After NAC, 24 patients (23.1%) out of 104 total patients had a pathological complete response (pCR). We found that changes in at least one biomarker were observed in 41 patients (51.2%), among 80 patients with RD. In patients with RD after NAC (n = 80), a subtype change was identified in 20 patients (25.0%). Any kind of change in the HER2 status was present 19 (23.7%) patients. The hormone receptor (HR)+/HER2+ subtype was significantly associated with better disease-free survival (DFS) (HR, 0.13; 95% CI, 0.02–0.99; p = 0.049). No change in p53 was associated with better DFS, and negative-to-positive change in p53 expression after NAC was correlated with worse DFS (p < 0.001). Negative-to-positive change in p53 was an independent, worse DFS factor in the multivariate analysis (HR,18.44; 95% CI, 1.86–182.97; p = 0.013). *Conclusions*: Biomarker change and subtype change after NAC were not infrequent, which can affect the further treatment strategy after surgery. The expression change of p53 might have a prognostic role. Overall, we suggest that the re-evaluation of biomarkers after NAC can provide a prognostic role and is needed for the best decision to be made on further treatment.

Keywords: breast cancers; neoadjuvant chemotherapy; breast cancer subtype; biomarker; p53; prognostic factor

Citation: Lee, S.; Kim, J.Y.; Lee, S.J.; Hwang, C.S.; Lee, H.J.; Kim, K.B.; Lee, J.H.; Shin, D.H.; Choi, K.U.; Lee, C.H.; et al. Impact of Neoadjuvant Chemotherapy (NAC) on Biomarker Expression in Breast Cancer. *Medicina* **2024**, *60*, 737. https://doi.org/10.3390/medicina60050737

Academic Editors: Valentin Titus Grigorean and Daniel Alin Cristian

Received: 9 April 2024
Revised: 24 April 2024
Accepted: 28 April 2024
Published: 29 April 2024

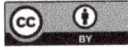

Copyright: © 2024 by the authors. Licensee MDPI, Basel, Switzerland. This article is an open access article distributed under the terms and conditions of the Creative Commons Attribution (CC BY) license (https://creativecommons.org/licenses/by/4.0/).

1. Introduction

Recently, neoadjuvant chemotherapy (NAC) has been considered a standard treatment for locally advanced breast cancer, and the use of NAC has increased [1].

Mohan et al. reported that the residual disease (RD) burden at the time of surgery after completion of NAC has been shown to have a significant effect on prognosis in all disease subtypes [2], but there is no agreement on the exact definition of RD or the pathological complete response (pCR). In the Miller–Payne grading system, the treatment response is estimated only as the reduction in primary invasive tumor cellularity and does not consider the presence or absence of ductal carcinoma in situ and lymph node metastasis [3]. In the residual cancer burden grading system, the treatment response is considered as the bidimensional diameter and cellularity of the invasive primary tumor, including lymph node metastasis, but the presence or absence of ductal carcinoma in situ is not considered [4]. The National Comprehensive Cancer Network (NCCN) guidelines, one of the most important guidelines, refers to pCR as no invasive and no in situ residual lesions in the breast and lymph nodes, and this concept can be used to best differentiate between patients with favorable and unfavorable outcomes [5]. Therefore, it is necessary to reach consensus on the evaluation criteria for the treatment response in patients with NAC to evaluate patient prognosis and establish a treatment standard in regard to NAC. One of the issues related to NAC is the biomarker status change. According to the NCCN guidelines, the biomarker status should be tested using the tumor core needle biopsy samples to determine the appropriate NAC, but it is not mandatory to repeat the biomarker status test using the resection samples to guide the adjuvant treatment choice. However, in prior studies, biomarker status was altered by NAC in some tumors. But biomarker status changes induced by NAC have been the focus of recent systemic and meta-analyses, and changes in the hormone receptor (HR) status induced by NAC can be used as a prognostic factor in breast cancer patients for predicting both overall survival (OS) and disease-free survival (DFS) [6,7]. Additionally, therapeutic options continue to be constrained in regard to pretreated advanced breast cancer patients, while several antibody–drug conjugates and immunotherapies are presently undergoing clinical trials [8,9]. Also, research is being conducted to investigate the effectiveness of combining various modalities in treatment and whether this effectiveness varies according to patient characteristics, such as gender [10]. It is anticipated that research will also explore which parameters will impact a patient's treatment and investigate the most effective combination of therapeutic modalities tailored to individual patient characteristics.

However, there is relatively little published data on the impact of change in the receptor status on survival outcomes following neoadjuvant chemotherapy in breast cancer, but it should be considered in some circumstances [11]. In Korea, the data on biomarker changes after NAC and on the correlation between biomarker change and patient prognosis are limited. Thus, investigating biomarker discordance induced by NAC in Korean patients is important for determining treatment methods after surgery and predicting the patient's progress.

The objective of this study was to explore biomarker discordance before and after NAC and to investigate ER, PR, HER2, p53, and Ki67 expression as a prognostic factor in RD patients after NAC.

2. Materials and Methods

2.1. Patients and Data Collection

We retrospectively evaluated 108 patients with invasive breast cancer who underwent surgery at Pusan National University Hospital from 2015 to July 2022. The patient was included if they: (1) received NAC prior to surgery, (2) underwent IHC biomarker testing on their core biopsy specimen at the time of diagnosis, (3) had paired immunohistochemistry biomarker testing on a surgical specimen. Among 108 patients, 4 patients were excluded because there was no paired testing. Clinical information was collected from electronic medical records, and pathologic information was collected from pathology reports. Exemption from informed consent after de-identification of the patients' information was approved by the institutional review board at Pusan National University Hospital (2209-024-119).

2.2. Neoadjuvant Chemotherapy

All included patients had inoperable breast cancer, or HER2-positive or triple-negative disease, at an operable early-stage state. Also, they were treated with neoadjuvant chemotherapy (NAC) at Pusan National University Hospital. Patients with HER2-negative disease received 4 cycles of AC (doxorubicin, cyclophosphamide) every 21 days, followed by 4 cycles of paclitaxel or docetaxel. Patients with HER2-positive disease received 6 cycles of TCHP (docetaxel, carboplatin, trastuzumab, and pertuzumab) every 21 days. After NAC, all patients received breast conservative surgery or a mastectomy.

2.3. Immunohistochemistry

Immunohistochemistry for the estrogen receptor (ER; SP1, prediluted, Ventana Medical Systems, Tuscon, AZ, USA), progesterone receptor (PR; 1E2, prediluted, Ventana Medical Systems), human epidermal growth factor receptor type 2 (HER2; 4B5, prediluted, Ventana Medical Systems), p53 (DO7, prediluted, Ventana Medical Systems), and Ki67 (30-9, prediluted, Ventana Medical Systems) was performed using a Benchmark Ultra instrument (Ventana Medical Systems). The thickness of the paraffin sections was 3 µm. ER, PR, and HER2 positivity was assessed according to the American Society of Clinical Oncology (ASCO) guidelines. Staining for HRs (ER and PR) was considered positive when it exceeded 1% of any nuclear staining. HER2 positivity was defined as an immunostaining score of 3 (circumferential membrane staining that is complete, intense, and observed in >10% of tumor cells), or as gene amplification confirmed by silver in situ hybridization (SISH), which was performed with a HER2/CEP17 chromosome dual probe (Ventana Medical Systems). Cases with a HER2 immunostaining score of 2 (equivocal; weak-to-moderate complete membrane staining observed in >10% of tumor cells) received SISH testing to verify the HER2 gene amplification. A HER2 low positive case was defined as 1+ HER2 immunostaining or 2+ HER2 immunostaining without gene amplification on SISH. Positive staining for p53 was defined as strong diffuse nuclear staining, which is considered the most common pattern associated with mutations [12]. The Ki67 proliferation index was calculated as the overall average percentage of positive nuclear staining. If there were clear hot spots of Ki67 staining, data from these samples were also included in the overall score. The Ki67 proliferation index was categorized as low (<20%) or high ($\geq$20%) for the purpose of the analysis.

Patients were categorized into four subtypes based on their HR (ER and PR) and HER2 expression status: (1) HR+/HER2−, (2) HR+/HER2+, (3) HR−/HER2+, and (4) HR−/HER2−.

2.4. Evaluation of NAC Response

We used the strict definition of pCR according to the NCCN guidelines. We defined RD as any presence of an invasive or in situ lesion in the breast or lymph nodes, except if there was only a lympho-vascular invasion [5].

2.5. Statistics

We analyzed the discordance in the biomarker status between the biopsy specimen and the surgical specimen using the Chi-square test. Kaplan–Meier analysis was used to study prognosis (OS rate and DFS rate). OS was defined as the time from diagnosis to death or the last follow-up date, and DFS was defined as the time from diagnosis to any recurrence, new metastasis, and death. Multivariable Cox regression analysis was used to estimate the effects of the clinical and pathological variables. All analyses were performed using the SPSS statistical software (version 18; IBM, Armonk, NY, USA). All tests were two-sided and $p < 0.05$ was considered statistically significant.

3. Results

3.1. Patient Characteristics

The clinico-pathological characteristics of the patients included in this study are shown in Table 1. The median age of the patients at diagnosis was 54 years (range 24–77). Of the total 104 patients, 24 patients (23.1%) had a pCR, and 80 patients (76.9%) were in RD status after NAC. The subtypes of the biopsy samples pre-NAC were as follows: 33 patients (31.7%) were HR+/HER2−, 17 patients (16.4%) were HR+/HER2+, 28 patients (26.9%) were HR−/HER2+, and 26 patients (25.0%) were HR−/HER2−.

Table 1. Clinico-pathological characteristics of study cohort.

	Age at Diagnosis	54 (24–77)	
NAC response	Pathological complete response (pCR)	24 (23.1)	
	Residual disease (RD)	80 (76.9)	
Pre-NAC subtypes (biopsy)	HR+/HER2−	33 (31.7)	
	HR+/HER2+	17 (16.4)	
	HR−/HER2+	28 (26.9)	
	HR−/HER2−	26 (25.0)	
Pre-NAC clinical stage (c stage, biopsy)	I	3 (2.9)	
	II	17 (16.3)	
	III	79 (76.0)	
	IV	5 (4.8)	
Pre-NAC nuclear grade (biopsy)	Low (grade 1, 2)	71 (68.3)	
	High (grade 3)	29 (27.9)	Total patients (n = 104)
	Not applicable	4 (3.8)	
Post-NAC pathological stage (yp stage, resection)	0	32 (30.8)	
	I	14 (13.5)	
	II	31 (29.8)	
	III	27 (26.0)	
Post-NAC lympho-vascular invasion (resection)	Absent	72 (69.2)	
	Present	32 (30.8)	
Post-NAC nuclear grade (resection)	Low (grade 1, 2)	35 (33.7)	
	High (grade 3)	33 (31.7)	
Post-NAC histological grade (resection)	Not applicable	36 (34.6)	
	Low (well, moderately)	39 (37.5)	
	High (poorly)	28 (26.9)	
Post-NAC subtypes (resection)	Not applicable	37 (35.6)	
	HR+/HER2−	36 (45.0)	Residual disease patients (n = 80)
	HR+/HER2+	7 (8.8)	
	HR−/HER2+	16 (20.0)	

The pathological characteristics of RD patients (n = 80), according to pre-NAC biopsy subtypes, are presented in Table 2. In patients with RD after NAC (n = 80), a subtype change was identified in 20 patients (25.0%). Among them, a subtype change occurred in three (15.0%) patients with the HR+/HER2− biopsy subtype, eight patients (40.0%) with the HR+/HER2+ biopsy subtype, six patients (30.0%) with the HR−/HER2+ biopsy subtype, and three patients (15%) with the HR−/HER2− biopsy subtype.

Table 2. Pathologic characteristics of residual disease patients, according to pre-NAC biopsy subtypes (n = 80).

		Pre-NAC Subtypes (Biopsy)			
		HR+/HER2− (n = 31)	HR+/HER2+ (n = 12)	HR−/HER2+ (n = 17)	HR−/HER2− (n = 20)
Pre-NAC nuclear grade (biopsy)	Low (grade 1, 2)	25 (80.6)	11 (91.7)	7 (41.2)	11 (55.0)
	High (grade 3)	4 (12.9)	1 (8.3)	10 (58.8)	8 (40.0)
	Not applicable	2 (6.5)	0 (0.0)	0 (0.0)	1 (5.0)
Pre-NAC clinical stage (c stage, biopsy)	I	3 (9.7)	0 (0.0)	0 (0.0)	0 (0.0)
	II	6 (19.4)	2 (16.7)	3 (17.6)	2 (10.0)
	III	20 (64.5)	9 (75.0)	13 (76.5)	17 (85.0)
	IV	2 (6.5)	1 (8.3)	1 (5.9)	1 (5.0)

Table 2. Cont.

		Pre-NAC Subtypes (Biopsy)			
		HR+/HER2− (n = 31)	HR+/HER2+ (n = 12)	HR−/HER2+ (n = 17)	HR−/HER2− (n = 20)
Post-NAC subtypes (resection)	HR+/HER2−	28 (90.3)	4 (33.3)	2 (11.8)	2 (10.0)
	HR+/HER2+	0 (0.0)	4 (33.3)	3 (17.6)	0 (0.0)
	HR−/HER2+	0 (0.0)	4 (33.3)	11 (64.7)	1 (5.0)
	HR−/HER2−	3 (9.7)	0 (0.0)	1 (5.9)	17 (85.0)
Post-NAC nuclear grade (resection)	Low (grade 1)	22 (71.0)	4 (33.3)	6 (35.3)	3 (15.0)
	High (grade 2, 3)	6 (19.4)	7 (58.3)	6 (35.3)	14 (70.0)
	Not applicable	3 (9.7)	1 (8.3)	5 (29.4)	3 (15.0)
Post-NAC pathological stage (yp stage, resection)	0	3 (9.7)	1 (8.3)	3 (17.6)	1 (5.0)
	I	5 (16.1)	2 (16.7)	6 (35.3)	1 (5.0)
	II	10 (32.3)	8 (66.7)	2 (11.8)	11 (55.0)
	III	13 (41.9)	1 (8.3)	6 (35.3)	7 (35.0)

3.2. Correlation between Clinico-Pathological Variables and NAC Response

The association between the clinico-pathological parameters and the NAC response is presented in Table 3. After NAC, 24 patients (23.1%) out of 104 total patients had a pCR. Their subtypes in regard to their biopsy samples before NAC are shown in Table 3. The pCR was most frequently observed in the HR−/HER2+ biopsy subtype (11, 45.8%) and at clinical stage III (20, 83.3%) (Table 3).

Table 3. Correlation between NAC response and pathologic variables in total patients (n = 104).

Variables		Pathological Complete Response (n = 24)	Residual Disease (n = 80)	p-Value
Age at Diagnosis		55.5 Years (29–71)	54 Years (24–77)	
Pre-NAC subtypes (biopsy)	HR+/HER2−	2 (8.3)	31 (38.8)	0.019
	HR+/HER2+	5 (20.8)	12 (15.0)	
	HR−/HER2+	11 (45.8)	17 (21.3)	
	HR−/HER2−	6 (25.0)	20 (25.0)	
Pre-NAC clinical stage (c stage, biopsy)	I	0 (0.0)	3 (3.8)	0.453
	II	4 (16.7)	13 (16.3)	
	III	20 (83.3)	59 (73.8)	
	IV	0 (0.0)	5 (6.3)	
Pre-NAC nuclear grade (biopsy)	Low (grade 1, 2)	17 (70.8)	54 (67.5)	0.926
	High (grade 3)	6 (25.0)	23 (28.8)	
	Not applicable	1 (4.2)	3 (3.8)	
Post-NAC pathological stage (yp stage, resection)	0	24 (100.0)	8 (10.0)	<0.001
	I	0 (0.0)	14 (17.5)	
	II	0 (0.0)	31 (38.8)	
	III	0 (0.0)	27 (33.8)	
Post-NAC lympho-vascular invasion (resection)	Absent	23 (95.8)	49 (61.3)	0.001
	Present	1 (4.2)	31 (38.8)	
Post-NAC nuclear grade (resection)	Low (grade 1, 2)	0 (0.0)	35 (43.8)	<0.001
	High (grade 3)	0 (0.0)	33 (41.3)	
	Not applicable	24 (100.0)	12 (15.0)	
Post-NAC histological grade (resection)	Low (well, moderately)	0 (0.0)	39 (48.8)	<0.001
	High (poorly)	0 (0.0)	28 (35.0)	
	Not applicable	24 (100.0)	13 (16.3)	

3.3. Changes in Each Biomarker Status after NAC

The changes in each biomarker status after NAC in 80 residual patients are shown in Figure 1. Most patients maintained stable expression of HRs, with 69 patients (86.3%) for

ER and 65 patients (81.3%) for PR, as well as 61 patients (76.3%) for HER2 and 73 patients (91.3%) for p53. Additionally, 54 patients (67.6%) exhibited consistent Ki67 expression. However, of all 80 patients with RD, changes in at least one biomarker were observed in 41 patients (51.2%) (Figure 2a).

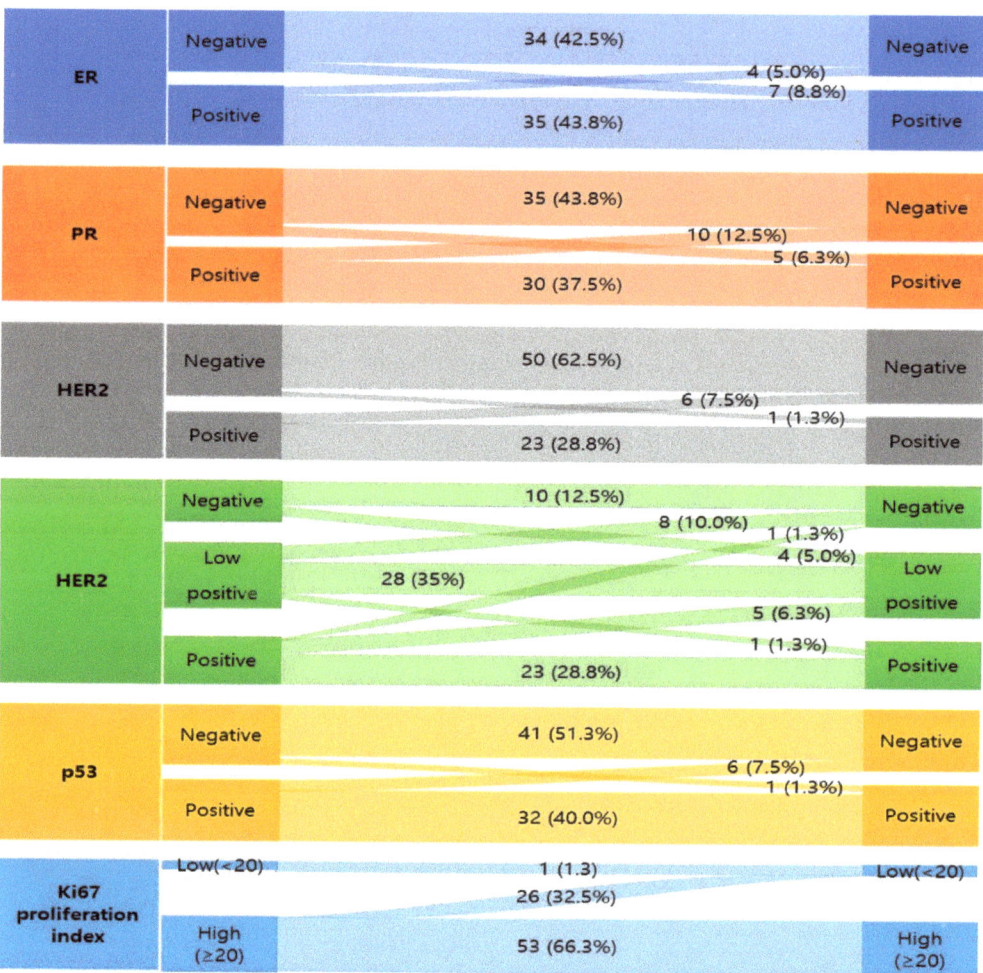

Figure 1. Biomarker changes after NAC (total residual patients, n = 80).

The biomarker status changes after NAC, according to the pre-NAC biopsy subtype, are presented in Figure 2b–e. The change in HER2 status, from positive to negative, was not identified in HR+/HER2− pre-NAC biopsy subtypes. Only positive to negative change in the HER2 status was identified in HER2+ subtypes (HR+/HER2+ and HR−/HER2+ subtypes). Notably, there was one case of negative to positive change in the HER2 status in HR−/HER2− subtypes and this case was a change from low positive to positive, which is described below (Figure 2e).

The HER2 status change, according to post-NAC resection subtypes, is presented in detail in Table 4. We found any kind of change in the HER2 status in 19 (23.7%) patients (Table 4). These changes include negative to low positive (4, 5.0%), low positive to negative (8, 10.0%), low positive to positive (1, 1.2%), positive to negative (1, 1.2%), and positive to low positive (5, 6.2%) (Table 4). Among them, five patients (6.2%) were HR+/HER2−

subtype, four (5.0%) were HR+/HER2+ subtype, two (2.5%) were HR−/HER2+, and the remaining eight (10.0%) were HR−/HER2− subtype. Overall, there were six cases of positive to negative in terms of changes to the HER2 status.

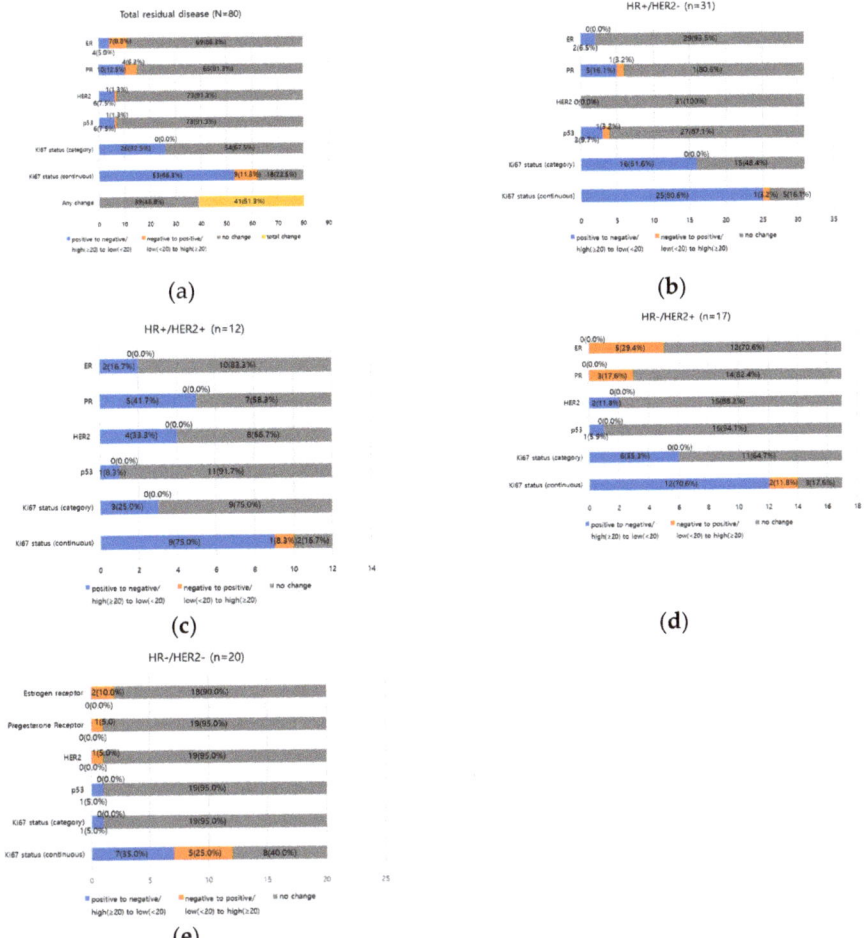

Figure 2. Biomarker changes after NAC according to biopsy subtype in residual disease patients (n = 80): (**a**) total residual patients (n = 80); (**b**) HR+/HER2− biopsy subtype (n = 31), (**c**) HR+/HER2+ biopsy subtype (n = 12); (**d**) HR−/HER2+ biopsy subtype (n = 17); (**e**) HR−/HER2− biopsy subtype (n = 20).

The change in p53 expression after NAC was present in seven cases (8.7%). One (14.3%) of them had a negative to positive change and the other six patients (85.7%) showed a positive to negative change in p53 expression (Figure 1). The subtypes of the cases showing a p53 expression change are presented in Table 5.

The change in the Ki67 proliferation index group from low to high after NAC was not identified (Figure 1). However, in regard to the Ki-67 proliferation index as a continuous variable, there were nine cases (11.3%) of increment in the proliferation index; although it did not lead to a group change from low to high (Figure 2).

Table 4. HER2 expression changes according to post-NAC subtypes in residual disease patients (n = 80).

		Total Residual (n = 80)				Post-NAC Subtypes (Resection)												
						HR+/HER2− (n = 31)				HR+/HER2+ (n = 12)				HR−/HER2+ (n = 17)				HR−/HER2− (n = 20)
		Negative	Low Positive	Positive	p-Value	Negative	Low Positive	Positive	p-Value	Negative	Low Positive	Positive	p-Value	Negative	Low Positive	Positive	p-Value	Negative	Low Positive	Positive	p-Value
Pre-NAC HER2 status (biopsy)	Negative	10 (52.6)	4 (10.8)	0 (0.0)	<0.001	5 (62.5)	2 (8.7)	0 (0.0)	0.002	0 (0.0)	0 (0.0)	0 (0.0)		0 (0.0)	0 (0.0)	0 (0.0)		5 (50.0)	2 (22.2)	0 (0.0)	0.337
	Low positive	8 (42.1)	28 (75.7)	1 (4.2)		3 (37.5)	21 (91.3)	0 (0.0)		1 (100.0)	3 (100.0)	0 (0.0)		0 (0.0)	0 (0.0)	0 (0.0)		5 (50.0)	7 (77.8)	1 (100.0)
	Positive	1 (5.3)	5 (13.5)	23 (95.8)		0 (0.0)	0 (0.0)	0 (0.0)		0 (0.0)	3 (100.0)	8 (100.0)		0 (0.0)	2 (100.0)	15 (100.0)		0 (0.0)	0 (0.0)	0 (0.0)

(a) HER2 expression in immunohistochemistry (IHC) 0; (b) HER2 expression in IHC 1+ or 2+ in the absence of HER2 gene amplification; (c) HER2 expression in IHC 2+ in the presence of HER2 gene amplification or IHC 3.

Table 5. Cases showing p53 expression change after NAC.

Case	Change Type	Pre-NAC Biopsy Subtype	Post-NAC Resection Subtype
5	Positive to negative	HR+/HER2−	HR+/HER2−
13	Negative to positive	HR+/HER2−	HR+/HER2−
19	Positive to negative	HR+/HER2+	HR+/HER2−
20	Positive to negative	HR−/HER2+	HR+/HER2+
39	Positive to negative	HR−/HER2−	HR−/HER2−
82	Positive to negative	HR+/HER2−	HR+/HER2−
91	Positive to negative	HR+/HER2−	HR−/HER2−

3.4. Overall Survival and Disease-Free Survival

The survival analyses are shown in Figure 3. The HR+/HER2− pre-NAC biopsy subtype had the worst DFS, followed by the HR−/HER2− subtype. Also, the HR+/HER2+ subtype had the best DFS ($p = 0.044$, Figure 3b). The change in p53 expression had a significant impact on the DFS ($p < 0.001$). A negative to positive change in p53 had the worst DFS, while no change in p53 showed the best DFS (Figure 3d). According to the p53 status before and after NAC, no change in p53 was associated with better DFS; positivity of p53 in both pre-NAC biopsy and post-NAC resection samples had the best DFS, followed by negativity of p53 in both pre-NAC biopsy and post-NAC resection samples. Negative-to-positive change in p53 expression had the worst DFS ($p < 0.001$, Figure 3f). In addition, advanced yp stage (including yp stage III) patients after NAC tended to have worse DFS than early yp stage (including yp stage 0, I, II) patients ($p = 0.085$, Figure 3h).

In the multivariate analysis, the HR+/HER2+ subtype was an independent factor for better DFS (HR, 0.13; 95% CI, 0.02–0.99; $p = 0.049$). Also, negative-to-positive change in p53 expression after NAC was an independent factor for worse DFS (HR, 18.44; 95% CI, 1.86–182.97; $p = 0.013$) (Table 6).

Table 6. Analysis of disease-free survival in residual disease patients (n = 80).

		Univariable		Multivariable	
		Hazard Ratio (95% CI)	*p*-Value	Hazard Ratio (95% CI)	*p*-Value
Pre-NAC subtypes (biopsy)	HR+/HER2−	1	0.086	1	0.131
	HR+/HER2+	0.12 (0.02–0.90)	0.039	0.13 (0.02–0.99)	0.049
	HR−/HER2+	0.37 (0.12–1.12)	0.079	0.41 (0.13–1.25)	0.115
	HR−/HER2−	0.69 (0.29–1.62)	0.387	0.74 (0.31–1.76)	0.49
Pre-NAC clinical stage (c Stage, biopsy)	Early (0, I, II)	1			
	Advanced (III, IV)	1.71 (0.59–4.94)	0.319		
Post-NAC pathologic stage (yp Stage, resection)	Early (0, I, II)	1			
	Advanced (III)	1.92 (0.90–4.08)	0.09		
Post-NAC histologic grade (resection)	Low (well, moderately)	0.75 (0.29–1.99)	0.567		
	High (poorly)	0.59 (0.21–1.66)	0.314		
	Not applicable	1	0.600		
ER change	No change	1	0.754		
	Positive to negative	1.44 (0.34–6.13)	0.620		
	Negative to positive	0.68 (0.16–2.88)	0.600		
PR change	No change	1	0.665		
	Positive to negative	1.63 (0.56–4.75)	0.371		
	Negative to positive	0.98 (0.23–4.17)	0.977		
HER2 change	No change	1	0.563		
	Positive to negative	0	0.978		
	Negative to positive	3.00 (0.40–22.46)	0.284		
P53 change	No change	1	0.008	1	0.03
	Positive to negative	2.34 (0.70–7.90)	0.170	1.972 (0.58–6.67)	0.275
	Negative to positive	28.26 (2.92–273.57)	0.004	18.44 (1.86–182.97)	0.013
Ki67 change	No change	1			
	High (≥20) to low (<20)	0.79 (0.35–1.80)	0.577		
	Low (<20) to high (≥20)				

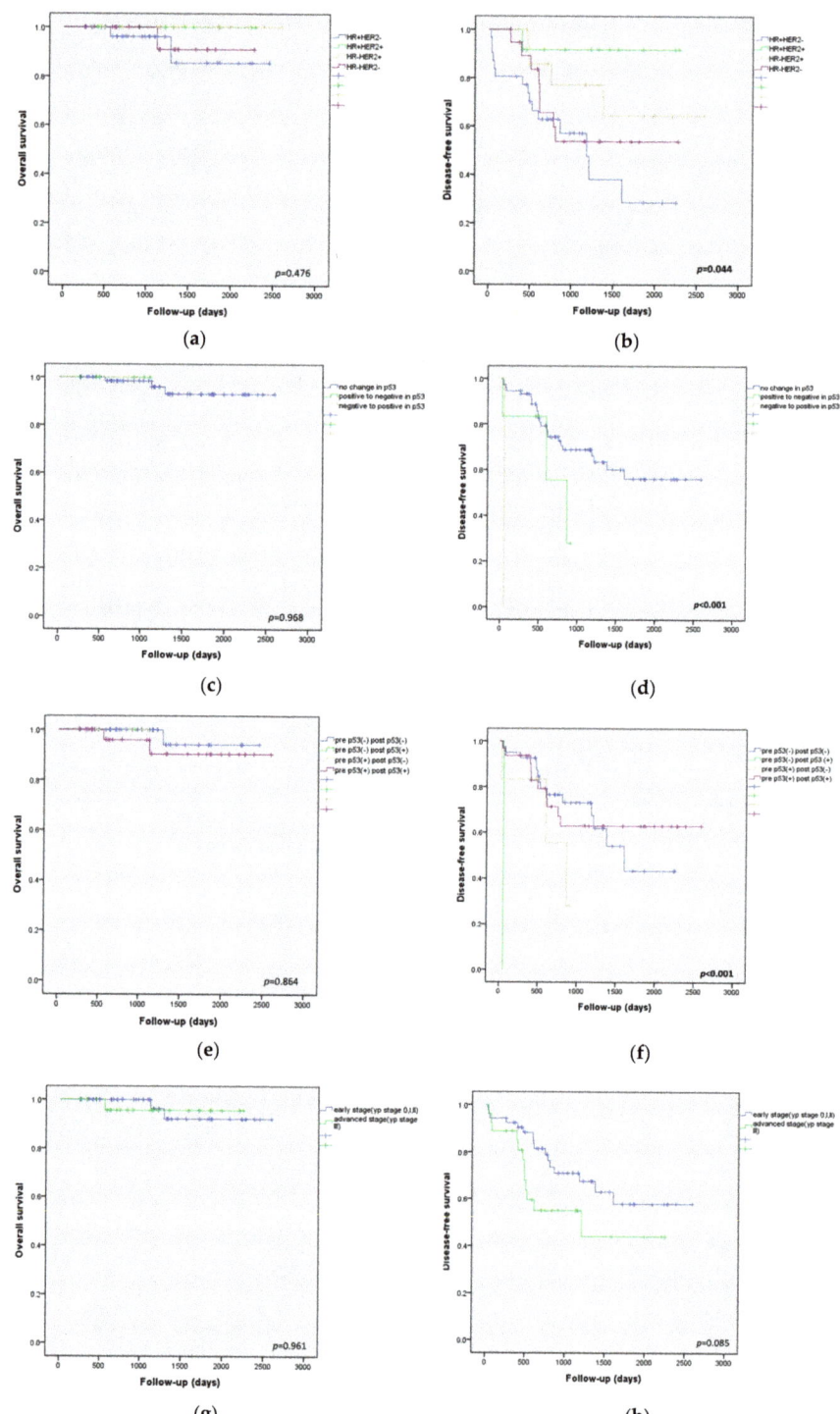

Figure 3. Kaplan–Meier estimates of overall survival and disease-free survival (residual disease patients, n = 80): (**a**) overall survival according to biopsy subtype (pre-NAC); (**b**) disease-free survival

according to biopsy subtype (pre-NAC); (**c**) overall survival according to changes in p53 expression status after NAC; (**d**) disease-free survival according to changes in p53 expression status after NAC; (**e**) overall survival according to p53 status before and after NAC; (**f**) disease-free survival according to p53 status before and after NAC; (**g**) overall survival according to yp stage (post-NAC); (**h**) disease-free survival according to yp stage (post-NAC).

4. Discussion

We found that biomarker change was common (51.2% of the RD patients) between specimens taken before and after NAC. A change in p53 expression after NAC was associated with a particularly poor prognosis in RD patients.

Biomarker change, according to NAC, in breast cancer patients appears in various ways, according to previous studies. Changes in biomarkers after NAC in breast cancer patients have been studied mainly in regard to Ki-67 [13–15] and it usually changes after adjusting the NAC [16,17]. Ki-67, a marker of cell proliferation, is expressed in all phases of the cell cycle, except G0 [18]. A decrease in Ki-67 after NAC was associated with a pCR and with better DFS and OS [13,15]. Rey-Vargas et al. observed no significant correlation between a Ki-67 decrease and the survival rate, but they reported a tendency of Ki-67 to decrease after NAC [14]. The same was true for this study, in which 26 patients (32.5%) showed a discordance of Ki-67 between pre-NAC and post-NAC specimens and all changes involved a decline, but these changes were not significantly correlated with the survival rate.

HER2 has been used as a treatment target over the past few decades since trastuzumab was developed. Recently, early-phase clinical trials have reported promising antiHER2 antibody–drug conjugates (ADCs), trastuzumab–deruxtecan and trastuzumab–duocarmazine, in HER2 low-positive patients [19,20]. Ahn et al. reported that positive-to-negative change in HER2 expression was more common than negative-to-positive change after NAC [21]. Also, Tural et al. showed that HER2 status change from positive to negative was an independent risk factor for worse DFS [22]. In this study, we did not reveal HER2 change as a prognostic factor after NAC. However, any change that can alter further treatment after NAC resection was significant in number, namely 19 patients (23.7%). Of note, four patients had negative HER2 expression in their pre-NAC biopsy sample and then showed HER2 low positive in their resection specimen after NAC. While it has not yet been established as the standard treatment protocol, the transition to HER2 low-positive status in patients following therapy suggests the potential diversification of treatment modalities in the future.

TP53, which encodes for the tumor suppressor protein p53, is the most frequently mutated gene in most types of human cancer, including breast cancer [23]. The role of p53 as a prognostic factor predicting pCR after NAC is controversial [24–26]. Bae et al. investigated, regardless of p53 expression, before NAC; the high expression of the p53 group after NAC indicated better OS in triple-negative breast cancer (TNBC) patients receiving NAC [27].

We found that no change in p53 expression after NAC was a significant predictor of improved prognosis. In particular, p53 positivity in both pre-NAC and post-NAC specimens was associated with the best improved prognosis. A few studies have shown that p53 positivity predicted chemotherapy-sensitive disease compared with p53 negative cases in TNBC [26,27]. In our study, patients with p53 positivity, both pre-NAC and post-NAC, had a better prognosis than those with negative p53 in both specimens.

In addition, we observed that any change in the p53 status was associated with worse prognosis than no change. In particular, a negative-to-positive change in p53 expression after NAC predicted a lower DFS. In patients who did not achieve a pCR, NAC resulted in a subpopulation of chemotherapy-resistant cells [28]. And diffuse nuclear positivity for p53 has previously been shown to be highly correlated with TP53 mutations [29]. Balko et al. molecularly profiled the RD remaining after NAC in a cohort of 111 TNBC. Alterations in

TP53 were identified in 89% of the samples [30]. MCL1 gene amplifications were seen in 54%, and MYC gene amplifications were seen in 35% of the samples [30]. These findings suggest that these alterations are present at high frequency in chemotherapy-treated TNBCs and may play a role in de novo or acquired therapeutic resistance [30]. Therefore, although this study was not limited to the triple-negative subtype, we could consider the possibility of the emergence of treatment resistance in patients with a p53 status alteration.

Patients with HR+ subtypes of breast cancer have the best prognosis, by contrast patients with HR− subtypes, especially those with triple-negative disease, have the worst prognosis, in part because of the lack of a receptor target [31,32]. We also observed that HR+/HER2+ patients who underwent NAC had improved DFS, in the multivariable analysis. Interestingly, however, among patients with NAC, the HR+HER2− subtype had worse prognosis than the HR−HER2− subtype. Luminal A breast cancers generally have a good prognosis and respond well to hormonal therapies, and patients with these cancers do not appear to benefit from the addition of the microtubule-targeted chemotherapy drug paclitaxel commonly used for NAC [33]. This may explain the poor therapeutic effect of NAC in luminal A breast cancer patients. In addition to this, after NAC, the residual tumors of most such patients had alterations in at least one of the clinically targetable pathways, resulting in therapeutic resistance [30]. These are the likely reasons why luminal A breast cancer patients had the worst prognosis in this study.

This study had several limitations. Firstly, it was conducted retrospectively, and this suggests the potential presence of confounding factors that were not considered. Secondly, the sample size was relatively small and data collection was carried out in a single institution. Thirdly, recent studies suggest that the distribution of residual disease, whether scattered or concerted, may impact patients' long-term survival [34,35]. Nevertheless, the distribution pattern of residual tumors was not considered in this study. However, it is important that the collected data can be used as a foundation for further research and provide insight on biomarker changes after NAC.

5. Conclusions

Our findings suggested that NAC has the potential to elicit alterations in biomarker expression and ultimately results in a subtype change after NAC, which was not common. In addition, p53 expression change may provide a prognostic role. Further studies are needed to clarify these issues and determine the need to re-evaluate biomarkers after NAC. This small and retrospective study provides a basis for future research investigating the prognostic and predictive role of biomarker re-evaluation.

Author Contributions: Conceptualization, S.L. and A.K.; methodology, S.L., A.K. and J.Y.K.; software, S.L. and A.K.; validation, S.L. and A.K.; formal analysis, S.L., A.K., S.J.L., K.B.K., C.S.H., H.J.L., J.H.L., D.H.S., K.U.C., C.H.L. and G.Y.H.; investigation, S.L., A.K., S.J.L., K.B.K., C.S.H., H.J.L. and J.H.L.; resources, S.L., A.K., J.Y.K., D.H.S., K.U.C., C.H.L. and G.Y.H.; data curation, S.L. and A.K.; writing—original draft preparation, S.L. and A.K.; writing—review and editing, S.L., A.K., S.J.L., C.S.H., H.J.L., J.H.L., J.Y.K., D.H.S., K.U.C., C.H.L. and G.Y.H.; visualization, S.L.; supervision, A.K.; project administration, A.K.; funding acquisition, A.K. All authors have read and agreed to the published version of the manuscript.

Funding: This work was supported by Pusan National University Research Grant, 2022 (202215760001).

Institutional Review Board Statement: This study was conducted according to the guidelines in the Declaration of Helsinki and approved by the institutional review board at Pusan National University Hospital (2209-024-119).

Informed Consent Statement: Patient consent was waived due to de-identification of the patients' information and the treatment outcomes did not result in any adverse consequences.

Data Availability Statement: The data presented in this study are available on request from the corresponding author due to ethical reasons.

Conflicts of Interest: The authors declare that there are no competing financial interests.

References

1. Thompson, A.M.; Moulder-Thompson, S.L. Neoadjuvant treatment of breast cancer. *Ann. Oncol.* **2012**, *23* (Suppl. 10), 231–236. [CrossRef] [PubMed]
2. Mohan, S.C.; Walcott-Sapp, S.; Lee, M.K.; Srour, M.K.; Kim, S.; Amersi, F.F.; Giuliano, A.E.; Chung, A.P. Alterations in Breast Cancer Biomarkers Following Neoadjuvant Therapy. *Ann. Surg. Oncol.* **2021**, *28*, 5907–5917. [CrossRef] [PubMed]
3. Cortazar, P.; Zhang, L.; Untch, M.; Mehta, K.; Costantino, J.P.; Wolmark, N.; Bonnefoi, H.; Cameron, D.; Gianni, L.; Valagussa, P.; et al. Pathological complete response and long-term clinical benefit in breast cancer: The CTNeoBC pooled analysis. *Lancet* **2014**, *384*, 164–172. [CrossRef] [PubMed]
4. Symmans, W.F.; Peintinger, F.; Hatzis, C.; Rajan, R.; Kuerer, H.; Valero, V.; Assad, L.; Poniecka, A.; Hennessy, B.; Green, M.; et al. Measurement of residual breast cancer burden to predict survival after neoadjuvant chemotherapy. *J. Clin. Oncol.* **2007**, *25*, 4414–4422. [CrossRef] [PubMed]
5. von Minckwitz, G.; Untch, M.; Blohmer, J.-U.; Costa, S.D.; Eidtmann, H.; Fasching, P.A.; Gerber, B.; Eiermann, W.; Hilfrich, J.; Huober, J.; et al. Definition and impact of pathologic complete response on prognosis after neoadjuvant chemotherapy in various intrinsic breast cancer subtypes. *J. Clin. Oncol.* **2012**, *30*, 1796–1804. [CrossRef] [PubMed]
6. Chen, X.; He, C.; Han, D.; Zhou, M.; Wang, Q.; Tian, J.; Li, L.; Xu, F.; Zhou, E.; Yang, K. The predictive value of Ki-67 before neoadjuvant chemotherapy for breast cancer: A systematic review and meta-analysis. *Future Oncol.* **2017**, *13*, 843–857. [CrossRef] [PubMed]
7. Li, C.; Fan, H.; Xiang, Q.; Xu, L.; Zhang, Z.; Liu, Q.; Zhang, T.; Ling, J.; Zhou, Y.; Zhao, X.; et al. Prognostic value of receptor status conversion following neoadjuvant chemotherapy in breast cancer patients: A systematic review and meta-analysis. *Breast Cancer Res. Treat.* **2019**, *178*, 497–504. [CrossRef] [PubMed]
8. Rizzo, A.; Cusmai, A.; Acquafredda, S.; Rinaldi, L.; Palmiotti, G. Ladiratuzumab vedotin for metastatic triple negative cancer: Preliminary results, key challenges, and clinical potential. *Expert Opin. Investig. Drugs* **2022**, *31*, 495–498. [CrossRef] [PubMed]
9. Emens, L.A. Breast Cancer Immunotherapy: Facts and Hopes. *Clin. Cancer Res.* **2018**, *24*, 511–520. [CrossRef]
10. Santoni, M.; Rizzo, A.; Mollica, V.; Matrana, M.R.; Rosellini, M.; Faloppi, L.; Marchetti, A.; Battelli, N.; Massari, F. The impact of gender on The efficacy of immune checkpoint inhibitors in cancer patients: The MOUSEION-01 study. *Crit. Rev. Oncol.* **2022**, *170*, 103596. [CrossRef]
11. Shaaban, A.M.; Provenzano, E. Receptor Status after Neoadjuvant Therapy of Breast Cancer: Significance and Implications. *Pathobiology* **2022**, *89*, 297–308. [CrossRef] [PubMed]
12. Yemelyanova, A.; Vang, R.; Kshirsagar, M.; Lu, D.; Marks, M.A.; Shih, I.M.; Kurman, R.J. Immunohistochemical staining patterns of p53 can serve as a surrogate marker for TP53 mutations in ovarian carcinoma: An immunohistochemical and nucleotide sequencing analysis. *Mod. Pathol.* **2011**, *24*, 1248–1253. [CrossRef] [PubMed]
13. Enomoto, Y.; Morimoto, T.; Nishimukai, A.; Higuchi, T.; Yanai, A.; Miyagawa, Y.; Miyoshi, Y. Impact of biomarker changes during neoadjuvant chemotherapy for clinical response in patients with residual breast cancers. *Int. J. Clin. Oncol.* **2016**, *21*, 254–261. [CrossRef] [PubMed]
14. Rey-Vargas, L.; Mejia-Henao, J.C.; Sanabria-Salas, M.C.; Serrano-Gomez, S.J. Effect of neoadjuvant therapy on breast cancer biomarker profile. *BMC Cancer* **2020**, *20*, 675. [CrossRef] [PubMed]
15. Tan, S.; Fu, X.; Xu, S.; Qiu, P.; Lv, Z.; Xu, Y.; Zhang, Q. Quantification of Ki67 Change as a Valid Prognostic Indicator of Luminal B Type Breast Cancer After Neoadjuvant Therapy. *Pathol. Oncol. Res.* **2021**, *27*, 1609972. [CrossRef] [PubMed]
16. Zhou, X.; Zhang, J.; Yun, H.; Shi, R.; Wang, Y.; Wang, W.; Lagercrantz, S.B.; Mu, K. Alterations of biomarker profiles after neoadjuvant chemotherapy in breast cancer: Tumor heterogeneity should be taken into consideration. *Oncotarget* **2015**, *6*, 36894–36902. [CrossRef] [PubMed]
17. Gianni, L.; Colleoni, M.; Bisagni, G.; Mansutti, M.; Zamagni, C.; Del Mastro, L.; Zambelli, S.; Bianchini, G.; Frassoldati, A.; Maffeis, I.; et al. Effects of neoadjuvant trastuzumab, pertuzumab and palbociclib on Ki67 in HER2 and ER-positive breast cancer. *npj Breast Cancer* **2022**, *8*, 1–7. [CrossRef] [PubMed]
18. Brown, J.R.; DiGiovanna, M.P.; Killelea, B.; Lannin, D.R.; Rimm, D.L. Quantitative assessment Ki-67 score for prediction of response to neoadjuvant chemotherapy in breast cancer. *Lab. Investig.* **2014**, *94*, 98–106. [CrossRef] [PubMed]
19. Banerji, U.; van Herpen, C.M.; Saura, C.; Thistlethwaite, F.; Lord, S.; Moreno, V.; Aftimos, P. Trastuzumab duocarmazine in locally advanced and metastatic solid tumours and HER2-expressing breast cancer: A phase 1 dose-escalation and dose-expansion study. *Lancet Oncol.* **2019**, *20*, 1124–1135. [CrossRef]
20. Modi, S.; Park, H.; Murthy, R.K.; Iwata, H.; Tamura, K.; Tsurutani, J.; Takahashi, S. Antitumor Activity and Safety of Trastuzumab Deruxtecan in Patients With HER2-Low-Expressing Advanced Breast Cancer: Results From a Phase Ib Study. *J. Clin. Oncol.* **2020**, *38*, 1887–1896. [CrossRef]
21. Ahn, S.; Woo, J.W.; Lee, K.; Park, S.Y. HER2 status in breast cancer: Changes in guidelines and complicating factors for interpretation. *J. Pathol. Transl. Med.* **2020**, *54*, 34–44. [CrossRef] [PubMed]
22. Tural, D.; Karaca MFau—Zirtiloglu, A.; Zirtiloglu AFau—MHacioglu, B.; MHacioglu BFau—Sendur, M.A.; Sendur Ma Fau—Ozet, A.; Ozet, A. Receptor discordances after neoadjuvant chemotherapy and their effects on survival. *J. BU ON* **2019**, *24*, 20–25.
23. Duffy, M.J.; Synnott, N.C.; Crown, J. Mutant p53 in breast cancer: Potential as a therapeutic target and biomarker. *Breast Cancer Res. Treat.* **2018**, *170*, 213–219. [CrossRef] [PubMed]

24. Darb-Esfahani, S.; Denkert, C.; Stenzinger, A.; Salat, C.; Sinn, B.; Schem, C.; Endris, V.; Klare, P.; Schmitt, W.; Blohmer, J.-U.; et al. Role of *TP53* mutations in triple negative and HER2-positive breast cancer treated with neoadjuvant anthracycline/taxane-based chemotherapy. *Oncotarget* **2016**, *7*, 67686–67698. [CrossRef]
25. Albinsaad, L.S.; Kim, J.; Chung, I.Y.; Ko, B.S.; Kim, H.J.; Lee, J.W.; Lee, S.B. Prognostic value of p53 expression in hormone receptor-positive and human epidermal growth factor receptor 2-negative breast cancer patients receiving neoadjuvant chemotherapy. *Breast Cancer Res. Treat.* **2021**, *187*, 447–454. [CrossRef] [PubMed]
26. Kim, T.; Han, W.; Kim, M.K.; Lee, J.W.; Kim, J.; Ahn, S.K.; Noh, D.Y. Predictive Significance of p53, Ki-67, and Bcl-2 Expression for Pathologic Complete Response after Neoadjuvant Chemotherapy for Triple-Negative Breast Cancer. *J. Breast Cancer* **2015**, *18*, 16–21. [CrossRef] [PubMed]
27. Bae, S.Y.; Lee, J.H.; Bae, J.W.; Jung, S.P. Differences in prognosis by p53 expression after neoadjuvant chemotherapy in triple-negative breast cancer. *Ann. Surg. Treat. Res.* **2020**, *98*, 291–298. [CrossRef] [PubMed]
28. Wein, L.; Loi, S. Mechanisms of resistance of chemotherapy in early-stage triple negative breast cancer (TNBC). *Breast* **2017**, *34* (Suppl. 1), S27–S30. [CrossRef] [PubMed]
29. Singh, N.; Piskorz, A.M.; Bosse, T.; Jimenez-Linan, M.; Rous, B.; Brenton, J.D.; Köbel, M. p53 immunohistochemistry is an accurate surrogate for TP53 mutational analysis in endometrial carcinoma biopsies. *J. Pathol.* **2020**, *250*, 336–345. [CrossRef]
30. Balko, J.M.; Giltnane, J.M.; Wang, K.; Schwarz, L.J.; Young, C.D.; Cook, R.S.; Arteaga, C.L. Molecular profiling of the residual disease of triple-negative breast cancers after neoadjuvant chemotherapy identifies actionable therapeutic targets. *Cancer Discov.* **2014**, *4*, 232–245. [CrossRef]
31. Howlader, N.; Cronin, K.A.; Kurian, A.W.; Andridge, R. Differences in Breast Cancer Survival by Molecular Subtypes in the United States. *Cancer Epidemiol. Biomark. Prev.* **2018**, *27*, 619–626. [CrossRef] [PubMed]
32. Tao, L.; Chu, L.; Wang, L.I.; Moy, L.; Brammer, M.; Song, C.; Green, M.; Kurian, A.W.; Gomez, S.L.; Clarke, C.A. Occurrence and outcome of de novo metastatic breast cancer by subtype in a large, diverse population. *Cancer Causes Control* **2016**, *27*, 1127–1138. [CrossRef] [PubMed]
33. Goldhirsch, A.; Wood, W.C.; Coates, A.S.; Gelber, R.D.; Thürlimann, B.; Senn, H.J. Strategies for subtypes--dealing with the diversity of breast cancer: Highlights of the St. Gallen International Expert Consensus on the Primary Therapy of Early Breast Cancer 2011. *Ann. Oncol.* **2011**, *22*, 1736–1747. [CrossRef] [PubMed]
34. Laws, A.; Pastorello, R.; Dey, T.; Grossmith, S.; King, C.; McGrath, M.; Schnitt, S.J.; Mittendorf, E.A.; King, T. Impact of the Histologic Pattern of Residual Tumor After Neoadjuvant Chemotherapy on Recurrence and Survival in Stage I–III Breast Cancer. *Ann. Surg. Oncol.* **2022**, *29*, 7726–7736. [CrossRef]
35. Tinterri, C.; Fernandes, B.; Zambelli, A.; Sagona, A.; Barbieri, E.; Di Maria Grimaldi, S.; Gentile, D. The Impact of Different Patterns of Residual Disease on Long-Term Oncological Outcomes in Breast Cancer Patients Treated with Neo-Adjuvant Chemotherapy. *Cancers* **2024**, *16*, 376. [CrossRef]

Disclaimer/Publisher's Note: The statements, opinions and data contained in all publications are solely those of the individual author(s) and contributor(s) and not of MDPI and/or the editor(s). MDPI and/or the editor(s) disclaim responsibility for any injury to people or property resulting from any ideas, methods, instructions or products referred to in the content.

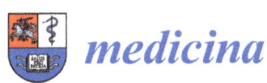 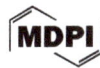

Article

Human Papillomavirus Is Rare and Does Not Correlate with p16^{INK4A} Expression in Non-Small-Cell Lung Cancer in a Jordanian Subpopulation

Ola Abu Al Karsaneh [1,*], Arwa Al Anber [2], Sahar AlMustafa [3], Hussien AlMa'aitah [3], Batool AlQadri [4], Abir Igbaria [4], Rama Tayem [4], Mustafa Khasawneh [4], Shaima Batayha [5], Tareq Saleh [2], Mohammad ALQudah [1] and Maher Sughayer [3,*]

1. Department of Microbiology, Pathology and Forensic Medicine, Faculty of Medicine, The Hashemite University, Zarqa 13133, Jordan; m.alqudah12@hu.edu.jo
2. Department of Pharmacology and Public Health, Faculty of Medicine, The Hashemite University, Zarqa 13133, Jordan; arwaa@hu.edu.jo (A.A.A.); tareq@hu.edu.jo (T.S.)
3. Department of Pathology and Laboratory Medicine, King Hussein Cancer Center, Amman 11941, Jordan; sa.15353@khcc.jo (S.A.); ha.11789@khcc.jo (H.A.)
4. Faculty of Medicine, Jordan University of Science and Technology, Irbid 22110, Jordan; bnalqadri17@med.just.edu.jo (B.A.); aaigbaria17@med.just.edu.jo (A.I.); rmtayem17@med.just.edu.jo (R.T.); mqkhasawneh171@med.just.edu.jo (M.K.)
5. Department of Pathology and Microbiology, Faculty of Medicine, Jordan University of Science and Technology, Irbid 22110, Jordan; sabatayha20@med.just.edu.jo
* Correspondence: olaa@hu.edu.jo (O.A.A.K.); msughayer@khcc.jo (M.S.); Tel.: +962-5-390-3333 (ext. 5577) (O.A.A.K.); +962-6-530-0460 (ext. 1551) (M.S.)

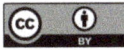

Abstract: *Background and Objectives*: Human papillomavirus (HPV) was previously investigated in lung cancer with wide inter-geographic discrepancies. p16^{INK4a} has been used as a surrogate for detecting high-risk HPV (HR-HPV) in some cancer types. This study assessed the evidence of HPV in non-small-cell lung cancer (NSCLC) among Jordanian patients, investigated the expression of p16^{INK4a}, and evaluated its prognostic value and association with HPV status. *Materials and Methods*: The archived samples of 100 patients were used. HPV DNA detection was performed by real-time polymerase chain reaction (RT-PCR). p16^{INK4a} expression was assessed by immunohistochemistry (IHC). The Eighth American Joint Committee on Cancer protocol (AJCC) of head and neck cancer criteria were applied to evaluate p16^{INK4a} positivity considering a moderate/strong nuclear/cytoplasmic expression intensity with a distribution in ≥75% of cells as positive. *Results*: HPV DNA was detected in 5% of NSCLC cases. Three positive cases showed HR-HPV subtypes (16, 18, 52), and two cases showed the probable HR-HPV 26 subtype. p16^{INK4a} expression was positive in 20 (20%) NSCLC cases. None of the HPV-positive tumors were positive for p16^{INK4a} expression. A statistically significant association was identified between p16^{INK4a} expression and the pathological stage ($p = 0.029$) but not with other variables. No survival impact of p16^{INK4a} expression was detected in NSCLC cases as a group; however, it showed a statistically significant association with overall survival (OS) in squamous cell carcinoma (SqCC) cases ($p = 0.033$). *Conclusions*: This is the first study to assess HPV and p16^{INK4a} expression in a Jordanian population. HPV positivity is rare in NSCLC among a Jordanian subpopulation. P16^{INK4a} reliability as a surrogate marker for HPV infection in lung cancer must be revisited.

Keywords: HPV; PCR; p16^{INK4a}; immunohistochemistry; NSCLC; Jordan

1. Introduction

Lung cancer is the leading cause of cancer-related morbidity and mortality in males and females worldwide [1]. Lung cancer pathogenesis is a complex process involving genetic and environmental factors [2]. Although smoking is the most significant causative agent for lung cancer, fewer than 20% of smokers develop lung cancer, and lung cancer remains the primary cause of death among never-smokers [3,4]. Other factors, such as genetic susceptibility, unfavorable occupational exposure, air pollution, and viral infections, are implicated in the development of lung cancer [5,6]. Human papillomavirus (HPV) is one of the viruses associated with lung cancer [7].

HPV is a DNA virus that belongs to the Papovaviridae family and is genotyped into three groups based on its oncogenic risk: high-risk group (HR-HPV) such as HPVs 16, 18, 31, 33, 35, 39, 45, 51, and 52, which can lead to cancerous transformation, probable/possible carcinogen such as HPVs 26, 53, 66, 68, 73, and 82, and low-risk- group (LR-HPV) such as HPVs 6, 11, 40, 42, 43, 44, 54, 61, and 72, which cause benign lesions [8]. The HPV DNA encodes for several proteins, including the early (E) E1-E2, E4-E7, and late (L), L1, and L2 proteins, that carry oncogenic potential [9].

The role of HPV in causing cervical cancer and a subset of anogenital and oropharyngeal cancers is established [10–12]. In this regard, a recent study detected a high frequency of HPV DNA (94.4%) in high-grade vaginal intraepithelial neoplasia, with 26.8% showing multiple infections [13]. Furthermore, these HPV-induced cancers show overexpression of the p16^{INK4a} protein, which is used as a surrogate for HPV status in these cancers [14,15]. The molecular pathways of HPV-induced cervical and head and neck carcinomas are linked to its two main oncogenes, E6 and E7, which deactivate the p53 and Rb tumor suppressor genes, respectively. After infection, the HPV-E7 protein binds to the Rb protein, causing its inactivation and leading to the release of E2F, which drives the expression of several pro-proliferative proteins. Several studies showed that Rb inactivation and the consequent E2F activation stimulate the expression of the tumor suppressor gene p16^{INK4a}, a cyclin-dependent kinase inhibitor (CDKI), through negative feedback [16–18]. Subsequently, p16^{INK4a} expression has been highly correlated with HR-HPV.

On the other hand, although several studies have also indicated that HR-HPV may have a role in the pathogenesis of lung cancer [2,7,19], this role has not been well established. The first report to suggest a connection between HPV and lung cancer was in 1979 by Syrjaanen et al., indicating the presence of histological changes similar to the HPV-linked condylomatous changes in the bronchial epithelium adjacent to squamous cell carcinoma [20]. Since then, several studies have been conducted and showed conflicting results regarding the relationship between HPV infection and lung cancer development, with inconsistency in the reported prevalence, possibly due to geographic differences and methodological variability. For example, in one meta-analysis, Srinivasan et al. found that the prevalence of HPV varied greatly between geographic areas and histological subtypes, with a global range of 0.0 to 78.3%. This meta-analysis, in addition, showed that Asian studies reported a higher HPV prevalence compared to European studies [4]. Unlike cervical and head and neck cancers, the relationship between HPV and p16^{INK4a} expression in NSCLC is not well established. Some studies failed to reveal a significant correlation between HPV infection and p16^{INK4a} expression in lung cancer [15,21]. In any case, p16^{INK4a} expression has been evaluated for its prognostic role in NSCLC regardless of the HPV status, and several studies showed that it had a significant prognostic value [22–25].

In Jordan, lung cancer is the leading cause of cancer-related deaths, and recent estimates expect an increasing burden of lung cancer on public health, particularly with increasing smoking habits. Further, the prevalence of HPV, despite being relatively low, seems to be increasing in Jordan [26]. However, to the best of our knowledge, there is no data that link lung cancer and HPV among Jordanian patients. This study aimed to evaluate the prevalence of HPV and p16^{INK4a} expression in NSCLC among a Jordanian subpopulation.

2. Materials and Methods

2.1. Patients and Tissue Samples

A total of 100 tumor tissue samples of patients who were surgically treated for their NSCLC between 2009 and 2022 at King Hussein Cancer Center (KHCC), Amman, Jordan, were obtained for this work. The cases were selected after a retrospective search of the archived cases at the Department of Pathology and Laboratory Medicine, KHCC. The patients' inclusion criteria included the following: patients with surgical resection of primary lung cancer, lack of preoperative chemotherapy or radiotherapy, negative history of other tumors at the time of diagnosis, particularly those derived from an HPV-driven anatomical area, and the presence of adequate tissue samples and clinical follow-up data. The patients' clinicopathological characteristics, including age, gender, smoking status, postoperative treatment history, histologic subtypes, pathologic stage, and survival data, were collected from the patients' medical records and pathological reports. The respective H&E-stained slides of the cases were evaluated by two pathologists (O.A.A.K. and S.A.) to confirm the pathological features. Tumor subtypes and grades were determined according to the World Health Organization (WHO) guidelines [27,28]. Grading of the adenocarcinoma (ADC) cases was determined based on the combination of the predominant and the worst architectural patterns. Squamous cell carcinoma (SqCC) grades were specified based on the degree of tumor keratinization. Tumor grades were divided into two categories: low-grade, which included well to moderately differentiated cancers, and high-grade, which included cancers with poor differentiation. The stages were determined according to the seventh and eighth editions of the American Joint Committee (AJC) on the Cancer TNM classification system, depending on the time of diagnosis [29,30]. Overall survival (OS) was measured from the time of surgery to the time of death or the last follow-up visit. Disease-free survival (DFS) was calculated from the time of surgery to the time of the first of two events: recurrence or death from any cause.

2.2. Extraction of DNA

FFPE tissue blocks were retrieved from the pathology department in KHCC. For each patient, 10 sections of 10 µm thickness were cut using the HistoCore BIOCUT manual rotary microtome, where the blade gently sweeps the sections after cutting to be stored in 2 mL microcentrifuge tubes positioned underneath. Once all sections had been collected, the tube was securely capped to prevent sample loss or contamination. DNA extraction was carried out using the ReliaPrep™ FFPE gDNA Miniprep System® Genomic DNA Kits (Promega, Madison, WI, USA) according to the manufacturer's instructions. Briefly, the FFPE sections were deparaffinized by adding 1 mL of 100% xylene to the samples with centrifuging for 2 min at maximum speed at room temperature to remove residual xylene, then adding 1 mL of 95–100% ethanol (100%) with centrifuging for 2 min at maximum speed at room temperature. After that, centrifuging for 30 s at maximum speed and drying the pellet for 5–15 min at 37 °C was performed to evaporate residual ethanol. Then, 200 µL of Lysis Buffer and 20 µL of Proteinase K were directly added to the samples and incubated at 56 °C for 1 h and at 80 °C for 4 h. Subsequently, 10 µL of RNAse A was added to the lysed sample and incubated at room temperature for 5 min. Then, 220 µL of BL Buffer and 240 µL of ethanol (95–100%) were added and mixed thoroughly, followed by the binding and column washing steps. Then, DNA was eluted by adding 50 µL of Elution Buffer, centrifuging at 16,000× g for 1 min, and storing at −30 to −10 °C for subsequent processing.

2.3. HPV Detection and Genotyping

HPV detection and genotyping were performed by real-time PCR (RT-PCR) using the HPV Genotypes 21 Real-TM Quant Kit (Sacace Biotechnologies, Como, Italy). The HPV Genotypes 21 Real-TM Quant Kit is capable of identifying 21 HPV subtypes, including three low-risk (HPV 6, 11, 44), six probable high-risk (HPV 26, 53, 66, 68, 73, 82), and 12 high-risk (HPV 16, 18, 31, 33, 35, 39, 45, 51, 52, 56, 58, 59). The kit amplifies a target of DNA sequence. The kit contains an artificial sequence of the HPV genome as a positive internal control (IC) to monitor the quality and efficiency of the PCR and the DNA amplification process and a PCR mix for the amplification of human genomic DNA (sample intake control (SIC)) that allows for the exclusion of preanalytical error. The kit also provides positive and negative controls. Briefly, 10.0 µL of Taq DNA Polymerase was added to each strip of PCR-mix 21 along with 5.0 µL of extracted DNA from the clinical samples. The negative and positive control strips received the same mix. After that, all strips were capped and spun for 2–3 s and transferred into the thermal cycler (Anatolia geneworks RT-PCR) and went through the following program: 1 cycle of 80 °C for 30 s followed by 94 °C for 90 s; 5 cycles of 94 °C for 30 s followed by 64 °C for 15 s; 45 cycles of 94 °C for 10 s followed by 64 °C for 25 s; and finally 1 cycle of 94 °C for 5 s. The PCR was considered valid if the positive controls showed a signal and the negative controls did not. Results interpretation was performed using the software of SLAN 8.3 RT-PCR system.

2.4. Immunohistochemistry (IHC)

The specimens were fixed in 10% neutral-buffered formalin (NBF) immediately or within 5 min of the resection, with a fixation duration between 12 and 28 h. Immunohistochemistry was performed using a BOND III autostainer and Detection Kit (DS9800; Leica Biosystems, Deer Park, TX, USA) according to the manufacturer's instructions. Briefly, tissue sections of 3 μm thickness were cut from the FFPE specimens using the HistoCore BIOCUT manual rotary microtome, prepared on IHC adhesive slides (TOMO®), and put in an oven for about 15 min at 65–70 °C to assist the sections adhering to the slides. Then, the sections were deparaffinized and rehydrated. Antigen retrieval was performed using Bond Epitope Retrieval Solution 1 (Citrate; pH 6.0) (AR9961; Leica Biosystems) for 20 min. Blocking was achieved with Peroxide 3–4% (vol/vol) hydrogen peroxide for 5 min at 100 °C. Slides were incubated at room temperature with the ready-to-use anti-p16 mouse monoclonal primary antibody for 20 min (clone INK4A/JC2, Cell Marque, Rocklin, CA, USA). Visualization was achieved using 3,3′-diaminobenzidine (DAB) staining and hematoxylin counterstaining (Leica Biosystems). Finally, the slides were dehydrated and cleared with xylene, then cover-slipped with dibutyl phthalate in xylene (D.P.X.) mounting media. Cervical squamous severe dysplasia known to be p16-positive was used as a positive control, and negative control was obtained by removing the primary antibody.

2.5. $p16^{INK4a}$ Protein Expression Scoring

The samples were assessed and scored independently by two pathologists (O.A.A.K. and S.A.) using a light microscope (Olympus BX53, Tokyo, Japan), and a consensus was obtained on all cases. All cases were scored for staining intensity in tumor cells as follows: 0: unstained, 1+: weak, 2+: moderate, 3+: strong. The distribution of staining in tumor cells was scored as follows: 0: no staining, 1+: 1–<25%, 2+: 25–<50%, 3+: 50–<75%, 4+: ≥75%. Then, following the 8th edition of the AJCC staging system for head and neck cancer, a positive $p16^{INK4a}$ expression was defined as cases with nuclear/cytoplasmic staining with intensity of 2+/3+ and a distribution of 4+ (cases with at least moderate staining intensity in ≥75% of tumor cells) [31,32]. Cases with cytoplasmic staining alone were considered negative [33].

2.6. Statistical Analysis

Categorical variables were summarized using counts and percentages. The Chi-square test or Fisher's exact test was used in a univariate study to discover relationships between $p16^{INK4a}$ expression and clinicopathological features. The Kaplan–Meier method was used to estimate the OS and DFS, and the log-rank test was performed to compare the results. All statistical analyses were undertaken with a two-tailed test. The threshold for statistical significance was set at *p*-values less than or equal to 0.05. Statistical analysis was performed using IBM SPSS Statistics software for Windows version 29 (IBM Corp., New York, NY, USA).

3. Results

3.1. Patients' Characteristics

Table 1 summarizes the primary features of the patients' sample. The cohort included 100 NSCLC patients who underwent surgical resection. Most patients underwent a lobectomy (84/100, 84%), ten patients underwent wedge resection, and six patients had a pneumonectomy. Six patients had positive bronchial or vascular margins. In terms of their histologic subtype, 59% of the cases were ADC, and 41% were SqCC. Most patients were older than 60 with a median age of 69 (range 46–86 years), and 85% were males. The vast majority of patients (~85%) were either current or former smokers. Most patients had high-grade tumors with poor differentiation (59%). The majority of cases were of early stages, and the distribution of the pathological stages was as follows: stage I (33%), stage II (36%), stage III (28%) and stage IV (3%). Most patients had a tumor size of more than 3 cm (64%), and 37% had positive lymph node metastasis. Regarding the architectural patterns of the ADC cases, the majority had an acinar predominant pattern (47.5%), followed by solid (25.4%), lepidic (23.7%), and micropapillary (3.4%).

Table 1. Patients' clinicopathological features according to $p16^{INK4a}$ expression.

Variables	Number (%)	$p16^{INK4a}$ Positive [b]	$p16^{INK4a}$ Negative	p Value *
Total	100 (100.0)	20 (20.0)	80 (80.0)	
Age (Years)				0.232
≤60	23 (23.0)	7 (35.0)	16 (20.0)	
>60	77 (77.0)	13 (65.0)	64 (80.0)	
Gender				0.072
Male	85 (85.0)	14 (70.0)	71 (88.7)	
Female	15 (15.0)	6 (30.0)	9 (11.3)	
Smoking history [a]				0.729
Current/former smoker	84 (84.8)	16 (80.0)	68 (86.1)	
Never smoker	15 (15.2)	4 (20.0)	11 (13.9)	
Histological subtype				1.000
Adenocarcinoma (ADC)	59 (59.0)	12 (60.0)	47 (58.8)	
Squamous cell carcinoma (SqCC)	41 (41.0)	8 (40.0)	33 (41.2)	
Grade				0.617
Low-grade (well and moderately differentiated)	41 (41.0)	7 (35.0)	34 (42.5)	
High-grade (poorly differentiated)	59 (59.0)	13 (65.0)	46 (57.5)	
Tumor size				0.193
≤3 cm	36 (36.0)	10 (50.0)	26 (32.5)	
>3 cm	64 (64.0)	10 (50.0)	54 (67.5)	
Lymph nodes metastasis				0.799
Positive	37 (37.0)	8 (40.0)	29 (36.3)	
Negative	63 (63.0)	12 (60.0)	51 (63.7)	
Pathological stage				**0.029**
I, II	69 (69.0)	18 (90.0)	51 (63.7)	
III, IV	31 (31.0)	2 (10.0)	29 (36.3)	
Predominant histological pattern (For ADC cases, 59 cases)				0.422
Lepidic	14 (23.7)	3 (25.0)	11 (23.4)	
Acinar	28 (47.5)	4 (33.3)	24 (51.1)	

Table 1. Cont.

Variables	Number (%)	p16^{INK4a} Positive [b]	p16^{INK4a} Negative	p Value *
Micropapillary	2 (3.4)	1 (8.3)	1 (2.1)	
Solid	15 (25.4)	4 (33.3)	11 (23.4)	
Papillary	0 (0.0)	0 (0.0)	0 (0.0)	
Recurrence/Progression				1.000
Present	34 (34.0)	7 (35.0)	27 (33.8)	
Absent	66 (66.0)	13 (65.0)	53 (66.3)	
HPV Status				
Positive	5 (5.0)	0 (0.0)	5 (6.3)	0.580
Negative	95 (95.0)	20 (100.0)	75 (93.7)	

[a] One patient was excluded due to the absence of smoking history. [b] p16^{INK4a} was considered positive by immunohistochemistry when it showed at least moderately strong nuclear and cytoplasmic staining in ≥75% of tumor cells. * 2-sided p-value, p-value ≤ 0.05 is considered significant (bold).

Regarding the postoperative treatment, 47 patients received no therapy, 38 patients received chemotherapy, 4 patients received radiotherapy, and 11 patients had a combination of chemoradiation therapy. About 34 patients developed disease recurrence or progression either in the form of locoregional recurrence or distant metastasis. Of these, four patients did not have any further therapy; nine patients had radiation therapy, five patients had chemotherapy, eight patients received chemoradiation therapy, three patients received a combination of chemotherapy with immunotherapy, one patient received a combination of chemotherapy and epidermal growth factor receptor (EGFR) tyrosine kinase inhibitor, one patient received EGFR tyrosine kinase inhibitor alone, one patient was treated with Anaplastic lymphoma kinase (ALK) inhibitor, one patient received immunotherapy, and one patient was treated with surgery alone. The status of the driver gene mutations was available for a limited number of cases. ALK1 was tested in 32 cases by an FDA-approved CDx grade IHC, and only 2 were positive. ROS1 was tested in six cases by IHC, and only one was positive. EGFR gene mutations were investigated in eleven cases, where only two cases showed exon 19 deletion and L858R mutation. The tumor proportion score of PD-L1 was available for 47 cases, where 28 cases were positive, with a score of 1% or more.

3.2. HPV Detection and Correlation with p16^{INK4a} Expression

Real-time PCR revealed that among the 100 NSCLC cases, 5 cases (5%) were positive for HPV. Three cases were positive for HR-HPV subtypes (16, 18, and 52), and two cases were positive for the probable HR-HPV 26 subtype (Table 2). Four of the positive cases were ADC, and only one case was of SqCC histological type. These positive cases were detected in three males and two females with a mean age of 70 (range: 56–78). Four cases occurred in patients with a smoking history and one in a non-smoker. Four of them also demonstrated low-grade disease, and one was high-grade. Three cases were of pathological stage I, 1 of stage II, and 1 of stage III. Only one of these positive cases showed a progression of the disease. The median follow-up time of the patients with HPV-positive tumors was 36 months (range: 24–70). Surprisingly, none of the HPV-positive cases were positive for p16^{INK4a} by IHC according to the followed criteria. However, all cases showed p16^{INK4a} expression ranging from 5 to 60% with weak to moderate intensity (Figure 1A–E). No statistically significant association was identified between the HPV status and other clinicopathological variables.

Table 2. Clinicopathological characteristics of HPV-positive tumors.

HPV-Positive Tumor	Age	Gender	Smoking History	Histological Subtype	Grade [a]	Pathological Stage	Recurrence/ Progression	p16^{INK4a} Expression [b]
HPV 16+	56	Female	Former smoker	ADC	High	Stage I	Absent	Negative
HPV 18+	74	Male	Smoker	ADC	Low	Stage II	Present	Negative
HPV 26+	72	Male	Smoker	SqCC	Low	Stage I	Absent	Negative
HPV 26+	78	Male	Smoker	ADC	Low	Stage III	Absent	Negative
HPV 52+	70	Female	Non-smoker	ADC	Low	Stage I	Absent	Negative

[a] Low-grade tumors include well- and moderately differentiated tumors. High-grade tumors include poorly differentiated tumors. [b] P16 was considered positive by immunohistochemistry when it showed at least moderately strong nuclear and cytoplasmic staining in ≥75% of tumor cells. Abbreviations: ADC: adenocarcinoma, SqCC: squamous cell carcinoma.

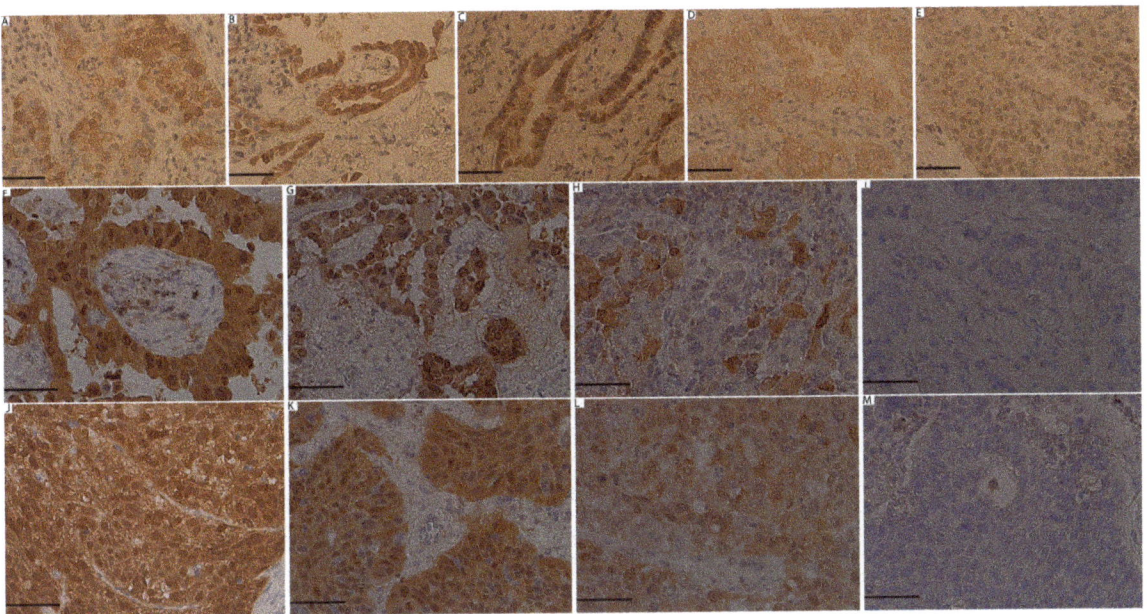

Figure 1. Representative images of p16^{INK4a} immunohistochemistry expression. (**A**) p16^{INK4a} expression in HPV-16-positive ADC case. (**B**) p16^{INK4a} expression in HPV-18-positive ADC case. (**C**) p16^{INK4a} expression in HPV-52-positive ADC case. (**D**) p16^{INK4a} expression in HPV-26-positive ADC case. (**E**) p16^{INK4a} expression in HPV-26-positive SqCC case. All HPV-positive cases showed negative p16^{INK4a} results with variable expression demonstrating weak to moderate intensity. (**F**) p16^{INK4a} expression showing score 3+ with strong nuclear and cytoplasmic expression in ADC. (**G**) p16^{INK4a} expression showing score 2+ with moderate nuclear and cytoplasmic expression in ADC. (**H**) p16^{INK4a} expression showing score 1+ with weak nuclear and cytoplasmic expression in ADC. (**I**) p16^{INK4a} expression showing score 0 with complete lack of staining in ADC. (**J**) p16^{INK4a} expression showing score 3+ with strong nuclear and cytoplasmic expression in SqCC. (**K**) p16^{INK4a} expression showing score 2+ with moderate nuclear and cytoplasmic expression in SqCC. (**L**) p16^{INK4a} expression showing score 1+ with weak nuclear and cytoplasmic expression in SqCC. (**M**) p16^{INK4a} expression showing a score of 0 with a complete lack of staining in SqCC. Abbreviations: ADC: adenocarcinoma, SqCC: squamous cell carcinoma. All images were obtained at 40× magnification. Scale bars = 5 μm.

3.3. p16^{INK4a} Expression Detection and Correlation with the Clinicopathological Features

In total, 20 out of 100 cases were positive for p16^{INK4a} expression. Of those, 12 cases were ADC (12/59, 20.3%), and 8 cases were SqCC (8/41, 19.5%). In both ADC and SqCC, p16^{INK4a} expression varied from being strongly positive to aberrant to completely negative (Figure 1F–M). Cases with non-specific cytoplasmic staining were considered negative. Analysis of p16^{INK4a} expression in correlation to the clinicopathological variables revealed a statistically significant association with the pathological stage ($p = 0.029$), where most of the cases with positive p16^{INK4a} expression were either stage I or II. No significant association was demonstrated with the other characteristics, including HPV status (Table 1).

3.4. Survival Analysis of p16^{INK4a} Expression and Other Clinicopathological Variables

The median overall survival (OS) for all patients was 35 months (mean 43.45 months), and the median disease-free survival (DFS) was 26.5 months (mean 36.11 months) following surgical resection. Survival analysis of all cases showed no statistically significant association between p16^{INK4a} expression and either OS ($p = 0.151$) or DFS ($p = 0.522$). However, by dividing the cases according to the histological subtypes, a statistically significant association was found between p16^{INK4a} expression and OS in SqCC cases, where cases with positive p16^{INK4a} expression exhibited a better overall survival ($p = 0.033$) but not in ADC cases ($p = 0.930$) (Figure 2A–D). Kaplan–Meier survival analysis showed that advanced pathological stages, positive lymph node metastasis, and tumor size > 3 cm were significantly associated with poor OS and DFS in p16^{INK4a} negative cases. In contrast, in p16^{INK4a} positive cases, only positive lymph node metastasis and advanced pathological stages were significantly associated with poor OS and DFS, respectively (Figure 3A–L).

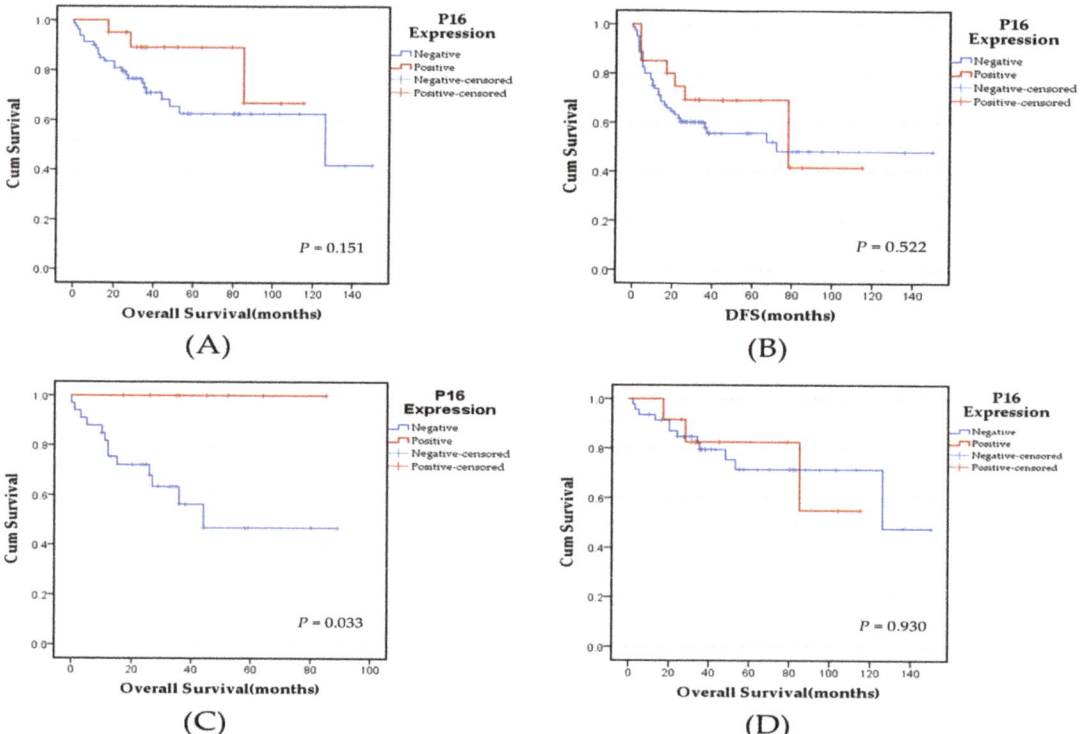

Figure 2. Kaplan–Meier survival curves according to p16^{INK4a} expression in NSCLC, ADC, and SqCC cases. (**A**) OS of p16^{INK4a}-positive and negative NSCLC tumors. (**B**) DFS of p16^{INK4a}-positive and

negative NSCLC tumors. (**C**) OS of p16^{INK4a}-positive and negative SqCC tumors. (**D**) OS of p16^{INK4a}-positive and negative ADC tumors. Abbreviations: NSCLC: non-small-cell lung cancer, ADC: adenocarcinoma, SqCC: squamous cell carcinoma, OS: overall survival, DFS: disease-free survival. *p*-values of ≤0.05 were regarded as statistically significant.

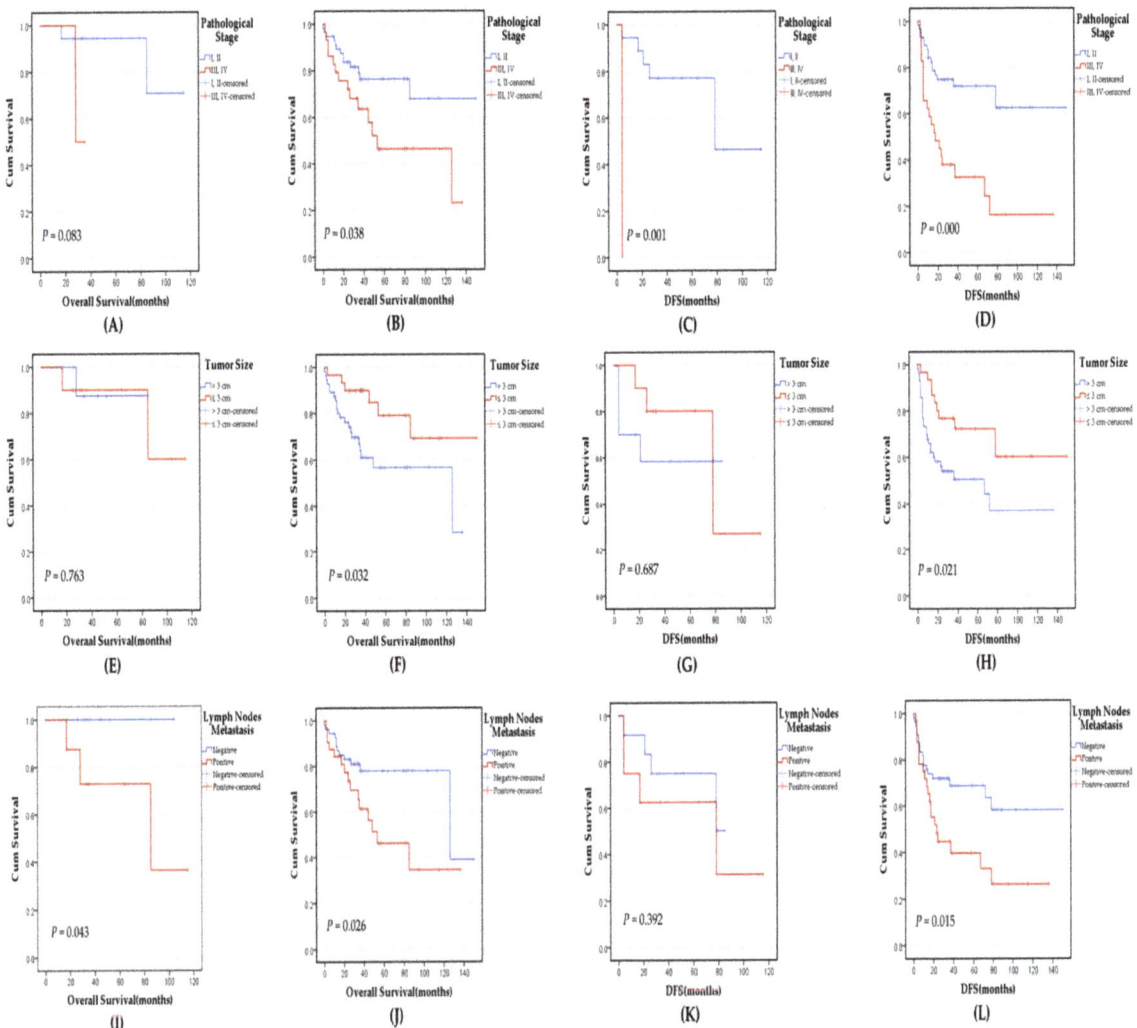

Figure 3. Kaplan–Meier survival curves of OS and DFS according to different clinicopathological variables based on p16^{INK4a} expression. (**A**,**B**) The correlation between the OS and different pathological tumor stages in p16^{INK4a}-positive and negative cases, respectively. (**C**,**D**) The correlation between the DFS and different pathological tumor stages in p16^{INK4a}-positive and negative cases, respectively. Tumor stages were divided into two groups, one composed of early stages I and II and another group comprised of late tumor stages III and IV. (**E**,**F**) The correlation between the OS and tumor sizes in p16^{INK4a}-positive and negative cases, respectively. (**G**,**H**) The correlation between the DFS and tumor sizes in p16^{INK4a}-positive and negative cases, respectively. (**I**,**J**) The correlation between the OS and

lymph node metastasis status in p16^{INK4a}-positive and negative cases, respectively. (**K,L**) The correlation between the DFS and lymph node metastasis status in p16^{INK4a}-positive and negative cases, respectively. Abbreviations: OS: overall survival, DFS: disease-free survival. *p*-values of ≤0.05 were regarded as statistically significant.

4. Discussion

The role of HPV as a causative agent in lung cancer has been previously suggested but with wide variability based on geographic and methodological differences [34]. This work represents the first study to investigate the prevalence of HPV infection in NSCLC among a Jordanian subpopulation. This study investigated 100 NSCLC cases, particularly ADC and SqCC types, from a central referral hospital in Jordan. All cases were assessed for the presence of 12 HR-HPV, 6 probable HR-HPV, and 3 LR-HPV genotypes. HPV prevalence in this study was 5%; four cases were of the ADC histological subtype, and one was of the SqCC subtype. Three cases were of high-risk subtypes, and two cases were of the probable high-risk HPV 26 subtype (40%, 2/5). Due to the rarity of studies investigating the relationship between HPV infection and lung cancer, locally and in the neighboring countries in the Middle East and North Africa (MENA) area, it was challenging to compare our findings with previous work. A study conducted by Nadji et al. in Iran investigated the presence of HPV DNA in 129 lung cancer cases and 90 non-cancer control subjects using nested PCR. The study found an HPV prevalence of 25.6% in lung cancer cases compared to 9% in control cases, with HR-HPV 16 and 18 subtypes being more prevalent in cancer cases than in control cases [35]. Interestingly, similar to our results, they detected only one HPV-26-positive lung cancer case. Another more recent study in an Iranian subpopulation investigated a relatively similar sample size to the one in this work, including 109 lung cancer cases and 52 control cases [36]. The study utilized RT-PCR to analyze the presence of HPV, assessed the expression of E2, E6, and E7 viral oncoproteins, the expression of p53 and Rb genes, and selected miRNAs and genes related to epithelial–mesenchymal transition (EMT). They reported a 51.4% prevalence of HPV among lung cancer cases and 23.1% among control samples, which is significantly higher than what was observed by our analysis. HPV 16 was the most detected type, both in cancer and control cases. Of interest, authors also suggested that HPV infection could play a role in EMT [36].

The prevalence of HPV among lung cancer cases had a higher frequency in Asian populations compared to European and North American populations, as reported by several meta-analyses [4,37,38]. The HPV frequency range has been found to be 0 to 78.3% (mean 33.9%) in Asia, 0 to 69.2% (mean 10.5%) in Europe, 27.8% to 29% (mean 28.6%) in South America and 0 to 22% (mean 10.2%) in North America [39]. Although our results revealed a low prevalence of HPV positivity in NSCLC among the Jordanian population, it falls within the worldwide range of 0.0 to 78.3%, and it shows partial agreement with some studies [4]. For example, Joh et al. investigated 51 frozen lung samples from 30 NSCLC patients to assess the presence of HPV using PCR and DNA sequencing [40]. HPV DNA was identified in 16.7% of NSCLC patients, all of which were of ADC histological type, with HPV 16 being the most prevalent genotype [40]. Another study investigated 176 lung SqCC and 128 lung ADC from eight Asian institutions for the presence of HPV using PCR and in situ hybridization (ISH). HPV infection was detected in 6.3% and 7% of patients with lung SqCC and lung ADC, respectively. Most of the HPV-positive cases were HPV 16/18 genotypes [41]. Similarly, Sarchianaki et al. investigated 100 NSCLC using RT-PCT and reported a prevalence of 19% for HPV with a higher frequency in ADC cases [2], which is similar to the current study. On the other hand, Yanagawa et al. assessed the presence of the HPV genotype in 336 primary NSCLC cases using PCR and ISH and detected a prevalence of 1.5% using both methods. All cases were of the HPV 16 genotype and were found in SqCC [39]. Similarly, de Oliveira et al. reported a higher frequency of HPV in lung SqCC compared to ADC cases. Inconsistent with these results, Silva et al. investigated the presence of HPV DNA in 62 NSCLC cases using multiplex PCR and HPV16-specific

RT-PCR, and none of the cases were positive for HPV [42]. Similar results of HPV negativity in lung cancer were reported in other two studies using different methods [43,44].

As suggested by previous studies, it seems that the heterogeneity in HPV prevalence is attributed to geographic differences, sociocultural differences, sensitivities of the methods used, sample size, and, finally, the histologic subtypes of the studied cases. Evidently, in Jordan, the prevalence of oncogenic HPV is relatively low in comparison to Western countries, with some studies reporting a general prevalence of 4% in a subpopulation of patients [45]. In this work, no statistically significant association was identified between the HPV status and other clinicopathological variables. This can be attributed to the very small number of HPV-positive cases detected. Similar to our results, some previous studies failed to find an association between HPV and other clinicopathological features in lung cancer [2,46,47].

$p16^{INK4a}$ overexpression has a strong correlation with HR-HPV infection in uterine cervix carcinoma and a subset of oropharyngeal SqCC and is frequently utilized as a surrogate for such cancers [43]. However, this link has not been adequately established in lung cancer. Therefore, we further assessed the expression of $p16^{INK4a}$ in the whole cohort of patients, trying to explore any correlation with the HPV status. $p16^{INK4a}$ overexpression was detected in 20% of cases; surprisingly, none of these cases were positive for HPV DNA, and further, none of the five HPV-positive cases were positive for $p16^{INK4a}$ overexpression considering at least a moderate intensity of staining in $\geq 75\%$ of tumor cells as positive. Still, all HPV-positive cases showed some degree of positive $p16^{INK4a}$ expression ranging from weak to moderate intensity. HPV-unrelated $p16^{INK4a}$ overexpression can be attributed to Rb gene inactivation by mechanisms other than HR-HPV E7 expression [48,49] or be part of tumor cell senescence, as reported previously in lung cancer [50–52]. Similarly, several previous studies failed to find a correlation between $p16^{INK4a}$ overexpression and HPV status in lung cancer [39,42,47]. For example, Bishop et al. assessed 220 cases of lung SqCC and found a prevalence of 24.5% of $p16^{INK4a}$ overexpression, considering a strong and diffuse nuclear and cytoplasmic staining present in $\geq 70\%$ of the tumor as positive, while only 5% of cases were positive for HR-HPV by ISH [21]. In agreement with that, Doxtader et al. reported a 35% positivity rate of $p16^{INK4a}$ in lung SqCC (considering a strong and diffuse nuclear and cytoplasmic staining present in $\geq 50\%$ of the tumor as positive), where all cases were negative for HR-HPV [15], and similarly considering a strong and diffuse nuclear and cytoplasmic staining present in $\geq 70\%$ of the tumor as positive, Chang et al. reported a strong diffuse expression of $p16^{INK4a}$ in 14.6% of NSCLC cases with negative results for HPV [43]. Subsequently, $p16^{INK4a}$ expression might not be a reliable surrogate for HPV infection in lung cancer. On the contrary, Robinson et al. investigated 70 NSCLC cases where $p16^{INK4a}$ expression significantly correlated with the presence of HPV [53]. Further, high $p16^{INK4a}$ expression may have provided more persuasive evidence that the virus has molecularly affected cellular proliferation, according to some studies [53,54].

Regardless of the HPV status, the correlation between the $p16^{INK4a}$ expression and other clinicopathological factors and its prognostic value in lung cancer is not clear. In this study, $p16^{INK4a}$ expression was significantly correlated with early-stage disease. In agreement with this, Bian et al. reported that negative $p16^{INK4a}$ expression by IHC has a statistically significant correlation with a higher pathological stage and lymph node metastasis but not with other variables such as age, gender, differentiation, and tumor size [55]. Another study revealed that $p16^{INK4a}$ overexpression is significantly associated with early-stage IA1 and IA2 disease [25]. Another exciting study used the same scoring criteria of $p16^{INK4a}$ expression as in this work and found that $p16^{INK4a}$ positivity is significantly associated with the N0 stage, while $p16^{INK4a}$ negativity is significantly associated with SqCC [24]. On the contrary, Zou et al. [47] and Silva et al. [42] did not find a significant correlation between $p16^{INK4a}$ expression and other clinicopathological features.

When all cases of NSCLC were analyzed, no significant impact of the $p16^{INK4a}$ expression on the OS ($p = 0.151$) or DFS ($p = 0.522$) was detected in this work. However, $p16^{INK4a}$ expression showed a statistically significant association with OS in patients with the SqCC histological subtype, where patients with positive p16^{INK4a} expression showed a better overall survival (p = 0.033). Further, poor OS and DFS were significantly associated with advanced pathological stages, positive lymph node metastasis, and tumor size >3 cm in p16^{INK4a} negative cases, while, in p16^{INK4a}-positive cases, only positive lymph node metastasis and advanced pathological stages were significantly associated with poor OS and DFS, respectively. Similarly, Huang et al. did not find a significant difference in five-year survival and p16^{INK4a} status in NSCLC; however, a worse OS rate of patients with negative p16^{INK4a} was established in early stages [33]. In contrast, Zhou et al. found that p16^{INK4a} expression was associated with a statistically significant favorable prognosis in ADC cases, whereas in SqCC, p16^{INK4a} expression showed a slightly worse median OS, albeit not statistically significant [47]. Bian et al. also reported that loss of p16^{INK4a} expression, tumor size, lymph node metastasis, and pathological stages are associated with significantly shorter OS in lung ADC [55]. On the other hand, An et al. indicated that negative p16^{INK4a} expression was significantly associated with shorter disease-specific survival and DFS, and similar to our results, advanced pathological tumor stages were significantly associated with poor survival [24]. Collectively, the evidence supports a prognostic role of p16^{INK4a} expression in lung cancer and the variability between different studies can be attributed to different methodological approaches, especially p16^{INK4a} scoring, different sample sizes, and different histological subtypes.

This study has some limitations. First, this retrospective study was performed in a single center and, thus, was amenable to selection bias. Second, it utilized a single modality to assess the presence of HPV in spite of the fact that PCR is a sensitive and specific method to investigate HPV in lung cancer. Further, we recognize that the mere presence of HPV in lung cancer does not provide sufficient evidence about its role in carcinogenesis, and this requires further investigations. Finally, the relatively small sample size may have affected the results.

5. Conclusions

This is the first study to assess the HPV status and p16^{INK4a} expression in lung cancer among a Jordanian subpopulation and one of the very few conducted in the MENA area. This study showed that HPV is rare in NSCLC among the Jordanian population, with a prevalence in the studied sample of 5%, all of the high-risk or probable high-risk groups. Although p16^{INK4a} expression was detected in 20% of cases, unlike other cancer types, its reliability as a surrogate for HPV infection in lung cancer requires further investigation. p16^{INK4a} expression carries a good prognostic value in SqCC lung cancer but not in ADC cases. Overall, the potential role of HPV and p16^{INK4a} in the carcinogenesis of lung cancer should be further studied.

Author Contributions: Conceptualization, O.A.A.K., B.A., A.I., R.T., M.K., S.B. and M.A.; methodology, O.A.A.K., S.A., H.A., B.A., A.I., R.T., M.K., S.B. and M.A.; software, A.A.A.; formal analysis, O.A.A.K. and A.A.A.; investigation, O.A.A.K., S.A. and H.A.; data curation, O.A.A.K., S.A. and T.S.; writing—original draft preparation, O.A.A.K.; writing—review and editing, O.A.A.K., A.A.A., S.A., H.A., B.A., A.I., R.T., M.K., S.B., M.A., T.S. and M.S.; supervision, O.A.A.K. and M.S.; project administration, O.A.A.K.; funding acquisition, O.A.A.K. All authors have read and agreed to the published version of the manuscript.

Funding: This research was funded by the Scientific Research Deanship, The Hashemite University, Zarqa, Jordan, Grant No. 935/57/2023, O.A.A.K.

Institutional Review Board Statement: The study was conducted in accordance with the Declaration of Helsinki and approved by the Institutional Review Boards of Hashemite University (No.28/5/2022/2023, on 10 April 2023) and King Hussein Cancer Center (No. 23 KHCC 99, on 26 September 2023).

Informed Consent Statement: Patient consent was waived by the Institutional Review Boards due to the retrospective nature of the study and as no patient identifications were used.

Data Availability Statement: The data collected and analyzed during the current study are available upon reasonable request from the corresponding author.

Conflicts of Interest: The authors declare no conflicts of interest. The funders had no role in the design of the study; in the collection, analyses, or interpretation of data; in the writing of the manuscript; or in the decision to publish the results.

Abbreviations

HPV	Human papillomavirus
HR-HPV	High-risk human papillomavirus
NSCLC	Non-small-cell lung cancer
IHC	Immunohistochemistry
FFPE	Formalin-fixed, paraffin-embedded
KHCC	King Hussein Cancer Center
RT-PCR	Real-time polymerase chain reaction
AJCC	American Joint Committee on Cancer protocol
ADC	Adenocarcinoma
SqCC	Squamous cell carcinoma
LR-HPV	Low-risk human papillomavirus
CDK	Cyclin-dependent kinase
WHO	World Health Organization
OS	Overall survival
DFS	Disease-free survival
EGFR	Epidermal growth factor receptor
ALK	Anaplastic lymphoma kinase
ISH	In situ hybridization

References

1. Torre, L.A.; Bray, F.; Siegel, R.L.; Ferlay, J.; Lortet-Tieulent, J.; Jemal, A. Global Cancer Statistics, 2012. *CA Cancer J. Clin.* **2015**, *65*, 87–108. [CrossRef] [PubMed]
2. Sarchianaki, E.; Derdas, S.P.; Ntaoukakis, M.; Vakonaki, E.; Lagoudaki, E.D.; Lasithiotaki, I.; Sarchianaki, A.; Koutsopoulos, A.; Symvoulakis, E.K.; Spandidos, D.A.; et al. Detection and Genotype Analysis of Human Papillomavirus in Non-Small Cell Lung Cancer Patients. *Tumor Biol.* **2014**, *35*, 3203–3209. [CrossRef] [PubMed]
3. Sun, S.; Schiller, J.H.; Gazdar, A.F. Lung Cancer in Never Smokers—A Different Disease. *Nat. Rev. Cancer* **2007**, *7*, 778–790. [CrossRef] [PubMed]
4. Srinivasan, M.; Taioli, E.; Ragin, C.C. Human Papillomavirus Type 16 and 18 in Primary Lung Cancers—A Meta-Analysis. *Carcinogenesis* **2009**, *30*, 1722–1728. [CrossRef]
5. Spyratos, D.; Zarogoulidis, P.; Porpodis, K.; Tsakiridis, K.; Machairiotis, N.; Katsikogiannis, N.; Kougioumtzi, I.; Dryllis, G.; Kallianos, A.; Rapti, A.; et al. Occupational Exposure and Lung Cancer. *J. Thorac. Dis.* **2013**, *5* (Suppl. S4), S44–S45. [CrossRef]
6. de Freitas, A.C.; Gurgel, A.P.; de Lima, E.G.; de França São Marcos, B.; do Amaral, C.M.M. Human Papillomavirus and Lung Cancinogenesis: An Overview. *J. Cancer Res. Clin. Oncol.* **2016**, *142*, 2415–2427. [CrossRef] [PubMed]
7. Zhai, K.; Ding, J.; Shi, H.-Z. HPV and Lung Cancer Risk: A Meta-Analysis. *J. Clin. Virol.* **2015**, *63*, 84–90. [CrossRef]
8. Bruni, L.; Albero, G.; Serrano, B.; Mena, M.; Collado, J.J.; Gómez, D.; Muñoz, J.; Bosch, F.X.; de Sanjosé, S. ICO/IARC Information Centre on HPV and Cancer (HPV Information Centre). Human Papillomavirus and Related Diseases in the World. Summary Report 10 March 2023. Available online: https://hpvcentre.net/statistics/reports/XWX.pdf (accessed on 16 March 2024).
9. Corneanu, L.M.; Stănculescu, D.; Corneanu, C. HPV and Cervical Squamous Intraepithelial Lesions: Clinicopathological Study. *Rom. J. Morphol. Embryol.* **2011**, *52*, 89–94. [PubMed]
10. Berman, T.A.; Schiller, J.T. Human Papillomavirus in Cervical Cancer and Oropharyngeal Cancer: One Cause, Two Diseases. *Cancer* **2017**, *123*, 2219–2229. [CrossRef]
11. Muñoz, N.; Castellsagué, X.; de González, A.B.; Gissmann, L. Chapter 1: HPV in the Etiology of Human Cancer. *Vaccine* **2006**, *24*, S1–S10. [CrossRef]
12. Gillison, M.L.; Koch, W.M.; Capone, R.B.; Spafford, M.; Westra, W.H.; Wu, L.; Zahurak, M.L. Evidence for a Causal Association Between Human Papillomavirus and a Subset of Head and Neck Cancers. *J. Natl. Cancer Inst.* **2000**, *92*, 709–720. [CrossRef]
13. Preti, M.; Boldorini, R.; Gallio, N.; Cavagnetto, C.; Borella, F.; Pisapia, E.; Ribaldone, R.; Bovio, E.; Bertero, L.; Airoldi, C.; et al. Human papillomavirus genotyping in high-grade vaginal intraepithelial neoplasia: A multicentric Italian study. *J. Med. Virol.* **2024**, *96*, e29474. [CrossRef]

14. Sano, T.; Oyama, T.; Kashiwabara, K.; Fukuda, T.; Nakajima, T. Immunohistochemical Overexpression of P16 Protein Associated with Intact Retinoblastoma Protein Expression in Cervical Cancer and Cervical Intraepithelial Neoplasia. *Pathol. Int.* **1998**, *48*, 580–585. [CrossRef] [PubMed]
15. Doxtader, E.E.; Katzenstein, A.-L.A. The Relationship between P16 Expression and High-Risk Human Papillomavirus Infection in Squamous Cell Carcinomas from Sites Other than Uterine Cervix: A Study of 137 Cases. *Hum. Pathol.* **2012**, *43*, 327–332. [CrossRef] [PubMed]
16. Khleif, S.N.; DeGregori, J.; Yee, C.L.; Otterson, G.A.; Kaye, F.J.; Nevins, J.R.; Howley, P.M. Inhibition of Cyclin D-CDK4/CDK6 Activity Is Associated with an E2F-Mediated Induction of Cyclin Kinase Inhibitor Activity. *Proc. Natl. Acad. Sci. USA* **1996**, *93*, 4350–4354. [CrossRef] [PubMed]
17. Munger, K.; Jones, D.L. Human Papillomavirus Carcinogenesis: An Identity Crisis in the Retinoblastoma Tumor Suppressor Pathway. *J. Virol.* **2015**, *89*, 4708–4711. [CrossRef] [PubMed]
18. McLaughlin-Drubin, M.E.; Crum, C.P.; Münger, K. Human Papillomavirus E7 Oncoprotein Induces KDM6A and KDM6B Histone Demethylase Expression and Causes Epigenetic Reprogramming. *Proc. Natl. Acad. Sci. USA* **2011**, *108*, 2130–2135. [CrossRef] [PubMed]
19. Cheng, Y.-W.; Wu, M.-F.; Wang, J.; Yeh, K.-T.; Goan, Y.-G.; Chiou, H.-L.; Chen, C.-Y.; Lee, H. Human Papillomavirus 16/18 E6 Oncoprotein Is Expressed in Lung Cancer and Related with P53 Inactivation. *Cancer Res.* **2007**, *67*, 10686–10693. [CrossRef]
20. Syrjänen, K.; Syrjänen, S.; Kellokoski, J.; Kärjä, J.; Mäntyjärvi, R. Human Papillomavirus (HPV) Type 6 and 16 DNA Sequences in Bronchial Squamous Cell Carcinomas Demonstrated by in Situ DNA Hybridization. *Lung* **1989**, *167*, 33–42. [CrossRef]
21. Bishop, J.A.; Ogawa, T.; Chang, X.; Illei, P.B.; Gabrielson, E.; Pai, S.I.; Westra, W.H. HPV Analysis in Distinguishing Second Primary Tumors From Lung Metastases in Patients With Head and Neck Squamous Cell Carcinoma. *Am. J. Surg. Pathol.* **2012**, *36*, 142–148. [CrossRef]
22. Myong, N.-H. Cyclin D1 Overexpression, P16 Loss, and pRb Inactivation Play a Key Role in Pulmonary Carcinogenesis and Have a Prognostic Implication for the Long-Term Survival in Non-Small Cell Lung Carcinoma Patients. *Cancer Res. Treat.* **2008**, *40*, 45–52. [CrossRef]
23. Sterlacci, W.; Tzankov, A.; Veits, L.; Zelger, B.; Bihl, M.P.; Foerster, A.; Augustin, F.; Fiegl, M.; Savic, S. A Comprehensive Analysis of P16 Expression, Gene Status, and Promoter Hypermethylation In Surgically Resected Non-Small Cell Lung Carcinomas. *J. Thorac. Oncol.* **2011**, *6*, 1649–1657. [CrossRef]
24. An, H.J.; Koh, H.M.; Song, D.H. New P16 Expression Criteria Predict Lymph Node Metastasis in Patients With Non-Small Cell Lung Cancer. *Vivo* **2019**, *33*, 1885–1892. [CrossRef] [PubMed]
25. Pezzuto, A.; Cappuzzo, F.; D'Arcangelo, M.; Ciccozzi, M.; Navarini, L.; Guerrini, S.; Ricci, A.; D'Ascanio, M.; Carico, E. Prognostic Value of P16 Protein in Patients With Surgically Treated Non-Small Cell Lung Cancer; Relationship With Ki-67 and PD-L1. *Anticancer Res.* **2020**, *40*, 983–990. [CrossRef] [PubMed]
26. Qaqish, A.; Abdo, N.; Abbas, M.M.; Saadeh, N.; Alkhateeb, M.; Msameh, R.; Tarawneh, S.; Al-Masri, M. Awareness and Knowledge of Physicians and Residents on the Non-Sexual Routes of Human Papilloma Virus (HPV) Infection and Their Perspectives on Anti-HPV Vaccination in Jordan. *PLoS ONE* **2023**, *18*, e0291643. [CrossRef] [PubMed]
27. Travis, W.D.; Brambilla, E.; Nicholson, A.G.; Yatabe, Y.; Austin, J.H.M.; Beasley, M.B.; Chirieac, L.R.; Dacic, S.; Duhig, E.; Flieder, D.B.; et al. The 2015 World Health Organization Classification of Lung Tumors. *J. Thorac. Oncol.* **2015**, *10*, 1243–1260. [CrossRef]
28. Nicholson, A.G.; Tsao, M.S.; Beasley, M.B.; Borczuk, A.C.; Brambilla, E.; Cooper, W.A.; Dacic, S.; Jain, D.; Kerr, K.M.; Lantuejoul, S.; et al. The 2021 WHO Classification of Lung Tumors: Impact of Advances Since 2015. *J. Thorac. Oncol.* **2022**, *17*, 362–387. [CrossRef]
29. Mirsadraee, S.; Oswal, D.; Alizadeh, Y.; Caulo, A.; van Beek, E.J. The 7th Lung Cancer TNM Classification and Staging System: Review of the Changes and Implications. *World J. Radiol.* **2012**, *4*, 128–134. [CrossRef]
30. Detterbeck, F.C. The Eighth Edition TNM Stage Classification for Lung Cancer: What Does It Mean on Main Street? *J. Thorac. Cardiovasc. Surg.* **2018**, *155*, 356–359. [CrossRef]
31. Würdemann, N.; Wagner, S.; Sharma, S.J.; Prigge, E.-S.; Reuschenbach, M.; Gattenlöhner, S.; Klussmann, J.P.; Wittekindt, C. Prognostic Impact of AJCC/UICC 8th Edition New Staging Rules in Oropharyngeal Squamous Cell Carcinoma. *Front. Oncol.* **2017**, *7*, 129. [CrossRef]
32. Machczyński, P.; Majchrzak, E.; Niewinski, P.; Marchlewska, J.; Golusiński, W. A Review of the 8th Edition of the AJCC Staging System for Oropharyngeal Cancer According to HPV Status. *Eur. Arch. Otorhinolaryngol.* **2020**, *277*, 2407–2412. [CrossRef] [PubMed]
33. Huang, C.-I.; Taki, T.; Higashiyama, M.; Kohno, N.; Miyake, M. P16 Protein Expression Is Associated with a Poor Prognosis in Squamous Cell Carcinoma of the Lung. *Br. J. Cancer* **2000**, *82*, 374–380. [CrossRef]
34. Syrjänen, K. Detection of Human Papillomavirus in Lung Cancer: Systematic Review and Meta-Analysis. *Anticancer Res.* **2012**, *32*, 3235–3250. [PubMed]
35. Nadji, S.A.; Mokhtari-Azad, T.; Mahmoodi, M.; Yahyapour, Y.; Naghshvar, F.; Torabizadeh, J.; Ziaee, A.A.; Nategh, R. Relationship between Lung Cancer and Human Papillomavirus in North of Iran, Mazandaran Province. *Cancer Lett.* **2007**, *248*, 41–46. [CrossRef]

36. Hussen, B.M.; Ahmadi, G.; Marzban, H.; Fard Azar, M.E.; Sorayyayi, S.; Karampour, R.; Nahand, J.S.; Hidayat, H.J.; Moghoofei, M. The Role of HPV Gene Expression and Selected Cellular MiRNAs in Lung Cancer Development. *Microb. Pathog.* **2021**, *150*, 104692. [CrossRef] [PubMed]
37. Klein, F.; Amin Kotb, W.F.M.; Petersen, I. Incidence of Human Papilloma Virus in Lung Cancer. *Lung Cancer* **2009**, *65*, 13–18. [CrossRef] [PubMed]
38. Hasegawa, Y.; Ando, M.; Kubo, A.; Isa, S.; Yamamoto, S.; Tsujino, K.; Kurata, T.; Ou, S.-H.I.; Takada, M.; Kawaguchi, T. Human Papilloma Virus in Non-Small Cell Lung Cancer in Never Smokers: A Systematic Review of the Literature. *Lung Cancer* **2014**, *83*, 8–13. [CrossRef] [PubMed]
39. Yanagawa, N.; Wang, A.; Kohler, D.; Santos, G.D.C.; Sykes, J.; Xu, J.; Pintilie, M.; Tsao, M.-S. Human Papilloma Virus Genome Is Rare in North American Non-Small Cell Lung Carcinoma Patients. *Lung Cancer* **2013**, *79*, 215–220. [CrossRef] [PubMed]
40. Joh, J.; Jenson, A.B.; Moore, G.D.; Rezazedeh, A.; Slone, S.P.; Ghim, S.; Kloecker, G.H. Human Papillomavirus (HPV) and Merkel Cell Polyomavirus (MCPyV) in Non Small Cell Lung Cancer. *Exp. Mol. Pathol.* **2010**, *89*, 222–226. [CrossRef]
41. Goto, A.; Li, C.-P.; Ota, S.; Niki, T.; Ohtsuki, Y.; Kitajima, S.; Yonezawa, S.; Koriyama, C.; Akiba, S.; Uchima, H.; et al. Human Papillomavirus Infection in Lung and Esophageal Cancers: Analysis of 485 Asian Cases. *J. Med. Virol.* **2011**, *83*, 1383–1390. [CrossRef]
42. Silva, E.M.; Mariano, V.S.; Pastrez, P.R.A.; Pinto, M.C.; Nunes, E.M.; Sichero, L.; Villa, L.L.; Scapulatempo-Neto, C.; Syrjanen, K.J.; Longatto-Filho, A. Human Papillomavirus Is Not Associated to Non-Small Cell Lung Cancer: Data from a Prospective Cross-Sectional Study. *Infect. Agent. Cancer* **2019**, *14*, 18. [CrossRef] [PubMed]
43. Chang, S.Y.; Keeney, M.; Law, M.; Donovan, J.; Aubry, M.-C.; Garcia, J. Detection of Human Papillomavirus in Non–Small Cell Carcinoma of the Lung. *Hum. Pathol.* **2015**, *46*, 1592–1597. [CrossRef] [PubMed]
44. Iwakawa, R.; Kohno, T.; Enari, M.; Kiyono, T.; Yokota, J. Prevalence of Human Papillomavirus 16/18/33 Infection and P53 Mutation in Lung Adenocarcinoma. *Cancer Sci.* **2010**, *101*, 1891–1896. [CrossRef] [PubMed]
45. Khasawneh, A.I.; Asali, F.F.; Kilani, R.M.; Abu-Raideh, J.A.; Himsawi, N.M.; Salameh, M.A.; Al Ghabbiesh, G.H.; Saleh, T. Prevalence and Genotype Distribution of Human Papillomavirus Among a Subpopulation of Jordanian Women. *Int. J. Womens Health* **2020**, *9*, 017–023. [CrossRef]
46. Ragin, C.; Obikoya-Malomo, M.; Kim, S.; Chen, Z.; Flores-Obando, R.; Gibbs, D.; Koriyama, C.; Aguayo, F.; Koshiol, J.; Caporaso, N.E.; et al. HPV-Associated Lung Cancers: An International Pooled Analysis. *Carcinogenesis* **2014**, *35*, 1267–1275. [CrossRef] [PubMed]
47. Zhou, Y.; Höti, N.; Ao, M.; Zhang, Z.; Zhu, H.; Li, L.; Askin, F.; Gabrielson, E.; Zhang, H.; Li, Q.K. Expression of P16 and P53 in Non-Small-Cell Lung Cancer: Clinicopathological Correlation and Potential Prognostic Impact. *Biomark. Med.* **2019**, *13*, 761–771. [CrossRef] [PubMed]
48. Gorgoulis, V.G.; Zacharatos, P.; Kotsinas, A.; Liloglou, T.; Kyroudi, A.; Veslemes, M.; Rassidakis, A.; Halazonetis, T.D.; Field, J.K.; Kittas, C. Alterations of the P16-pRb Pathway and the Chromosome Locus 9p21–22 in Non-Small-Cell Lung Carcinomas. *Am. J. Pathol.* **1998**, *153*, 1749–1765. [CrossRef]
49. Romagosa, C.; Simonetti, S.; López-Vicente, L.; Mazo, A.; Lleonart, M.E.; Castellvi, J.; Ramon Y Cajal, S. p16Ink4a Overexpression in Cancer: A Tumor Suppressor Gene Associated with Senescence and High-Grade Tumors. *Oncogene* **2011**, *30*, 2087–2097. [CrossRef]
50. Paez-Ribes, M.; González-Gualda, E.; Doherty, G.J.; Muñoz-Espín, D. Targeting Senescent Cells in Translational Medicine. *EMBO Mol. Med.* **2019**, *11*, e10234. [CrossRef]
51. Domen, A.; Deben, C.; De Pauw, I.; Hermans, C.; Lambrechts, H.; Verswyvel, J.; Siozopoulou, V.; Pauwels, P.; Demaria, M.; Van De Wiel, M.; et al. Prognostic Implications of Cellular Senescence in Resected Non-Small Cell Lung Cancer. *Transl. Lung Cancer Res.* **2022**, *11*, 1526–1539. [CrossRef]
52. Saleh, T.; Bloukh, S.; Hasan, M.; Al Shboul, S. Therapy-Induced Senescence as a Component of Tumor Biology: Evidence from Clinical Cancer. *Biochim. Biophys. Acta Rev. Cancer* **2023**, *1878*, 188994. [CrossRef] [PubMed]
53. Robinson, L.A.; Jaing, C.J.; Pierce Campbell, C.; Magliocco, A.; Xiong, Y.; Magliocco, G.; Thissen, J.B.; Antonia, S. Molecular Evidence of Viral DNA in Non-Small Cell Lung Cancer and Non-Neoplastic Lung. *Br. J. Cancer* **2016**, *115*, 497–504. [CrossRef] [PubMed]
54. Marcos, B.F.S.; De Oliveira, T.H.A.; Do Amaral, C.M.M.; Muniz, M.T.C.; Freitas, A.C. Correlation between HPV PCNA, P16, and P21 Expression in Lung Cancer Patients. *Cell. Microbiol.* **2022**, *2022*, 9144334. [CrossRef]
55. Bian, C.; Li, Z.; Xu, Y.; Wang, J.; Xu, L.; Shen, H. Clinical Outcome and Expression of Mutant P53, P16, and Smad4 in Lung Adenocarcinoma: A Prospective Study. *World J. Surg. Oncol.* **2015**, *13*, 128. [CrossRef]

Disclaimer/Publisher's Note: The statements, opinions and data contained in all publications are solely those of the individual author(s) and contributor(s) and not of MDPI and/or the editor(s). MDPI and/or the editor(s) disclaim responsibility for any injury to people or property resulting from any ideas, methods, instructions or products referred to in the content.

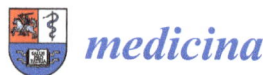 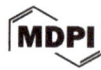

Article

Retrospective Evaluation of the Efficacy of Total Neoadjuvant Therapy and Chemoradiotherapy Neoadjuvant Treatment in Relation to Surgery in Patients with Rectal Cancer

Lucian Dragoș Bratu [1,2], Michael Schenker [2,3,*], Puiu Olivian Stovicek [2,4,*], Ramona Adriana Schenker [2], Alina Maria Mehedințeanu [2], Tradian Ciprian Berisha [1,2], Andreas Donoiu [1,5] and Stelian Ștefăniță Mogoantă [5,6]

[1] Doctoral School, University of Medicine and Pharmacy of Craiova, 200349 Craiova, Romania; berishatc.sfn@gmail.com (T.C.B.); donoiuandreas@yahoo.com (A.D.)
[2] Sf. Nectarie Oncology Center, 200347 Craiova, Romania; ramona_schenker@yahoo.com (R.A.S.); alina.maria591@gmail.com (A.M.M.)
[3] Department of Oncology, University of Medicine and Pharmacy of Craiova, 200349 Craiova, Romania
[4] Department of Pharmacology, Faculty of Nursing, Târgu Jiu Subsidiary, Titu Maiorescu University, 040441 Bucharest, Romania
[5] 3rd General Surgery Clinic, Emergency County Hospital, 200642 Craiova, Romania; stelian.mogoanta@umfcv.ro
[6] Department of Surgery, University of Medicine and Pharmacy of Craiova, 200349 Craiova, Romania
* Correspondence: michael.schenker@umfcv.ro (M.S.); olivian_sfn@yahoo.com (P.O.S.); Tel.: +40-727774974 (M.S.)

Citation: Bratu, L.D.; Schenker, M.; Stovicek, P.O.; Schenker, R.A.; Mehedințeanu, A.M.; Berisha, T.C.; Donoiu, A.; Mogoantă, S.Ș. Retrospective Evaluation of the Efficacy of Total Neoadjuvant Therapy and Chemoradiotherapy Neoadjuvant Treatment in Relation to Surgery in Patients with Rectal Cancer. *Medicina* **2024**, *60*, 646. https://doi.org/10.3390/medicina60040656

Academic Editor: Seung-Gu Yeo

Received: 8 April 2024
Revised: 14 April 2024
Accepted: 16 April 2024
Published: 19 April 2024

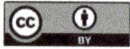

Copyright: © 2024 by the authors. Licensee MDPI, Basel, Switzerland. This article is an open access article distributed under the terms and conditions of the Creative Commons Attribution (CC BY) license (https://creativecommons.org/licenses/by/4.0/).

Abstract: *Background and Objective*: In the therapeutic strategy of rectal cancer, radiotherapy has consolidated its important position and frequent use in current practice due to its indications as neoadjuvant, adjuvant, definitive, or palliative treatment. In recent years, total neoadjuvant therapy (TNT) has been established as the preferred regimen compared to concurrent neoadjuvant chemoradiotherapy (CRT). In relation to better outcomes, the percentage of patients who achieved pathological complete response (pCR) after neoadjuvant treatment is higher in the case of TNT. This study aimed to analyze the response to TNT compared to neoadjuvant CRT regarding pCR rate and the change in staging after surgical intervention. *Materials and Methods*: We performed a retrospective study on 323 patients with rectal cancer and finally analyzed the data of 201 patients with neoadjuvant treatment, selected based on the inclusion and exclusion criteria. Patients received CRT neoadjuvant therapy or TNT neoadjuvant therapy with FOLFOX or CAPEOX. *Results*: Out of 157 patients who underwent TNT treatment, 19.74% had pathological complete response, whereas in the group with CRT (*n* = 44), those with pCR were 13.64%. After neoadjuvant treatment, the most frequent TNM classifications were ypT2 (40.30%) and ypN0 (79.10%). The statistical analysis of the postoperative disease stage, after neoadjuvant therapy, showed that the most frequent changes were downstaging (71.14%) and complete response (18.41%). Only four patients (1.99%) had an upstaging change. The majority of patients (88.56%) initially presented clinical evidence of nodal involvement whereas only 20.9% of the patients still presented regional disease at the time of surgical intervention. *Conclusions*: By using TNT, a higher rate of stage reduction is obtained compared to the neoadjuvant CRT treatment. The post-neoadjuvant-treatment imagistic evaluation fails to accurately evaluate the response. A better response to TNT was observed in young patients.

Keywords: rectal cancer; neoadjuvant therapy; total neoadjuvant therapy; chemoradiotherapy; tumor stage

1. Introduction

Worldwide, colorectal cancer represents a challenge due to its high incidence (third place) and mortality (second place). In our country, colorectal cancer ranks first in terms of incidence (13.541 cases/year) and second in terms of mortality (7.381 deaths/year), according to Globocan 2022 (data for Romania) [1]. With reference to rectal cancer, it represents approximately one third of all patients with colorectal cancer, which maintains its positioning among the most frequently encountered types of cancer in medical practice. The most critical prognosis indicators for rectal cancer are the tumor regression grade following neoadjuvant therapy and the pathological staging [2]. A recent analysis of the Surveillance, Epidemiology, and End Results (SEER) database showed an increase in the incidence of rectal cancer in patients under 50 years of age, but the reason for this increase has not yet been explained [3].

In view of the high incidence and mortality of this type of cancer, there is a major and constant interest in the development and improvement of diagnostic and treatment methods. In recent years, due to intensive research on improving treatments for rectal cancer, the recommendations of international guidelines have been modified relatively frequently; one of them is the introduction of total neoadjuvant therapy (TNT) as a type of therapeutic approach. Although TNT is recognized for its therapeutic benefits, long-term side effects have not been well documented [4]. In the therapeutic strategy of rectal cancer, radiotherapy has consolidated its important position and frequent use in current practice due to its indications as neoadjuvant, adjuvant, definitive, or palliative treatment [5]. Neoadjuvant radiotherapy is performed according to the recommendations of international guidelines using one of the following two fractionation regimens: "short-course" radiotherapy (25 Gy/5 fractions) or "long-course" radiotherapy (50.4 Gy/28 fractions) [6]. Based on the results of the German CAO/ARO/AIO 94 study, neoadjuvant chemoradiotherapy (CRT) is included in international guidelines as a treatment for patients with T3-4N0 or N+ rectal cancer [7]. Related to the choice of concomitant radiosensitization chemotherapy, there has been debate regarding the benefits and risks of using 5-Fluorouracil (5-FU) or capecitabine. The results of the NSABP R-04 study [8] and that of Hofheinz et al. [9] demonstrated the equivalence of the two regimens. Several studies demonstrated better outcome in patients who achieved a better pathological response to neoadjuvant treatment. In a retrospective analysis of 566 patients with pathologic complete response (pCR) after neoadjuvant CRT Capirci reported a 5-year disease-free survival (DFS) of 85% and a 5-year overall survival (OS) of 90% [10]. A meta-analysis of the results of 3015 patients from 14 studies showed an important improvement in local recurrence, disease-free survival (DFS), and overall survival (OS) in the 16% of patients who achieved pathological complete response after neoadjuvant treatment [11]. Phase III clinical trials looked at possible benefits of adding oxaliplatin to preoperative chemotherapy with 5-FU or capecitabine. In the CAO/ARO/AIO-04 study, the addition of oxaliplatin to 5-FU significantly increased the percentage of patients with pathological complete response (17% vs. 13%, $p = 0.031$) without a significant impact on grade 3 toxicity (23% vs. 22%) [12,13].

In recent years, total neoadjuvant therapy (TNT) has been established as preferable to concurrent neoadjuvant CRT [6] due to the better results obtained in the studies that analyzed the results of this type of treatment [14–16]. In relation to better outcomes, the percentage of patients who achieved pathological complete response after neoadjuvant treatment is higher in the case of TNT [4,17]. By using TNT, not only a higher pathological complete response rate (pCR), but also a better systemic control of the disease is obtained [15].

It is not clearly established whether it is better to start with chemotherapy, then follow with CRT (induction TNT), or the other way around (consolidation TNT), when following a TNT approach [6].

Clinical trials in which neoadjuvant CRT was performed demonstrated better results when surgery was carried out after a time interval of several weeks after the completion of radiation therapy. Data from the Lyon R90-01 study show that the chances of down-staging increase when this period is longer than 2 weeks [18]. Sloothaak et al., in a retrospective analysis of 1593 patients treated with preoperative CRT, showed that an interval of 16 weeks from the completion of radiotherapy to surgery was required to achieve a maximal percentage of 16% of pathological complete response among operated patients [19]. In the past, the recommended interval for performing surgery was 4–6 weeks after the completion of neoadjuvant treatment, but this time interval increased to 6–10 weeks in recent clinical trials [20].

Preoperative CRT may have a potential anal sphincter-preserving benefit in low rectal cancers. The results of some prospective analysis carried out by the collective from the Memorial Sloan Kettering Cancer Center showed similar 3-year local control rates for operations with resection margins greater than 2cm, less than 2cm, greater than 1cm, and less than 1cm [21,22]. Similar data have been reported by other investigators [23]. The most recommended chemotherapeutic regimens used in TNT for rectal cancer are CAPEOX (capecitabine plus oxaliplatin) and FOLFOX (5-fluorouracil, oxaliplatin, and leucovorin). The multicenter phase III CONVERT study demonstrated the efficacy and safety of CAPEOX as neoadjuvant chemotherapy for patients with rectal cancer, decreasing the incidence of perioperative distant metastases and preventive ileostomy [24]. The effectiveness of FOLFOX in the unadjuvated treatment of rectal cancer was highlighted in the phase III study PROSPECT NCT01515787 [25].

Neoadjuvant radiotherapy also has long-term benefits in patients with rectal cancer. Patients who received preoperative radiotherapy had a much lower recurrence rate compared to those operated without neoadjuvant treatment (12% vs. 27%; $p < 0.001$), and also an improved 5-year survival (58% vs. 48%; $p = 0.004$). The significant improvement was maintained at 13 years (38% vs. 30%; $p = 0.008$) [26].

The results of the STAR-01 [27], ACCORD [28–30], NSABP R-04 [31], and PETACC-6 [32] studies showed that the combination of oxaliplatin did not bring therapeutic benefits nor did it increase the toxicity of the treatment.

The administration of FOLFOX or CAPEOX as neoadjuvant therapy associated with RT, followed by surgery, reduces the occurrence of metastatic disease, increases the interval of disease-free survival, and has an implicit positive effect on the patient's prognosis, survival, and quality of life [33]. However, additional data are needed regarding the patients' evolution over time.

In this context, this study aimed to analyze the response to neoadjuvant CRT compared to total neoadjuvant treatment (TNT) regarding the modification of the staging evaluated by means of the pathological result after the surgical intervention, and particularly the determination of the pathological complete response rate (pCR) after neoadjuvant treatment.

2. Materials and Methods

2.1. Patient Selection, Inclusion and Exclusion Criteria

We conducted a single-institution, retrospective study of 323 patients with rectal cancer admitted to the Radiotherapy Department of Sf. Nectarie Oncology Center, Craiova, Romania, between July 2020 and June 2023, and we analyzed data of 201 patients with neoadjuvant treatment based on the inclusion and exclusion criteria. Patient data were recorded, including age, sex, the histopathological result of the biopsy and surgical specimen, clinical and pathological TNM (8th edition) staging [34], information on the systemic treatment administered prior to surgery, dose and fractionation used in radiotherapy, the result of the post-treatment imaging examination, and information on whether or not surgery was performed. The primary endpoint of our study was to compare pathologic downstaging rate after neoadjuvant CRT vs. TNT. The secondary endpoint was the correlation between imagistic post-therapeutic evaluation and pathological report findings.

The change in the pathological staging compared to the initial (clinical) staging was followed in response to the neoadjuvant treatment with the classification of this change in 4 subtypes: "unchanged"—no modification of the stage; "upstaging"—increasing the stage of the disease; "downstaging"—reducing the stage of the disease; and "complete response (pCR)"—no signs of disease.

For the inclusion of patients in the study and the performance of the statistical analysis, the following specific criteria were established.

Inclusion criteria: age over 18 years; indication for neoadjuvant radiotherapy; the patient's informed consent to the oncological records regarding treatment and the processing of medical data for research purposes; the patient's option for surgery after neoadjuvant treatment; the diagnosis of adenocarcinoma based on the histopathological examination on sample biopsy; and concurrent CRT with capecitabine or total neoadjuvant therapy (TNT) with CAPEOX or FOLFOX.

Exclusion criteria: "short-course" neoadjuvant radiotherapy; patients without chemotherapy as neoadjuvant treatment (refusal or contraindications); patients who have not completed the neoadjuvant treatment; patients without imaging investigations after neoadjuvant treatment; or patients who did not undergo surgery after neoadjuvant treatment.

From the total number of 323 patients with rectal cancer who presented to radiotherapy consultations, those who did not have an indication for radiotherapy according to NCCN international guidelines and internal hospital protocols were excluded (n = 29) as well those who refused radiotherapy or did not show up for the start of treatment (n = 5), thus leaving a total number of 289 patients with rectal neoplasm who benefited from radiotherapy during the mentioned period. Of the total number of treated patients, 230 benefited from neoadjuvant radiotherapy, while the rest (n = 59) had an indication for adjuvant, palliative, or definitive radiotherapy. From the 230 patients who received neoadjuvant radiotherapy, according to the study criteria, were excluded patients who had another histopathological form of rectal cancer besides adenocarcinoma (n = 1, squamous carcinoma), patients who did not benefit from neoadjuvant chemotherapy (n = 4), patients who received "short-course" neoadjuvant radiotherapy (n = 3), those who did not complete radiotherapy (n = 3), patients who did not show up for imaging control (n = 6), and patients (n = 12) who were not operated upon after radiotherapy (3 patients who refused surgery and 9 patients with unresectable tumors). Finally, the data of 201 treated patients were analyzed (Figure 1).

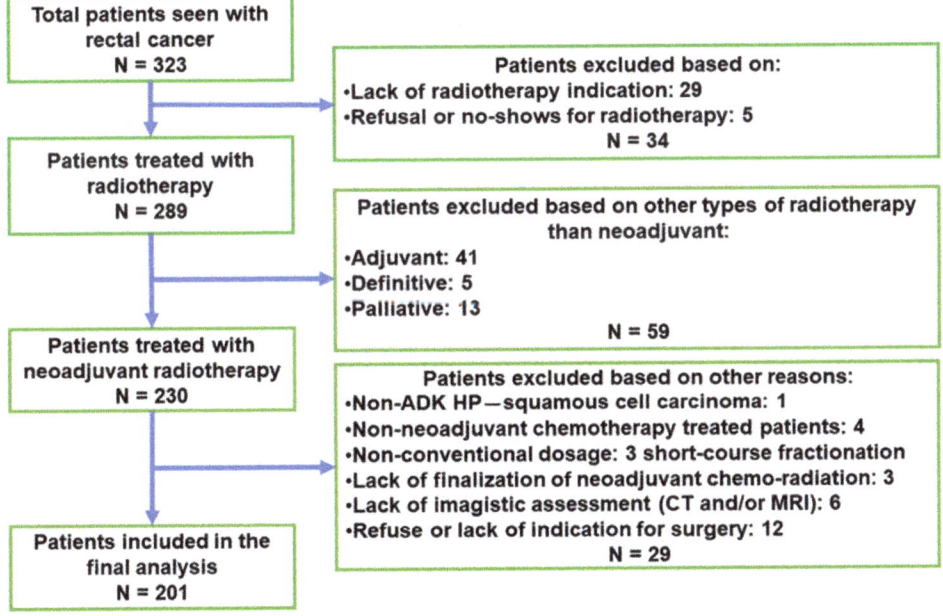

Figure 1. Flow diagram for the inclusion of patients in the study.

2.2. Indications for Neoadjuvant Therapy

Neoadjuvant treatment was indicated after tumor board analysis based on clinical staging for T1-2 N1-2, T3/T4 cases and at the surgeon's indication (initially considered unresectable tumors). In patients with oligometastatic disease, the decision regarding inclusion in the study was based on the assessment of the possibility of resection of synchronous hepatic or pulmonary metastases. Thus, 10 patients with stage IVA, who had potentially resectable synchronous hepatic or pulmonary metastases, benefited from neoadjuvant treatment. The association of chemotherapy in the form of TNT or neoadjuvant CRT was proposed by the treating oncologist, and the therapeutic conduct in all analyzed cases was established within the tumor board multidisciplinary oncological team.

Capecitabine treatment was used as part of CRT and TNT: 825 mg/m^2, oral administration, two times a day (BID), from Monday to Friday, on days of radiation treatment only, throughout the duration of RT. In the cases where TNT was administered, the chemotherapy was of the CAPEOX type: oxaliplatin 130 mg/m^2 intravenously day 1 and capecitabine 1000 mg/m^2 oral administration, BID, for 14 days every 3 weeks; or FOLFOX: oxaliplatin 85 mg/m^2 intravenously, day 1, leucovorin 400 mg/m^2 intravenously day 1 and 5-FU 400 mg/m^2 intravenously bolus on day 1, followed by 1200 mg/m^2/day × 2 days (total 2400 mg/m^2 over 46–48 h) continuous infusion. The administration of chemotherapy (CAPEOX or FOLFOX) before CRT was carried out over a period of 12–16 weeks. Patients who performed at least 4 cycles of CAPEOX or 6 cycles of FOLFOX were included in this study. These chemotherapy regimens are recommended by international guidelines [6]. In our institution, the administration of chemotherapy before CRT (induction TNT) was preferred for earlier treatment initiation. In this study, all patients who benefited from TNT underwent chemotherapy before CRT (induction TNT).

2.3. Performing Neoadjuvant Radiotherapy

After signing the informed consent, the patients underwent computed tomography scan for the treatment plan. The delineation of target volumes and organs at risk was performed based on the clinical data of the patients and the recommendations of the contouring guidelines [35–38]. The fractionation used during neoadjuvant radiotherapy was "long-course" 50.4 Gy/28 fractions. The treatment was performed using the Halcyon linear accelerator (manufactured by Varian Pablo Alto, CA, USA). Patients who completed neoadjuvant radiotherapy were recommended to perform imaging control (abdominal-pelvic MRI/CT examination with contrast) at an interval of 4–8 weeks after the completion of treatment. After performing the imaging control, the patients were sent to the surgery service to determine the opportunity of the surgical intervention and its type. Anorectoscopy or anorectal endoscopic ultrasound examinations were performed on surgeon demand for a better surgery planning. The data of the anatomical-pathological examination were collected based on the surgical excision.

2.4. Data Analysis

The statistical analysis was performed based on the data obtained from a sample of 201 subjects with rectal cancer. Demographic data and medical characteristics of the study sample were collected as categorical variables and expressed as frequencies and percentages. The comparative analysis of the differences between the 2 groups was carried out by using t-tests, chi-square tests, and proportionality tests, because the number of subjects in each group was unequal. The threshold for statistical significance in hypothesis testing was $p < 0.05$. p-values were the results of proportionality tests on each scale. The collected data were analyzed using the statistical processing program R v3.5, and the Microsoft Excel application from the Microsoft Office 365 package was used for the descriptive analysis.

3. Results

In the analyzed group (N = 201), most patients were men (57.71%) and were aged between 50 and 69 years (52.73%). The average age of the patients was 64.02 years, with standard deviation SD = 10.71 years. The minimum registered age was 34 years and the maximum age was 85 years. The comparative analysis between the ages and the gender of the patients showed that there is no statistically significant difference, suggesting that the age does not differ significantly between the two gender groups (t = 1.289; p = 0.199).

From a clinicopathological point of view, most rectal tumors were located in the middle rectum (43.28%) and predominantly had a G2 grade (44.78%). From the point of view of TNM classification, the most frequent classifications were T3 (64.68%), N1b (42.29%), and M0 (95.02%) (Table 1).

Table 1. Distribution of patients according to demographic and clinicopathological characteristics.

Characteristics		Total Group		CAPEOX		FOLFOX		CRT	
Demographic Characteristics		N	%	N	%	N	%	N	%
Gender	M	116	57.71	75	59.52	17	54.84	24	0
	F	85	42.29	51	40.48	14	45.16	20	100
Age (years)	34–49	22	10.95	18	14.29	2	6.45	2	5
	50–69	106	52.73	66	52.38	19	61.29	10	50
	70+	73	36.32	42	33.33	10	32.26	21	45
Clinicopathological characteristics		N	%	N	%	N	%	N	%
Rectal tumor location	Inferior	75	37.31	50	39.68	8	25.81	17	38.64
	Superior	39	19.41	51	40.48	14	45.16	22	50
	Middle	87	43.28	25	19.84	9	29.03	5	11.36
Tumor differentiation grade	G1	65	32.34	41	32.54	10	32.26	14	31.82
	G2	90	44.78	58	46.03	14	45.16	18	40.91
	G3	46	22.88	27	21.43	7	22.58	12	27.27
T	T1	6	2.98	3	2.38	0	0	3	6.82
	T2	36	17.91	24	19.05	2	6.45	10	22.73
	T3	130	64.68	82	65.08	22	70.97	26	59.09
	T4a	21	10.45	13	10.32	4	12.90	4	9.09
	T4b	8	3.98	4	3.17	3	9.68	1	2.27
N	N0	23	11.44	12	9.52	5	16.13	6	13.64
	N1a	26	12.94	18	14.29	2	6.45	6	13.64
	N1b	85	42.29	52	41.27	11	35.48	22	50
	N2a	46	22.89	31	24.60	7	22.58	8	18.18
	N2b	21	10.44	13	10.32	6	19.35	2	4.55
M	M0	191	95.02	119	94.44	28	90.32	44	100
	M1a	10	4.98	7	5.56	3	9.68	0	0
Stage at diagnosis	IIA	18	8.95	10	7.94	4	12.90	4	9.09
	IIB	5	2.49	2	1.59	1	3.23	2	4.55
	IIIA	28	13.93	16	12.70	2	6.45	10	22.73
	IIIB	108	53.73	71	56.35	12	38.71	25	56.82
	IIIC	32	15.92	20	15.87	9	29.03	3	6.82
	IVA	10	4.98	6	4.76	3	9.68	0	0

After neoadjuvant treatment, the most frequent TNM classifications were ypT2 (40.30%) and ypN0 (79.10%). Imaging evaluation performed before surgery compared with baseline showed that most cases had partial response (PR) (36.81%) and stable disease (SD) (45.27%). The statistical analysis of the postoperative disease stage, after neoadjuvant therapy, showed that the most common stage was stage I (39.80%), compared to zero cases at the initial evaluation. Also, 18.41% of cases had the pCR stage. The most frequent stage changes were downstaging (71.14%) and complete response (18.41%). Only four patients (1.99%) had an upstaging change (Table 2).

Table 2. Distribution of patients according to clinical, radiological, and pathological characteristics after radiotherapy.

Clinicopathological Characteristics		N	%
TNT	YES	157	78.11
	NO	44	21.89
ypT	ypT0	33	16.42
	ypT1	21	10.45
	ypT2	81	40.30
	ypT3	52	25.87
	ypT4a	11	5.47
	ypT4b	3	1.49
ypN	ypN0	159	79.10
	ypN1a	20	9.95
	ypN1b	9	4.48
	ypN1c	5	2.49
	ypN2a	6	2.98
	ypN2b	2	1
Postoperative stage (pathologic evaluation)	I	80	39.80
	IIA	37	18.41
	IIB	4	1.99
	IIC	1	0.50
	IIIA	14	6.96
	IIIB	22	10.95
	IIIC	6	2.98
	pCR	37	18.41
Stage change (according to pathologic report) Total lot N = 201	Complete response (pCR)	37	18.41
	Upstaging	4	1.99
	Downstaging	143	71.14
	Unchanged	17	8.46
Stage change TNT CAPEOX N = 126	Complete response (pCR)	28	22.22
	Upstaging	2	1.59
	Downstaging	88	69.84
	Unchanged	8	6.35

Table 2. Cont.

Clinicopathological Characteristics		N	%
Stage change TNT FOLFOX N = 31	Complete response (pCR)	3	9.68
	Upstaging	1	3.23
	Downstaging	23	74.19
	Unchanged	4	12.90
Stage change CRT N = 44	Complete response (pCR)	6	13.64
	Upstaging	1	2.27
	Downstaging	32	72.73
	Unchanged	5	11.36
Imagistic post-neoadjuvant evaluation Total lot N = 201	Complete Response	18	8.96
	Progressive Disease	18	8.96
	Partial Response	74	36.81
	Stable Disease	91	45.27
Imagistic post-neoadjuvant evaluation TNT CAPEOX N = 126	Complete Response	13	10.32
	Progressive Disease	12	9.52
	Partial Response	48	38.10
	Stable Disease	53	42.06
Imagistic post-neoadjuvant evaluation TNT FOLFOX N = 31	Complete Response	2	6.45
	Progressive Disease	4	12.90
	Partial Response	13	41.94
	Stable Disease	12	38.71
Imagistic post-neoadjuvant evaluation CRT N = 44	Complete Response	3	6.82
	Progressive Disease	2	4.55
	Partial Response	13	29.55
	Stable Disease	26	59.09

The statistical analysis between patient gender and treatment response indicated that there is no statistically significant association between patient gender and imaging response criteria ($\chi^2 = 3.502$, $p = 0.321$). This suggests that response to treatment, as assessed through imaging, does not depend on patient gender.

The Spearman correlation between patients' age and treatment response revealed that there is a weak but statistically significant negative correlation between patients' age and treatment response (correlation coefficient = -0.211, $p = 0.0027$), meaning that younger patients tend to have better responses to treatment than older patients.

The Kruskal–Wallis test to compare the treatment response between different tumor grades (G1, G2, and G3) showed that there are no statistically significant differences between the treatment responses of patients with different tumor grades (H = 1.479, $p = 0.477$). The evaluation of ages in relation to the different stages of the disease did not reveal statistically significant differences (H = 10.455, $p = 0.0633$).

The statistical analysis indicated that there is no statistically significant difference between the tumor grade and the initial stage of the disease ($\chi^2 = 16.795$, $p = 0.157$) nor between the tumor grade and the postoperative stage of the disease ($\chi^2 = 8.889$, $p = 0.838$). These results emphasize the complexity of the relationships between tumor characteristics and disease progression.

For categorical variables (gender, location, grade, TNM classification, and initial stage), all p-values are greater than 0.05, suggesting no statistically significant differences between treatment groups for these characteristics. This indicates a relatively homogeneous distribution of demographic and clinicopathological characteristics between the groups. For the continuous variable (age), the p-value is 0.02085, which is below the significance threshold of 0.05, indicating the existence of significant statistical differences between the treatment groups in terms of patient age.

From the group of patients treated with CAPEOX, 69.84% of cases presented downstaging and 22.22% complete response. For the arm with FOLFOX, the highest percentages were for downstaging (74.19%) and unchanged (12.9%). In the case of conventional treatment, 72.73% of patients presented downstaging and 13.64% pathological complete response (Figure 2).

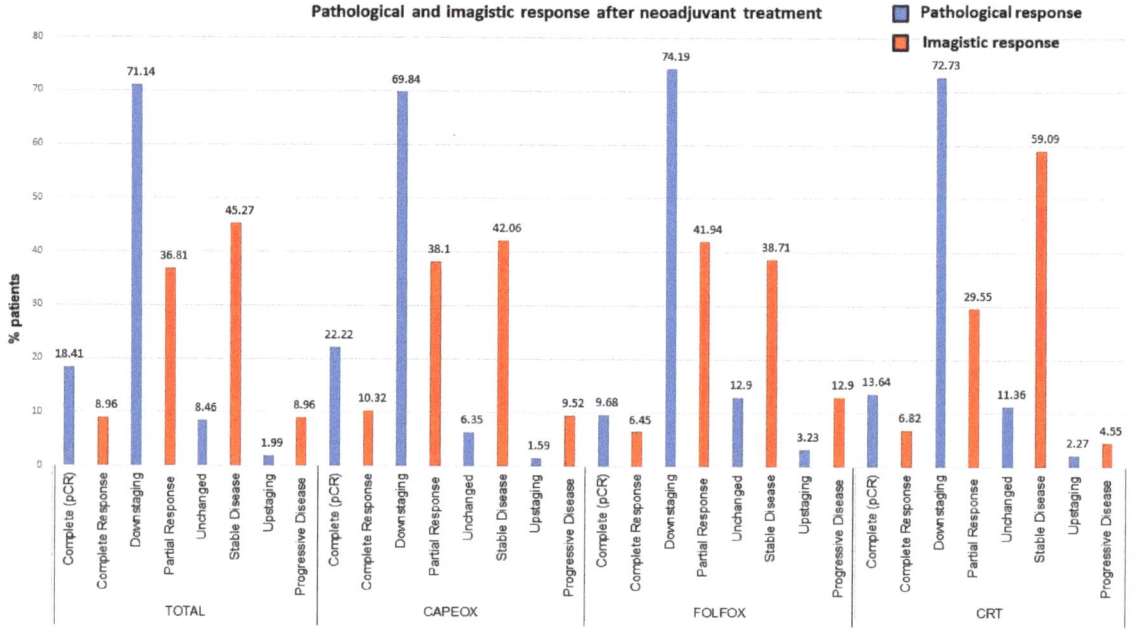

Figure 2. Pathological and imagistic response after neoadjuvant treatment.

Out of the total number of patients who underwent TNT treatment, 19.74% had a pathological complete response, whereas in the group with CRT, there were 13.64% cases with pCR. The statistical analysis cannot highlight statistically significant differences considering the large difference between the number of patients in each treatment group.

For this reason, the statistical analysis was descriptive, to provide a better understanding of the distributions for the initial and final stage, the imaging response, and the change in pathological stage within each treatment group (CAPEOX, FOLFOX, and CRT). From an imaging point of view, in patients treated with CAPEOX the results were as follows: complete response 13 patients (10.32%), progressive disease 12 patients (9.52%), partial response 48 patients (38.10%), and stable disease 53 patients (42.06%). In the case of the group treated with FOLFOX, it was observed that 2 patients (6.45%) had complete response, 4 patients (12.90%) progressive disease, 13 patients (41.94%) partial response, and 12 patients (38.71%) stable disease. In the case of the CRT group, 3 patients had complete response (6.82%), 2 patients progressive disease (4.55%), 13 patients partial response (29.55%), and 26 patients stable disease (59.09%). The descriptive analysis highlighted large differences between imaging and histopathological evaluation, after neoadjuvant treatment, both in the total group and in each treatment arm (Figure 3).

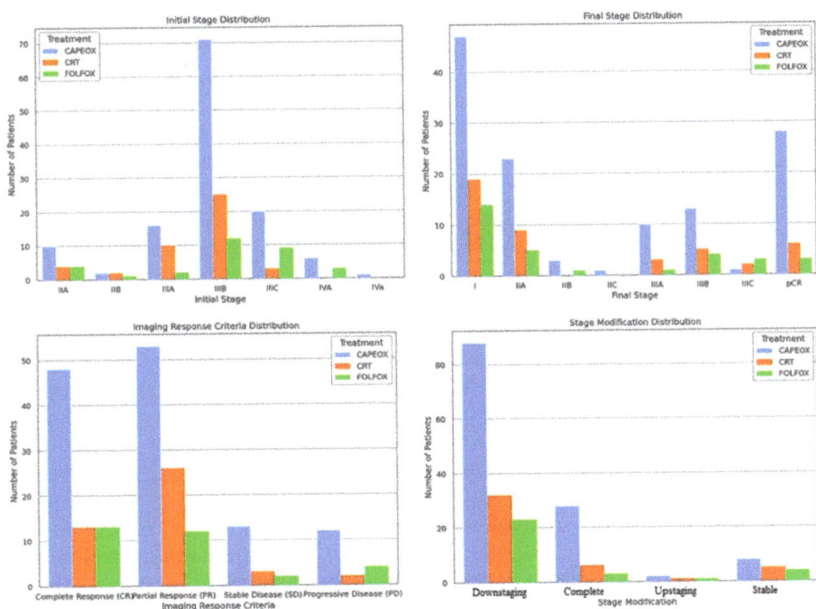

Figure 3. Distribution of patients in the initial stage, the final stage, the imaging response, and the change in the pathological stage, depending on each type of treatment.

The analysis of the relationship between cancer location and treatment types for 201 patients (87 with median, 75 with lower, and 39 with upper locations) revealed no significant difference in treatment distribution or in the independence between cancer location and treatment choice ($p = 0.171$). Similarly, imaging response and stage changes showed no significant variance across different rectal cancer locations, with imaging response p-value closely nearing significance ($p = 0.087$). However, a statistically significant difference was observed in post-treatment tumor classification (ypT) by location ($p = 0.022$), suggesting location may impact treatment response. Despite this, direct comparisons between locations using the Mann–Whitney test did not yield significant differences, likely due to reduced statistical power in individual tests for small sample sizes. No significant differences were found in post-treatment lymph node classification (ypN, $p = 0.744$) or in the final cancer stage ($p = 0.118$), though the latter approached significance.

4. Discussion

In the USA, the male–female incidence ratio of rectal cancer is estimated to be 1.39:1, and the median age at diagnosis is in the seventh decade of life [39]. The results of our study are consistent with these epidemiological data, with the male–female ratio being 1.36:1 and the average age being 64.02 years.

TNT in rectal cancer is a relatively new treatment strategy that involves the administration of a combination of neoadjuvant chemotherapy and radiotherapy before surgery. This approach is used to treat the tumor before surgery, with the aim of improving the chances of success of the surgery, facilitating the surgical removal of the tumor, and reducing the risk of recurrence. After the administration of neoadjuvant treatment, surgery is performed to remove the rest of the tumor and assess the pathological stage of the disease.

Patients who underwent TNT treatment had chemotherapy options with FOLFOX and CAPEOX. This therapeutic combination determined positive results for the patients when evaluating the postoperative stage (complete response 18.41%, downstaging 71.14%). Only 7.64% of patients had unchanged stage and 1.91% had upstaging.

A similar efficacy of TNT was demonstrated in another study in patients who received FOLFOX and chemoradiotherapy (50.4 Gy in 28 fractions) before surgery. Half of the patients received chemotherapy first, and the other half received radiation therapy. Consolidation resulted in better adherence to radiation (97% vs. 91%) but worse adherence to chemotherapy compared with induction (85% vs. 92%). However, the pCR percentage was better (25%) in the consolidation group compared to induction (17%) [40].

Among the patients included in our study, only 11.44% were in stage II of the disease (IIA and IIB), with the majority (88.56%) being diagnosed in advanced stages of the disease (III and IVA). The distribution of postoperative stage after neoadjuvant therapy was substantially changed, with only 20.89% of patients remaining in locally advanced stages (IIIA, IIIB, and IIIC) and 20.9% in stage II (A–C), while a percentage of 39, 8% of the patients were classified as stage I of the disease, and 18.41% of the total analyzed patients obtained a pathological complete response.

It should be noted that in the present study, patients (n = 10) with metastatic disease (stage IVA, potentially resectable synchronous liver or lung metastases) also benefited from neoadjuvant treatment, in which the evaluation of the change in stage took into account only the loco-regional response (ypT and ypN); all these patients showed downstaging after surgery. This fact reinforces the idea that certain patients with oligometastatic disease may benefit from curative treatment, with a possible positive impact on survival [41].

The majority of patients (88.56%) in this analysis initially presented clinical evidence of nodal involvement, and the analysis of the results after the surgical intervention shows that only 20.9% of the patients still presented regional disease.

In this study, differences related to patient gender and parameters such as staging or evolution were not statistically significant. Even if the incidence is higher in men, with an age distribution of 59–60 years, the differences are statistically insignificant correlated with the staging of the cancer at diagnosis and postoperatively. These results correlate with the fact that no gender differences were observed in the diagnosis of more advanced disease and the age-standardized 5-year survival is similar between the sexes [42].

The absence of notable correlations between the tumor grade and the initial disease stage, as well as between the tumor grade and the postoperative stage and treatment response, underscores the complexity of this localized disease. It emphasizes the necessity to explore additional factors, such as specific molecular markers, to better predict the potential response to neoadjuvant treatment.

Older people may have a reduced tolerance to chemotherapy treatments and side effects may be more pronounced. However, it is essential to assess each patient's situation individually. Some older patients may tolerate treatment well, while others may need dose adjustments or the choice of other therapeutic options. The better response of young patients to neoadjuvant therapy is an additional argument for starting treatment as early as possible from the moment of oncological diagnosis, and thus the application of screening measures for rectal cancer is very important [43].

Data from the literature regarding the pathological complete response rate (pCR) after neoadjuvant treatment in rectal cancer in relation with the age of the patients are contradictory. Some authors present results that show a better response to treatment in the case of young people [44], whereas in other studies the results are worse [45,46]. Possible mechanisms to explain these differences are given by means of molecular and clinical characteristics. Lieu et al. found that in microsatellite stable tumors, TP53 and CTNNB1 alterations were more common in younger patients while APC, KRAS, BRAF, and FAM123B were more commonly altered in older patients. Although rates of alterations in microsatellite genes were similar between young and old patients, when focusing on MSI-H tumors, alterations in APC and KRAS were more common in younger patients, while BRAF alterations were more common in older patients [47]. These differences might partially explain differences in pCR rates [44].

Another possible mechanism to explain this difference in response would be a possible better oxygenation at the tumor level (reduced areas of hypoxia), which leads to an increase in the effectiveness of neoadjuvant radiotherapy in the case of young people.

Considering that patients have a great fear regarding the side effects of chemotherapy and radiotherapy, psychological counseling was necessary. The discussions with the psycho-oncologist facilitated the patient's communication with the members of the multidisciplinary team, including the clinical pharmacologist [48–51].

In our study, the lack of significant statistical correlations between the treatment response assessed by means of the imaging investigation and that objectivized by the histopathological examination of the surgical excision is not unexpected. Even if they are frequently used in medical practice to assess the response to neoadjuvant treatment, CT and MRI examinations are not reliable to assess the change in the stage of the disease by reducing the size and invasion of the tumor, the disappearance or reduction of regional adenopathy, nor regarding the pathological complete response (pCR). This fact is supported by the results of meta-analyses that assessed this subject [52,53]. Several clinical studies have shown an important reduction in FDG capture when examining PET-CT in patients who responded to neoadjuvant treatment compared to those who did not respond [54]. The current favorable situation in Romania regarding the possibility of performing the PET-CT exam more frequently, due to the emergence of several medical imaging centers that offer this type of examination, could help us in the future to conduct a study on the accuracy of the PET-CT examination concerning the response to neoadjuvant treatment in patients with rectal cancer.

Since our study is a retrospective one, we must also acknowledge several limitations, starting with the unbalanced arms of neoadjuvant CRT vs. TNT. Also, the short follow-up period did not allow an evaluation of long-term results. Another important issue that we identified while collecting data was the presence of inadequate/incomplete/unstandardized pathologic reports since the patients included in the study addressed different surgical services and, consequently, different pathologic laboratories. The most frequent reporting error was related to the status of margins through the use of a vague statement like "uninvaded margins" without specifying which margins were evaluated. On the other hand, our study "observes" the introduction of TNT approach for rectal cancer in a real-world environment away from the controlled conditions of a trial.

5. Conclusions

Neoadjuvant therapy has a major role in downstaging patients with rectal cancer, allowing a better surgical approach. Our results show that by using TNT, a higher rate of the stage reduction is obtained compared to the neoadjuvant CRT treatment, and in particular, a higher percentage of patients obtained pathological complete response (pCR) in the case of TNT versus CRT. The post-neoadjuvant treatment imagistic evaluation fails to accurately evaluate the response since fibrosis or post-radiotherapy lesions might be confounded with neoplastic extensions that do not have a pathologic correspondence on resected specimens. For a more accurate evaluation of the post-therapeutic results, the standardization of pathologic reports of the resected specimen is mandatory. The better response to TNT observed in our study in young patients underscores the need to expand screening limits to younger ages, as these patients may benefit from an early evaluation, diagnosis, initiation of TNT, and surgery.

Author Contributions: Conceptualization, L.D.B. and S.Ș.M.; methodology, L.D.B., M.S., P.O.S. and S.Ș.M.; formal analysis and investigation, L.D.B., M.S., P.O.S., R.A.S., A.M.M., A.D. and T.C.B.; writing—original draft preparation, L.D.B., M.S., P.O.S., R.A.S., A.M.M., A.D. and T.C.B.; writing—review and editing, L.D.B., M.S., P.O.S. and S.Ș.M.; visualization, L.D.B., M.S., P.O.S. and S.Ș.M.; supervision, L.D.B., M.S. and S.Ș.M. All authors have read and agreed to the published version of the manuscript.

Funding: This research received no external funding.

Institutional Review Board Statement: This study was conducted according to the guidelines of the Declaration of Helsinki, and approved by the Ethics Committee of Sf. Nectarie Oncology Center, Craiova, according to decision number 003 from 7 February 2021.

Informed Consent Statement: Patient consent was waived due to the retrospective nature of the study. At the time of treatment, all patients signed a written consent that stated that all their medical data can be used anonymously by the medical staff of Sf. Nectarie Oncology Center for research and medical quality improvement purposes.

Data Availability Statement: Data are contained within the article. All data are available by request to the corresponding authors.

Conflicts of Interest: The authors declare no conflicts of interest.

References

1. Ferlay, J.; Ervik, M.; Lam, F.; Laversanne, M.; Colombet, M.; Mery, L.; Piñeros, M.; Znaor, A.; Soerjomataram, I.; Bray, F. *Global Cancer Observatory: Cancer Today*; International Agency for Research on Cancer: Lyon, France, 2024; Available online: https://gco.iarc.who.int/today (accessed on 7 April 2024).
2. Lotfollahzadeh, S.; Kashyap, S.; Tsoris, A.; Recio-Boiles, A.; Babiker, H.M. Rectal Cancer. In *StatPearls [Internet]*; StatPearls Publishing: Treasure Island, FL, USA, 2024. Available online: https://www.ncbi.nlm.nih.gov/books/NBK493202 (accessed on 7 April 2024).
3. Bailey, C.E.; Hu, C.Y.; You, Y.N.; Bednarski, B.K.; Rodriguez-Bigas, M.A.; Skibber, J.M.; Cantor, S.B.; Chang, G.J. Increasing disparities in the age-related incidences of colon and rectal cancers in the United States, 1975–2010. *JAMA Surg.* **2015**, *150*, 17–22. [CrossRef]
4. Kasi, A.; Abbasi, S.; Handa, S.; Al-Rajabi, R.; Saeed, A.; Baranda, J.; Sun, W. Total Neoadjuvant Therapy vs Standard Therapy in Locally Advanced Rectal Cancer: A Systematic Review and Meta-analysis. *JAMA Netw. Open* **2020**, *3*, e2030097. [CrossRef] [PubMed]
5. Feeney, G.; Sehgal, R.; Sheehan, M.; Hogan, A.; Regan, M.; Joyce, M.; Kerin, M. Neoadjuvant radiotherapy for rectal cancer management. *World J. Gastroenterol.* **2019**, *25*, 4850–4869. [CrossRef]
6. The National Comprehensive Cancer Network. NCCN Guidelines with Evidence Blocks—Rectal Cancer Version 1. 2024. Available online: https://www.nccn.org/guidelines/recently-published-guidelines (accessed on 7 April 2024).
7. Sauer, R.; Becker, H.; Hohenberger, W.; Rödel, C.; Wittekind, C.; Fietkau, R.; Martus, P.; Tschmelitsch, J.; Hager, E.; Hess, C.F.; et al. Preoperative versus postoperative chemoradiotherapy for rectal cancer. *N. Engl. J. Med.* **2004**, *351*, 1731–1740. [CrossRef] [PubMed]
8. O'Connell, M.J.; Colangelo, L.H.; Beart, R.W.; Petrelli, N.J.; Allegra, C.J.; Sharif, S.; Pitot, H.C.; Shields, A.F.; Landry, J.C.; Ryan, D.P.; et al. Capecitabine and oxaliplatin in the preoperative multimodality treatment of rectal cancer: Surgical end points from National Surgical Adjuvant Breast and Bowel Project trial R-04. *J. Clin. Oncol. Off. J. Am. Soc. Clin. Oncol.* **2014**, *32*, 1927–1934. [CrossRef]
9. Hofheinz, R.; Wenz, F.K.; Post, S.; Matzdorff, A.; Laechelt, S.; Hartmann, J.T.; Muller, L.; Link, H.; Moehler, M.H.; Kettner, E.; et al. Capecitabine (Cape) versus 5-fluorouracil (5-FU) based (neo)adjuvant chemoradiotherapy (CRT) for locally advanced rectal cancer (LARC): Long term results of a randomized, phase III trial. *J. Clin. Oncol.* **2011**, *29*, 3504. [CrossRef]
10. Capirci, C.; Valentini, V.; Cionini, L.; De Paoli, A.; Rodel, C.; Glynne-Jones, R.; Coco, C.; Romano, M.; Mantello, G.; Palazzi, S.; et al. Prognostic value of pathologic complete response after neoadjuvant therapy in locally advanced rectal cancer: Long-term analysis of 566 ypCR patients. *Int. J. Radiat. Oncol. Biol. Phys.* **2008**, *72*, 99–107. [CrossRef]
11. Maas, M.; Nelemans, P.J.; Valentini, V.; Das, P.; Rödel, C.; Kuo, L.J.; Calvo, F.A.; García-Aguilar, J.; Glynne-Jones, R.; Haustermans, K.; et al. Long-term outcome in patients with a pathological complete response after chemoradiation for rectal cancer: A pooled analysis of individual patient data. *Lancet Oncol.* **2010**, *11*, 835–844. [CrossRef] [PubMed]
12. Rödel, C.; Graeven, U.; Fietkau, R.; Hohenberger, W.; Hothorn, T.; Arnold, D.; Hofheinz, R.D.; Ghadimi, M.; Wolff, H.A.; Lang-Welzenbach, M.; et al. Oxaliplatin added to fluorouracil-based preoperative chemoradiotherapy and postoperative chemotherapy of locally advanced rectal cancer (the German CAO/ARO/AIO-04 study): Final results of the multicentre, open-label, randomised, phase 3 trial. *Lancet Oncol.* **2015**, *16*, 979–989. [CrossRef]
13. Rödel, C.; Liersch, T.; Becker, H.; Fietkau, R.; Hohenberger, W.; Hothorn, T.; Graeven, U.; Arnold, D.; Lang-Welzenbach, M.; Raab, H.R.; et al. Preoperative chemoradiotherapy and postoperative chemotherapy with fluorouracil and oxaliplatin versus fluorouracil alone in locally advanced rectal cancer: Initial results of the German CAO/ARO/AIO-04 randomised phase 3 trial. *Lancet Oncol.* **2012**, *13*, 679–687. [CrossRef]
14. Garcia-Aguilar, J.; Chow, O.S.; Smith, D.D.; Marcet, J.E.; Cataldo, P.A.; Varma, M.G.; Kumar, A.S.; Oommen, S.; Coutsoftides, T.; Hunt, S.R.; et al. Effect of adding mFOLFOX6 after neoadjuvant chemoradiation in locally advanced rectal cancer: A multicentre, phase 2 trial. *Lancet Oncol.* **2015**, *16*, 957–966. [CrossRef] [PubMed]

15. Bahadoer, R.R.; Dijkstra, E.A.; van Etten, B.; Marijnen, C.A.M.; Putter, H.; Kranenbarg, E.M.; Roodvoets, A.G.H.; Nagtegaal, I.D.; Beets-Tan, R.G.H.; Blomqvist, L.K.; et al. Short-course radiotherapy followed by chemotherapy before total mesorectal excision (TME) versus preoperative chemoradiotherapy, TME, and optional adjuvant chemotherapy in locally advanced rectal cancer (RAPIDO): A randomised, open-label, phase 3 trial. *Lancet Oncol.* **2021**, *22*, 29–42. [CrossRef] [PubMed]
16. Conroy, T.; Bosset, J.F.; Etienne, P.L.; Rio, E.; François, É.; Mesgouez-Nebout, N.; Vendrely, V.; Artignan, X.; Bouché, O.; Gargot, D.; et al. Neoadjuvant chemotherapy with FOLFIRINOX and preoperative chemoradiotherapy for patients with locally advanced rectal cancer (UNICANCER-PRODIGE 23): A multicentre, randomised, open-label, phase 3 trial. *Lancet Oncol.* **2021**, *22*, 702–715. [CrossRef] [PubMed]
17. Petrelli, F.; Trevisan, F.; Cabiddu, M.; Sgroi, G.; Bruschieri, L.; Rausa, E.; Ghidini, M.; Turati, L. Total Neoadjuvant Therapy in Rectal Cancer: A Systematic Review and Meta-analysis of Treatment Outcomes. *Ann. Surg.* **2020**, *271*, 440–448. [CrossRef] [PubMed]
18. Francois, Y.; Nemoz, C.J.; Baulieux, J.; Vignal, J.; Grandjean, J.P.; Partensky, C.; Souquet, J.C.; Adeleine, P.; Gerard, J.P. Influence of the interval between preoperative radiation therapy and surgery on downstaging and on the rate of sphincter-sparing surgery for rectal cancer: The Lyon R90-01 randomized trial. *J. Clin. Oncol. Off. J. Am. Soc. Clin. Oncol.* **1999**, *17*, 2396. [CrossRef] [PubMed]
19. Sloothaak, D.A.; Geijsen, D.E.; van Leersum, N.J.; Punt, C.J.; Buskens, C.J.; Bemelman, W.A.; Tanis, P.J.; Dutch Surgical Colorectal Audit. Optimal time interval between neoadjuvant chemoradiotherapy and surgery for rectal cancer. *Br. J. Surg.* **2013**, *100*, 933–939. [CrossRef] [PubMed]
20. Tepper, J.E.; Foote, R.L.; Michalski, J.M. *Gunderson & Tepper's Clinical Radiation Oncology*, 5th ed.; Elsevier: Philadelphia, PA, USA, 2021; Chapter 58; pp. 1021–1022.
21. Guillem, J.G.; Chessin, D.B.; Shia, J.; Suriawinata, A.; Riedel, E.; Moore, H.G.; Minsky, B.D.; Wong, W.D. A prospective pathologic analysis using whole-mount sections of rectal cancer following preoperative combined modality therapy: Implications for sphincter preservation. *Ann. Surg.* **2007**, *245*, 88–93. [CrossRef] [PubMed]
22. Moore, H.G.; Riedel, E.; Minsky, B.D.; Saltz, L.; Paty, P.; Wong, D.; Cohen, A.M.; Guillem, J.G. Adequacy of 1-cm distal margin after restorative rectal cancer resection with sharp mesorectal excision and preoperative combined-modality therapy. *Ann. Surg. Oncol.* **2003**, *10*, 80–85. [CrossRef]
23. Bujko, K.; Rutkowski, A.; Chang, G.J.; Michalski, W.; Chmielik, E.; Kusnierz, J. Is the 1-cm rule of distal bowel resection margin in rectal cancer based on clinical evidence? A systematic review. *Ann. Surg. Oncol.* **2012**, *19*, 801–808. [CrossRef]
24. Hattori, N.; Nakayama, G.; Uehara, K.; Aiba, T.; Ishigure, K.; Sakamoto, E.; Tojima, Y.; Kanda, M.; Kobayashi, D.; Tanaka, C.; et al. Phase II study of capecitabine plus oxaliplatin (CapOX) as adjuvant chemotherapy for locally advanced rectal cancer (CORONA II). *Int. J. Clin. Oncol.* **2020**, *25*, 118–125. [CrossRef]
25. Schrag, D.; Shi, Q.; Weiser, M.R.; Gollub, M.J.; Saltz, L.B.; Musher, B.L.; Goldberg, J.; Al Baghdadi, T.; Goodman, K.A.; McWilliams, R.R.; et al. Preoperative Treatment of Locally Advanced Rectal Cancer. *N. Engl. J. Med.* **2023**, *389*, 322–334. [CrossRef] [PubMed]
26. Birgisson, H.; Pahlman, L.; Gunnarsson, U.; Glimelius, B. Adverse effects of preoperative radiation therapy for rectal cancer: Long-term follow-up of the Swedish Rectal Cancer Trial. *J. Clin. Oncol.* **2005**, *23*, 8697–8705. [PubMed]
27. Aschele, C.; Cionini, L.; Lonardi, S.; Pinto, C.; Cordio, S.; Rosati, G.; Artale, S.; Tagliagambe, A.; Ambrosini, G.; Rosetti, P.; et al. Primary tumor response to preoperative chemoradiation with or without oxaliplatin in locally advanced rectal cancer: Pathologic results of the STAR-01 randomized phase III trial. *J. Clin. Oncol. Off. J. Am. Soc. Clin. Oncol.* **2011**, *29*, 2773–2780. [CrossRef] [PubMed]
28. Gérard, J.P.; Azria, D.; Gourgou-Bourgade, S.; Martel-Laffay, I.; Hennequin, C.; Etienne, P.L.; Vendrely, V.; François, E.; de La Roche, G.; Bouché, O.; et al. Comparison of two neoadjuvant chemoradiotherapy regimens for locally advanced rectal cancer: Results of the phase III trial ACCORD 12/0405-Prodige 2. *J. Clin. Oncol. Off. J. Am. Soc. Clin. Oncol.* **2010**, *28*, 1638–1644. [CrossRef] [PubMed]
29. Gérard, J.P.; Azria, D.; Gourgou-Bourgade, S.; Martel-Lafay, I.; Hennequin, C.; Etienne, P.L.; Vendrely, V.; François, E.; de La Roche, G.; Bouché, O.; et al. Clinical outcome of the ACCORD 12/0405 PRODIGE randomized trial in rectal cancer. *J. Clin. Oncol.* **2012**, *36*, 4558–4565. [CrossRef]
30. Memon, S.; Lynch, A.C.; Akhurst, T.; Ngan, S.Y.; Warrier, S.K.; Michael, M.; Heriot, A.G. Systematic review of FDG-PET prediction of complete pathological response and survival in rectal cancer. *Ann. Surg. Oncol.* **2014**, *21*, 3598–3607. [CrossRef]
31. Allegra, C.J.; Yothers, G.; O'Connell, M.J.; Roh, M.S.; Lopa, S.H.; Petrelli, N.J.; Beart, R.W.; Sharif, S.; Wolmark, N. Final results from NSABP protocol R-04: Neoadjuvant chemoradiation (RT) comparing continuous infusion (CIV) 5-FU with capecitabine (Cape) with or without oxaliplatin (Ox) in patients with stage II and III rectal cancer. *J. Clin. Oncol.* **2014**, *32*, 3603. [CrossRef]
32. Schmoll, H.J.; Stein, A.; Van Cutsem, E.; Price, T.; Hofheinz, R.D.; Nordlinger, B.; Daisne, J.F.; Janssens, J.; Brenner, B.; Reinel, H.; et al. Pre- and Postoperative Capecitabine Without or With Oxaliplatin in Locally Advanced Rectal Cancer: PETACC 6 Trial by EORTC GITCG and ROG, AIO, AGITG, BGDO, and FFCD. *J. Clin. Oncol. Off. J. Am. Soc. Clin. Oncol.* **2021**, *39*, 17–29. [CrossRef]
33. Iv, A.A.; Koprowski, M.A.; Nabavizadeh, N.; Tsikitis, V.L. The evolution of rectal cancer treatment: The journey to total neoadjuvant therapy and organ preservation. *Ann. Gastroenterol.* **2022**, *35*, 226–233. [CrossRef]
34. American Joint Committee on Cancer (AJCC). *TNM Staging Classification for Rectal Cancer*, 8th ed.; AJCC: Chicago, IL, USA, 2017.
35. Lee, N.Y.; Riaz, N.; Lu, J.J. Chapter Rectal Cancer. In *Target Volume Delineation for Conformal and Intensity-Modulated Radiation Therapy*; Springer International Publishing: Cham, Switzerland, 2014; Part IV; pp. 307–308.

36. Myerson, R.J.; Garofalo, M.C.; El Naqa, I.; Abrams, R.A.; Apte, A.; Bosch, W.R.; Das, P.; Gunderson, L.L.; Hong, T.S.; Kim, J.J.; et al. Elective clinical target volumes for conformal therapy in anorectal cancer: A radiation therapy oncology group consensus panel contouring atlas. *Int. J. Radiat. Oncol. Biol. Phys.* **2009**, *74*, 824–830. [CrossRef]
37. Taylor, A.; Rockall, A.G.; Reznek, R.H.; Powell, M.E. Mapping pelvic lymph nodes: Guidelines for delineation in intensity-modulated radiotherapy. *Int. J. Radiat. Oncol. Biol. Phys.* **2005**, *63*, 1604–1612. [CrossRef] [PubMed]
38. Daly, M.E.; Murphy, J.D.; Mok, E.; Christman-Skieller, C.; Koong, A.C.; Chang, D.T. Rectal and bladder deformation and displacement during preoperative radiotherapy for rectal cancer: Are current margin guidelines adequate for conformal therapy? *Pract. Radiat. Oncol.* **2011**, *1*, 85–94. [CrossRef] [PubMed]
39. Gaffney, D.K.; Shrieve, D.C.; Hitchcock, Y.J.; Tward, J.D. Section 5 Gastrointestinal System. In *Radiation Oncology: Imaging and Treatment*; Amirsys: Salt Lake City, UT, USA, 2013; pp. 5–54.
40. Johnson, G.G.R.J.; Park, J.; Helewa, R.M.; Goldenberg, B.A.; Nashed, M.; Hyun, E. Total neoadjuvant therapy for rectal cancer: A guide for surgeons. *Can. J. Surg. J. Can. Chir.* **2023**, *66*, E196–E201. [CrossRef] [PubMed]
41. Lim, A.R.; Rim, C.H. Oligometastasis: Expansion of Curative Treatments in the Field of Oncology. *Medicina* **2023**, *59*, 1934. [CrossRef] [PubMed]
42. White, A.; Ironmonger, L.; Steele, R.J.C.; Ormiston-Smith, N.; Crawford, C.; Seims, A. A review of sex-related differences in colorectal cancer incidence, screening uptake, routes to diagnosis, cancer stage and survival in the UK. *BMC Cancer* **2018**, *18*, 906. [CrossRef] [PubMed]
43. Kanth, P.; Inadomi, J.M. Screening and prevention of colorectal cancer. *BMJ (Clin. Res. Ed.)* **2021**, *374*, n1855. [CrossRef] [PubMed]
44. Suarez, J.; Alsina, M.; Castro, N.; Marin, G.; Llanos, C.; Oronoz, B.; Mata, E.; Aznárez, R.; Jiménez, G.; Martínez, M.I.; et al. Higher rate of pathologic complete response in patients with early-onset locally advanced rectal cancer. *ESMO Gastrointest. Oncol.* **2024**, *3*, 100033. [CrossRef]
45. Zhang, Y.; Yan, L.; Wu, Y.; Xu, M.; Liu, X.; Guan, G. Worse treatment response to neoadjuvant chemoradiotherapy in young patients with locally advanced rectal cancer. *BMC Cancer* **2020**, *20*, 854. [CrossRef] [PubMed]
46. Foppa, C.; Maroli, A.; Luberto, A.; La Raja, C.; Spaggiari, P.; Bonifacio, C.; De Zanet, S.; Montorsi, M.; Piscuoglio, S.; Terracciano, L.M.; et al. Early Age of Onset Is an Independent Predictor for a Worse Response to Neoadjuvant Therapies in Sporadic Rectal Cancer Patients. *Cancers* **2023**, *15*, 3750. [CrossRef]
47. Lieu, C.H.; Golemis, E.A.; Serebriiskii, I.G.; Newberg, J.; Hemmerich, A.; Connelly, C.; Messersmith, W.A.; Eng, C.; Eckhardt, S.G.; Frampton, G.; et al. Comprehensive genomic landscapes in early and later onset colorectal cancer. *Clin. Cancer Res.* **2019**, *25*, 5852–5858.
48. Seol, K.H.; Bong, S.H.; Kang, D.H.; Kim, J.W. Factors Associated with the Quality of Life of Patients with Cancer Undergoing Radiotherapy. *Psychiatry Investig.* **2021**, *18*, 80–87. [CrossRef] [PubMed]
49. Yang, Y.; Wen, Y.; Bedi, C.; Humphris, G. The relationship between cancer patient's fear of recurrence and chemotherapy: A systematic review and meta-analysis. *J. Psychosom. Res.* **2017**, *98*, 55–63. [CrossRef]
50. Neibart, S.S.; Manne, S.L.; Jabbour, S.K. Quality of Life After Radiotherapy for Rectal and Anal Cancer. *Curr. Color. Cancer Rep.* **2020**, *16*, 1–10. [CrossRef] [PubMed]
51. Tezcan, S.; İzzettin, F.V.; Sancar, M.; Turhal, N.S.; Yumuk, P.F. Role of clinical oncology pharmacist in determination of pharmaceutical care needs in patients with colorectal cancer. *Eur. J. Hosp. Pharm. Sci. Pract.* **2018**, *25*, e17–e20. [CrossRef] [PubMed]
52. De Jong, E.A.; ten Berge, J.C.; Dwarkasing, R.S.; Rijkers, A.P.; van Eijck, C.H. The accuracy of MRI, endorectal ultrasonography, and computed tomography in predicting the response of locally advanced rectal cancer after preoperative therapy: A metaanalysis. *Surgery* **2016**, *159*, 688–699. [CrossRef] [PubMed]
53. Sclafani, F.; Brown, G.; Cunningham, D.; Wotherspoon, A.; Mendes, L.S.T.; Balyasnikova, S.; Evans, J.; Peckitt, C.; Begum, R.; Tait, D.; et al. Comparison between MRI and pathology in the assessment of tumour regression grade in rectal cancer. *Br. J. Cancer* **2017**, *117*, 1478–1485. [CrossRef]
54. Joye, I.; Deroose, C.M.; Vandecaveye, V.; Haustermans, K. The role of diffusion-weighted MRI and (18)F-FDG PET/CT in the prediction of pathologic complete response after radiochemotherapy for rectal cancer: A systematic review. *Radiother. Oncol. J. Eur. Soc. Ther. Radiol. Oncol.* **2014**, *113*, 158–165. [CrossRef]

Disclaimer/Publisher's Note: The statements, opinions and data contained in all publications are solely those of the individual author(s) and contributor(s) and not of MDPI and/or the editor(s). MDPI and/or the editor(s) disclaim responsibility for any injury to people or property resulting from any ideas, methods, instructions or products referred to in the content.

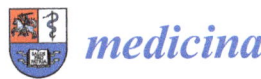 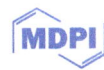

Article

A Potential Radiomics–Clinical Model for Predicting Failure of Lymph Node Control after Definite Radiotherapy in Locally Advanced Head and Neck Cancer

Seunghak Lee [1], Sunmin Park [2], Chai Hong Rim [2], Young Hen Lee [3], Soon Young Kwon [4], Kyung Ho Oh [4] and Won Sup Yoon [2,*]

[1] Core Research and Development Center, Korea University Ansan Hospital, Ansan 15355, Republic of Korea; victor87822@gmail.com
[2] Department of Radiation Oncology, College of Medicine, Korea University Ansan Hospital, 123 Jeokgeum-ro, Danwon-gu, Ansan 15355, Republic of Korea; sunmini815@gmail.com (S.P.); crusion3@naver.com (C.H.R.)
[3] Department of Radiology, Korea University Ansan Hospital, Ansan 15355, Republic of Korea; younghen@korea.ac.kr
[4] Department of Otolaryngology, Korea University Ansan Hospital, Ansan 15355, Republic of Korea; entkwon@korea.ac.kr (S.Y.K.); ohkyungho@korea.ac.kr (K.H.O.)
* Correspondence: irionyws@korea.ac.kr; Tel.: +82-31-412-6850; Fax: +82-31-412-4214

Abstract: *Background and Objectives*: To optimally predict lymph node (LN) failure after definite radiotherapy (RT) in head and neck cancer (HNC) with LN metastases, this study examined radiomics models extracted from CT images of different periods during RT. *Materials and Methods*: This study retrospectively collected radiologic and clinical information from patients undergoing definite RT over 60 Gy for HNC with LN metastases from January 2010 to August 2021. The same largest LNs in each patient from the initial simulation CT (CTpre) and the following simulation CT (CTmid) at approximately 40 Gy were indicated as regions of interest. LN failure was defined as residual or recurrent LN within 3 years after the end of RT. After the radiomics features were extracted, the radiomics alone model and the radiomics plus clinical parameters model from the set of CTpre and CTmid were compared. The LASSO method was applied to select features associated with LN failure. *Results*: Among 66 patients, 17 LN failures were observed. In the radiomics alone model, CTpre and CTmid had similar mean accuracies (0.681 and 0.697, respectively) and mean areas under the curve (AUC) (0.521 and 0.568, respectively). Radiomics features of spherical disproportion, size zone variance, and log minimum 2 were selected for CTpre plus clinical parameters. Volume, energy, homogeneity, and log minimum 1 were selected for CTmid plus clinical parameters. Clinical parameters including smoking, T-stage, ECE, and regression rate of LN were important for both CTpre and CTmid. In the radiomics plus clinical parameters models, the mean accuracy and mean AUC of CTmid (0.790 and 0.662, respectively) were more improved than those of CTpre (0.731 and 0.582, respectively). *Conclusions*: Both models using CTpre and CTmid were improved by adding clinical parameters. The radiomics model using CTmid plus clinical parameters was the best in predicting LN failure in our preliminary analyses.

Keywords: radiomics; radiotherapy; head and neck cancer; lymph node

Citation: Lee, S.; Park, S.; Rim, C.H.; Lee, Y.H.; Kwon, S.Y.; Oh, K.H.; Yoon, W.S. A Potential Radiomics–Clinical Model for Predicting Failure of Lymph Node Control after Definite Radiotherapy in Locally Advanced Head and Neck Cancer. *Medicina* **2024**, *60*, 92. https://doi.org/10.3390/medicina60010092

Academic Editors: Valentin Titus Grigorean and Daniel Alin Cristian

Received: 17 November 2023
Revised: 21 December 2023
Accepted: 30 December 2023
Published: 3 January 2024

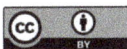

Copyright: © 2024 by the authors. Licensee MDPI, Basel, Switzerland. This article is an open access article distributed under the terms and conditions of the Creative Commons Attribution (CC BY) license (https://creativecommons.org/licenses/by/4.0/).

1. Introduction

Definite radiotherapy (RT) is widely used in advanced head and neck cancer (HNC) with regional lymph node (LN) metastases. Although the prognosis differs depending on the details of disease progression, loco-regional recurrence generally occurs in 10–20% for better sub-sites such as the nasopharynx or human papillomavirus (HPV)-positive oropharynx [1,2] and in up to 30–40% for worse sub-sites such as the HPV-negative oropharynx, oral cavity, larynx, and hypopharynx [3,4]. Loco-regional recurrence is quite an important issue in HNC as it not only affects survival but also affects quality of life. It ultimately requires salvage treatment.

To increase loco-regional control, an advanced RT technique has been developed. The simultaneous integrated boost (SIB) technique can add radiation doses to risky areas such as gross tumors and hypoxic regions [5,6]. Various combinations with chemo-regimen and schedule have been studied [7]. As a part of the treatment to control HNC by preserving function, induction chemotherapy is of great interest [8]. However, whether the response could be assessed in advance remains unclear. If the response prediction in the middle of definite RT is judged to be radio-resistant, early surgical resection could be considered before fibrosis occurs due to full-dose radiation. Alternatively, clinical trials on additional chemotherapy for high-risk groups with incomplete response after definite RT could also be attempted. As a result, it would be possible to perform a multidisciplinary approach in a more comprehensive way.

Radiomics is a research method that can extract various features from images using detailed image analysis, convert phenotypes into numerical values, and predict certain results. A study including advanced HNC has shown that overall survival, progression-free survival, and local control can be well predicted with radiomics features extracted from computer tomography (CT) [9]. Another study has shown that radiomics features are as good as clinical factors for predicting disease-free survival and successfully dividing patients into low- and high-risk groups [10]. Although these previous studies have shown the potential of radiomics as an imaging biomarker, both studies were conducted based on work-ups performed before definite therapy. RT could cause various tumor microenvironment (TME) changes in response to radiation [11]. However, studies focusing on TME changes during definite RT are limited. We hypothesize that intrinsic resistance could be predicted more accurately than previous methods if TME changes during RT could be reflected in radiomics.

Thus, this study evaluated the applicability of an LN failure model with radiomics extracted from different periods of initial CT images and other CT images in the middle of RT in advanced HNC with LN metastases. The improvement in each model after adding clinical parameters was then examined. An optimal model of LN failure was then suggested.

2. Materials and Methods

2.1. Patient Information

This study was conducted on patients who underwent definite RT for HNC with LN metastases from January 2010 to August 2021. The inclusion criteria were as follows: (1) HNC was initially confirmed with a pathologic evaluation; (2) LN metastases were confirmed with structural or functional images with a diameter of the short axis > 7 mm; (3) fractionated conventional RT or concurrent chemoradiotherapy (CRT) was planned; (4) an Eastern Cooperative Oncology Group performance score of 0 or 1; and (5) image sets of simulation CT were acquired before and during RT. The exclusion criteria were as follows: (1) an LN was excised before RT or infiltrated to the skin; (2) HNC originated from the skin, paranasal sinus, salivary gland, or unknown primary site; (3) the second simulation CT was delayed over one week compared with the planned schedule; (4) RT was incompletely finished with a dose less than 60 Gy; and (5) patients who had arbitrarily follow-up loss within 2 years. This study was approved by the Institutional Review Board (K-2021AS0138). Written informed consent was waived due to the retrospective nature of this study.

2.2. CT Imaging and Radiotherapy

Our institutional principle of CT simulation of HNC had generally been unchanged in the study period. After laying the patients down with a suitable headrest and fixing them with aquaplast to cover from head to shoulder, the patients' images were acquired using a Big Bore CT simulation (Philips Medical System, Amsterdam, The Netherlands). The thickness of the CT image was 3 mm for 3D conformal RT (3DCRT) and 2 mm for intensity-modulated RT (IMRT). Iodine contrast (70 mL) for CT was injected at 1 mL/s. Images were taken 70 s after injection. After the initial plan for 3DCRT, cone-down was performed at about 40 Gy and 60 Gy excluding low- and intermediate-risk areas, respectively. High-risk areas including at least a margin of 3 mm from the gross primary tumor and LN were irradiated at up to 70 Gy. For IMRT, the same SIB technique of 2.2 Gy and 2 Gy per fraction, cone-down was performed at about 44 Gy. Low-, intermediate-, and high-risk areas were irradiated with 40 Gy, 64 Gy, and 70.4 Gy, respectively. We collected a pretreatment set of CT images (CTpre) and a mid-treatment set of CT images (CTmid). These CT images were taken 1 week before and 3.5 weeks after starting RT, respectively (Figure 1).

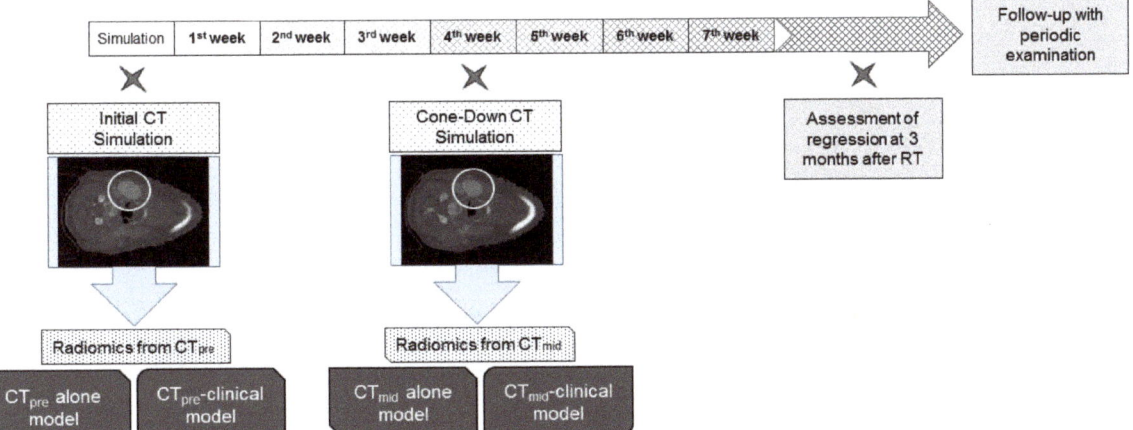

Figure 1. Diagram of the sequence of this study. Initial simulation CT (CTpre) and cone-down simulation CT were acquired prior to RT and in the middle of RT at 4 weeks, respectively. Lymph node within the white circle indicated the region of interest in this study.

2.3. Radiomics Feature Extraction and Clinical Features

For radiomics analyses, regions of interest (ROIs) of the largest LN were drawn on CT-pre and CTmid after matching the same lymph node. If the largest LN was conglomerated with circumferential LNs without a distinct border, the ROIs included all adjacent LNs. A radiation oncologist with over 20 years of experience performed 3D ROI segmentation using a semi-automated method (MRIcro).

A total of 70 radiomics features were extracted from each CT image. These features were divided into the following four categories: (1) histogram-based features ($N = 19$), which were computed using the voxel intensity of the tumor; (2) shape-based features ($N = 11$), which were calculated based on 2D and 3D ROIs; (3) texture-based features ($N = 13$), which were computed using GLCM (gray-level co-occurrence matrix) and GLSZM (gray-level size zone matrix); and (4) filtered-based features ($N = 27$), which were calculated using 3D Laplacian of Gaussian. A total of 70 radiomics features were extracted using a combination of PyRadiomics (ver. 3.0.)- and MATLAB (Math Works, Inc., Portola Valley, CA, USA)-based in-house code. Detailed descriptions of all features are given in Supplementary Table S1.

Clinical information on age, sex, primary site, smoking history, viral infection history, and disease stage according to the 7th AJCC stage were collected. In addition, specific information for the main LN such as size, degree of response during treatment, extracapsular extension (ECE), central necrosis (CN), multiplicity, bi-laterality, and level of lymph nodes was examined.

2.4. Radiomics Feature Selection

Radiomics analysis involves selecting features from the extracted feature set to effectively explain the intended clinical variables of interest. We applied the LASSO (Least Absolute Shrinkage and Selection Operator) method to select features associated with LN control. We applied cross-validation to the LASSO method for feature selection. After ten repetitions of the LASSO analysis, we selected features that were chosen five or more times as the final set (signature).

2.5. Statistical Test

Our endpoint was the failure of LN control with residual or recurrent LN of an ROI after RT or CRT. Our study restricted the observation period to be 3 years considering median follow-up of disease-free patients. Residual disease was confirmed with pathologic findings of LNs or biopsy and clinical progression. If the residual LN was totally regressed in pathologic findings with a stable status continued during follow-up examination, it was defined as successful LN control. If the recurrence of ROIs sequentially progressed over a window period of 3 months after the primary recurrence or distant metastases, those cases were excluded from our radiomics analyses. If the ROI was aggravated over 3 years after the end of RT or CRT, it was excluded from our radiomics analyses (Figure 2).

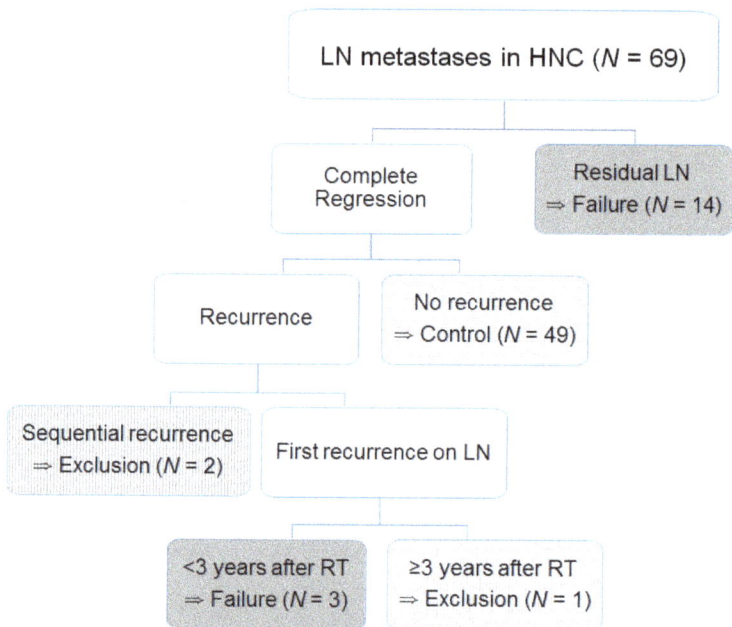

Figure 2. The flow of the selection process for the entire cohort. After excluding sequential recurrence following primary lesion and recurrence over 3 years (vertical line), a total of 17 LN control failures (gray color) were considered in 66 cases for radiomics analyses.

Survival was evaluated on the last follow-up day or event occurrence from the start of RT. All survival rates were calculated with Kaplan–Meyer methods.

The selected final signature set was input into a Random Forest (RF) model to predict LN control. We used 200 decision trees, which were trained using the training set and evaluated using the test set. The training and test sets were split at a 7:3 ratio. Patients were randomly selected for each iteration, and we repeated the performance tests 20 times. We measured AUC (area under the curve), sensitivity, specificity, and accuracy for objective performance evaluation. All statistical analysis procedures were performed using MATLAB.

We compared predictive performances using the same method across a total of five categories: CTpre, CTmid, clinical parameters alone, CTpre plus clinical parameters, and CTmid plus clinical parameters.

3. Results

3.1. Survival and Failure of LN Control

A total of 69 patients were analyzed. Table 1 provides detailed characteristics of the patients. Three-year disease-free survival and overall survival (standard error) were 53.3%

(6.2%) and 73.2% (5.4%), respectively (Figure 3). Progression of primary site and distant metastases occurred in 15 and 20 patients, respectively. Among 21 patients with failure of LN control, two cases of LN recurrence were developed after 11 and 18 months of primary site recurrence and one case was developed 61 months after CRT. After excluding these three patients from the radiomics analyses, a total of 66 patients were enrolled with 17 LN control failures.

Table 1. Distribution of clinical parameters ($N = 69$).

Category	Sub-Category	
Sex	Male: female	58:11
Age (years)	Median (range)	55 (26–84)
Primary site	Nasopharynx:oropharynx:larynx:oral cavity: hypopharynx	25:31:3:1:9
Virus status	EBV:HPV:negative:unknown	21:17:11:20
Smoking	Never, ex-smoker, current smoker ≤10:>10 (pack years)	24:17:28 30:39
Primary tumor T-stage Size	T1–2: T3–4 ≤2:2.1–4:>4 (cm)	39:30 15:35:19
Lymph node (LN) N-Stage Size Multiplicity Laterality Extra capsular extension Central necrosis	N1:N2–3 ≤3:3.1–6:>6 ≤2:>2 (lymph node stations) Unilateral: bilateral No:yes No:yes	15: 54 27:38:4 29:40 33:36 29:40 27:42
Total radiation dose	<70:≥70 (Gy)	9:60
Concurrent chemotherapy	No:yes	2:67
Regression of the largest LN size (long diameter CT_{mid}/CT_{pre})	Median (range)	0.762 (0.436–1.250)

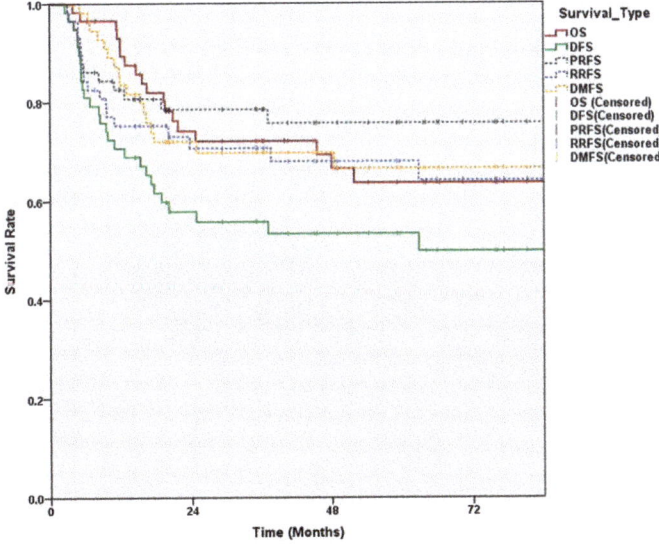

Figure 3. Survival curve of our cohort. OS: overall survival; DFS: disease-free survival; DMFS: distant metastases-free survival; RRFS: regional recurrence-free survival; PRFS: primary recurrence-free survival.

3.2. Feature Selection

In the CTpre alone model, out of a total of 75 radiomics features, two features were selected: size zone variance (GLSZM-based) and log minimum 2 (filtered-based). In the

CTmid alone model, five features were selected: uniformity (histogram-based), volume (shape-based), energy (GLCM-based), homogeneity (GLCM-based), and log minimum 1 (filtered-based). In the clinical parameters alone model, age, virus status, LN size, ECE, and CN were important. In the CTpre plus clinical parameters model, out of 96 features including clinical parameters and radiomics features, 8 features were selected: spherical disproportion (shape-based), size zone variance (GLSZM-based), and log minimum 2 (filtered-based) of radiomics features and age, smoking, T-stage, ECE, and regression rate of LN. In the CTmid plus clinical parameters model, a total of eight features were selected: volume (shape-based), energy (GLCM-based), homogeneity (GLCM-based), log minimum 1 (filtered-based), smoking, T-stage, ECE, and regression rate of LN.

3.3. Performance Test

The predictive model of CTpre and CTmid consisted of two and five different radiomics features, respectively. Clinical parameters including smoking, T-stage, ECE, and diameter regression rate during RT were commonly used for both models. Age was additionally used for the CTpre model. The mean accuracies (standard deviation) of the models with CTpre, CTmid, and clinical parameters were 0.681 (0.069), 0.698 (0.089), and 0.726 (0.089), respectively (Figure 4). These mean values of CTpre and CTmid plus clinical parameters became 0.731 (0.100) and 0.790 (0.095), respectively. Mean areas under the curve (AUC) of the models with CTpre, CTmid, and clinical parameters were 0.521 (0.080), 0.568 (0.093), and 0.593 (0.085), respectively. These mean values of CTpre and CTmid became 0.582 (0.088) and 0.662 (0.133) when the clinical parameters were included. These results are summarized in Table 2.

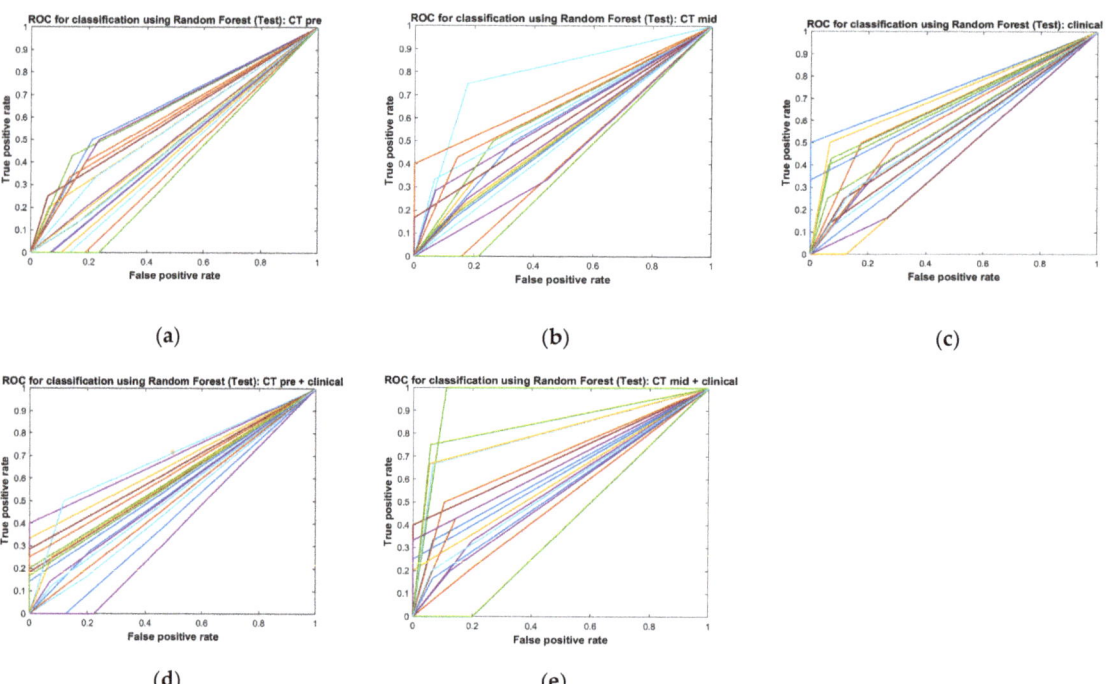

Figure 4. Visualization of receiver operating characteristic (ROC) curves. Each line represents the visualization of an ROC curve during the performance test, with a total of 20 repetitions. Each color line means the outcome of independent performance test. Each figure corresponds to (**a**) the CT_{pre} alone model, (**b**) the CT_{mid} alone model, (**c**) the clinical parameters alone model, (**d**) the CT_{pre} plus clinical parameters model, and (**e**) the CT_{mid} plus clinical parameters model.

Table 2. Values (mean ± standard deviation) of ACC and AUC according to various radiomics models.

	CT_{pre}	CT_{mid}	Clinical Parameters	CT_{pre} Plus Clinical Parameters	CT_{mid} Plus Clinical Parameters
ACC	0.681 ± 0.069	0.698 ± 0.089	0.726 ± 0.089	0.731 ± 0.100	0.790 ± 0.095
AUC	0.521 ± 0.008	0.568 ± 0.093	0.593 ± 0.085	0.582 ± 0.088	0.662 ± 0.133

ACC: accuracy; AUC: area under the curve.

3.4. Feature Importance

We evaluated the importance of features for each model that underwent performance testing using the out-of-bag method. The importance of each feature is visualized in Figure 5.

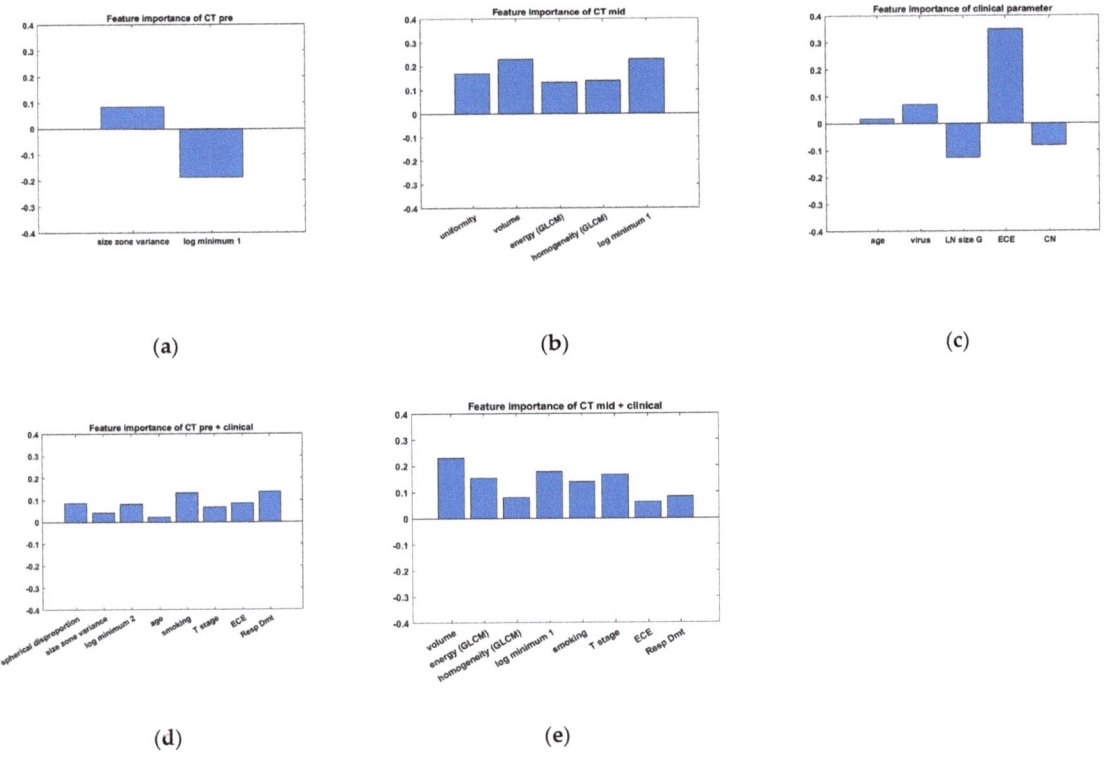

Figure 5. Visualization of the importance of each feature calculated using out-of-bag with a histogram. Each figure corresponds to (**a**) the CT_{pre} alone model, (**b**) the CT_{mid} alone model, (**c**) the clinical parameters alone model, (**d**) the CT_{pre} plus clinical parameters model, and (**e**) the CT_{mid} plus clinical parameters model that underwent performance testing using the out-of-bag method.

4. Discussion

This study aimed to suggest a model to predict LN control failure after definite RT in advanced HNC with regional LN metastases. It was designed to determine whether radiomics differentiate the intrinsic sensitivity of LN to radiation doses and whether clinical parameters have a synergic effect over radiomics alone. LNs were targeted as ROIs in our study. Since LNs have a round or oval shape different from a primary tumor, the physician could more readily conduct ROI delineation. Another benefit is the reproducibility of CTmid images since LNs maintain a consistent shape despite regression during treatment. Lastly, as shown in the recurrence pattern of our study, the LN was a common first recurrence site in locally advanced HNC and an important factor in determining the success of definite RT. The radiomics alone model for both CTpre and CTmid showed a moderate ACC to predict LN control failure. The predictability of radiomics was improved after adding clinical parameters.

A previous radiomics study of LN regression for 374 LNs from 113 patients showed an AUC of 0.71 in external validation [12]. Although our study differed from the above study in that only the largest lymph node was selected and analyzed in each patient, the outcomes of our study fell short with an ACC of 0.698 and an AUC of 0.568 in the CTmid set. In addition, a high ECE rate (58.0%) showed that our cohort consisted of more advanced LN metastases.

In our study, node regression rates during RT, ECE, T-stage, and heavy smoking were significant clinical parameters that could intensify the accuracy and AUC of radiomics. Previous studies have found that clinical–radiomics models show improved predictability, similar to our study. The radiomics features from MRI combined with clinical information improved the predictability of DFS and OS [13]. One report showed that combining genetic information on the hedgehog pathway and E2F transcriptional targets can potentially improve a radiomics model [14]. For lung cancer, dosimetric parameters of stereotactic body RT could improve the predictability of local control in addition to the clinical–radiomics model [15]. Thus, the radiomics model could be improved by adding other fields or omics information related to prognoses.

In the CTpre alone and the CTpre plus clinical parameters models, size zone variance and log minimum ($\sigma = 2$) were consistently chosen. Size zone variance measures how diverse the sizes of identical texture regions are within the ROI, reflecting texture heterogeneity. The log minimum is primarily observed at a tumor's edge and is sensitive to subtle texture changes within the tumor. In the CTmid alone and the CTmid plus clinical parameters models, volume, energy (GLCM-based), homogeneity (GLCM-based), and log minimum were consistently selected. Volume, representing the size of the tumor projected in the image, was deemed crucial for predicting LN failure in this study. Energy (GLCM-based), signifying the degree of brightness variation within an ROI, indicates texture heterogeneity, expressing a tumor's complexity and contributing as an important predictive factor of LN failure. Homogeneity, similar to energy, measures a tumor's consistency and assesses the tumor's unseen uniformity, thus playing a significant role in predicting LN control failure. The log minimum ($\sigma = 1$), a feature common with CTpre, was chosen again, reinforcing its role as a predictive feature of LN control failure in this study. Our research results encompass various aspects such as tumor texture, size, and brightness changes. By considering these factors collectively, we anticipate enhancing the accuracy of the LN control failure.

In terms of TME changes during RT, the radiomics at about 40 Gy was another key point of our study. For TME in HNC, there have been studies performed to distinguish subtypes of HNC using radiomics. One study showed that radiomics analysis could identify biologic features of tumors such as HPV status and T-cell infiltration [16]. Another study using 12 radiomics features more efficiently differentiated HPV-positive tumors in HNC [17]. Radiomics was also useful in distinguishing atypical, basal, classical, and mesenchymal subtypes of HNC [14]. These research studies suggest that intrinsic TME during RT could be detected with radiomics. In our study, the radiomics of mid-treatment at 40 Gy was better than the radiomics at pretreatment, suggesting that intrinsic sensitivity to radiation could be more efficiently presented during RT. Due to the limitations of a retrospective study, changes were observed once in the fourth week during RT. Therefore, the optimal timing to observe radiation effects should be examined in further studies. In one study using 18F-FDG-PET/CT, the cluster of metabolic radiomics at 20 Gy showed a significant relation with recurrence-free survival in oropharyngeal cancer [18]. In another study using 18F-FMISO-PET to assess hypoxia of intra-tumor, radiomics at 2 weeks and 5 weeks showed higher predictability of the treatment response with an AUC of approximately 0.8 in HNC [19]. It would be necessary to combine metabolic images and enhanced CT images to improve the predictive model of intrinsic sensitivity.

Delta radiomics can be used to analyze paired images and observe changes in TME. In the case of tumors, it was difficult to control the image itself through deformation because regression during treatment occurred and the ROI was deformed. It was also hard to judge the appropriateness of the values of delta features by subtracting or fractionating from one to another. Therefore, delta radiomics was not used in our study. Normal tissues such as salivary glands would be beneficial to examine the change with delta radiomics because the contour of the ROI is preserved [20]. In nasopharyngeal cancer, delta radiomics has been attempted using MRI. Three image sets at pretreatment and after induction chemotherapy and CRT were used, and the AUC to predict the efficacy of definite therapy was improved with delta radiomics [21]. Using cone-beam CT to originally check inter-fractional variation during RT is another method applied in delta radiomics. The model using radiomics features including coarseness and hemoglobin level moderately predicted tumor response in HNC in delta radiomics of cone-beam CT [22]. However, since the image quality is lower than helical CT images, its practical application still has limitations.

This study was based on retrospectively collected image data over about 10 years. Although the protocol for acquiring CT images for HNC has not changed, a few biases might have developed. Some artifacts from the immobilization device of aquaplast and head rest and prosthetics of teeth especially affected the LN in level IIa. This is an important problem that must be solved for radiomics studies using simulation CT images of RT. Efforts should be made to secure appropriate image quality in actual practice in future studies. Second, our study consisted of various kinds of primary sites originating from epithelial cells in HNC. Since it is important to analyze a certain number of patients as a preliminary radiomics study, examinations according to each sub-primary site were not performed. In addition, there were no data on HPV in some patients at the beginning of this study. Therefore, it was not sufficiently analyzed as an important clinical parameter. Based on this study, future research will be conducted targeting a more refined patient group by recruiting multiple institutions. Lastly, the RT technique was changed from 3DCRT to IMRT, although patients received sufficient radiation doses for ROIs regardless of the RT technique.

5. Conclusions

This preliminary study presented radiomics results of CT images for pretreatment and mid-treatment to predict LN control failure after definite RT in HNC with LN metastases. Both models were improved by adding clinical parameters. The model of CTmid plus clinical parameters was the best in our analyses. However, the results shown in our study still lacked predictive power to determine significant modification of treatment methods during definite RT. To activate radiomics research in HNC, efforts are needed to acquire high-quality images with minimum artifacts in actual clinical practice. In addition, future studies should combine various omics methods using other kinds of images, biomarkers, and genetic information.

Supplementary Materials: The following supporting information can be downloaded at: https://www.mdpi.com/article/10.3390/medicina60010092/s1, Table S1: Detailed descriptions of all radiomics features.

Author Contributions: Conception and design, S.L. and W.S.Y.; data acquisition: Y.H.L., S.P., C.H.R. and W.S.Y.; statistical analysis: S.L. and W.S.Y.; interpretation of data: K.H.O., S.Y.K., S.L. and W.S.Y.; drafting: S.P., S.L. and W.S.Y. All authors have read and agreed to the published version of the manuscript.

Funding: This research was funded by Korea University Ansan Hospital, grant number K-2010971.

Institutional Review Board Statement: This study was conducted in accordance with the Declaration of Helsinki and approved by the Institutional Review Board of Korea University Ansan Hospital (K-2021AS0138 was approved on 11 May 2021).

Informed Consent Statement: Written informed consent was waivered by the Institutional Review Board of Ansan Hospital, Korea University, due to the retrospective observational nature of this study using clinical information from patients who completed therapy, which posed minimal risk to the subjects.

Data Availability Statement: The original contributions presented in this study are included in this article/Supplementary Material. Further inquiries can be directed to the corresponding authors.

Conflicts of Interest: The authors declare that this research was conducted in the absence of any commercial or financial relationships that could be construed as a potential conflict of interest.

References

1. Sun, Y.; Li, W.F.; Chen, N.Y.; Zhang, N.; Hu, G.Q.; Xie, F.Y.; Sun, Y.; Chen, X.Z.; Li, J.G.; Zhu, X.D.; et al. Induction chemotherapy plus concurrent chemoradiotherapy versus concurrent chemoradiotherapy alone in locoregionally advanced nasopharyngeal carcinoma: A phase 3, multicentre, randomised controlled trial. *Lancet Oncol.* **2016**, *17*, 1509–1520. [CrossRef] [PubMed]
2. Lee, N.C.J.; Kelly, J.R.; Park, H.S.; An, Y.; Judson, B.L.; Burtness, B.A.; Husain, Z.A. Patterns of failure in high-metastatic node number human papillomavirus-positive oropharyngeal carcinoma. *Oral. Oncol.* **2018**, *85*, 35–39. [CrossRef] [PubMed]
3. Pagh, A.; Grau, C.; Overgaard, J. Failure pattern and salvage treatment after radical treatment of head and neck cancer. *Acta Oncol.* **2016**, *55*, 625–632. [CrossRef] [PubMed]
4. Deshmukh, J.; Chatterjee, A.; Dora, T.K.; Bose, S.; Goel, A.; Kakade, A.; Saini, A.; Pahwa, S.; Singh, A.; Laskar, S.G.; et al. Recurrence pattern with respect to two different dose fractionations in patients with locally advanced head and neck cancer treated with chemoradiation using image-guided volumetric arc therapy. *Head Neck* **2022**, *44*, 1690–1701. [CrossRef] [PubMed]
5. Lopes, S.; Ferreira, S.; Caetano, M. PET/CT in the Evaluation of Hypoxia for Radiotherapy Planning in Head and Neck Tumors: Systematic Literature Review. *J. Nucl. Med. Technol.* **2021**, *49*, 107–113. [CrossRef] [PubMed]
6. Grover, A.; Soni, T.P.; Patni, N.; Singh, D.K.; Jakhotia, N.; Gupta, A.K.; Sharma, L.M.; Sharma, S.; Gothwal, R.S. A randomized prospective study comparing acute toxicity, compliance and objective response rate between simultaneous integrated boost and sequential intensity-modulated radiotherapy for locally advanced head and neck cancer. *Radiat. Oncol. J.* **2021**, *39*, 15–23. [CrossRef] [PubMed]
7. Pignon, J.P.; le Maitre, A.; Bourhis, J.; Group, M.-N.C. Meta-Analyses of Chemotherapy in Head and Neck Cancer (MACH-NC): An update. *Int. J. Radiat. Oncol. Biol. Phys.* **2007**, *69*, S112–S114. [CrossRef]
8. Forastiere, A.A.; Zhang, Q.; Weber, R.S.; Maor, M.H.; Goepfert, H.; Pajak, T.F.; Morrison, W.; Glisson, B.; Trotti, A.; Ridge, J.A.; et al. Long-term results of RTOG 91-11: A comparison of three nonsurgical treatment strategies to preserve the larynx in patients with locally advanced larynx cancer. *J. Clin. Oncol.* **2013**, *31*, 845–852. [CrossRef] [PubMed]
9. Cozzi, L.; Franzese, C.; Fogliata, A.; Franceschini, D.; Navarria, P.; Tomatis, S.; Scorsetti, M. Predicting survival and local control after radiochemotherapy in locally advanced head and neck cancer by means of computed tomography based radiomics. *Strahlenther. Onkol.* **2019**, *195*, 805–818. [CrossRef]
10. Zhai, T.T.; Langendijk, J.A.; van Dijk, L.V.; Halmos, G.B.; Witjes, M.J.H.; Oosting, S.F.; Noordzij, W.; Sijtsema, N.M.; Steenbakkers, R.J.H.M. The prognostic value of CT-based image-biomarkers for head and neck cancer patients treated with definitive (chemo-)radiation. *Oral. Oncol.* **2019**, *95*, 178–186. [CrossRef]
11. Van den Bossche, V.; Zaryouh, H.; Vara-Messler, M.; Vignau, J.; Machiels, J.P.; Wouters, A.; Schmitz, S.; Corbet, C. Microenvironment-driven intratumoral heterogeneity in head and neck cancers: Clinical challenges and opportunities for precision medicine. *Drug Resist. Updat.* **2022**, *60*, 100806. [CrossRef]
12. Zhai, T.T.; Wesseling, F.; Langendijk, J.A.; Shi, Z.; Kalendralis, P.; van Dijk, L.V.; Hoebers, F.; Steenbakkers, R.J.; Dekker, A.; Wee, L.; et al. External validation of nodal failure prediction models including radiomics in head and neck cancer. *Oral. Oncol.* **2021**, *112*, 105083. [CrossRef]
13. Alfieri, S.; Romano, R.; Bologna, M.; Calareso, G.; Corino, V.; Mirabile, A.; Ferri, A.; Bellanti, L.; Poli, T.; Marcantoni, A.; et al. Prognostic role of pre-treatment magnetic resonance imaging (MRI)-based radiomic analysis in effectively cured head and neck squamous cell carcinoma (HNSCC) patients. *Acta Oncol.* **2021**, *60*, 1192–1200. [CrossRef]
14. Rabasco Meneghetti, A.; Zwanenburg, A.; Linge, A.; Lohaus, F.; Grosser, M.; Baretton, G.B.; Kalinauskaite, G.; Tinhofer, I.; Guberina, M.; Stuschke, M.; et al. Integrated radiogenomics analyses allow for subtype classification and improved outcome prognosis of patients with locally advanced HNSCC. *Sci. Rep.* **2022**, *12*, 16755. [CrossRef]
15. Luo, L.M.; Huang, B.T.; Chen, C.Z.; Wang, Y.; Su, C.H.; Peng, G.B.; Zeng, C.B.; Wu, Y.X.; Wang, R.H.; Huang, K.; et al. A Combined Model to Improve the Prediction of Local Control for Lung Cancer Patients Undergoing Stereotactic Body Radiotherapy Based on Radiomic Signature Plus Clinical and Dosimetric Parameters. *Front. Oncol.* **2021**, *11*, 819047. [CrossRef]
16. Katsoulakis, E.; Yu, Y.; Apte, A.P.; Leeman, J.E.; Katabi, N.; Morris, L.; Deasy, J.O.; Chan, T.A.; Lee, N.Y.; Riaz, N.; et al. Radiomic analysis identifies tumor subtypes associated with distinct molecular and microenvironmental factors in head and neck squamous cell carcinoma. *Oral. Oncol.* **2020**, *110*, 104877. [CrossRef]
17. Bagher-Ebadian, H.; Lu, M.; Siddiqui, F.; Ghanem, A.I.; Wen, N.; Wu, Q.; Liu, C.; Movsas, B.; Chetty, I.J. Application of radiomics for the prediction of HPV status for patients with head and neck cancers. *Med. Phys.* **2020**, *47*, 563–575. [CrossRef]

18. Lafata, K.J.; Chang, Y.; Wang, C.; Mowery, Y.M.; Vergalasova, I.; Niedzwiecki, D.; Yoo, D.S.; Liu, J.; Brizel, D.M.; Yin, F. Intrinsic radiomic expression patterns after 20 Gy demonstrate early metabolic response of oropharyngeal cancers. *Med. Phys.* **2021**, *48*, 3767–3777. [CrossRef]
19. Carles, M.; Fechter, T.; Grosu, A.L.; Sorensen, A.; Thomann, B.; Stoian, R.G.; Wiedenmann, N.; Rühle, A.; Zamboglou, C.; Ruf, J.; et al. ^{18}F-FMISO-PET Hypoxia Monitoring for Head-and-Neck Cancer Patients: Radiomics Analyses Predict the Outcome of Chemo-Radiotherapy. *Cancers* **2021**, *13*, 3449. [CrossRef]
20. Berger, T.; Noble, D.J.; Shelley, L.E.A.; McMullan, T.; Bates, A.; Thomas, S.; Carruthers, L.J.; Beckett, G.; Duffton, A.; Paterson, C.; et al. Predicting radiotherapy-induced xerostomia in head and neck cancer patients using day-to-day kinetics of radiomics features. *Phys. Imaging Radiat. Oncol.* **2022**, *24*, 95–101. [CrossRef]
21. Xi, Y.; Ge, X.; Ji, H.; Wang, L.; Duan, S.; Chen, H.; Wang, M.; Hu, H.; Jiang, F.; Ding, Z. Prediction of Response to Induction Chemotherapy Plus Concurrent Chemoradiotherapy for Nasopharyngeal Carcinoma Based on MRI Radiomics and Delta Radiomics: A Two-Center Retrospective Study. *Front. Oncol.* **2022**, *12*, 824509. [CrossRef] [PubMed]
22. Sellami, S.; Bourbonne, V.; Hatt, M.; Tixier, F.; Bouzid, D.; Lucia, F.; Pradier, O.; Goasduff, G.; Visvikis, D.; Schick, U. Predicting response to radiotherapy of head and neck squamous cell carcinoma using radiomics from cone-beam CT images. *Acta Oncol.* **2022**, *61*, 73–80. [CrossRef] [PubMed]

Disclaimer/Publisher's Note: The statements, opinions and data contained in all publications are solely those of the individual author(s) and contributor(s) and not of MDPI and/or the editor(s). MDPI and/or the editor(s) disclaim responsibility for any injury to people or property resulting from any ideas, methods, instructions or products referred to in the content.

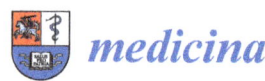

Article

Germline DNA Damage Response Gene Mutations in Localized Prostate Cancer

Tomas Januskevicius [1], Ieva Vaicekauskaite [2,3], Rasa Sabaliauskaite [2,3], Augustinas Matulevicius [3,4], Alvydas Vezelis [5], Albertas Ulys [5], Sonata Jarmalaite [2,3] and Feliksas Jankevicius [1,4,*]

1. Clinic of Gastroenterology, Nephro-Urology and Surgery, Institute of Clinical Medicine, Faculty of Medicine, Vilnius University, M. K. Ciurlionio St. 21/27, LT-03101 Vilnius, Lithuania
2. Laboratory of Genetic Diagnostic, National Cancer Institute, Santariskiu St. 1, LT-08406 Vilnius, Lithuania
3. Division of Human Genome Research Centre, Institute of Biomedical Sciences, Life Sciences Center, Vilnius University, Sauletekio Ave. 7, LT-10257 Vilnius, Lithuania
4. Urology Centre, Vilnius University Hospital Santaros Klinikos, Santariskiu St. 2, LT-08661 Vilnius, Lithuania
5. Oncourology Department, National Cancer Institute, Santariskiu St. 1, LT-08660 Vilnius, Lithuania
* Correspondence: feliksas.jankevicius@santa.lt

Abstract: *Background and Objectives*: Germline DNA damage response (DDR) gene mutations correlate with increased prostate cancer (PCa) risk and a more aggressive form of the disease. DDR mutation testing is recommended for metastatic PCa cases, while eligible information about the mutations' burden in the early-stage localized PCa is still limited. This study is aimed at the prospective detection of DDR pathway mutations in cases with localized PCa and correlation with clinical, histopathological, and radiological data. A comparison to the previously assessed cohort of the advanced PCa was performed. *Materials and Methods*: Germline DDR gene mutations were assessed prospectively in DNA samples from 139 patients, using a five-gene panel (*BRCA1*, *BRCA2*, *ATM*, *CHEK2*, and *NBN*) targeted next-generation sequencing. *Results*: This study revealed an almost three-fold higher risk of localized PCa among mutation carriers as compared to non-carriers (OR 2.84 and 95% CI: 0.75–20.23, $p = 0.16$). The prevalence of germline DDR gene mutations in PCa cases was 16.8% (18/107) and they were detected only in cases with PI-RADS 4/5 lesions. *BRCA1/BRCA2/ATM* mutation carriers were 2.6 times more likely to have a higher (>1) cISUP grade group compared to those with a *CHEK2* mutation ($p = 0.27$). However, the number of cISUP > 1-grade patients with a *CHEK2* mutation was significantly higher in advanced PCa than in localized PCa: 66.67% vs. 23.08% ($p = 0.047$). *Conclusions*: The results of our study suggest the potential of genetic screening for selected DDR gene mutations for early identification of cases at risk of aggressive PCa.

Keywords: DNA damage response; germline mutation; localized prostate cancer; next-generation sequencing

Citation: Januskevicius, T.; Vaicekauskaite, I.; Sabaliauskaite, R.; Matulevicius, A.; Vezelis, A.; Ulys, A.; Jarmalaite, S.; Jankevicius, F. Germline DNA Damage Response Gene Mutations in Localized Prostate Cancer. *Medicina* **2024**, *60*, 73. https://doi.org/10.3390/medicina60010073

Academic Editors: Valentin Titus Grigorean and Daniel Alin Cristian

Received: 1 December 2023
Revised: 23 December 2023
Accepted: 28 December 2023
Published: 30 December 2023

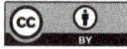

Copyright: © 2023 by the authors. Licensee MDPI, Basel, Switzerland. This article is an open access article distributed under the terms and conditions of the Creative Commons Attribution (CC BY) license (https://creativecommons.org/licenses/by/4.0/).

1. Introduction

Prostate cancer (PCa) is one of the most common problems faced by the male population in the oncology field. Based on the data from the European Cancer Information System, PCa is the most frequently occurring cancer in men; it was responsible for 23.2% of new cancer cases in men in 2020 [1]. Low-risk localized PCa patients may benefit from active surveillance or can be treated by surgery or radiotherapy, usually resulting in complete remission. Intermediate and high-risk localized PCa patients might suffer from disease progression regardless of the primary treatment. In some patients with inherited specific genetic mutations, PCa may manifest in a more severe course, and resistance to conventional treatment develops earlier [2,3]. The transition of next-generation sequencing (NGS) from research to clinical practice revealed new possibilities in the detection of PCa-specific mutations. Due to progress in genomic technologies, mutation status can be verified not only in tumor tissue but also in human body liquids, and it is more widely used in genetic counseling. Blood-based testing of PCa-specific mutations in metastatic PCa patients became increasingly promising, while considering these alterations' detection for localized PCa is still limited and not widely adopted in clinical practice.

Despite various genetic and epigenetic alterations detectable in PCa, inheritance of PCa risk is mainly attributed to genetic alterations of the DNA damage response (DDR) pathway [4]. This molecular pathway is responsible for the maintenance of the genomic integrity of the cell, and the main players of this pathway are proteins encoded by *BRCA1*, *BRCA2*, *ATM*, *ATR*, *TP53*, *CHEK1*, *CHEK2*, and some other genes. The proteins of the DDR pathway sense DNA damage, induce cell cycle arrest and DNA repair, and protect cells from deleterious genetic alteration accumulation. Inactivation of the DDR pathway leads to genomic instability, uncontrolled cell growth, and malignization. Strong enrichment of mutations in the genes of the DDR pathway is detectable in PCa tissue, especially in metastatic cases [5,6], while a systemic review of the largest PCa studies [7] suggests even higher median prevalence of these mutations in the germline profile of PCa. *BRCA1*, *BRCA2*, *ATM*, *CHEK2*, and *NBN* genes are some of the most important alterations in the PCa genetic evaluation process and are frequently included in extensive PCa gene panels.

Most guidelines suggest DDR pathway mutation screening for familial and metastatic PCa, aiming at personalized therapy with poly-ADP ribose polymerase inhibitors (PARPi) [8]. According to the systemic review median prevalence rate for germline DDR gene mutations in general (unselected) PCa is higher than in the metastatic disease (18.6% vs 11.6%), suggesting a higher burden of these mutations than expected [7]. However, quite a few studies analyzed the DDR gene mutation rate in localized or locally advanced PCa and detected a prevalence of 1.44–9.5% [9–13]. In PCa, germline DDR mutations seem to have a higher prevalence than somatic ones and, due to the low penetrance of some mutations, remain undetected in families until manifestation in aggressive forms of cancer [7]. It was shown that patients with inherited pathogenic mutations of several DDR genes are at increased risk of developing more aggressive forms of the disease, while *BRCA2* mutations are directly associated with poor survival in metastatic PCa [14–16]. Metastatic PCa patients with mutant DDR genes already benefit from targeted therapies with PARPi, while patients with the localized disease could be evaluated for the risk of early recurrence or take advantage of personalized treatment options in the future; however, such observations need further investigation. Early detection of DDR mutation carriers is also vital for family members' consultation due to the high risk of aggressive breast, ovarian, and some other tumors [17]. Since at least a quarter of PCa patients identified with germline mutations lack a cancer-related family history, and the mutations possibly evolve de novo [18], it is important to develop algorithms for the meaningful selection of PCa patients for germline mutation testing.

Our prospective, single-center cohort study aimed to assess the prevalence of germline DDR gene mutations (*BRCA1*, *BRCA2*, *ATM*, *CHEK2*, and *NBN*) in patients with localized PCa that was diagnosed based on positive findings of multiparametric magnetic resonance and ultrasound imaging (mpMRI/UG) fusion-guided targeted biopsy. Associations between mutation status and clinical, histopathological, and radiological data were analyzed and a comparison to the previously assessed advanced PCa cohort [19] was performed.

2. Materials and Methods

2.1. Patient Cohort

Between 2019 and 2023, a total of 150 patients with suspected PCa were enrolled in this study at the National Cancer Institute (Vilnius, Lithuania). Prostate mpMRI was performed on all study patients and was reported using the Prostate Imaging Reporting & Data System version 2.1 (PI-RADSv2.1) [20]. A positive mpMRI scan was characterized by the presence of PI-RADS lesions with a score ≥ 3. Patients with a positive prostate mpMRI scan, in accordance with their medical history, clinical data, and/or elevated (>3.0 ng/mL) prostate-specific antigen (PSA) level, underwent mpMRI/US fusion-guided targeted biopsy. PSA density was defined as total PSA (ng/mL) divided by mpMRI calculated prostate volume (mL). Biopsy results were evaluated based on the International Society of Urological Pathology (cISUP) grading system. Low-risk localized, intermediate-risk localized, and high-risk localized/locally advanced diseases were defined by the European Association of Urology (EAU) risk stratification groups for biochemical recurrence [21]. This study was performed in line with the principles of the Declaration of Helsinki. This study was approved by the Regional Bioethics Committee (05.11.2019/No: 2019/11-1166-654) and written informed consent was obtained from all participants.

2.2. Sample Collection and NGS

Blood samples were collected prospectively into EDTA blood collection tubes according to the standardized clinical procedures. The collected buffy coat was frozen and stored at a temperature of −80 °C. The DNA extraction was performed by using a GeneJET Genomic DNA Purification kit (Thermo Fisher Scientific, Vilnius, Lithuania), following the manufacturer's instructions. DNA concentration and purity were determined using the NanoDrop 2000 spectrophotometer (Thermo Scientific, Wilmington, DE, USA) as well as Qubit™ dsDNA BR Assay Kit on a Qubit™ 2.0 Fluorimeter (Invitrogen, TFS, Eugene, OR, USA) and stored at −20 °C until use. Targeted DNA sequencing was performed on the Ion Torrent™ Ion S5™ system, and for the library preparation, Ion AmpliSeq™ Library Kit 2.0 and custom On-Demand Panel (consisting of *BRCA1*, *BRCA2*, *CHEK2*, *ATM*, and *NBN* genes) (from Life Technologies (LT), Carlsbad, CA, USA) were used under conditions provided by the manufacturer's protocol. Sequencing results were analyzed in the Ion ReporterTM Software (version 5.20.2.0) system (Life Technologies, Carlsbad, CA, USA), verified manually in the Integrative Genomics Viewer (IGV, version 2.6.3) tool (Broad Institute, Cambridge, MA, USA), and compared to the hg19 reference human genome sequence. The pathogenic and likely pathogenic mutations were confirmed if the mutation was listed in the clinical variant base ClinVar, as well as visualized on the Integrative Genomics Viewer 2.4.8 tool.

2.3. Statistical Analysis

Statistical analysis was performed using R Version 4.1.1 on R Studio version 2022.07.0 (R Core Team, Vienna, Austria). Oncoprint was created using ComplexHeatmap R package version 2.11.1 [22]. Mutation associations with clinical data were assessed by Fisher exact test, Chi-square test, or *t*-test where appropriate. The odds ratio (OR) was computed by analyzing two-by-two tables. The statistical significance of the OR was evaluated using Fisher exact tests. Results were considered statistically significant if the *p*-value was <0.05.

3. Results

3.1. Characteristics of Study Group

In a study cohort of 150 patients, 11 cases were excluded from further analysis due to clinical or sample quantity reasons. After mpMRI/US fusion-guided targeted biopsy, all patients ($n = 139$) were divided into two groups: 107 were histologically confirmed with localized PCa, and 32 patients without PCa diagnosis were assigned to the control group. Based on the presence or absence of pathogenic mutation in the analyzed genes, the patients were divided into mutation-positive–DDR(+) and mutation-negative–DDR(−) groups.

PCa patients ($n = 107$) revealed PI-RADS lesions ranging from 3 to 5, with a dominance of PI-RADS 4 lesions (67/107, 62.62%). Also, different cISUP grade groups were observed: the most prevalent cISUP grade group was 1 (68/107, 63.55%), followed by grade group 2 (24/107, 22.43%), grade group 3 (11/107, 10.28%), and grade group 4 (4/107, 3.74%). According to EAU risk groups [21], patients with PCa revealed low-risk disease as the most common: 58/107, 54.20%. Intermediate- and high-risk diseases were detected in 44 (41.12%) and 5 (4.68%) patients, respectively. The main clinicopathological characteristics and mpMRI features of PCa patients are shown in Table 1.

Table 1. Clinicopathological characteristics and mpMRI features of localized PCa patients.

Variable	DDR(+), n = 18	DDR(−), n = 89	p Value
Age at PCa diagnosis, years (mean ± SD)	61.56 (±5.66)	63.69 (±7.70)	0.268
PSA level at PCa diagnosis, ng/mL (median (IQR))	5.79 (4.31)	5.90 (3.73)	0.739
Prostate volume, mL (median (IQR))	55.77 (50.57)	44.16 (20.63)	0.057
PSA density (median (IQR))	0.11 (0.07)	0.14 (0.12)	0.170
cISUP grade group			
<3, n (%)	15 (83.33%)	77 (86.62%)	0.714
≥3, n (%)	3 (16.67%)	12 (13.48%)	
PI-RADS category based on the prostate mpMRI			
PI-RADS 3, n (%)	0 (0.00%)	4 (4.50%)	
PI-RADS 4, n (%)	12 (66.66%)	55 (61.79%)	1.000
PI-RADS 5, n (%)	6 (33.34%)	30 (33.70%)	
EAU risk groups			
Low-risk PCa, n (%)	9 (50.00%)	49 (55.06%)	0.694
Intermediate- or high-risk PCa, n (%)	9 (50.00%)	40 (44.94%)	

Abbreviations: PCa—prostate cancer; PSA—prostate-specific antigen; cISUP—International Society of Urological Pathology grade group; mpMRI—multiparametric magnetic resonance imaging; PI-RADS—Prostate Imaging Reporting & Data System; EAU—European Association of Urology; SD—standard deviation; IQR—interquartile range.

3.2. DDR Gene Mutations Rates

Out of 139 cases, 14.4% (n = 20) were identified with germline mutations of selected DDR genes (*BRCA1, BRCA2, ATM, CHEK2,* and *NBN*) in the blood cells (Figure 1). The mutation rate in the group of cases with PCa diagnosis was 16.8% (18/107), and 19 alterations in DDR genes were found, with one case showing multiple alterations in the *CHEK2* gene: *CHEK2* c.470T>C and *CHEK2* c.1100delC (Figure 2). *BRCA1* mutation was detected in one PCa patient (0.93%), *BRCA2*—3 (2.8%), *ATM*—1 (0.93%), and *CHEK2*—13 (12.15%). None of the cases were identified with *NBN* mutation.

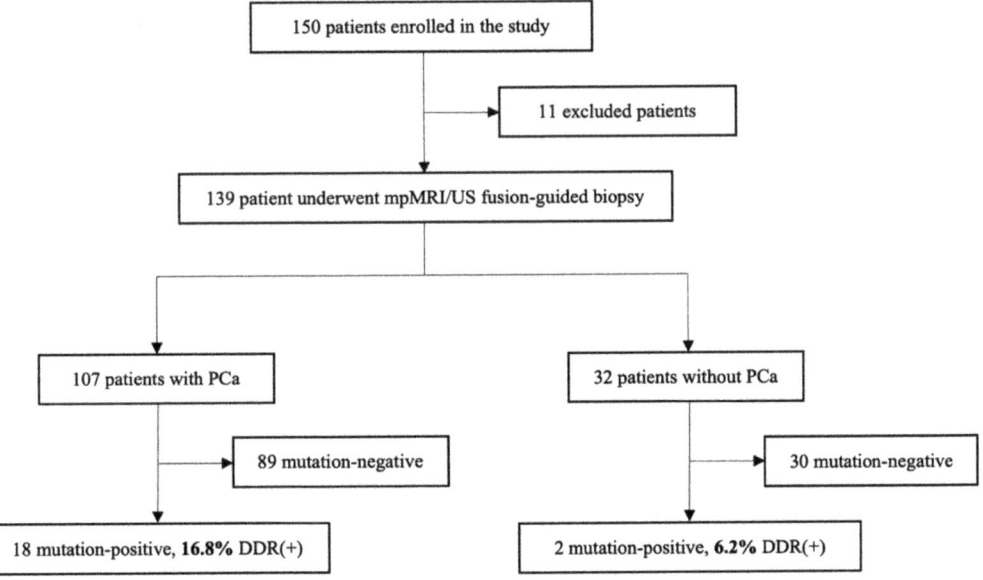

Figure 1. Flowchart of the patient cohort included in the study. Abbreviations: mpMRI—multiparametric magnetic resonance imaging; US—ultrasound; DDR—DNA damage response; PCa—prostate cancer.

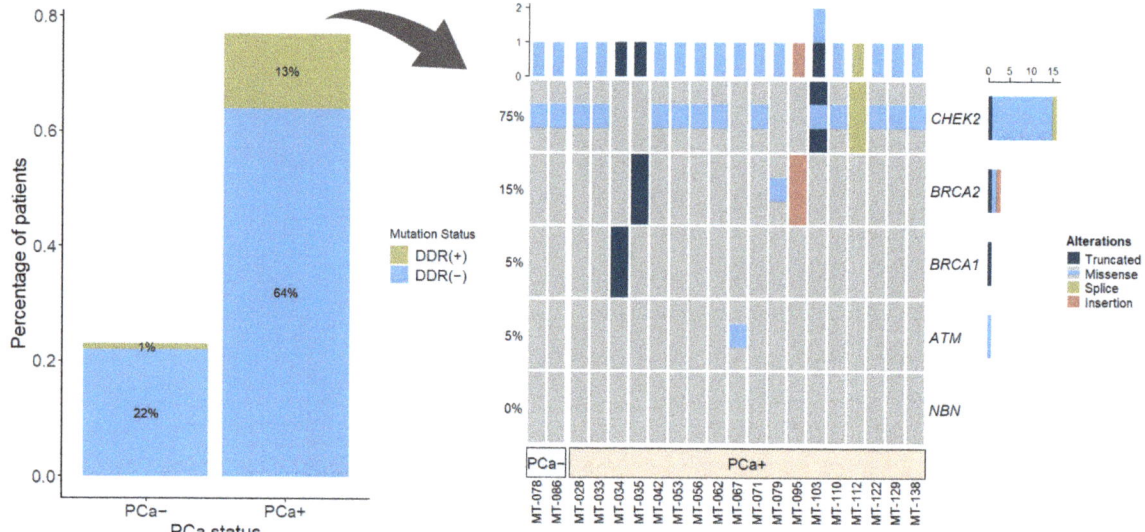

Figure 2. Percentage of patients (n = 107) with and without DDR gene mutations: overall (barplot) and according to each selected gene (oncoprint). Abbreviations: DDR—DNA damage response; PCa+—prostate cancer, PCa−—controls.

In the control group of 32 cases without confirmed PCa diagnosis, only two *CHEK2* gene mutations were detected (2/32; 6.2%). Comparison of localized PCa to control group revealed an almost three-fold higher risk of localized PCa among DDR gene mutation carriers as compared to non-carriers (OR 2.84 and 95% CI: 0.75–20.23, p = 0.16), and *CHEK2* mutation was responsible for the doubling in risk of localized PCa (OR 1.95, 95% CI: 0.49–14.18, p = 0.51). Due to the small number of cases with DDR gene mutations, the OR comparison did not reach statistical significance.

Comparison to the advanced PCa cohort from our previous study [19] revealed a higher rate of the DDR gene (*BRCA1/BRCA2/ATM/CHEK2*) mutations in the localized PCa than in the advanced disease (16.8% vs. 14.8%, p = 0.70).

3.3. Clinical Characteristics of DDR Mutation-Positive PCa

Analysis in the localized PCa group (n = 107) revealed that the DDR(+) cases (n = 18) were younger compared to DDR(−) cases (61.56 vs. 63.69 years, p = 0.27) and were presented with slightly lower PSA concentration and PSA density (Table 1). However, prostate volume was higher in the DDR(+) PCa group (55.77 vs. 44.16, p = 0.06) (Table 1). Importantly, *BRCA1/BRCA2/ATM* mutation carriers were markedly younger in the localized PCa cohort than in the advanced PCa group from our previous study [19]: 61.20 vs. 68.30 years; p = 0.06.

The localized PCa cases with DDR gene mutations were most frequently identified with PI-RADS 4 (12/18, 66.66%) lesions (Table 1), and the combined occurrence of any DDR gene mutation in PI-RADS 4/5 lesions reached 17.47%. The highest mutation rate was detected in cISUP grade group 4 and accounted for 25.00%. *BRCA1/BRCA2/ATM* mutation carriers (n = 5) revealed higher cISUP grade group scores (cISUP > 1 vs. cISUP = 1) compared to those with *CHEK2* mutation (n = 13) and the overall group of patients with mutations: (n = 18)—60.00% vs. 23.08%, p = 0.27 and 60.00% vs. 33.33%, p = 0.34, respectively. There were no statistically significant differences in mutation frequency according to risk groups divided by low-risk and intermediate/high-risk disease (Table 1).

The DDR gene mutations rate was also high in the cISUP > 1-grade group scores among advanced PCa cases [19] and exceeded mutation prevalence in the localized cISUP > 1 disease (59.10% vs. 33.33%, *p* = 0.13), and the number of cISUP > 1-grade group patients with *CHEK2* mutation was markedly higher in mCRPC as compared to localized PCa: 66.67% vs. 23.08% (*p* = 0.047) (Figure 3).

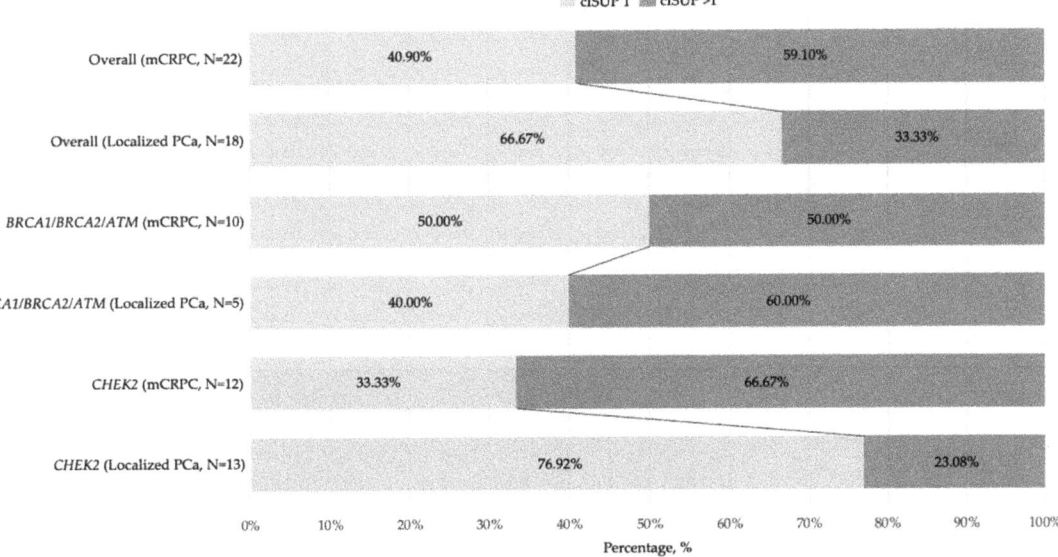

Figure 3. Bar graphs showing a prevalence of various DDR(+) mutations by cISUP grade group in localized and advanced prostate cancer groups, N. Abbreviations: cISUP—International Society of Urological Pathology grade group; mCRPC—metastatic castration-resistant prostate cancer; PCa—prostate cancer.

4. Discussion

Currently, PCa in the localized setting is characterized by its heterogeneous nature, whereas standard treatment options are generally well-established and approved by various guidelines worldwide. Nonetheless, in this PCa stage, there remains a significant knowledge gap regarding the significance of germline DDR pathway mutations in the management of the disease. Until the development of castration resistance or the diagnosis of distant-spread diseases, the range of follow-up means or specific treatment possibilities for patients with the alterations remains limited, and the weight of various mutations on the disease aggressiveness remains obscure.

In this study, prospective five DDR gene mutation testing was performed in 139 men who underwent mpMRI/US fusion-guided targeted prostate biopsy. We detected a substantial rate of genetic alterations in histologically confirmed PCa patients, reaching a prevalence of 16.8% (18/107). In comparison, our previous study on advanced castration-resistant PCa (mCRPC) revealed a germline mutation prevalence of 14.8% in the same genes (*BRCA1*, *BRCA2*, *ATM*, and *CHEK2*) [19]. Our data support observations of previous studies [9–13], i.e., that mutation rates can be relatively high in localized PCa in comparison with metastatic disease. This observation suggests that DDR gene mutations are probably early events in the evolution of aggressive prostate tumors and emphasizes the significance of conducting germline testing from the early stages of PCa.

To our knowledge, limited data exist on the association of mpMRI lesions and the presence of DDR gene mutations in localized PCa studies, usually aiming at a radiological nodal status. When analyzing the prevalence of the DDR gene mutations based on the PI-RADSv2.1 scoring system, we found that the combined occurrence of any DDR gene mutation in PI-RADS 4/5 lesions reached 17.47%. Meanwhile, no DDR gene mutations were detected in cases with lower-category (PI-RADS ≤ 3) lesions. Although these results are arguable because of their clinical application, their potential benefit might be seen in the future, when different strategies of germline testing can be adopted in patients with suspicious PCa.

In our study, the DDR pathway mutations were highly specific to cases, and only two controls without confirmed PCa were identified with *CHEK2* gene mutations. In our cohort, DDR gene mutations were associated with an almost three-fold, while *CHEK2* mutations were associated with a two-fold, increase in localized PCa risk. Positive DDR mutation status may not only help to identify PCa but it also is associated with an aggressive course [14,15] and can help verify localized PCa cases that demand timely treatment.

In our cohort, *CHEK2* alteration was found to be the most prevalent (12.15%) in localized PCa, and missense alteration *c.470T>C* was the predominant type of mutation (12/19). Most notably, Wang, Y. et al. [23], revealed that *CHEK2 c.470T>C* significantly increased the PCa risk: OR 1.80, 95% CI: 1.51–2.14, $p < 0.0001$. The significant association between *CHEK2* mutations and PCa risk (OR 1.9, 95% CI: 1.6–2.2, $p < 0.0001$) was also found in a study by Cybulski, C. et al. [24]. Specifically, they observed that truncating *CHEK2* variants was associated with higher risk when compared to missense mutations such as *c.470T>C* [24]. Our study results, in comparison with our previous study [19], revealed a predominance of *CHEK2* mutations in high cISUP grade mCRPC, but not in localized PCa ($p = 0.047$). This encourages further studies of the impact of various *CHEK2* mutation types on the aggressiveness of PCa.

The combination of alterations in *BRCA1/BRCA2* and *ATM* genes is associated with more aggressive PCa and is widely investigated in extensive mCRPC trials with PARPi [25–27]. In our cohort, *BRCA1/BRCA2* and *ATM* mutations accounted for a percentage of 4.67. The prevalence of *BRCA1/BRCA2* and *ATM* mutations was found to be greater than the reported rates of low-risk localized PCa patients by Na, R. et al. [9], i.e., 1.44%, and is consistent with the findings in the cohort analyzed by Marshall, C.H. et al. [10]—5.4%. When comparing these alterations individually, with the European ancestry patients from the large study by Lee, D.J. et al. [13], we identified higher mutation rates in *BRCA1* (0.93% vs. 0.77%), *BRCA2* (2.8% vs. 1.0%), and *ATM* (0.93% vs. 0.51%). The Cancer Genome Atlas (TCGA) [5] analysis of 333 primary prostate tumors revealed *BRCA2* and *BRCA1* mutation rates that were quite similar to our study (3% and 1%, respectively), while *ATM* mutations were slightly more frequent than in our study (4% in TCGA vs. 1% in our study). Looking closer at this study on cBioPortal [28], when excluding somatic mutations in this particular cohort, the *BRCA1* mutation rate was 1% and the *BRCA2* was 1.5%, and there were no germline mutations noted in any of the other six genes (*ATM*, *NBN*, and *CHEK2* from our study, and *CDK12*, *FANCD2*, and *RAD51c* from the TCGA study).

In our study, the DDR pathway alterations were less common in low-risk PCa patients than in intermediate- or high-risk diseases compared to non-carriers. DDR gene mutation carriers with *BRCA1/BRCA2* and *ATM* alterations were 2.6 and 1.8 times more likely to have a higher (>1) cISUP grade group, compared to those with *CHEK2* mutation and with all mutated cases, respectively. Taken together, our data and the data of other authors [2,3,14,15] suggest that these DDR gene mutations can significantly contribute to a more aggressive course of PCa.

There are several limitations of this study. Although our findings revealed a high percentage of DDR gene mutation carriers among localized PCa patients, the sample size with DDR mutations remains relatively small and reduces the statistical power of the study. Also, only five genes were included in the analysis, and the *NBN* mutation was not detected at all. Several other DDR pathway genes are associated with genetic risk of PCa and may also be important in localized disease. In our analysis, we did not include the family cancer history of the study patients, because family histories were incomplete or inaccurate in a majority of the cases. In addition, we did not investigate how the mutation status may affect clinical outcomes, though this facet merits further studies.

The high prevalence of DDR alterations in localized PCa observed in our and other studies suggests that these mutations are an early event in prostate carcinogenesis. Since

DDR deficiency may be associated with an aggressive cancer phenotype, knowledge of DDR gene status in localized stage disease may be critical, requiring more accurate decision-making in various clinical settings, such as choosing active surveillance over radical therapy or surgery over radiation, assessing the optimal timing of salvage radiotherapy after radical prostatectomy, and many other. In addition, DDR gene mutation testing in early-stage localized PCa can provide a better understanding of the molecular biology of PCa and optimize genetic testing strategies for familial cancer management. The impact on clinicopathological data and the correlation between mpMRI findings and mutation status revealed in our study provides additional arguments for wider DDR gene mutation testing in PCa.

5. Conclusions

Results of our study display a quite high rate of germline DDR mutations in localized PCa with certain implications on clinical outcomes suggesting a potential benefit of targeted genetic testing for the early identification of mutation carriers at risk of aggressive PCa.

Author Contributions: Conceptualization, S.J. and F.J.; formal analysis, I.V.; investigation, T.J., I.V. and R.S.; data curation, T.J., R.S., A.M., A.V. and A.U.; writing—original draft preparation, T.J., I.V. and R.S.; visualization, T.J., I.V. and R.S.; supervision, S.J. and F.J.; funding acquisition, S.J. and F.J. All authors have read and agreed to the published version of the manuscript.

Funding: This research received no external funding.

Institutional Review Board Statement: This study was conducted in accordance with the Declaration of Helsinki and approved by the Regional Bioethics Committee (No: 2019/11-1166-654) (5 November 2019).

Informed Consent Statement: Written informed consent was obtained from all participants involved in this study.

Data Availability Statement: The data are not publicly available due to privacy or ethical restrictions.

Acknowledgments: We would like to thank the Future Biomedicine Charity Fund (Lithuania) for the donation of materials used in the study.

Conflicts of Interest: The authors declare no conflicts of interest.

References

1. Cancer Burden Statistics and Trends across Europe | ECIS. Available online: https://ecis.jrc.ec.europa.eu/ (accessed on 30 October 2023).
2. Castro, E.; Goh, C.; Olmos, D.; Saunders, E.; Leongamornlert, D.; Tymrakiewicz, M.; Mahmud, N.; Dadaev, T.; Govindasami, K.; Guy, M.; et al. Germline BRCA mutations are associated with higher risk of nodal involvement, distant metastasis, and poor survival outcomes in prostate cancer. *J. Clin. Oncol.* **2013**, *31*, 1748–1757. [CrossRef] [PubMed]
3. Leongamornlert, D.; Saunders, E.; Dadaev, T.; Tymrakiewicz, M.; Goh, C.; Jurgnauth-Little, S.; Kozarewa, I.; Fenwick, K.; Assiotis, I.; Barrowdale, D.; et al. Frequent germline deleterious mutations in DNA repair genes in familial prostate cancer cases are associated with advanced disease. *Br. J. Cancer* **2014**, *110*, 1663–1672. [CrossRef] [PubMed]
4. Lozano, R.; Castro, E.; Aragón, M.I.; Cendón, Y.; Cattrini, C.; López-Casas, P.P.; Olmos, D. Genetic aberrations in DNA repair pathways: A cornerstone of precision oncology in prostate cancer. *Br. J. Cancer* **2021**, *124*, 552–563. [CrossRef] [PubMed]
5. Abeshouse, A.; Ahn, J.; Akbani, R.; Ally, A.; Amin, S.; Andry, C.D.; Annala, M.; Aprikian, A.; Armenia, J.; Arora, A.; et al. The Molecular Taxonomy of Primary Prostate Cancer. *Cell* **2015**, *163*, 1011–1025. [CrossRef] [PubMed]
6. Robinson, D.; Van Allen, E.M.; Wu, Y.M.; Schultz, N.; Lonigro, R.J.; Mosquera, J.M.; Montgomery, B.; Taplin, M.E.; Pritchard, C.C.; Attard, G.; et al. Integrative clinical genomics of advanced prostate cancer. *Cell* **2015**, *161*, 1215–1228. [CrossRef] [PubMed]
7. Lang, S.H.; Swift, S.L.; White, H.; Misso, K.; Kleijnen, J.; Quek, R.G.W. A systematic review of the prevalence of DNA damage response gene mutations in prostate cancer. *Int. J. Oncol.* **2019**, *55*, 597–616. [CrossRef] [PubMed]
8. Antonarakis, E.S.; Gomella, L.G.; Petrylak, D.P. When and How to Use PARP Inhibitors in Prostate Cancer: A Systematic Review of the Literature with an Update on On-Going Trials. *Eur. Urol. Oncol.* **2020**, *3*, 594–611. [CrossRef]
9. Na, R.; Zheng, S.L.; Han, M.; Yu, H.; Jiang, D.; Shah, S.; Ewing, C.M.; Zhang, L.; Novakovic, K.; Petkewicz, J.; et al. Germline Mutations in ATM and BRCA1/2 Distinguish Risk for Lethal and Indolent Prostate Cancer and are Associated with Early Age at Death. *Eur. Urol.* **2017**, *71*, 740–747. [CrossRef]

10. Marshall, C.H.; Fu, W.; Wang, H.; Baras, A.S.; Lotan, T.L.; Antonarakis, E.S. Prevalence of DNA repair gene mutations in localized prostate cancer according to clinical and pathologic features: Association of Gleason score and tumor stage. *Prostate Cancer Prostatic Dis.* **2018**, *22*, 59–65. [CrossRef]
11. Wu, Y.; Yu, H.; Li, S.; Wiley, K.; Zheng, S.L.; LaDuca, H.; Gielzak, M.; Na, R.; Sarver, B.A.J.; Helfand, B.T.; et al. Rare Germline Pathogenic Mutations of DNA Repair Genes Are Most Strongly Associated with Grade Group 5 Prostate Cancer. *Eur. Urol. Oncol.* **2020**, *3*, 224–230. [CrossRef]
12. Berchuck, J.E.; Zhang, Z.; Silver, R.; Kwak, L.; Xie, W.; Lee, G.-S.M.; Freedman, M.L.; Kibel, A.S.; Van Allen, E.M.; McKay, R.R.; et al. Impact of Pathogenic Germline DNA Damage Repair alterations on Response to Intense Neoadjuvant Androgen Deprivation Therapy in High-risk Localized Prostate Cancer. *Eur. Urol.* **2021**, *80*, 295–303. [CrossRef] [PubMed]
13. Lee, D.J.; Hausler, R.; Le, A.N.; Kelly, G.; Powers, J.; Ding, J.; Feld, E.; Desai, H.; Morrison, C.; Doucette, A.; et al. Association of Inherited Mutations in DNA Repair Genes with Localized Prostate Cancer. *Eur. Urol.* **2022**, *81*, 559–567. [CrossRef] [PubMed]
14. Cheng, H.H.; Pritchard, C.C.; Montgomery, B.; Lin, D.W.; Nelson, P.S. Prostate Cancer Screening in a New Era of Genetics. *Clin. Genitourin. Cancer* **2017**, *15*, 625–628. [CrossRef] [PubMed]
15. Marino, F.; Totaro, A.; Gandi, C.; Bientinesi, R.; Moretto, S.; Gavi, F.; Pierconti, F.; Iacovelli, R.; Bassi, P.; Sacco, E. Germline mutations in prostate cancer: A systematic review of the evidence for personalized medicine. *Prostate Cancer Prostatic Dis.* **2023**, *26*, 655–664. [CrossRef] [PubMed]
16. Castro, E.; Romero-Laorden, N.; del Pozo, A.; Lozano, R.; Medina, A.; Puente, J.; Piulats, J.M.; Lorente, D.; Saez, M.I.; Morales-Barrera, R.; et al. Prorepair-B: A Prospective Cohort Study of the Impact of Germline DNA Repair Mutations on the Outcomes of Patients with Metastatic Castration-Resistant Prostate Cancer. *J. Clin. Oncol.* **2019**, *37*, 490–503. [CrossRef] [PubMed]
17. Parker, C.; Castro, E.; Fizazi, K.; Heidenreich, A.; Ost, P.; Procopio, G.; Tombal, B.; Gillessen, S.; ESMO Guidelines Committee. Prostate cancer: ESMO Clinical Practice Guidelines for diagnosis, treatment and follow-up. *Ann. Oncol.* **2020**, *31*, 1119–1134. [CrossRef] [PubMed]
18. Nombela, P.; Lozano, R.; Aytes, A.; Mateo, J.; Olmos, D.; Castro, E. BRCA2 and Other DDR Genes in Prostate Cancer. *Cancers* **2019**, *11*, 352. [CrossRef] [PubMed]
19. Januskevicius, T.; Sabaliauskaite, R.; Dabkeviciene, D.; Vaicekauskaite, I.; Kulikiene, I.; Sestokaite, A.; Vidrinskaite, A.; Bakavicius, A.; Jankevicius, F.; Ulys, A.; et al. Urinary DNA as a tool for germline and somatic mutation detection in castration-resistant prostate cancer patients. *Biomedicines* **2023**, *11*, 761. [CrossRef]
20. Turkbey, B.; Rosenkrantz, A.B.; Haider, M.A.; Padhami, A.R.; Villeirs, G.; Macura, K.J.; Tempany, C.M.; Choyke, P.L.; Cornud, F.; Margolis, D.J.; et al. Prostate Imaging Reporting and Data System Version 2.1: 2019 Update of Prostate Imaging Reporting and Data System Version 2. *Eur. Urol.* **2019**, *76*, 340–351. [CrossRef]
21. Mottet, N.; van den Bergh, R.C.N.; Briers, E.; Van den Broeck, T.; Cumberbatch, M.G.; Santis, M.D.; Fanti, S.; Fossati, N.; Gandaglia, G.; Gillessen, S.; et al. EAU-EANM-ESTRO-ESUR-SIOG Guidelines on Prostate Cancer-2020 Update. Part 1: Screening, Diagnosis, and Local Treatment with Curative Intent. *Eur. Urol.* **2021**, *79*, 243–262. [CrossRef]
22. Gu, Z.; Eils, R.; Schlesner, M. Complex Heatmaps Reveal Patterns and Correlations in Multidimensional Genomic Data. *Bioinformatics* **2016**, *32*, 2847–2849. [CrossRef] [PubMed]
23. Wang, Y.; Dai, B.; Ye, D. CHEK2 Mutation and Risk of Prostate Cancer: A Systematic Review and Meta-Analysis. *Int. J. Clin. Exp. Med.* **2015**, *8*, 15708. Available online: https://www.ncbi.nlm.nih.gov/pmc/articles/PMC4658955 (accessed on 14 November 2023). [PubMed]
24. Cybulski, C.; Wokolorczyk, D.; Kluzniak, W.; Jakubowska, A.; Gorski, B.; Gronwald, J.; Huzarski, T.; Kashyap, A.; Byrski, T.; Debniak, T.; et al. An Inherited NBN Mutation Is Associated with Poor Prognosis Prostate Cancer. *Br. J. Cancer* **2012**, *108*, 461–468. [CrossRef] [PubMed]
25. de Bono, J.; Mateo, J.; Fizazi, K.; Saad, F.; Shore, N.; Sandhu, S.; Chi, K.N.; Sartor, O.; Agarwal, N.; Olmos, D.; et al. Olaparib for Metastatic Castration-Resistant Prostate Cancer. *N. Engl. J. Med.* **2020**, *382*, 2091–2102. [CrossRef]
26. Fizazi, K.; Piulats, J.M.; Reaume, M.N.; Ostler, P.; McDermott, R.; Gingerich, J.R.; Pintus, E.; Sridhar, S.S.; Bambury, R.M.; Emmenegger, U.; et al. Rucaparib or Physician's Choice in Metastatic Prostate Cancer. *N. Engl. J. Med.* **2023**, *388*, 719–732. [CrossRef]
27. Bryce, A.H.; Piulats, J.M.; Reaume, P.J.; Ostler, R.S.; McDermott, J.R.; Gingerich, E.; Pintus, S.S.; Sridhar, W.; Abida, G.; Daugaard, A.; et al. Rucaparib for metastatic castration-resistant prostate cancer (mCRPC): TRITON3 interim overall survival and efficacy of rucaparib vs docetaxel or second-generation androgen pathway inhibitor therapy. *J. Clin. Oncol.* **2023**, *41* (Suppl. S6), 18. [CrossRef]
28. Cerami, E.; Gao, J.; Dogrusoz, U.; Gross, B.E.; Sumer, S.O.; Aksoy, B.A.; Jacobsen, A.; Byrne, C.J.; Heuer, M.L.; Larsson, E.; et al. The cBio cancer genomics portal: An open platform for exploring multidimensional cancer genomics data. *Cancer Discov.* **2012**, *2*, 401–404. [CrossRef]

Disclaimer/Publisher's Note: The statements, opinions and data contained in all publications are solely those of the individual author(s) and contributor(s) and not of MDPI and/or the editor(s). MDPI and/or the editor(s) disclaim responsibility for any injury to people or property resulting from any ideas, methods, instructions or products referred to in the content.

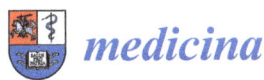

Article

Evaluation of Changes in Circulating Cell-Free DNA as an Early Predictor of Response to Chemoradiation in Rectal Cancer—A Pilot Study

Wee Liam Ong [1], Sorinel Lunca [1,2,*,†], Stefan Morarasu [1,2,*,†], Ana-Maria Musina [1,2], Alina Puscasu [1,2], Stefan Iacob [1,2], Irina Iftincai [3], Andreea Marinca [3], Iuliu Ivanov [4], Cristian Ena Roata [1,2], Natalia Velenciuc [1,2] and Gabriel Dimofte [1,2]

[1] 2nd Department of Surgical Oncology, Regional Institute of Oncology (IRO), 700483 Iasi, Romania; william05021990@gmail.com (W.L.O.); musina.anamaria@gmail.com (A.-M.M.); alinaioanapuscasu@yahoo.com (A.P.); dr.iacobstefan@yahoo.com (S.I.); roatacristianene@gmail.com (C.E.R.); velenciucn@gmail.com (N.V.); gdimofte@gmail.com (G.D.)

[2] Department of Surgery, University of Medicine and Pharmacy "Grigore T. Popa", 700115 Iasi, Romania

[3] Radiotherapy Department, Regional Institute of Oncology (IRO), 700483 Iasi, Romania; irina_iftincai@yahoo.com (I.I.); andreea.marinca@gmail.com (A.M.)

[4] "TRANSCEND" Centre for Fundamental Research and Experimental Development in Translational Medicine, Regional Institute of Oncology (IRO), 700483 Iasi, Romania; iuliuic@gmail.com

* Correspondence: sdlunca@yahoo.com (S.L.); morarasu.stefan@gmail.com (S.M.); Tel.: +40-744-437-305 (S.L.); +40-754-490-870 (S.M.)

† These authors contributed equally to this work.

Abstract: *Background and Objectives:* The objective of this study was to investigate quantitative changes in cell-free DNA (cfDNA) found in the bloodstream of patients with locally advanced rectal cancer who received neoadjuvant long-course chemoradiation, assuming a change in DNA fragments release during therapeutic stress. *Materials and Methods:* This was a prospective observational study that involved 49 patients who had three distinct pathologies requiring neoadjuvant chemoradiation: 18 patients with breast cancer, 18 patients with cervical cancer, and 13 patients with rectal cancer. Both breast cancer and cervical cancer patients were used as a control groups. Breast cancer patients were used as a control group as irradiation targeted healthy tissue after the tumor resection (R0), while cervical cancer patients were used as a control group to evaluate the effect of chemoradiation regarding cfDNA in a different setting (squamous cell carcinomas) and a different tumor burden. Rectal cancer patients were the study group, and were prospectively evaluated for a correlation between fragmentation of cfDNA and late response to chemoradiation. Blood samples were collected before the initiation of treatment and after the fifth radiation dose delivery. cfDNA was quantified in peripheral blood and compared with the patients' clinicopathological characteristics and tumor volume. *Conclusion:* Thirteen patients with locally advanced rectal cancer (T3/T4/N+/M0) were included in the study, and all of them had their samples analyzed. Eight were male (61.54%) and five were female (38.46%), with an average age of 70.85 years. Most of the patients had cT3 (53.85%) or cT4 (46.15%) tumors, and 92.31% had positive lymph nodes (N2–3). Of the thirteen patients, only six underwent surgery, and one of them achieved a pathological complete response (pCR). The mean size of the tumor was 122.60 mm^3 [35.33–662.60 mm^3]. No significant correlation was found between cfDNA, tumor volume, and tumor regression grade. cfDNA does not seem to predict response to neoadjuvant chemoradiotherapy and it is not correlated to tumor volume or tumor regression grade.

Keywords: rectal cancer; radiotherapy; DNA; neoadjuvant therapy; prognosis

Citation: Ong, W.L.; Lunca, S.; Morarasu, S.; Musina, A.-M.; Puscasu, A.; Iacob, S.; Iftincai, I.; Marinca, A.; Ivanov, I.; Roata, C.E.; et al. Evaluation of Changes in Circulating Cell-Free DNA as an Early Predictor of Response to Chemoradiation in Rectal Cancer—A Pilot Study. *Medicina* **2023**, *59*, 1742. https://doi.org/10.3390/medicina59101742

Academic Editors: Valentin Titus Grigorean and Daniel Alin Cristian

Received: 2 September 2023
Revised: 22 September 2023
Accepted: 26 September 2023
Published: 28 September 2023

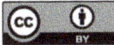

Copyright: © 2023 by the authors. Licensee MDPI, Basel, Switzerland. This article is an open access article distributed under the terms and conditions of the Creative Commons Attribution (CC BY) license (https:// creativecommons.org/licenses/by/ 4.0/).

1. Introduction

Recent advancements in the multimodal treatment of locally advanced rectal cancer have resulted in impressive rates of clinical complete response (cCR) [1,2]. In a comprehensive systematic review conducted by Hartley et al., involving a total of 3157 patients, the overall pathological complete response (pCR) rate was estimated at 13.5% [3]. Notably, consistently higher response rates have been associated with high-dose radiotherapy [4]. The Rectal Cancer and Preoperative Induction Therapy Followed by Dedicated Operation (RAPIDO) trial, in particular, demonstrated that patients undergoing Total Neoadjuvant Therapy (TNT) achieved a significantly higher pCR rate (28.4%) compared to those receiving standard radiochemotherapy (14.3%, $p < 0.0001$) [5].

Furthermore, a strategy centered on watchful waiting (W&W), with the aim of organ preservation, has emerged as a viable option for patients who achieve clinical complete response (cCR) following neoadjuvant (chemo)radiotherapy [6]. This W&W approach, initially proposed by Habr-Gama, has received recent support from the International Watch and Wait Database, which reported a 2-year cumulative local regrowth incidence of 25.2%. In contrast, it is worth noting that even the pathologic complete response (pCR) rate, classified as Dworak TRG 4, reached as high as 28.4%. In the same study, the favorable responders, categorized as Dworak TRG 2–3, constituted 52.7% of the cases, while the poor-to-non-responders, classified as Dworak TRG 0–1, comprised 38.2% [7].

The current standard approach for locally advanced rectal cancer (T3/T4 N+) involves long-course radiotherapy, typically utilizing conventionally fractionated radiotherapy. This entails administering doses of 180 to 200 centi-Gray per fraction, delivered in 25 to 28 daily fractions (five days per week), resulting in a cumulative dose ranging from 4500 to 5040 centi-Gray. Concurrently, chemotherapy is administered, with the most commonly used cytostatic agents being capecitabine at a dose of 825 mg/m^2 twice daily or 5-fluorouracil at a dose of 1200 mg/m^2 daily [2,5]. Surgery is usually scheduled for 4 to 12 weeks following the conclusion of radiotherapy, typically in the sixth or seventh week, resulting in a total treatment duration of 3–4 months. Importantly, this timeframe does not account for waiting periods associated with initiating radiation therapy and surgical treatment.

The next crucial step in modern rectal cancer treatment is to establish standardized biomarkers [8] capable of estimating response rates and defining individualized neoadjuvant protocols [9]. Currently, there is no universally accepted "gold standard" for distinguishing between individuals who respond positively to treatment and those who do not. The aspiration is to identify specific biomarkers that can assist in differentiating potential good responders, who would benefit from radiochemotherapy, from those who may not respond as favorably. Such differentiation can play a pivotal role in sparing the latter group from enduring an extended treatment regimen with limited potential for tumor size reduction or downstaging, thereby mitigating the risk of undue toxicity and further tumor progression.

More recently, the selection of mismatch repair-deficient (dMMR) [8] patients for neoadjuvant immunotherapy with PD-1 blockers has shown impressive results in a small cohort of cases [2,10,11]. Trials such as NICHE (pCR 13/32—69%) and PICC (pCR 4/17—88%) have demonstrated the potential of this approach. DNA mismatch repair deficiency is already an established predictor, as is Immunoscore [12], which has been shown to predict survival and response rates to neoadjuvant therapy. In addition to tumor biopsies, readily available biomarkers harvested from peripheral blood [13] are under intense study and proposed as simpler alternatives. Immune cell ratios, CRP (C-reactive protein), and CD8+ T cells have all been described as potential predictors, although results have been conflicting [12].

Another potential biomarker under consideration is cell-free DNA (cfDNA). CfDNA comprises DNA fragments ranging in length from 50 to 200 base pairs. These fragments are released by cells and enter the bloodstream, typically as a result of apoptosis or necrosis [14]. The term "circulating tumor DNA" (ctDNA) specifically refers to cfDNA originating from cancer cells in cancer patients [15]. Mandel and Metais were the pioneers who first described cfDNA in 1948 [16]. It has recently gained recognition as a promising biomarker, particularly for diagnosing advanced malignancies [13]. Individuals with rectal cancer can exhibit cfDNA levels up to 50 times higher compared to those in a healthy state. During neoadjuvant therapy, these levels are expected to increase due to tumor necrosis [17,18].

Numerous studies have produced promising results regarding the utility of cfDNA in diagnosing, monitoring, and prognosticating rectal cancer. Both Zitt et al. and Agostini et al. have concluded that responders to treatment exhibit a significant reduction in circulating DNA, whereas non-responders tend to experience a notable increase in circulating DNA levels following radiochemotherapy [19,20]. Truelsen et al. have proposed circulating cell-free DNA as a predictor of pathological complete response, providing potential value in monitoring patients with a complete clinical response within watch-and-wait (W&W) strategies [7].

For the above reasons, our aim was to investigate quantitative changes in cfDNA found in the bloodstream of patients with locally advanced rectal cancer who received neoadjuvant long-course chemoradiation, assuming changes in DNA fragment release during therapeutic stress, particularly early after the fifth session of radiation.

2. Materials and Methods

2.1. Design and Setting

This was a single-center, observational, prospective study of three groups of patients who had three distinct cancers requiring neoadjuvant chemoradiation: breast cancer, cervical cancer, and rectal cancer. All patients underwent standard oncological work-up and management based on multidisciplinary meetings. All patients were treated and followed at our institution. Informed consent was gained for each patient included in the study. This study was approved by our Institutions Ethics Committee (REGISTRATION NUMBER. 227/26 August 2019).

Rectal cancer patients were the study group, and were prospectively evaluated for a correlation between fragmentation of cfDNA and late response to chemoradiation. Breast cancer patients were used as a control group as irradiation targeted healthy tissue after the complete tumor resection, while cervical cancer patients were used as a control group to evaluate the effect of chemoradiation on cfDNA in a different histological type and a different tumor burden.

2.2. Inclusion and Exclusion Criteria

Patients with confirmed histology and full oncological work-up were included. Only patients with curative intent were included. Patients with other synchronous cancers were excluded. Patients with previous malignancies were excluded.

2.3. Experimental Protocol

Blood samples were collected before the initiation of treatment and after the 5th radiation dose delivery. The need for an early prediction of response cannot be overemphasized and the 5th dose was chosen because surgical treatment can still be initiated, in patients considered non-responders, within a week after the 5th dose, while continuation of treatment may only result in toxicity and prolong by 2 months the time for surgical procedure. Two samples were collected from each patient, one before radiotherapy and the other after the fifth dose. Within four hours of collection, DNA from the plasma was extracted using the Cobas cfDNA Sample Extraction Kit® (Roche Diagnostic GmbH, Mannheim, Germany) and stored at a temperature of $-20\ °C$. Once all the samples were collected, we measured the amount of cfDNA using the Agilent 2100 Bioanalyzer (Agilent Technologies, Waldbroan, Germany) with High Sensitivity DNA Kit® (Agilent Technologies, Waldbroan, Germany). The Agilent 2100 Bioanalyzer system is an established microfluidics-based automated electrophoresis solution for the sample quality control of biomolecules.

After obtaining the concentrations of cfDNA from all the samples, we proceeded to input the data into XLSTAT for a comprehensive analysis. This analysis encompassed the examination of differences (i.e., cfDNA concentration after the 5th radiation session minus cfDNA concentration before radiation) and ratios (i.e., cfDNA concentration after the 5th radiation session divided by cfDNA concentration before radiation) between each sample collected before radiation and after the 5th radiation session of the same patient. For these data sets, we computed the range (defined as the difference between the smallest and largest values), the average (which included the average cfDNA concentration before radiation, after radiation, as well as the averages of the calculated differences and ratios), and variance (calculated using the Variance.P function). Additionally, employing the software, we generated linear regression plots and Box and Whisker graphs to facilitate a comparative analysis between the control group (comprising cases of breast and cervical cancer) and the target group (consisting of rectal cancer cases).

Response to chemoradiation was assessed 8 weeks after completion of radiation therapy through pelvic MRI. Data on tumor volume were collected, including gross tumor target volume (GTV) and planning target volume (PTV) from the archive of treatment plan from the radiotherapy department. Tumor response was extracted from the pathological response rating (Dworak grading). Descriptive variables are reported as percentages, mean, and range for clinicopathologic characteristics and tumor measurements. The association between cfDNA distribution and tumor volume and tumor regression grade (TRG) was evaluated using the Pearson correlation coefficient test. A p value < 0.05 was considered statistically significant. XLSTAT software (Version 2309 Build 16.0.16827.20014) was used for statistical analysis.

3. Results

3.1. Patient Characteristics

This prospective study investigated 98 samples (from 49 patients). Specifically, all 18 patients with breast cancer had their samples analyzed, along with 18 patients from the cervical cancer group and 13 patients from the rectal cancer group.

Thirteen patients with locally advanced rectal cancer (T3/T4/N+/M0) were included in the study, and all of them had their samples analyzed; eight were male (61.54%) and five were female (55.56%), with an average age of 70.92 years. Most patients had cT3 (53.85%) or cT4 (46.15) tumors, and 92.31% had positive lymph nodes (N1–2). The disease stage was IIIc for nine patients, IIIb for three patients, and IIb for one patient. Of the thirteen patients, only six underwent surgery, and one of them achieved a pathological complete response (pCR). Two of the seven patients who did not have surgery were deemed inoperable due to metastasis or advanced disease and five patients died of other causes (Figure 1). All patients that received the standard concurrent chemoradiotherapy protocol were reevaluated after 8 weeks, and underwent surgical resection with total mesorectal excision (TME). Of six patients who underwent surgical resection, five patients (Dworak 1–2) showed poor response and one patient showed pathological complete response (Dworak 4). Table 1 summarizes the findings.

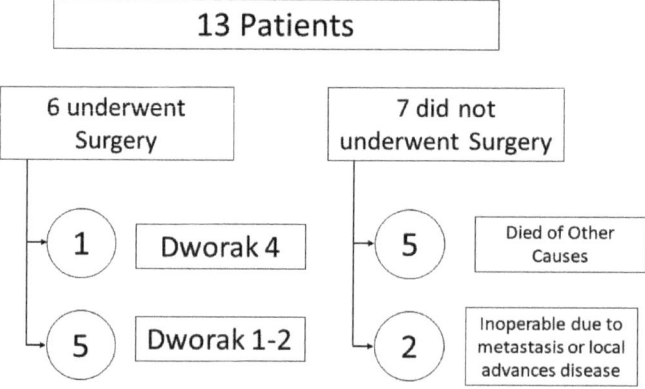

Figure 1. Diagram depicting management and response in the thirteen rectal cancer patients.

Table 1. Characteristics of included rectal cancer patients.

Clinical Variable	No. (%)
Sex:	
Male	8 (61.54)
Female	5 (38.46)
Age:	
<65	3 (23.07)
>65	10 (46.15)
Clinical TNM Staging	
Tumor	
cT3	7 (53.85)
cT4	6 (46.15)
Node	
cN0	1 (7.69)
cN1	3 (23.08)
cN2	9 (69.23)
Metastasis	
cM0	13 (100)
cM1	0 (0)
Clinical AJCC Staging	
IIb	1 (7.6)
IIIa	0 (0)
IIIb	3 (23.07)
IIIc	9 (69.23)
Management	
Operated	6 (46.1)
Not operated	7 (53.8)
Metastasis or locally advanced	2 (28.57)
Other causes	5 (71.42)
Pathology Staging	
Tumor	
ypT0	1 (16.67)
ypT1	0 (0)
ypT2	2 (33.33)
ypT3	3 (50.00)
Node	
ypN0	5 (83.33)
ypN1	1 (16.67)
Pathological Response	
Dworak TRG system	
1 (poor response)	3 (50.00)
2 (poor response)	2 (33.33)
3 (good response)	0 (0)
4 (Complete Responds)	1 (16.67)

3.2. Tumour Measurements

Thirteen patients were analyzed with regard to the mean size of the gross target volume (GTV), which measured 122.60 mm^3 (ranging from 35.33 mm^3 to 662.6 mm^3). The planning target volume (PTV) for these patients was determined to be 1839.75 mm^3, with a range of 1122.18 mm^3 to 2910 mm^3. To further investigate the correlation between tumor volume and tumor regression grade, a subgroup was established for patients who had undergone surgery, totaling six individuals. In this subgroup, the mean size of the gross target tumor volume was 75.25 mm^3, ranging from 60.92 mm^3 to 86.54 mm^3. Additionally, the planning target volume (PTV) was calculated as 2067.27 mm^3, ranging from 1463.40 mm^3 to 2910 mm^3 (Table 2).

Table 2. Tumor measurements in the rectal cancer cohort that underwent surgical treatment. Key: GTV, gross target volume; PTV, planning target volume; cTN, clinical tumor node staging; ypTN, pathological tumor node staging; TRG, tumor regression grade.

Sample	GTV (mm³)	PTV (mm³)	cTN	ypTN	TRG
R42	69.87	2177.66	cT3N2	ypT0N0	4
R50	86.54	1502.27	cT3N1	ypT3N0	1
R51	66.73	1633.77	cT3N1	ypT3N0	1
R52	60.92	1463.4	cT3N2	ypT2N0	2
R53	83.79	2910.00	cT3N1	ypT2N1	2
R61	83.63	2716.5	cT4N2	ypT3N0	1
Average	75.25	2067.27			

3.3. Quantification of cfDNA

In total, 98 samples were gathered and examined from 49 patients, (including 18 from the breast cancer group, 18 from the cervical cancer group, and 13 patients from the rectal cancer group).

Figure 2 displays an illustration of the outcome produced by utilizing the Agilent 2100 Bioanalyzer along with the High Sensitivity DNA Kit. The X-axis illustrates the concentration detected in seconds (s), while the Y-axis represents the concentration in picograms per microliter (pg/μL). The final result was computed through automated calculations using the Agilent 2100 Expert software(ver. B.02.08.SI648 [SR 1]) provided by Agilent 2100 Bioanalyzer. The kit is designed to accurately quantify and determine the size of DNA fragments and smears that fall within the range of 50 to 7000 bp. The red line represents the result prior to radiotherapy, while the blue line represents the outcome after the fifth dose of radiotherapy. We evaluated the area under the curve, which allowed us to estimate the total quantity of DNA fragments between the two collections and determine the ratio and differences between them.

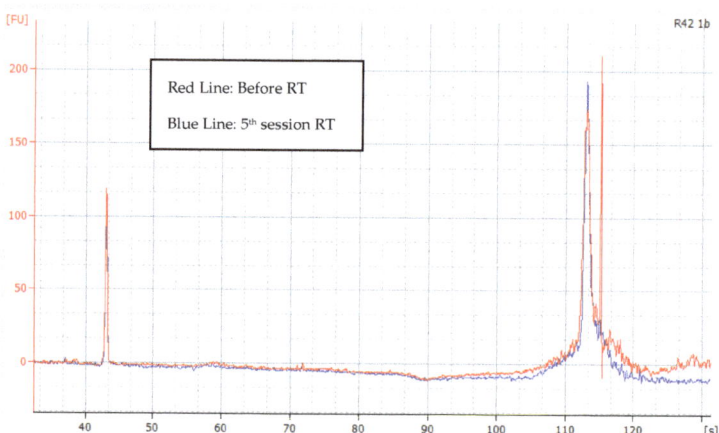

Figure 2. Example of result for cfDNA before and after 5th session of radiotherapy.

3.4. Distribution of cfDNA

Table 3 displays the mean value and variability of each sample group. For the target group (consisting of thirteen rectal cancer patients), the mean volume of cfDNA fragments collected from plasma was 455.45 pg/μL (with a range of 70.90–1013.80 pg/μL) before radiotherapy, and the mean volume on the 5th day of radiotherapy was 816.92 pg/μL (with a range of 72.50–3336.30 pg/μL). In the breast cancer control group, 18 samples were collected both before and on the 5th day of radiotherapy. The median value before treatment was 1494.92 pg/μL (with a range of 133.90–10,241.20 pg/μL), while the mean on the 5th day of radiotherapy was 1049.72 pg/μL (with a range of 62.3–6196.50 pg/μL). For cervical cancer patients, the mean concentration of cfDNA before radiotherapy was 3063.26 pg/μL (with a range of 300.80–22,660.00 pg/μL), and the mean value on the 5th day was 2192.03 pg/μL (with a range of 176.80–13,106.90 pg/μL). Figure 3 depicts the Box and Whisker plot of all samples. The overall data exhibited several outliners, and no discernible pattern or correlation was observed.

Table 3. Average and variance of cfDNA.

		Range	Average	Variance
Rectal Cancer	Before:	70.90—1013.80	455.45	116,860.18
	5th:	72.50–3336.30	816.92	789,032.72
	Difference:	−741.80–2427.00	361.48	737,937.48
	Ratio:	0.13–14.37	3.42	18.93
Breast Cancer	Before:	133.90–10,241.20	1494.92	5,206,590.66
	5th:	62.30–6196.50	1049.72	2,763,380.14
	Difference:	−10,083.00–4604.60	−445.20	7,669,628.27
	Ratio:	0.02–3.89	0.90	1.12
Cervical Cancer	Before:	300.80–22,660.00	3063.26	28,769,505.87
	5th:	176.80–13,105.90	2192.03	12,388,219.88
	Difference:	−22,203.40–11,347.80	−871.23	40,621,472.94
	Ratio:	0.02–7.45	1.39	2.82

Before: before radiotherapy; 5th: after 5th day of radiotherapy; Difference: difference between 5th day of radiotherapy and before radiotherapy; Ratio: ratio between 5th day of radiotherapy and before radiotherapy.

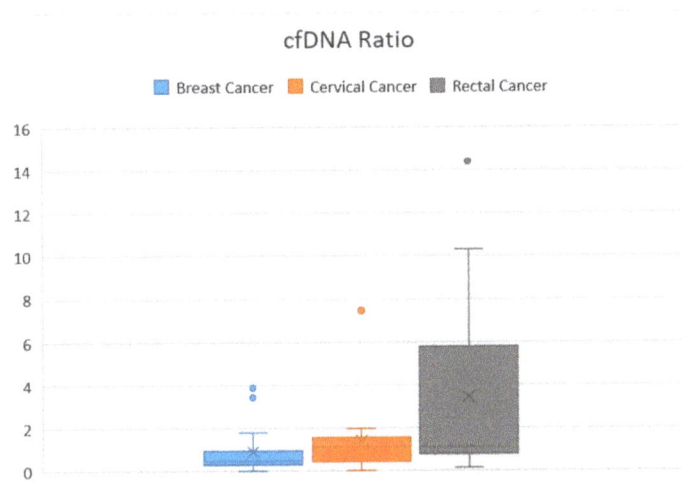

Figure 3. Box and Whisker plot of cfDNA ratio between samples.

3.5. Regression and Pearson Correlation Coefficient Test

Figure 4 displays a regression graph illustrating the cfDNA ratio within all three patient groups. Notably, rectal cancer ($r^2 = 0.1372$) and cervical cancer ($r^2 = 0.064$) show a positive regression trend, while breast cancer exhibits a negative regression, with an r^2 value of 0.003. It is important to emphasize that the Pearson test did not identify any significant correlations among cfDNA levels (measured both before and on the 5th day of radiotherapy), tumor volumes (GTV, PTV), and tumor regression grades (TRG), as outlined in Table 4.

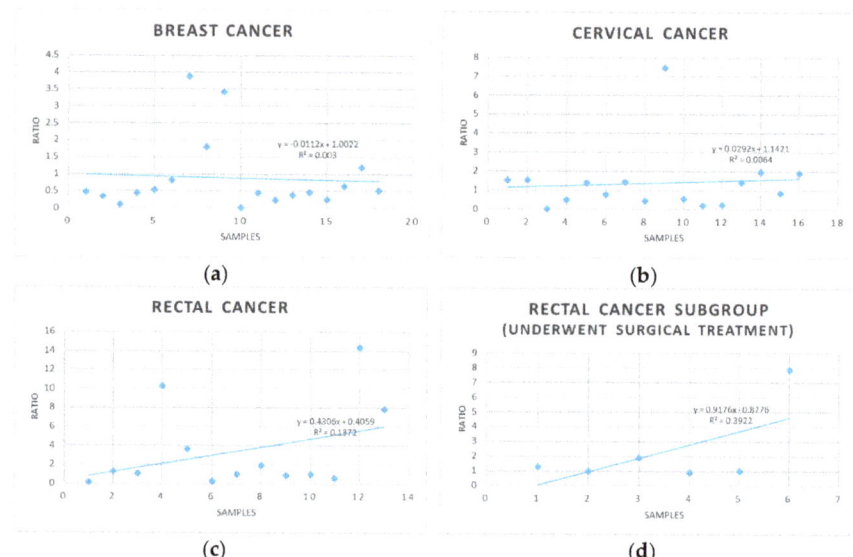

Figure 4. cfDNA ratio regression graph in all three groups of patients: (**a**) breast cancer group, (**b**) cervical cancer group, (**c**) rectal cancer group, (**d**) rectal cancer subgroup (underwent surgical treatment).

Table 4. Pearson correlation coefficient between cfDNA, tumor volume and TRG. (Key: cfDNA, cell-free DNA; pre-RT, before radiotherapy; GTV, gross target volume; PTV, planning target volume; TRG, tumor regression grade; Difference, difference between cfDNA after the fifth session of RT and cfDNA before RT).

	Pearson Correlation Coefficient (r)	*p* Value
cfDNA pre-RT—PTV	0.05	0.92
cfDNA pre-RT—GTV	0.49	0.31
Difference—GTV	0.04	0.94
cfDNA after 5th session RT—GTV	0.41	0.42
cfDNA after 5th session RT—PTV	0.41	0.92
Difference—TRG	0.50	0.31

4. Discussion

In this pilot study, we successfully demonstrated the extraction and standardized quantification of cfDNA from peripheral blood. However, in this specific experiment, a significant correlation was not observed between cfDNA levels and tumor response. This raises questions about the predictive role of cfDNA, which in turn prompts the need for further research and debate concerning the timing and methodology of cfDNA quantification, as its distribution may vary during neoadjuvant therapy.

As previously mentioned, a minor quantity of circulating free DNA (cfDNA) is typically detected in healthy individuals. Quantitative studies have shown that in healthy individuals, cfDNA concentrations usually fall within the range of 0–100 ng/mL of blood, with an average of 30 ng/mL, whereas in the blood of cancer patients, cfDNA concentrations exhibit a broader variation, ranging from 0 to 1000 ng/mL, with an average of 180 ng/mL [1,14,18].

Numerous studies have generated promising findings regarding the utility of circulating cell-free DNA (cfDNA) in monitoring the response to radiochemotherapy in patients with locally advanced rectal cancer. In a study conducted by M. Zitt et al., responders exhibited a reduction in cfDNA to 2.2 ng/mL (with a range of 1.5 to 2.9 ng/mL), while non-responders showed an increase to 5.1 ng/mL (with a range of 3.8 to 10.3 ng/mL) ($p = 0.006$) [19].

Furthermore, a separate investigation led by W. Sun et al. revealed a significant decline in the concentration of 400-base pair fragment DNA following chemoradiotherapy, particularly within the group exhibiting a favorable treatment response (TRG 0, 1, 2 group, $p = 0.17$; TRG 3, 4 group, $p < 0.01$) [21]. Additionally, another study demonstrated a noteworthy association between the levels of cell-free DNA and the presence of recurrent disease. Patients with recurrent disease displayed a median level of 13,000 copies/mL, in contrast to the 5200 copies/mL observed in non-recurrent patients ($p = 0.08$). This investigation also established a correlation between the total cell-free DNA levels and both the pathological stage and nodal involvement [22].

In our study, we established a control group comprising breast cancer patients undergoing adjuvant radiation therapy (RT). Our hypothesis was that following neoadjuvant therapy and mastectomy, most tumor cells would be eliminated. Adjuvant RT was then administered to irradiate healthy breast tissue with minimal residual tumor cells. Our study highlights a distinction between the breast cancer group, characterized by a limited tumor burden, and the cervical cancer group, which exhibits a more substantial tumor burden and is known for its favorable response to chemoradiation.

Before radiation therapy, cfDNA levels in the breast cancer group ranged from 133.90 to 10,241.20 pg/μL, with an average of 1494.92 pg/μL. In the cervical cancer group, the range was from 300.80 to 22,660.00 pg/μL, with an average of 3063.26 pg/μL. On the 5th day post-treatment, cfDNA levels in the breast cancer group ranged from 62.30 to 6196.50 pg/μL, while the cervical cancer group exhibited a wider range and a higher average (range: 176.80–13,105.90 pg/μL, average: 2192.03 pg/μL).

The objective of our study was to investigate quantitative variations in circulating free DNA (cfDNA) in patients diagnosed with locally advanced rectal cancer who underwent neoadjuvant long-course chemoradiation. We hypothesize that there may be changes in DNA fragment release during therapeutic stress. To achieve our goal, we established two control groups representing the upper and lower limits of cfDNA levels. Our aim is to differentiate between patients who will respond favorably to neoadjuvant long-course chemoradiation and those who will not. To accomplish this, we worked to establish a correlation between the difference in cfDNA levels before and on the 5th day of radiation treatment and the tumor regression grade (TRG) determined through pathological examination of surgically removed tumor specimens.

Unfortunately, among the initial cohort of thirteen patients who initiated neoadjuvant radiochemotherapy, only six patients ultimately underwent surgical resection. Notably, one patient exhibited a complete pathological response classified as Dworak 4, while the remaining patients demonstrated suboptimal responses, with three patients categorized as Dworak 1 and two patients as Dworak 2. Among the seven patients who did not undergo surgery, three were deemed ineligible for surgical intervention due to the presence of metastasis or locally advanced disease, while the unfortunate outcome was observed in four patients who succumbed to causes unrelated to their oncological condition.

Truelsen et al. from Elsevier propose that circulating cell-free DNA (cfDNA) can serve as a valuable biomarker and complementary tool to imaging in identifying candidates for a Wait and Watch (W&W) strategy among patients who have achieved a clinical complete response (cCR). They suggest that patients characterized as "cfDNA responders" may have an association with achieving a pathological complete response (pCR). In their investigation, cfDNA samples were collected at baseline, during the midpoint of therapy, and at the conclusion of treatment [7].

In contrast, our study adopted a different approach by collecting cfDNA samples before the initiation of radiation therapy and after the fifth session of radiation. The primary objective was to acquire early results that could assist in distinguishing patients who are unlikely to respond favorably to chemoradiation therapy. This approach sought to identify poor or non-responders at an early stage and to mitigate treatment-related toxicity [23] and reduce the extended waiting period, typically spanning 6–8 weeks after neoadjuvant therapy, before commencing surgical intervention.

In the subgroup of our study (Tables 2 and 5), in one patient who achieved a pathological complete response (pCR) before undergoing radiation therapy, the cfDNA level was measured at 137.80 pg/μL before treatment and a slight increase to 175.70 pg/μL after the fifth session, resulting in a difference of 37.90 pg/μL and a ratio of 1.28. For patients classified as Dworak 1 and 2, the cfDNA levels ranged from 70.90 pg/μL to 828.50 pg/μL before radiation therapy, with an average of 470.64 pg/μL. The average difference in cfDNA levels was 210.14 pg/μL, and the ratio was 2.54. Among patients who did not undergo surgery due to the presence of metastasis or locally advanced disease, baseline cfDNA levels ranged from 136.20 pg/μL to 327.50 pg/μL, with an average of 231.85 pg/μL. After the fifth session of radiation therapy, cfDNA levels ranged from 359.50 pg/μL to 1957.2 pg/μL, with an average of 1158.35 pg/μL. The average ratio was 7.73 and the average difference was 926.5 pg/μL. Noticeably, higher differences and ratios were observed in patients who were not eligible for surgical treatment. However, due to the limited size of our cohort, our study was unable to establish statistically significant results.

Table 5. Data between cfDNA (pg/μL), tumor volume (mm^3) and TRG. Key: RT, radiation therapy; GTV, gross target volume; PTV, planning target volume; TRG, tumor regression grade.

Sample	Pathological Response	cfDNA before RT	cfDNA 5th Day RT	Difference between cfDNA 5th Day RT and cfDNA before RT	GTV	PTV
R42	Complete respond TRG 4	137.80	175.70	37.90	68.87	2177.66
R50	Dworak TRG1	828.50	818.80	−9.70	86.54	1502.27
R51	Dworak TRG 1	595.70	1150.10	554.40	66.73	1633.77
R52	Dworak TRG2	80.60	72.50	−8.10	60.92	1463.40
R53	Dworak TRG2	777.50	804.00	26.50	83.79	2910.00
R61	Dworak TRG 1	70.90	558.50	487.60	83.63	2716.50

Cellular necrosis and apoptosis represent the primary sources of circulating cell-free DNA in plasma following radiation. Another plausible hypothesis involves exploring the correlation between cfDNA, tumor volume and the planning target volume. Several studies have yielded positive findings regarding the relationship between cfDNA levels and tumor size. All of our locally advanced rectal cancer patients underwent long-course radiotherapy (50.4 Gy/28F/5w), either with or without concomitant capecitabine at 850 mg/m^2 twice daily (BID). By maintaining this control variable, we aimed to establish a positive association between tumor size (GTV), planning target volume (PTV), and cfDNA quantity after the initiation of radiation.

Regrettably, despite all patients experiencing a reduction in tumor size following neoadjuvant chemoradiotherapy, no clear relationship between cfDNA and gross tumor volume (GTV), planning target volume (PTV), and tumor regression grade (TRG) was discerned [24]. This lack of correlation may be attributed to the insufficient number of samples and the timing of sample collection. It is conceivable that, on the 5th day post-radiotherapy, a substantial quantity of cfDNA has not yet been released, necessitating a more extended monitoring period to capture a significant release of cfDNA during and after the completion of radiotherapy. This consideration aligns with evidence indicating that tumors continue to respond to radiotherapy for at least two months after treatment completion. Other studies have taken a weekly sampling approach during radiotherapy, correlating the cumulative cfDNA levels with TRG or distinguishing between complete responders and non-responders [25]. Similarly, Truelsen et al. collected cfDNA samples at the onset, midpoint, and conclusion of radiotherapy, subsequently comparing the mean values of these samples using ROC curve analysis in relation to TRG [7].

This study recognizes the need for further research to address the current limitations of cfDNA analysis and enhance its prognostic utility in rectal cancer. It underscores the importance of conducting larger, more comprehensive studies to validate these findings and optimize cfDNA analysis as a prognostic tool for rectal cancer.

5. Conclusions

cfDNA does not seem to predict response to neoadjuvant chemoradiotherapy and it is not correlated to tumor volume or tumor regression grade.

Author Contributions: Conceptualization, W.L.O. and G.D.; Methodology, I.I. (Iuliu Ivanov); Software, A.-M.M.; Validation, N.V., S.L. and G.D.; Formal Analysis, S.M., S.I.; Investigation, A.P. and C.E.R.; Resources, I.I. (Irina Iftincai) and A.M.; Data Curation, A.-M.M. and G.D.; Writing—Original Draft Preparation, W.L.O.; Writing—Review and Editing, S.M. and G.D.; Visualization, G.D.; Supervision, G.D. and S.L.; Project Administration, W.L.O. and S.M.; Funding Acquisition, G.D. All authors have read and agreed to the published version of the manuscript.

Funding: The authors disclosed receipt of the following financial support for the research, authorship, and/or publication of this article: Roche Romania SRL.

Institutional Review Board Statement: The study was approved by the Ethics Committee of Regional Institute of Oncology (IRO), Iasi, Romania (protocol code REGISTRATION NUMBER. 227/26 August 2019).

Informed Consent Statement: Informed consent was obtained from all subjects involved in the study. Written informed consent has been obtained from the patient(s) to publish this paper.

Data Availability Statement: The data that support the findings of this study are available on request from the corresponding author, S.M.

Conflicts of Interest: The authors declare no conflict of interest. The funders had no role in the design of the study; in the collection, analyses, or interpretation of data; in the writing of the manuscript; or in the decision to publish the results.

References

1. Yan, Y.Y.; Guo, Q.R.; Wang, F.H.; Adhikari, R.; Zhu, Z.Y.; Zhang, H.Y.; Zhou, W.M.; Yu, H.; Li, J.Q.; Zhang, J.Y. Cell-Free DNA: Hope and Potential Application in Cancer. *Front. Cell Dev. Biol.* **2021**, *9*, 639233.
2. Kasi, A.; Abbasi, S.; Handa, S.; Al-Rajabi, R.; Saeed, A.; Baranda, J.; Sun, W. Total Neoadjuvant Therapy vs Standard Therapy in Locally Advanced Rectal Cancer. *JAMA Netw. Open* **2020**, *3*, e2030097. [PubMed]
3. Hartley, A.; Ho, K.F.; McConkey, C.; Geh, J.I. Pathological complete response following pre-operative chemoradiotherapy in rectal cancer: Analysis of phase II/III trials. *Br. J. Radiol.* **2005**, *78*, 934–938. [CrossRef] [PubMed]
4. Ceelen, W.; Fierens, K.; Van Nieuwenhove, Y.; Pattyn, P. Preoperative chemoradiation versus radiation alone for stage II and III resectable rectal cancer: A systematic review and meta-analysis. *Int. J. Cancer* **2009**, *124*, 2966–2972. [CrossRef]
5. Johnson, G.G.; Park, J.; Helewa, R.M.; Goldenberg, B.A.; Nashed, M.; Hyun, E. Total neoadjuvant therapy for rectal cancer: A guide for surgeons. *Can. J. Surg.* **2023**, *66*, E196–E201. [CrossRef]
6. Vymetalkova, V.; Cervena, K.; Bartu, L.; Vodicka, P. Circulating Cell-Free DNA and Colorectal Cancer: A Systematic Review. *Int. J. Mol. Sci.* **2018**, *19*, 3356. [CrossRef]
7. Truelsen, C.G.; Kronborg, C.S.; Sørensen, B.S.; Callesen, L.B.; Spindler, K.-L.G. Circulating cell-free DNA as predictor of pathological complete response in locally advanced rectal cancer patients undergoing preoperative chemoradiotherapy. *Clin. Transl. Radiat. Oncol.* **2022**, *36*, 9–15.
8. Li, M.; Xiao, Q.; Venkatachalam, N.; Hofheinz, R.D.; Veldwijk, M.R.; Herskind, C.; Ebert, M.P.; Zhan, T. Predicting response to neoadjuvant chemoradiotherapy in rectal cancer: From biomarkers to tumor models. *Ther. Adv. Med. Oncol.* **2022**, *14*, 17588359221077972. [CrossRef]
9. Peled, M.; Agassi, R.; Czeiger, D.; Ariad, S.; Riff, R.; Rosenthal, M.; Lazarev, I.; Novack, V.; Yarza, S.; Mizrakli, Y.; et al. Cell-free DNA concentration in patients with clinical or mammographic suspicion of breast cancer. *Sci. Rep.* **2020**, *10*, 14601.
10. Cercek, A.; Lumish, M.; Sinopoli, J.; Weiss, J.; Shia, J.; Lamendola-Essel, M.; El Dika, I.H.; Segal, N.; Shcherba, M.; Sugarman, R.; et al. PD-1 Blockade in Mismatch Repair–Deficient, Locally Advanced Rectal Cancer. *N. Engl. J. Med.* **2022**, *386*, 2363–2376.
11. De Rosa, N.; Rodriguez-Bigas, M.A.; Chang, G.J.; Veerapong, J.; Borras, E.; Krishnan, S.; Bednarski, B.; Messick, C.A.; Skibber, J.M.; Feig, B.W.; et al. DNA Mismatch Repair Deficiency in Rectal Cancer: Benchmarking Its Impact on Prognosis, Neoadjuvant Response Prediction, and Clinical Cancer Genetics. *J. Clin. Oncol.* **2016**, *34*, 3039–3046. [CrossRef] [PubMed]

12. Deschoolmeester, V.; Baay, M.; Lardon, F.; Pauwels, P.; Peeters, M. Immune Cells in Colorectal Cancer: Prognostic Relevance and Role of MSI. *Cancer Microenviron.* **2011**, *4*, 377–392. [CrossRef] [PubMed]
13. Morais, M.; Pinto, D.M.; Machado, J.C.; Carneiro, S. ctDNA on liquid biopsy for predicting response and prognosis in locally advanced rectal cancer: A systematic review. *Eur. J. Surg. Oncol.* **2022**, *48*, 218–227. [CrossRef] [PubMed]
14. Shtumpf, M.; Piroeva, K.V.; Agrawal, S.P.; Jacob, D.R.; Teif, V.B. NucPosDB: A database of nucleosome positioning in vivo and nucleosomics of cell-free DNA. *Chromosoma* **2022**, *131*, 19–28. [CrossRef]
15. Dang, D.K.; Park, B.H. Circulating tumor DNA: Current challenges for clinical utility. *J. Clin. Investig.* **2022**, *132*, e154941. [CrossRef]
16. Mandel, P.; Metais, P. Nuclear Acids in Human Blood Plasma. *Comptes Rendus des Seances de la Soc. de Biol. et de ses Fil.* **1948**, *142*, 241–243.
17. Bhangu, J.S.; Taghizadeh, H.; Braunschmid, T.; Bachleitner-Hofmann, T.; Mannhalter, C. Circulating cell-free DNA in plasma of colorectal cancer patients—A potential biomarker for tumor burden. *Surg. Oncol.* **2017**, *26*, 395–401. [CrossRef]
18. Hu, Z.; Chen, H.; Long, Y.; Li, P.; Gu, Y. The main sources of circulating cell-free DNA: Apoptosis, necrosis and active secretion. *Crit. Rev. Oncol. Hematol.* **2021**, *157*, 103166. [CrossRef]
19. Zitt, M.; Müller, H.M.; Rochel, M.; Schwendinger, V.; Zitt, M.; Goebel, G.; DeVries, A.; Margreiter, R.; Oberwalder, M.; Zeillinger, R.; et al. Circulating Cell-Free DNA in Plasma of Locally Advanced Rectal Cancer Patients Undergoing Preoperative Chemoradiation: A Potential Diagnostic Tool for Therapy Monitoring. *Dis. Markers* **2008**, *25*, 159–165. [CrossRef]
20. Agostini, M.; Pucciarelli, S.; Enzo, M.V.; Del Bianco, P.; Briarava, M.; Bedin, C.; Maretto, I.; Friso, M.L.; Lonardi, S.; Mescoli, C.; et al. Circulating Cell-Free DNA: A Promising Marker of Pathologic Tumor Response in Rectal Cancer Patients Receiving Preoperative Chemoradiotherapy. *Ann. Surg. Oncol.* **2011**, *18*, 2461–2468. [CrossRef]
21. Sun, W.; Sun, Y.; Zhu, M.; Wang, Z.; Zhang, H.; Xin, Y.; Jiang, G.; Guo, X.; Zhang, Z.; Liu, Y. The role of plasma cell-free DNA detection in predicting preoperative chemoradiotherapy response in rectal cancer patients. *Oncol. Rep.* **2014**, *31*, 1466–1472. [CrossRef] [PubMed]
22. Van Rees, J.M.; Wullaert, L.; Grüter, A.A.J.; Derraze, Y.; Tanis, P.J.; Verheul, H.M.W.; Martens, J.W.M.; Wilting, S.M.; Vink, G.; van Vugt, J.L.A.; et al. Circulating tumour DNA as biomarker for rectal cancer: A systematic review and meta-analyses. *Front. Oncol.* **2023**, *13*, 1083285. [CrossRef] [PubMed]
23. Kumar, A.R.; Sanford, N.N. Toxicity Management in the Era of Changing Treatment Paradigms for Locally Advanced Rectal Cancer. *Curr. Color. Cancer Rep.* **2022**, *18*, 55–59. [CrossRef] [PubMed]
24. Bredno, J.; Lipson, J.; Venn, O.; Aravanis, A.M.; Jamshidi, A. Clinical correlates of circulating cell-free DNA tumor fraction. *PLoS ONE* **2021**, *16*, e0256436. [CrossRef] [PubMed]
25. Kageyama, S.I.; Nihei, K.; Karasawa, K.; Sawada, T.; Koizumi, F.; Yamaguchi, S.; Kato, S.; Hojo, H.; Motegi, A.; Tsuchihara, K.; et al. Radiotherapy increases plasma levels of tumoral cell-free DNA in non-small cell lung cancer patients. *Oncotarget* **2018**, *9*, 19368–19378. [CrossRef]

Disclaimer/Publisher's Note: The statements, opinions and data contained in all publications are solely those of the individual author(s) and contributor(s) and not of MDPI and/or the editor(s). MDPI and/or the editor(s) disclaim responsibility for any injury to people or property resulting from any ideas, methods, instructions or products referred to in the content.

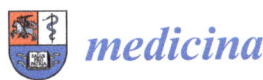

Article

Comparison of Open versus Laparoscopic Approaches in Salvage Hepatectomy for Recurrent Hepatocellular Carcinoma after Radiofrequency Ablation

Yeshong Park, Jai Young Cho *, Ho-Seong Han, Yoo-Seok Yoon, Hae Won Lee, Boram Lee, MeeYoung Kang and Jinju Kim

Department of Surgery, Seoul National University Bundang Hospital, Seoul National University College of Medicine, Seoul 03080, Republic of Korea; 82637@snubh.org (M.K.)
* Correspondence: jychogs@gmail.com; Tel.: +82-31-787-7096

Abstract: *Background and Objectives*: Although radiofrequency ablation (RFA) is widely used as an effective local treatment for hepatocellular carcinoma (HCC), evidence on salvage hepatectomy for local recurrence after RFA is limited. This study aims to compare open and laparoscopic approaches in salvage hepatectomy for recurrent HCC after RFA. *Materials and Methods*: Among patients who underwent hepatectomy between January 2004 and August 2022 at a single tertiary referral center, 55 patients who underwent salvage hepatectomy for marginal recurrence after RFA were selected. An open approach was used in 23 (41.8%) patients, while 32 (58.2%) patients underwent laparoscopic surgery. Short-term and long-term outcomes were compared between the two groups. *Results*: Major hepatectomy was more often performed in the open group (9 [39.1%] vs. 4 [12.5%], $p = 0.022$). Intraoperative blood loss was also greater in the open group (450 [325–750] vs. 300 [200–600], $p = 0.034$). Operation time ($p = 0.144$) and postoperative morbidity rates ($p = 0.639$) were similar, and there was no postoperative mortality in either group. Postoperative hospital stay was significantly longer in the open group compared to the laparoscopy group (8 [6–11] days vs. 5 [4–7] days, $p = 0.028$). The 1-, 3-, and 5-year disease-free survival rates showed no difference between the two groups (44.6% vs. 62.5%, 16.5% vs. 13.5%, and 8.3% vs. 13.5%, respectively; $p = 0.154$). The 1-, 3-, and 5-year overall survival rates between the two groups were also similar (85.7% vs. 96.8%, 79.6% vs. 86.0%, and 79.6% vs. 79.4%, respectively; $p = 0.480$). *Conclusions*: Laparoscopic salvage hepatectomy shows oncologic outcomes comparable to the open approach with faster postoperative recovery rates. Considering that recurrence rates are high after RFA, the laparoscopic approach should be considered as a first-line option in selected patients.

Keywords: hepatocellular carcinoma; radiofrequency ablation; salvage hepatectomy; laparoscopic liver resection

Citation: Park, Y.; Cho, J.Y.; Han, H.-S.; Yoon, Y.-S.; Lee, H.W.; Lee, B.; Kang, M.; Kim, J. Comparison of Open versus Laparoscopic Approaches in Salvage Hepatectomy for Recurrent Hepatocellular Carcinoma after Radiofrequency Ablation. *Medicina* **2023**, *59*, 1243. https://doi.org/10.3390/medicina59071243

Academic Editors: Valentin Titus Grigorean and Daniel Alin Cristian

Received: 1 June 2023
Revised: 24 June 2023
Accepted: 3 July 2023
Published: 4 July 2023

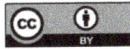

Copyright: © 2023 by the authors. Licensee MDPI, Basel, Switzerland. This article is an open access article distributed under the terms and conditions of the Creative Commons Attribution (CC BY) license (https://creativecommons.org/licenses/by/4.0/).

1. Introduction

Treatment selection for hepatocellular carcinoma (HCC) is based on various factors including disease stage, underlying liver condition, and the performance status of the patient. Local ablation techniques including radiofrequency ablation (RFA) are accepted as curative therapeutic options for very early and early-stage HCC [1–3]. However, marginal recurrence after RFA has been reported in 2% to 36% of patients, and high recurrence rates are generally known to affect long-term survival after RFA [4,5].

Most patients experiencing recurrence after RFA are treated with repeated local ablation or transcatheter arterial chemoembolization (TACE) [6]. Surgical treatment for recurred tumors, referred to as salvage hepatectomy, has also been reported as an acceptable treatment option [4,7–9]. Previous studies found the survival benefit of salvage hepatectomy to be comparable to primary hepatic resection with similar overall survival rates [4,7]. Yet the technical feasibility of salvage hepatectomy has been challenged; RFA procedures might cause dense adhesions that render the approach for liver mobilization extremely difficult, and more extensive resections might be necessary due to advanced-stage tumors [7,8].

Since its introduction, laparoscopic liver resection has been associated with better short-term outcomes and similar oncologic survival compared to the open approach [10–12]. Due to advances in minimally invasive techniques and surgical strategies, the indication for laparoscopic surgery has been extended to tumors in difficult locations, underlying advanced cirrhosis, and elderly patients with multiple comorbidities [13–15]. Yet the role of laparoscopic surgery in salvage hepatectomy for local recurrence after RFA has never been addressed. The aim of this study was to compare the short-term and long-term outcomes of open and laparoscopic salvage hepatectomy for recurrent HCC after RFA.

2. Materials and Methods

2.1. Study Population

Between January 2004 and August 2022, 1235 patients underwent hepatectomy for HCC at Seoul National University Bundang Hospital (SNUBH), a tertiary referral hospital in Korea. Among them, 60 consecutive patients who underwent salvage hepatectomy for marginal recurrence after RFA were selected. Five patients who underwent open conversion were excluded from the analysis. Finally, 23 patients who underwent open salvage hepatectomy and 32 patients who received laparoscopic salvage hepatectomy were compared (Figure 1). This study was approved by the institutional review boards of SNUBH and conducted in compliance with the STROBE guidelines for cohort studies.

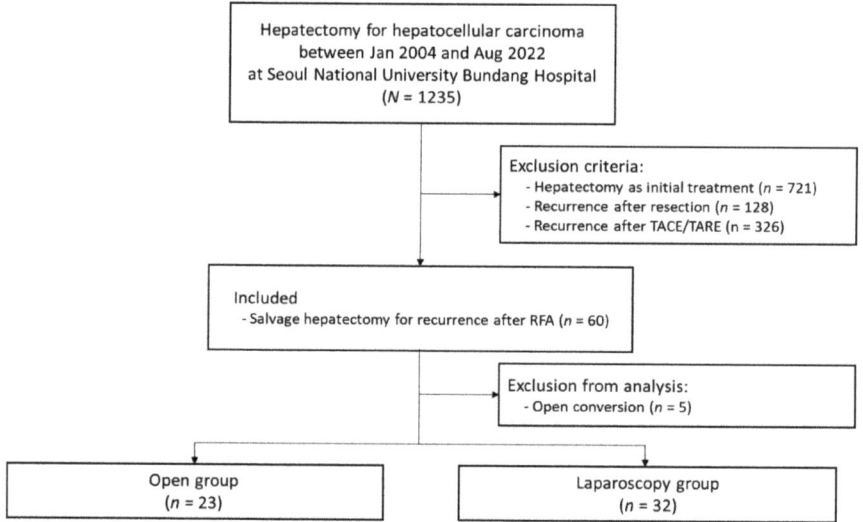

Figure 1. Flowchart diagram for patient selection.

2.2. Data Collection and Definitions

Demographic information, information related to operative data, information on pathological features, and survival data were collected from medical records. The terminology used for the hepatectomy procedures was based on Couinaud's classification [16]. Major hepatectomy was defined as the resection of three or more liver segments, and minor hepatectomy was defined as sectionectomy, segmentectomy, or non-anatomical liver wedge resection. Estimated blood loss was based on visual estimation at the end of surgery by both the surgeon and the anesthesiologist. Morbidities were graded by the Clavien–Dindo classification system [17]. In-hospital death was defined as death at any time during hospital stay.

2.3. Surgical Procedure

The decision on surgical approach was made individually based on tumor characteristics including size, number, and location and patient factors including liver cirrhosis, underlying disease, and history of previous abdominal operations. Open and laparoscopic salvage hepatectomies were performed by the same team with standardized operation procedures that were not influenced by the surgical approach. In open hepatectomy, the patient was placed in the supine position under general anesthesia. An upper midline incision with a right extension was used. Intraoperative ultrasound examinations were utilized to confirm the location and size of the tumor and its location in relation to major vessels. A Cavitron ultrasonic surgical aspirator (CUSA; Valleylab, Boulder, CO, USA) was used for liver parenchymal transection. Hemostasis was pursued through the use of monopolar or bipolar electrocautery, argon beam, or sutures. Abdominal drains were routinely placed at the hepatic resection margin.

In laparoscopic hepatectomy, the patient was placed in the lithotomy position. A subumbilical 12 mm trocar was used as the camera port. All operations were performed with a three-dimensional flexible tip laparoscope. Three to four additional working ports were placed in consideration of the tumor's location and size. Ultrasound examination was performed in the same manner as for the open approach. An ultrasonic dissector (Harmonic; Ethicon, Cincinnati, OH, USA) was used for adhesiolysis, liver mobilization, and superficial liver parenchymal transection; for deeper dissection, CUSA was used as in open hepatectomy. Hemostasis was performed with monopolar electrocautery, metal clips, or sutures. The liver specimen was delivered through an extension of the subumbilical incision. Abdominal drains were placed using the 5 mm trocar sites at the hepatic resection margin.

2.4. Follow-Up

All of the patients underwent regular follow-up with clinical examination, measurement of serum tumor markers including α-fetoprotein (AFP) and des-γ-carboxyprothrombin (DCP), and imaging studies including computed tomography (CT) or gadoxetic-acid-enhanced magnetic resonance imaging (MRI). Recurrence was defined as the appearance of a new lesion with radiologic features typical of HCC. The median time to recurrence after RFA was 9 months. Disease-free survival was defined as the interval between the operation and the date of first recurrence. Overall survival was defined as the interval between the operation and the date of cancer-related death or the last follow-up. The median follow-up duration was 33 months.

2.5. Statistical Analysis

All statistical analyses were performed using SPSS (version 25.0, IBM Inc., Armonk, NY, USA). Categorical data were expressed as frequency (percentage). Continuous variables were expressed as the mean ± standard deviation for normally distributed variables or as the median (interquartile range) for non-normally distributed variables. Continuous variables were compared using Student's t-test or the Mann–Whitney U test; categorical variables were compared using Pearson's chi-square test or Fisher's exact test. Survival analysis was conducted with the Kaplan–Meier method and log-rank test. Prognosis factors for survival were investigated using univariable and multivariable Cox regression analyses. All p-values were two-sided, and $p < 0.05$ was considered statistically significant.

3. Results

3.1. Patient Characteristics

The clinical characteristics of the study participants are summarized in Table 1. The open and laparoscopic salvage hepatectomy groups showed no statistically significant difference in age, sex, body mass index (BMI), and operation history. Baseline liver functions including Child–Pugh class, Model for End-Stage Liver Disease (MELD) score, platelet count, prothrombin time, and serum albumin level were similar between the two groups. Tumor marker levels also showed no difference.

Table 1. Baseline characteristics of the study participants.

	Open (n = 23)	Laparoscopy (n = 32)	Total (n = 55)	p-Value
Age (years)	61 (53–69)	63 (54–68)	62 (54–68)	0.755
Sex (male:female)	21:2	28:4	49:6	0.999
BMI (kg/m^2, mean ± SD)	24.0 ± 3.6	24.9 ± 2.6	24.6 ± 3.1	0.276
Hypertension	11 (47.8)	13 (40.6)	24 (43.6)	0.798
Diabetes	5 (21.7)	12 (37.5)	17 (30.9)	0.341
Cardiovascular disease	1 (4.3)	1 (3.1)	2 (3.6)	>0.999
Hepatitis B	18 (78.3)	27 (84.4)	45 (81.8)	0.726
Hepatitis C	4 (17.4)	2 (6.3)	6 (10.9)	0.223
Alcoholic	3 (13.0)	5 (15.6)	8 (14.5)	>0.999
Previous abdominal operation	8 (34.8)	12 (37.5)	20 (36.4)	>0.999
Child–Pugh class				0.418
A	22 (95.7)	32 (100)	54 (98.2)	
B	1 (4.3)	0	1 (1.8)	
MELD score	7.2 (6.8–8.4)	7.2 (6.8–8.2)	7.2 (6.8–8.4)	0.746
Platelet count (10^4/uL)	180 (100–242)	158 (117–194)	161 (113–226)	0.379
Prothrombin time (INR)	1.03 (1.01–1.11)	1.05 (1.00–1.10)	1.04 (1.01–1.10)	0.850
Total bilirubin (mg/dL)	0.76 (0.50–1.11)	0.71 (0.62–1.10)	0.71 (0.60–1.10)	0.374
Serum albumin (g/dL)	4.3 (4.1–4.7)	4.3 (3.9–4.5)	4.3 (4.0–4.6)	0.276
AFP (ng/mL)	18.5 (2.8–137.5)	4.5 (3.2–51.0)	7.1 (3.0–59.3)	0.256
DCP (AU/mL)	27 (19–65)	24 (16–77)	25 (17–69)	0.836

BMI, body mass index; SD, standard deviation; MELD, Model for End-Stage Liver Disease; INR, international normalized ratio; AFP, alpha-fetoprotein; DCP, des-gamma-carboxy prothrombin. The values are presented as the median (interquartile range) or n (%) unless otherwise indicated.

3.2. Operative Parameters

The operative parameters were compared between the open and laparoscopy groups (Table 2). Major hepatectomy was more frequently performed during open salvage hepatectomy (9 [39.1%] vs. 4 [12.5%], p = 0.049). There was no difference in anatomical resection rate, operation time, and duration of the Pringle maneuver. The open conversion rate in the laparoscopic group was 13.5% (5/37), with severe adhesion in three patients, intraoperative vital instability in one patient, and difficulty in securing the resection margin in one patient. Estimated blood loss was greater in the open group (450 (325–750) vs. 300 (200–600), p = 0.034), but the intraoperative transfusion rates were similar between the two groups.

Table 2. Comparison of operative parameters.

	Open (n = 23)	Laparoscopy (n = 32)	Total (n = 55)	p-Value
Operative extent				0.049
Major resection	9 (39.1)	4 (12.5)	13 (23.6)	
Minor resection	14 (60.9)	28 (87.5)	42 (76.4)	
Anatomical resection	12 (52.2)	11 (34.4)	23 (41.8)	0.297
Deviation from the initial plan				0.604
More extensive resection	10 (43.5)	10 (31.3)	20 (36.4)	
Less extensive resection	1 (4.3)	1 (3.1)	2 (3.6)	
Operation time (min)	230 (163–308)	153 (108–293)	220 (125–305)	0.144
Pringle time (min)	20 (15–30)	40 (23–60)	30 (15–45)	0.111
Estimated blood loss (cc)	450 (325–750)	300 (200–600)	350 (300–700)	0.034
RBC transfusion	3 (13.0)	3 (9.4)	6 (10.9)	>0.999

RBC, red blood cell. The values are presented as median (interquartile range) or n (%) unless otherwise indicated.

3.3. Pathologic Features and Postoperative Outcomes

When pathological data of the two groups were compared, there was no difference in tumor location, tumor number, tumor grade, vascular invasion rate, or margin status (Table 3). The tumor size was larger in the open salvage hepatectomy group (3.0 [1.9–3.5] vs. 2.0 [1.2–3.0], $p = 0.049$). In the analysis of postoperative outcomes, no statistically significant difference in postoperative complication rates or intensive care unit admission was found. There were no in-hospital deaths in either group. Postoperative hospital stay was significantly shorter in the laparoscopy group (8 [6–11] vs. 5 [4–7], $p = 0.028$).

Table 3. Comparison of pathological features and postoperative outcomes.

	Open ($n = 23$)	Laparoscopy ($n = 32$)	Total ($n = 55$)	p-Value
Tumor location				0.655
Anterolateral	16 (69.6)	24 (75.0)	40 (72.7)	
Posterosuperior	7 (30.4)	8 (25.0)	15 (27.3)	
Tumor number	1 (1–1)	1 (1–1)	1 (1–1)	0.592
Tumor size (cm)	3.0 (1.9–3.5)	2.0 (1.2–3.0)	2.6 (1.5–3.2)	0.049
Edmonson grade				0.555
1	0	1 (3.4)	1 (1.8)	
2	8 (40.0)	8 (27.6)	16 (29.1)	
3	8 (40.0)	16 (55.2)	24 (43.6)	
4	4 (20.0)	4 (13.8)	8 (14.5)	
Vascular invasion				
Macrovascular	5 (21.7)	2 (6.9)	7 (12.7)	0.251
Microvascular	11 (47.8)	10 (34.5)	21 (38.2)	0.491
Margin status				>0.999
R0	20 (87.0)	26 (89.7)	46 (88.5)	
R1	3 (13.0)	3 (10.3)	6 (11.5)	
Liver cirrhosis	10 (43.5)	17 (53.1)	27 (49.1)	0.480
Complication	4 (17.4)	3 (9.4)	7 (13.2)	0.639
Angina	0	1 (3.1)	1 (1.7)	
Pleural effusion	2 (8.7)	0	3 (5.0)	
Pulmonary thromboembolism	1 (4.3)	0	1 (1.7)	
Bile leakage	2 (8.7)	2 (6.2)	5 (8.3)	
Post-hepatectomy liver failure	1 (4.3)	0	1 (1.7)	
Ileus	0	1 (3.1)	1 (1.7)	
Clavien–Dindo grade ≥ IIIa complication	3 (14.3)	1 (3.1)	4 (7.5)	0.289
Intensive care unit stay	1 (4.8)	3 (9.4)	4 (7.5)	0.999
In-hospital death	0	0	0	-
Postoperative hospital stay (day)	8 (6–11)	5 (4–7)	6 (5–9)	0.028
Follow-up (months)	28 (16–95)	36 (19–74)	33 (18–74)	0.999
Recurrence				
Local recurrence	11 (47.8)	21 (65.6)	32 (58.2)	0.187
Systemic recurrence	11 (47.8)	9 (28.1)	20 (36.4)	0.134
Cancer-related death	5 (21.7)	8 (25.0)	13 (23.6)	0.779

The values are presented as the median (interquartile range) or n (%) unless otherwise indicated.

3.4. Survival Outcomes

The overall 1-, 3-, and 5-year DFS rates of the study population were 48.7, 32.5%, and 26.2%, respectively. The recurrence rates showed no statistically significant difference between the open and laparoscopic salvage hepatectomy groups for either local recurrence (11 [47.8%] vs. 21 [65.6%], $p = 0.187$) or systemic recurrence (11 [47.8%] vs. 9 [28.1%], $p = 0.134$). There was no difference in the 1-, 3-, and 5-year DFS rates between the two groups (44.6% vs. 62.5%, 16.5% vs. 13.5%, and 8.3% vs. 13.5%, respectively; $p = 0.154$). The overall 1-, 3-, and 5-year OS rates of the study population were 93.0%, 81.9%, and 78.0%, respectively. The cancer-related death rates were similar between the two groups (5 [21.7%] vs. 8 [25.0%], $p = 0.779$). The difference in the 1-, 3-, and 5-year overall survival rates between the two groups was also not statistically significant (85.7% vs. 96.8%, 79.6% vs. 86.0%, and 79.6% vs. 79.4%, respectively; $p = 0.480$). The cumulative disease-free and overall survival curves are shown in Figure 2.

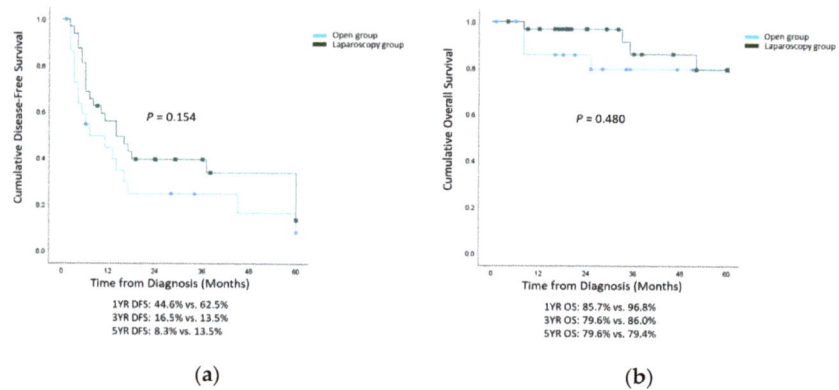

(a) (b)

Figure 2. Kaplan–Meier survival curves for disease-free and overall survival. (**a**) 5-year disease-free survival and (**b**) 5-year overall survival.

3.5. Risk Factor Analysis for Recurrence after RFA

Cox regression analysis was conducted to analyze risk factors for recurrence after RFA (Table 4). Tumor number was the only significant predictor for recurrence (hazard ratio [HR] 3.05, $p = 0.009$). In the univariable Cox regression analysis of risk factors for cancer-related death, Child–Pugh class, tumor number, tumor grade, and vascular invasion were found to be significant. In the multivariable analysis, tumor number (HR 8.34, $p = 0.009$), tumor grade (HR 17.98, $p = 0.008$), and vascular invasion (HR 8.19, $p = 0.014$) remained as prognostic factors.

Table 4. Cox regression analyses for recurrence and cancer-related death after RFA.

	Disease-Free Survival		Overall Survival			
	Univariable		Univariable		Multivariable	
	HR (95% CI)	*p*-Value	HR (95% CI)	*p*-Value	HR (95% CI)	*p*-Value
Sex						
Male	Ref.		Ref.			
Female	0.86 (0.30–2.42)	0.768	0.72 (0.09–5.53)	0.751		
Age (years)						
<60	Ref.		Ref.			
≥60	1.41 (0.71–2.80)	0.332	1.29 (0.42–3.96)	0.655		
Child–Pugh class						
A	Ref.		Ref.		Ref.	
B	4.44 (0.57–34.37)	0.154	11.58 (1.29–104.25)	0.029	7.59 (0.62–92.41)	0.112
AFP (ng/mL)						
<200	Ref.		Ref.			
≥200	0.94 (0.33–2.67)	0.912	1.45 (0.32–6.53)	0.633		
Operative method						
Open	Ref.		Ref.			
Laparoscopic	0.62 (0.32–1.18)	0.145	0.94 (0.31–2.88)	0.913		

Table 4. Cont.

	Disease-Free Survival		Overall Survival			
	Univariable		Univariable		Multivariable	
	HR (95% CI)	p-Value	HR (95% CI)	p-Value	HR (95% CI)	p-Value
Operative extent						
Minor resection	Ref.		Ref.			
Major resection	0.84 (0.38–1.84)	0.660	1.43 (0.39–5.26)	0.592		
Tumor location						
Anterolateral	Ref.		Ref.			
Posterosuperior	1.06 (0.53–2.16)	0.864	0.43 (0.10–1.95)	0.275		
Tumor number						
<3	Ref.		Ref.		Ref.	
≥3	3.05 (1.31–7.08)	0.009	3.41 (1.11–10.44)	0.032	8.34 (1.70–40.92)	0.009
Tumor size (cm)						
<3.0	Ref.		Ref.			
≥3.0	0.85 (0.44–1.64)	0.620	0.40 (0.12–1.32)	0.131		
Tumor grade						
Good/moderate	Ref.		Ref.		Ref.	
Poor	2.00 (0.92–4.34)	0.079	8.57 (1.51–48.78)	0.015	17.98 (2.15–150.59)	0.008
Vascular invasion						
No	Ref.		Ref.		Ref.	
Yes	1.38 (0.53–3.60)	0.508	3.47 (1.04–11.55)	0.043	8.19 (1.54–43.45)	0.014
Resection status						
R0	Ref.		Ref.			
R1	2.80 (0.84–9.36)	0.095	5.11 (0.53–49.14)	0.158		

HR, hazard ratio; CI, confidence interval.

4. Discussion

HCC is the fourth leading cause of cancer mortality worldwide and the second most common cause of cancer mortality in Korea [18]. RFA is an effective treatment strategy for early HCC, especially in patients with limited liver functional reserve [19]. However, post-RFA recurrence is relatively common, and locally recurrent tumors show more aggressive behavior compared to primary tumors [20–22]. Studies on the treatment strategies and long-term outcomes of local recurrence after RFA are limited [6]. Previous studies have shown that salvage hepatectomy could be a therapeutic option for recurrence after RFA, yet most results are based on retrospective cohort studies from single centers with limited sample sizes [4,7–9]. Due to such limitations, the effect of the surgical approach in salvage hepatectomy has never been addressed. To our knowledge, this is the first study to compare short-term and long-term outcomes of open and laparoscopic salvage hepatectomy for local recurrence after RFA.

Salvage hepatectomy for local recurrence after RFA has been associated with more technical difficulties compared to primary liver resection. One of the advantages of RFA over surgical resection is its less invasive nature, which allows for repeated procedures in case of recurrence; for such reasons, patients referred for salvage hepatectomy are likely to be those for whom repeated RFA was technically difficult [23,24]. Also, RFA might cause dense adhesions around the liver, which renders liver mobilization and approach to the tumor even more challenging. Previous studies showed that salvage hepatectomy was associated with longer operation times, more intraoperative blood loss, and higher transfusion rates compared to patients undergoing primary liver resection [4,7]. Yamashita et al. also found postoperative morbidity rates to be higher in the salvage hepatectomy group compared to a matched control group who underwent hepatectomy as initial treatment [8]. However, when salvage hepatectomy for recurrence after RFA was compared with secondary liver resection for recurrence after surgery, short-term outcomes including operative data and postoperative complications showed no statistically significant difference [25].

In all previous studies, salvage hepatectomy for recurrence after RFA was performed exclusively by the open approach. Therefore, the effect of the surgical approach on postoperative outcomes after salvage hepatectomy could not be analyzed. In the current study, 58.2% of all patients received laparoscopic surgery. Short-term outcomes including intraoperative blood loss, transfusion rates, operation time, and postoperative complication rates were comparable to previous studies. We also found that the laparoscopic approach was associated with less blood loss and shorter postoperative hospital stays. These results suggest that laparoscopic salvage hepatectomy is safe and technically feasible if performed by experienced surgeons. Yet the tumor size was larger in the open group, and major hepatectomy was more often performed by the open approach. Decision on the surgical approach, either open or laparoscopic, was made independently by the individual surgeon based on various factors including tumor size and location. It is possible that operators tended to use the open approach more often when major liver resection was necessary. This difference in tumor size and major hepatectomy rate could have influenced the postoperative outcomes including operation time, intraoperative blood loss, and postoperative hospital stay. Still, the results of the current study suggest that laparoscopic salvage hepatectomy could be performed safely in patients who are determined to be suitable for minimally invasive liver resection. In patients with large recurrent tumors requiring major hepatectomy or concurrent extrahepatic resection, open surgery should be considered. Further large-scale prospective studies are necessary to establish practical guidelines for performing laparoscopic salvage hepatectomy.

Reports on the long-term survival outcomes after salvage hepatectomy for recurrence after RFA vary between studies. Sugo et al. found no significant difference in overall survival between patients who underwent salvage hepatectomy and those who underwent primary hepatectomy, with a 5-year survival rate of 67% in the salvage hepatectomy group [4]. Yet the 1-, 3-, and 5-year disease-free survival rates were significantly worse in the salvage group. Another study from Japan found the 5-year overall survival rate of patients undergoing salvage hepatectomy to be 58.3%, which was equivalent to the Japanese nationwide survey of HCC [9]. On the contrary, Yamamoto et al. reported that cumulative survival rates were only 9.5% at 5 years in patients undergoing salvage hepatectomy, which was worse than the known survival rates after surgery as the initial treatment in Japanese HCC patients [26]. An Italian study on salvage hepatic resection for incomplete ablation of primary and secondary liver tumors reported that both 2-year disease-free survival rates (salvage hepatectomy 28.5% vs. primary hepatectomy 83.1%, $p = 0.003$) and overall survival rates (salvage hepatectomy 44.4% vs. primary hepatectomy 87.1%, $p < 0.001$) were worse in the salvage hepatectomy group [7].

In the current study, the 5-year overall survival rate of patients undergoing salvage hepatectomy was 78.0%, which was superior to previous studies. There was no difference in overall survival between the open and laparoscopy groups, which suggested that the survival outcomes were comparable between the two approaches. However, in accordance with previous literature, recurrence after salvage hepatectomy was relatively common. Systemic recurrence rates were especially high, which reflected the aggressive behavior of recurrent HCC after RFA. Disease-free survival rates between open and laparoscopic salvage hepatectomy showed no statistically significant difference. This result suggested that the relatively high recurrence rates after salvage hepatectomy should be attributed to the tumor biology itself, rather than the surgical approach.

Local recurrence after RFA has shown a correlation with various clinicopathological factors. Previous studies found that large tumor size, multiple nodules, high serum tumor marker levels, insufficient tumor margin, tumor location near the liver surface, and decreased expertise of the performing physician were associated with an increased risk of local recurrence [20,21,27–31]. In the current study, we found tumor number to be the only independent risk factor. The surgical approach had no prognostic effect, which suggested that laparoscopic salvage hepatectomy can be performed with favorable oncologic outcomes. Considering the relatively high recurrence rates after salvage hepatectomy, there is a high possibility that these patients might need additional treatment including local ablation, TACE, or even repeated surgical resection. In such cases, patients are likely to benefit from laparoscopic surgery, which allows for faster recovery, lower morbidity rates, and a higher chance for safe reoperation.

This study has certain limitations. First, this was a retrospective study conducted at a single institution. Second, the decision on the surgical approach was made by the individual surgeon, considering both patient factors and tumor characteristics. Although the baseline characteristics between the open and laparoscopy groups showed no statistically significant difference, it is possible that a selection bias existed between the two groups. Future large-scale prospective studies are necessary to further validate the effect of the surgical approach in salvage hepatectomy for local recurrence after RFA.

5. Conclusions

Salvage hepatectomy is an acceptable treatment option for recurrence after RFA with an overall survival benefit. Laparoscopic salvage hepatectomy shows oncologic outcomes comparable to the open approach with less intraoperative blood loss and faster postoperative recovery. Considering that recurrence rates are high after RFA and repetitive treatment may be necessary, the laparoscopic approach should be considered as a safe and feasible option in patients eligible for surgical resection.

Author Contributions: Conceptualization, Y.-S.Y. and H.W.L.; methodology, B.L.; formal analysis, Y.P.; resources, M.K. and J.K.; data curation, M.K. and J.K.; writing—original draft preparation, Y.P.; writing—review and editing, J.Y.C.; supervision, H.-S.H.; project administration, J.Y.C. All authors have read and agreed to the published version of the manuscript.

Funding: This research received no external funding.

Institutional Review Board Statement: The study was conducted in accordance with the Declaration of Helsinki and approved by the Institutional Review Board of SNUBH (B-2306-836-103).

Informed Consent Statement: Patient consent was waived because of the retrospective nature of the study and the analysis using only anonymous clinical data.

Data Availability Statement: The data presented in this study are available from the corresponding author upon request.

Conflicts of Interest: The authors declare no conflict of interest.

References

1. Reig, M.; Forner, A.; Rimola, J.; Ferrer-Fàbrega, J.; Burrel, M.; Garcia-Criado, Á.; Kelley, R.K.; Galle, P.R.; Mazzaferro, V.; Salem, R.; et al. BCLC strategy for prognosis prediction and treatment recommendation: The 2022 update. *J. Hepatol.* **2022**, *76*, 681–693. [CrossRef]
2. Lau, W.Y.; Lai, E.C. The current role of radiofrequency ablation in the management of hepatocellular carcinoma: A systematic review. *Ann. Surg.* **2009**, *249*, 20–25. [CrossRef]
3. Korean Liver Cancer Association (KLCA); National Cancer Center (NCC) Korea. 2022 KLCA-NCC Korea practice guidelines for the management of hepatocellular carcinoma. *Clin. Mol. Hepatol.* **2022**, *28*, 583–705. [CrossRef]
4. Sugo, H.; Ishizaki, Y.; Yoshimoto, J.; Imamura, H.; Kawasaki, S. Salvage hepatectomy for local recurrent hepatocellular carcinoma after ablation therapy. *Ann. Surg. Oncol.* **2012**, *19*, 2238–2245. [CrossRef]
5. Nault, J.C.; Sutter, O.; Nahon, P.; Ganne-Carrié, N.; Séror, O. Percutaneous treatment of hepatocellular carcinoma: State of the art and innovations. *J. Hepatol.* **2018**, *68*, 783–797. [CrossRef]
6. Xie, X.; Jiang, C.; Peng, Z.; Liu, B.; Hu, W.; Wang, Y.; Lin, M.; Lu, M.; Kuang, M. Local Recurrence after Radiofrequency Ablation of Hepatocellular Carcinoma: Treatment Choice and Outcome. *J. Gastrointest. Surg.* **2015**, *19*, 1466–1475. [CrossRef]
7. Torzilli, G.; Del Fabbro, D.; Palmisano, A.; Marconi, M.; Makuuchi, M.; Montorsi, M. Salvage hepatic resection after incomplete interstitial therapy for primary and secondary liver tumours. *Br. J. Surg.* **2007**, *94*, 208–213. [CrossRef]
8. Yamashita, S.; Aoki, T.; Inoue, Y.; Kaneko, J.; Sakamoto, Y.; Sugawara, Y.; Hasegawa, K.; Kokudo, N. Outcome of salvage hepatic resection for recurrent hepatocellular carcinoma after radiofrequency ablation therapy. *Surgery* **2015**, *157*, 463–472. [CrossRef]
9. Imai, K.; Beppu, T.; Chikamoto, A.; Mima, K.; Okabe, H.; Hayashi, H.; Nitta, H.; Ishiko, T.; Baba, H. Salvage treatment for local recurrence of hepatocellular carcinoma after local ablation therapy. *Hepatol. Res.* **2014**, *44*, e335–e345. [CrossRef]

10. Troisi, R.I.; Berardi, G.; Morise, Z.; Cipriani, F.; Ariizumi, S.; Sposito, C.; Panetta, V.; Simonelli, I.; Kim, S.; Goh, B.K.P.; et al. Laparoscopic and open liver resection for hepatocellular carcinoma with Child-Pugh B cirrhosis: Multicentre propensity score-matched study. *Br. J. Surg.* **2021**, *108*, 196–204. [CrossRef]
11. Ciria, R.; Cherqui, D.; Geller, D.A.; Briceno, J.; Wakabayashi, G. Comparative short-term benefits of laparoscopic liver resection: 9000 cases and climbing. *Ann. Surg.* **2016**, *263*, 761–777. [CrossRef]
12. Cheung, T.T.; Dai, W.C.; Tsang, S.H.; Chan, A.C.; Chok, K.S.; Chan, S.C.; Lo, C.M. Pure laparoscopic hepatectomy versus open hepatectomy for hepatocellular carcinoma in 110 patients with liver cirrhosis: A propensity analysis at a single center. *Ann. Surg.* **2016**, *264*, 612–620. [CrossRef]
13. Schmelzle, M.; Krenzien, F.; Schöning, W.; Pratschke, J. Laparoscopic liver resection: Indications, limitations, and economic aspects. *Langenbecks Arch. Surg.* **2020**, *405*, 725–735. [CrossRef]
14. Beard, R.E.; Wang, Y.; Khan, S.; Marsh, J.W.; Tsung, A.; Geller, D.A. Laparoscopic liver resection for hepatocellular carcinoma in early and advanced cirrhosis. *HPB* **2018**, *20*, 521–529. [CrossRef]
15. Delvecchio, A.; Conticchio, M.; Riccelli, U.; Ferraro, V.; Ratti, F.; Gelli, M.; Anelli, F.M.; Laurent, A.; Vitali, G.C.; Magistri, P.; et al. Laparoscopic versus open liver resection for hepatocellular carcinoma in elderly patients: A propensity score matching analysis. *HPB* **2022**, *24*, 933–941. [CrossRef]
16. Strasberg, S.M.; Belghiti, J.; Clavien, P.A.; Gadzijev, E.; Garden, J.O.; Lau, W.Y.; Makuuchi, M.; Strong, R.W. The Brisbane 2000 Terminology of Liver Anatomy and Resections. *HPB* **2000**, *2*, 333–339. [CrossRef]
17. Dindo, D.; Demartines, N.; Clavien, P.A. Classification of surgical complications: A new proposal with evaluation in a cohort of 6336 patients and results of a survey. *Ann. Surg.* **2004**, *240*, 205–213. [CrossRef]
18. Chon, Y.E.; Park, S.Y.; Hong, H.P.; Son, D.; Lee, J.; Yoon, E.; Kim, S.S.; Ahn, S.B.; Jeong, S.W.; Jun, D.W. Hepatocellular carcinoma incidence is decreasing in Korea but increasing in the very elderly. *Clin. Mol. Hepatol.* **2023**, *29*, 120–134. [CrossRef]
19. Ogihara, M.; Wong, L.L.; Machi, J. Radiofrequency ablation versus surgical resection for single nodule hepatocellular carcinoma: Long-term outcomes. *HPB* **2005**, *7*, 214–221. [CrossRef]
20. Mulier, S.; Ni, Y.; Jamart, J.; Ruers, T.; Marchal, G.; Michel, L. Local recurrence after hepatic radiofrequency coagulation: Multivariate meta-analysis and review of contributing factors. *Ann. Surg.* **2005**, *242*, 158–171. [CrossRef]
21. Lam, V.W.; Ng, K.K.; Chok, K.S.; Cheung, T.T.; Yuen, J.; Tung, H.; Tso, W.K.; Fan, S.T.; Poon, R.T. Risk factors and prognostic factors of local recurrence after radiofrequency ablation of hepatocellular carcinoma. *J. Am. Coll. Surg.* **2008**, *207*, 20–29. [CrossRef]
22. Lee, J.; Jin, Y.J.; Shin, S.K.; Kwon, J.H.; Kim, S.G.; Suh, Y.J.; Jeong, Y.; Yu, J.H.; Lee, J.W.; Kwon, O.S.; et al. Surgery versus radiofrequency ablation in patients with Child-Pugh class-A/single small (≤3 cm) hepatocellular carcinoma. *Clin. Mol. Hepatol.* **2022**, *28*, 207–218. [CrossRef]
23. Yamagishi, S.; Midorikawa, Y.; Nakayama, H.; Higaki, T.; Moriguchi, M.; Aramaki, O.; Yamazaki, S.; Tsuji, S.; Takayama, T. Liver resection for recurrent hepatocellular carcinoma after radiofrequency ablation therapy. *Hepatol. Res.* **2019**, *49*, 432–440. [CrossRef]
24. Rossi, S.; Ravetta, V.; Rosa, L.; Ghittoni, G.; Viera, F.T.; Garbagnati, F.; Silini, E.M.; Dionigi, P.; Calliada, F.; Quaretti, P.; et al. Repeated radiofrequency ablation for management of patients with cirrhosis with small hepatocellular carcinomas: A long-term cohort study. *Hepatology* **2011**, *53*, 136–147. [CrossRef]
25. Yokoyama, K.; Anan, A.; Iwata, K.; Nishizawa, S.; Morihara, D.; Ueda, S.; Sakurai, K.; Iwashita, H.; Hirano, G.; Sakamoto, M.; et al. Limitation of repeated radiofrequency ablation in hepatocellular carcinoma: Proposal of a three (times) × 3 (years) index. *J. Gastroenterol. Hepatol.* **2012**, *27*, 1044–1050. [CrossRef]
26. Yamamoto, N.; Okano, K.; Kushida, Y.; Deguchi, A.; Yachida, S.; Suzuki, Y. Clinicopathology of recurrent hepatocellular carcinomas after radiofrequency ablation treated with salvage surgery. *Hepatol. Res.* **2014**, *44*, 1062–1071. [CrossRef]
27. Shiina, S.; Tateishi, R.; Arano, T.; Uchino, K.; Enooku, K.; Nakagawa, H.; Asaoka, Y.; Sato, T.; Masuzaki, R.; Kondo, Y.; et al. Radiofrequency ablation for hepatocellular carcinoma: 10-year outcome and prognostic factors. *Am. J. Gastroenterol.* **2012**, *107*, 569–577. [CrossRef]
28. Komorizono, Y.; Oketani, M.; Sako, K.; Yamasaki, N.; Shibatou, T.; Maeda, M.; Kohara, K.; Shigenobu, S.; Ishibashi, K.; Arima, T. Risk factors for local recurrence of small hepatocellular carcinoma tumors after a single session, single application of percutaneous radiofrequency ablation. *Cancer* **2003**, *97*, 1253–1262. [CrossRef]
29. Yamanaka, Y.S.K.; Miyashita, K.; Inoue, T.; Kawakita, T.; Yamaguchi, Y.; Saitou, Y.; Yamamoto, N.; Nakano, T.; Nakatsuka, A.; Yamakado, K.; et al. Risk factors for the recurrence of hepatocellular carcinoma after radiofrequency ablation of hepatocellular carcinoma in patients with hepatitis C. *World J. Gastroenterol.* **2005**, *11*, 2174–2178. [CrossRef]
30. Kei, S.K.; Rhim, H.; Choi, D.; Lee, W.J.; Lim, H.K.; Kim, Y.S. Local tumor progression after radiofrequency ablation of liver tumors: Analysis of morphologic pattern and site of recurrence. *Am. J. Roentgenol.* **2008**, *190*, 1544–1551. [CrossRef]
31. Hori, T.; Nagata, K.; Hasuike, S.; Onaga, M.; Motoda, M.; Moriuchi, A.; Iwakiri, H.; Uto, H.; Kato, J.; Ido, A.; et al. Risk factors for the local recurrence of hepatocellular carcinoma after a single session of percutaneous radiofrequency ablation. *J. Gastroenterol.* **2003**, *38*, 977–981. [CrossRef] [PubMed]

Disclaimer/Publisher's Note: The statements, opinions and data contained in all publications are solely those of the individual author(s) and contributor(s) and not of MDPI and/or the editor(s). MDPI and/or the editor(s) disclaim responsibility for any injury to people or property resulting from any ideas, methods, instructions or products referred to in the content.

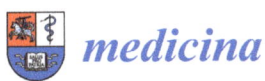

Article

The Conditioning of Adjuvant Chemotherapy for Stage II and III Rectal Cancer Determined by Postoperative Pathological Characteristics in Romania

Horia-Dan Liscu [1,2], Bogdan-Radu Liscu [2], Ruxandra Mitre [3], Ioana-Valentina Anghel [1], Ionut-Lucian Antone-Iordache [1], Andrei Balan [1], Simona Coniac [3], Andreea-Iuliana Miron [1,3,*] and Georgian Halcu [4]

1. Discipline of Oncological Radiotherapy and Medical Imaging, University of Medicine and Pharmacy "Carol Davila", 020021 Bucharest, Romania; horia-dan.liscu@drd.umfcd.ro (H.-D.L.)
2. Radiotherapy Department, Colțea Clinical Hospital, 030167 Bucharest, Romania
3. Medical Oncology Department, Colțea Clinical Hospital, 030167 Bucharest, Romania
4. Discipline of Pathological Anatomy, University of Medicine and Pharmacy "Carol Davila", 020021 Bucharest, Romania
* Correspondence: andreea-iuliana.miron@drd.umfcd.ro

Abstract: The management of locally advanced rectal cancer (LARC) suffered changes thanks to the development of improved surgical procedures, radiation delivery, and chemotherapy. Although treatment options improved individually, the optimal order is still debated. Neoadjuvant chemoradiotherapy followed by total mesorectal excision (TME) has been the "golden standard" for locally advanced rectal cancer. There is no common ground in international guidelines on the indications of adjuvant chemotherapy (ADJCHT), with differences between the American, European, and Japanese guidelines. This paper studies the preferences of Romanian oncologists in prescribing ADJCHT. We conducted a single-institution, retrospective study of all nonmetastatic, ECOG 0-1 LARC patients staged II-III who underwent TME and were admitted to the Oncology or Radiotherapy Department of Colțea Clinical Hospital, Bucharest between January 2017 and March 2021. A total of 186 patients were included in the study. A positive correlation was found between ADJCHT and each of the following: (y)pT > 2, (y)pN > 0, and the presence of perineural invasion (PNI+). A strong positive correlation was found between ADJCHT and the presence of at least one risk factor: (y)pT > 2, (y)pN > 0, PNI+, lymphovascular invasion, positive margins, or tumor grade > 1. Tumor downstaging decreased the risk of metastases in the first 2 years and was associated with the use of neoadjuvant radiotherapy, while adding neoadjuvant chemotherapy increased the chance of nodal downstaging. ADJCHT practice for LARC in Romania follows either NCCN or ESMO guidelines, at the discretion of the oncologist, due to the lack of national guideline.

Keywords: adjuvant chemotherapy; neoadjuvant radiotherapy; neoadjuvant radiochemotherapy; rectal cancer; tumor downstage; Romanian oncologists

1. Introduction

1.1. Overview

Locally advanced rectal cancer is most often treated with the three pillars of oncology: surgery, radiotherapy, and chemotherapy, with the classic order being neoadjuvant radiochemotherapy, followed by surgery, and finally by systemic therapy. Adjuvant chemotherapy (ADJCHT) after neoadjuvant treatment in rectal cancer is recommended by the American National Comprehensive Cancer Network [1], European Society for Medical Oncology [2], and Japanese Society for Cancer of the Colon and Rectum [3] guidelines on a routine basis for patients who have been treated with standard neoadjuvant treatment short-course radiotherapy (SCRT) or long-course radiochemotherapy (LCRCT) for stage

Citation: Liscu, H.-D.; Liscu, B.-R.; Mitre, R.; Anghel, I.-V.; Antone-Iordache, I.-L.; Balan, A.; Coniac, S.; Miron, A.-I.; Halcu, G. The Conditioning of Adjuvant Chemotherapy for Stage II and III Rectal Cancer Determined by Postoperative Pathological Characteristics in Romania. *Medicina* 2023, 59, 1224. https://doi.org/10.3390/medicina59071224

Academic Editors: Valentin Titus Grigorean, Daniel Alin Cristian and Konstantinos Dimas

Received: 30 May 2023
Revised: 17 June 2023
Accepted: 28 June 2023
Published: 29 June 2023

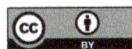

Copyright: © 2023 by the authors. Licensee MDPI, Basel, Switzerland. This article is an open access article distributed under the terms and conditions of the Creative Commons Attribution (CC BY) license (https://creativecommons.org/licenses/by/4.0/).

III. In the case of stage II rectal cancer, however, there are differences between the NCCN guideline, which recommends the use of adjuvant chemotherapy systematically, versus the ESMO and JSCCR guidelines, which recommend the use of adjuvant chemotherapy only in the presence of an increased risk of relapse [4].

In Romania, there is no national guideline for the treatment of colorectal cancer, with each oncologist having the possibility to follow international protocols and use free judgment in the decision to administer adjuvant chemotherapy. In 2021, a political initiative to promote a national cancer plan [5] emerged, which aims to improve the management of oncological diseases. A guideline was proposed that monitors the colorectal cancer patient pathway and recommends the use of adjuvant chemotherapy for all stage II and III rectal cancers, rather than mimicking the NCCN treatment guideline, without presenting its own nationally conducted studies.

This study aims to identify the criteria chosen by Romanian oncologists to administer adjuvant chemotherapy in patients with locally advanced rectal cancer, in the absence of a national guideline that clearly indicates this. The secondary objective is to analyze the relationships between the use of neoadjuvant treatment, the rate of tumor or nodal downstage, and the rate of recurrence or metastasis at 2 years.

1.2. Background

The oncological treatment of locally advanced rectal cancer has undergone many changes in recent decades, with it now using all three major oncological therapeutic options: radiotherapy, chemotherapy, and surgery. However, colorectal cancer still remained the second leading cause of mortality globally in 2020 [6] and has an increasing incidence in Central and Eastern Europe, including Romania, where more than 4800 new cases of rectal cancer were diagnosed in 2020 [7]. The appropriate administration order of the therapeutic methods was studied at the end of the 20th century, adding radiotherapy and chemotherapy to the neoadjuvant treatment scheme and establishing the total mesorectal excision (TME) technique as the gold-standard surgical procedure [8,9]. The 5-year local recurrence rate ranged from 15 to 40% [10,11] in the 1980s, decreasing to 4–15% in recent years with technological advances and the optimization of cancer treatment [12–14]. However, the reported metastasis rate (MR) for stage II-III rectal cancer is as high as 25%, with a slight improvement after the introduction of neoadjuvant radiosensitizing chemotherapy [15,16].

In recent years, the possibility of total neoadjuvant treatment (TNT) including short-course radiotherapy or long-course radiochemotherapy, given before or after 3–4 months of fluoropyrimidine and oxaliplatin chemotherapy, has been studied, with superior results for achieving a complete pathological response (pCR) and better disease-free survival (DFS) and overall survival (OS) [17,18]. The RAPIDO trial [19] shows an improvement in the rate of local recurrence and metastasis rate, and the OPRA trial [20] even proposes the "watch and wait" organ preservation strategy and omitting surgery in patients with complete response [21].

The total neoadjuvant treatment strategy is not yet recommended for all stages of locally advanced rectal neoplasm (LARC) [1] and is not adopted in all centers, which is why standard neoadjuvant treatment using short-course radiotherapy or long-course radiochemotherapy remains the basic indication in locally advanced rectal cancer.

In the case of adjuvant chemotherapy, the EORTC 22921 study indicated, at the first analysis, a benefit of adjuvant chemotherapy for local control [22], but at the 10-year analysis, it actually showed no survival benefit [23]. Another reference study is the Italian study published in 2014 showing no benefit of adjuvant fluoropyrimidine monotherapy for overall survival [24]. A large meta-analysis comprised of four studies concluded that adjuvant chemotherapy does not benefit overall survival, disease-free survival, or metastasis rate, except for upper rectal cancers [25]. The ADORE study also added oxaliplatin to the adjuvant treatment regimen and obtained better results for disease-free survival at 6 years (68% vs. 57% HR 0.63, 95% CI 0.43–0.93), with no difference in survival [26,27].

2. Materials and Methods

2.1. Patients and Design

We conducted a retrospective study on 186 patients with clinically or pathologically diagnosed locally advanced rectal cancer in stages II or III who presented to the Radiotherapy or Medical Oncology Department of Colțea Clinical Hospital, Bucharest between January 2017 and March 2021. All patients included in the study underwent surgery using the TME technique via the low anterior or abdominoperineal approach and had an ECOG performance status of 0 or 1 at the time of surgery.

Epidemiological information was collected on gender, age, and tumor location described by the surgeon during colonoscopy at the lower rectal, middle rectal, upper rectal, or rectosigmoid junction. All patients were clinically and pathologically staged, and the following histopathological report data were analyzed: tumor and nodal stage (pT and pN), resection margins (Postop), histopathological grade (Grade), and the presence/absence of lymphovascular (LVI) and perineural invasion (PNI). The extent of extramural invasion was not analyzed as not all preoperative MRIs provided this information. The tumor marker CEA was not routinely recorded in all patients and was excluded from the statistical analysis.

2.2. Treatment

Patients with locally advanced rectal cancer who received neoadjuvant treatment underwent long-course external pelvic radiotherapy with doses between 45 and 50.4 Gy, using the 3D or IMRT techniques +/− chemotherapy with capecitabine at a dose of 825 mg/m^2 twice daily during radiotherapy. TME surgery was performed for all patients 8–12 weeks after neoadjuvant treatment.

In the case of upper rectal cancer with sigmoid extension, some patients were treated with surgery per primam, followed by adjuvant treatment according to the postoperative pathological report.

Patients who received adjuvant chemotherapy received between 6 and 8 cycles (of 3 weeks each) of 1000 mg/m^2 capecitabine twice daily on days 1–14, concurrently with 130 mg/m^2 oxaliplatin on day 1, or 1250 mg/m^2 capecitabine monotherapy twice daily on days 1–14 if biological constants did not allow platinum administration.

2.3. Follow-Up

Patients were followed up by the attending medical oncologist or radiation oncologist every 3 months and CT or MRI imaging investigations were performed for locoregional evaluation, as per the clinic protocol. Follow-up data from the first 2 years were analyzed for all patients and any local recurrences or distant metastasis were recorded.

2.4. Statistical Analysis

Statistical analysis was performed using IBM SPSS Statistics v29 software, applying Pearson correlations and t-test statistical significance tests between the use of adjuvant chemotherapy and each of the histopathological criteria: (y)pT, (y)pN, LVI, PNI, Postop, and Grade. The same correlation algorithm was applied to identify the link between the use of neoadjuvant radiotherapy (NEORT) or radiochemotherapy (NEOCHTRT), the occurrence of local recurrence (relapse2y) or metastatic disease (metastasis2y) in the first 2 years, and the occurrence of tumor (T.downstage) and nodal (N.downstage) downstaging.

3. Results

Of the total 186 patients included in the study, 53.2% of patients (n = 99) were male (B) and 46.8% (n = 87) were female (F) (Table 1; Figure 1).

Table 1. Descriptive gender analysis.

		Gender Descriptive Statistics			
		Frequency	Percent	Valid Percent	Cumulative Percent
Valid	B	99	53.2	53.2	53.2
	F	S87	46.8	46.8	100.0
	Total	186	100.0	100.0	

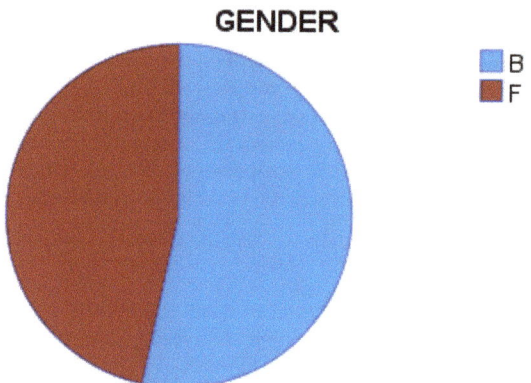

Figure 1. Pie chart for gender.

The mean age of the patients was 67.42 years with a standard deviation of 11.07 years. A majority distribution of patients was observed in the 60–80 years age range (Figure 2).

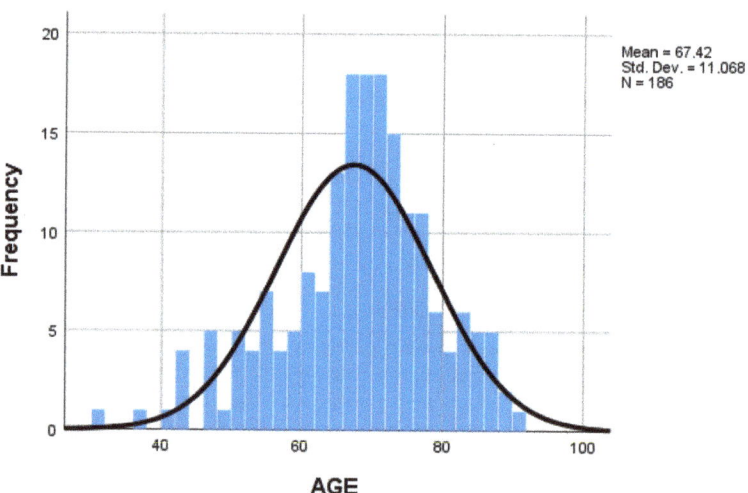

Figure 2. Histogram of age distribution.

The location of the tumor was at the lower rectal (RI) level in 29.25% of cases (n = 43), at the middle rectal (RM) level in 40.14% of cases (n = 59), at the upper rectal (RS) level in 26.53% of cases (n = 49), and at the rectosigmoid junction (JONC) in 30.61% of cases (n = 45). Most of the patients had tumors located in the middle rectum (Table 2, Figure 3).

Table 2. Location of tumor formation.

		\multicolumn{4}{c}{LOCALIZATION}			
		Frequency	Percent	Valid Percent	Cumulative Percent
Valid	JONC	45	24.2	24.2	24.2
	RI	43	23.1	23.1	47.3
	RM	59	31.7	31.7	79.0
	RS	39	21.0	21.0	100.0
	Total	186	100.0	100.0	

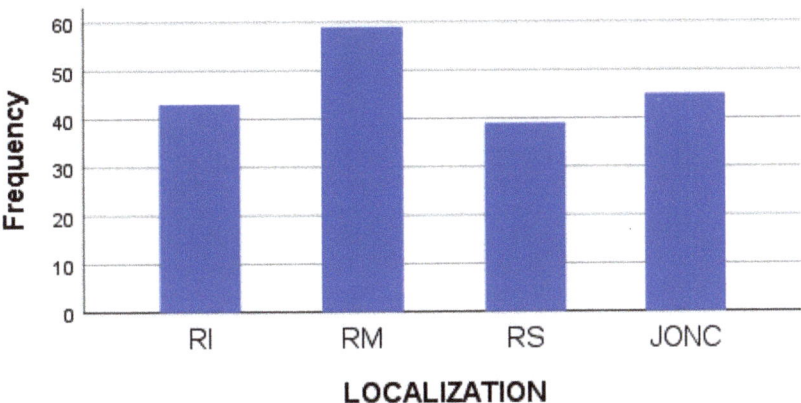

Figure 3. Bar chart showing the location of the tumor formation.

Compared to other rectal cancer studies, our study included patients with rectal tumors located higher up at the rectosigmoid junction, as some of them received neoadjuvant long-course radiochemotherapy treatment similar to standard rectal cancer treatment.

Pretreatment clinical staging includes 6.01% stage I patients (n = 11), 25.14% stage II patients (n = 46) and 68.85% stage III patients (n = 126) (Figure 4).

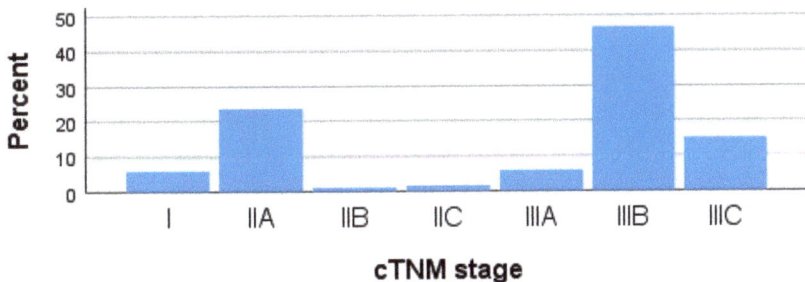

Figure 4. Bar chart with clinical staging cTNM of patients.

When it comes to clinical substages, most stage II patients were found in substage IIA (rectal tumor penetrating the muscularis propria and invading the colorectal tissues, without clinically detectable adenopathy). Of the stage III patients, most could be clinically substaged in IIIB (rectal tumor invading or penetrating its own muscle, with the presence of up to six clinically detectable malign lymph nodes).

Pathological staging performed after surgery was composed of 2.69% stage 0 patients with pathological complete response after neoadjuvant treatment (n = 5), 9.68% stage I patients (n = 18), 34.95% stage II patients (n = 65), and 52.69% stage III patients (n = 98) (Figure 5).

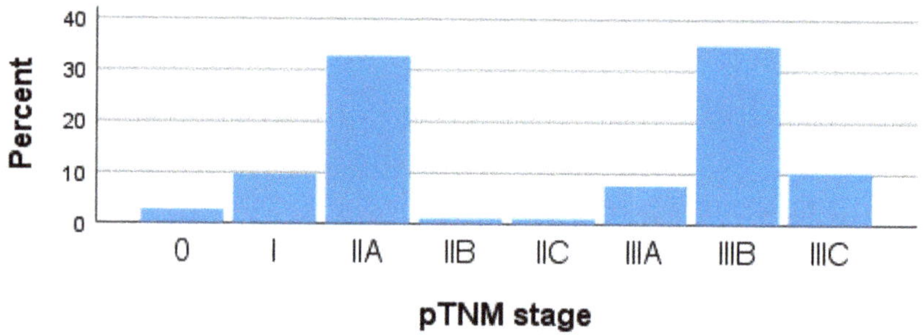

Figure 5. Bar chart with pathological staging pTNM of patients.

The substaging of patients in pathological stage II showed a clear majority of over 30% of patients in stage IIA. For stage III patients, most were pathologically substage IIIB, but with a significant 10% patients in stage IIIC.

We analyzed the correlation between adjuvant chemotherapy treatment and histopathology bulletin results by using the Pearson correlation coefficient and applying the two-tailed significance t-test. The correlation between adjuvant chemotherapy and a pathological T staging greater than 2 (y)pT > 2 (Figure 6) and between adjuvant chemotherapy and a positive pathological N staging (y)pN > 0 was tested. Other risk factors from the histopathology report that were taken into account were the presence of lymphovascular invasion LVI+ (Figure 7), the presence of perineural invasion PNI+ (Figure 8), positive resection margins Postop+, or a histopathological grade greater than 1 Grade > 1.

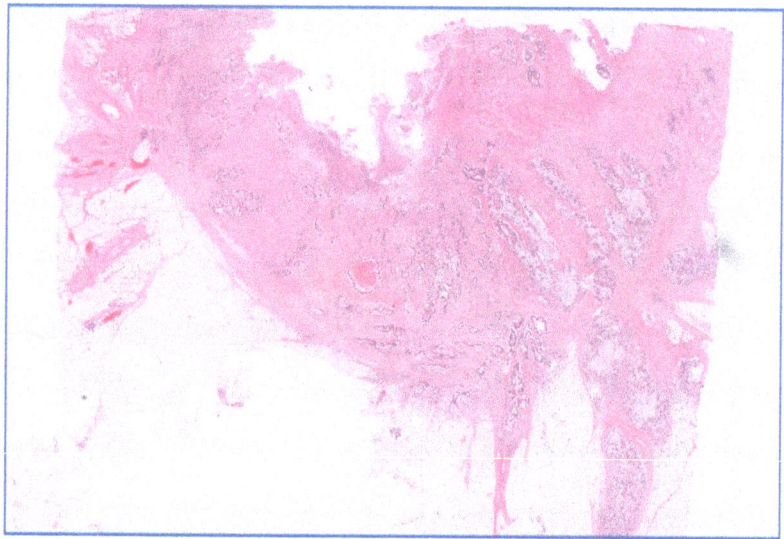

Figure 6. Persistent rectal adenocarcinoma after neoadjuvant radiochemotherapy; ypT3 with invasion in subserosal adipose tissue. HE stain × 0.5 magnification.

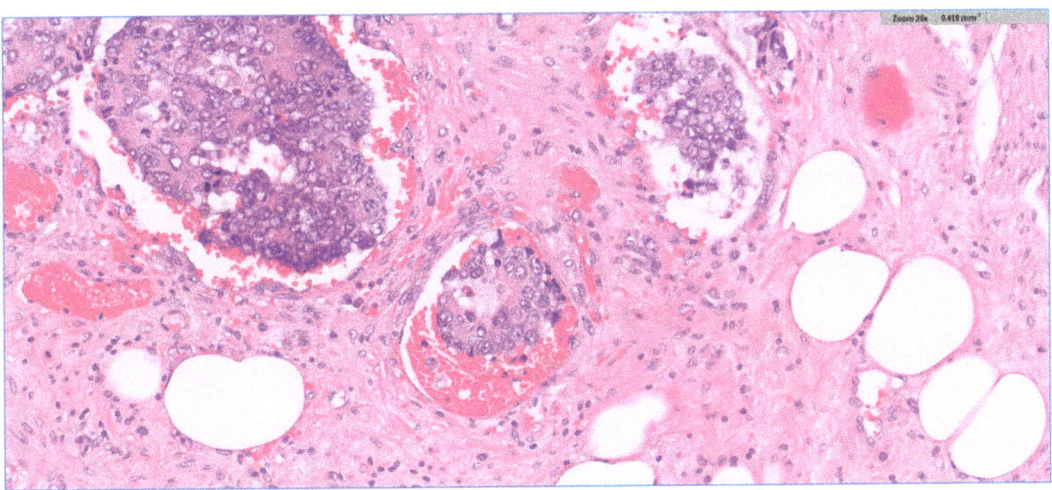

Figure 7. Depiction of extramural lymphovascular invasion; carcinomatous emboli of rectal adenocarcinoma. HE stain × 20 magnification.

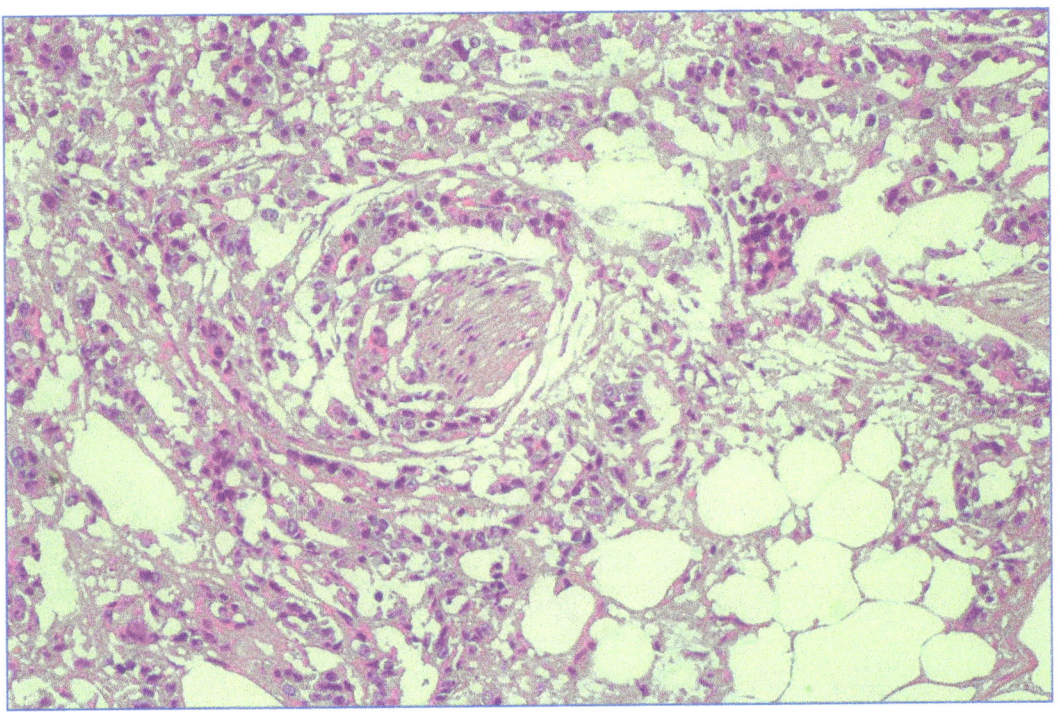

Figure 8. Depiction of perineural invasion; rectal adenocarcinoma. HE stain × 5 magnification.

Adjuvant chemotherapy is positively correlated with a moderate score of 0.432 for a histopathological stage (y)pT3 or (y)pT4 (Table 3). A moderate positive correlation score of 0.462 is also valid for the presence of nodal invasion (y)pN > 0. Both results are statistically significant with a score of $p < 0.001$.

Table 3. Correlation between adjuvant chemotherapy and pathological stages T and N.

		Correlations ADJCHT—pT and pN		
		ADJCHT	pT > 2	pN > 0
ADJCHT	Pearson correlation	1	0.432 **	0.462 **
	Sig. (two-tailed)		<0.001	<0.001
	N	186	186	186
pT > 2	Pearson correlation	0.432 **	1	0.120
	Sig. (two-tailed)	<0.001		0.104
	N	186	186	186
pN > 0	Pearson correlation	0.462 **	0.120	1
	Sig. (two-tailed)	<0.001	0.104	
	N	186	186	186

**—correlation is significant at the 0.01 level (2-tailed).

Analyzing the relationship between adjuvant chemotherapy, the presence of lymphovascular invasion, the presence of perineural invasion, the tumor grade, and the postoperative resection margins, the results show a very weak positive correlation between them, with a statistically significant p only in the case of the correlation between adjuvant chemotherapy and the presence of perineural invasion $p = 0.01$ (Table 4). In the case of lymphovascular invasion, positive resection margins, and histopathological grade greater than 1, the correlation with adjuvant treatment was very weak and statistical significance did not exist.

Table 4. Correlation between adjuvant chemotherapy, lymphovascular invasion, perineural invasion, resection margins, and differentiation grade.

		Correlations ADJCHT—LVI, PNI, Postop, and Grade				
		ADJCHT	LVI+	PNI+	Postop+	Grade > 1
ADJCHT	Pearson correlation	1	0.135	0.188 *	0.064	0.114
	Sig. (two-tailed)		0.065	0.010	0.388	0.123
	N	186	186	186	186	186
LVI+	Pearson correlation	0.135	1	0.563 **	0.262 **	0.154 *
	Sig. (two-tailed)	0.065		<0.001	<0.001	0.036
	N	186	186	186	186	186
PNI+	Pearson correlation	0.188 *	0.563 **	1	0.236 **	0.255 **
	Sig. (two-tailed)	0.010	<0.001		0.001	<0.001
	N	186	186	186	186	186
Postop+	Pearson correlation	0.064	0.262 **	0.236 **	1	0.164 *
	Sig. (two-tailed)	0.388	<0.001	0.001		0.025
	N	186	186	186	186	186
Grade > 1	Pearson correlation	0.114	0.154 *	0.255 **	0.164 *	1
	Sig. (two-tailed)	0.123	0.036	<0.001	0.025	
	N	186	186	186	186	186

*—correlation is significant at the 0.05 level (2-tailed); **—correlation is significant at the 0.01 level (2-tailed).

In the case of correlation analysis between the use of adjuvant chemotherapy and at least one risk factor for relapse, the Pearson score is highly positive (+0.633) with statistically significant $p < 0.001$, suggesting that in the presence of at least one risk factor for relapse, the oncologist would decide to administer adjuvant chemotherapy (Table 5, Figure 9). The risk factor may represent any of the following: histopathological stage pT3 or pT4, the presence of lymphatic invasion (pN > 0), the presence of lymphovascular invasion, the presence of perineural invasion, positive resection margins, or histopathological grade 2 or 3.

Table 5. Correlation between adjuvant chemotherapy and minimum 1 risk factor for relapse.

	Correlations ADJCHT—Min. 1 Risk Factor		
		ADJCHT	Min1RF
ADJCHT	Pearson correlation	1	0.633 **
	Sig. (two-tailed)		<0.001
	N	186	186
Min1RF	Pearson correlation	0.633 **	1
	Sig. (two-tailed)	<0.001	
	N	186	186

**—correlation is significant at the 0.01 level (2-tailed).

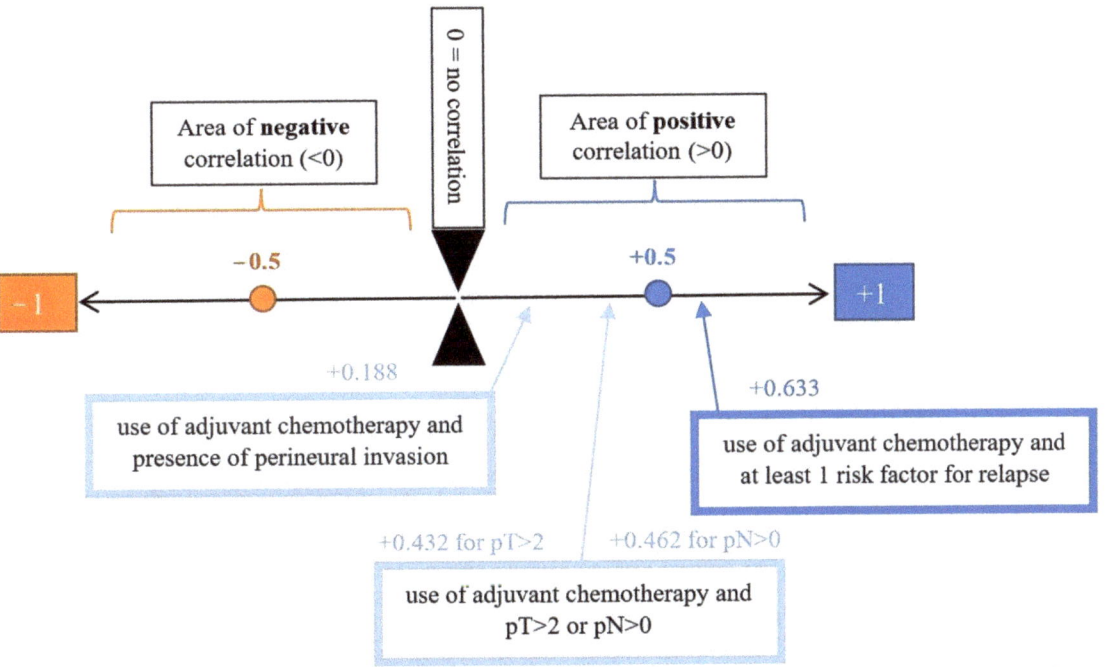

Figure 9. Graphical representation of the correlation between adjuvant chemotherapy and presence of perineural invasion; pT > 2 or pN > 0; minimum 1 risk factor for relapse.

Last but not least, the hypothesis that Romanian oncologists would administer adjuvant chemotherapy if neoadjuvant treatment is omitted was verified. There is a weak but statistically significant correlation supporting the omission of neoadjuvant treatment as an argument for adjuvant treatment ($p = 0.11$ for NEOCHTRT and $p = 0.009$ for NEORT) (Table 6).

Table 6. Correlation between adjuvant chemotherapy, neoadjuvant radiochemotherapy, and neoadjuvant radiotherapy.

		Correlations between ADJCHT, NEOCHTRT, and NEORT		
		ADJCHT	NEOCHTRT	NEORT
ADJCHT	Pearson correlation	1	−0.187 *	−0.190 **
	Sig. (two-tailed)		0.011	0.009
	N	186	186	186
NEOCHTRT	Pearson correlation	−0.187 *	1	0.746 **
	Sig. (two-tailed)	0.011		0.000
	N	186	186	186
NEORT	Pearson correlation	−0.190 **	0.746 **	1
	Sig. (two-tailed)	0.009	0.000	
	N	186	186	186

*—correlation is significant at the 0.05 level (2-tailed); **—correlation is significant at the 0.01 level (2-tailed).

Standard neoadjuvant treatment, LCRCT, was positively correlated with the occurrence of tumor and nodal downstaging, with the latter being more significant with a correlation score of 0.436 and statistical significance at $p < 0.001$. RT alone given in neoadjuvant regimen yielded similar results for tumor downstaging, but weaker ones for nodal downstaging (Table 7, Figure 10).

Table 7. Correlation between neoadjuvant treatment, downstaging for T and N, and metastasis or local recurrence at 2 years.

		Correlations between Neoadjuvant Treatment, Downstaging, and Metastasis/Relapse at 2y					
		NEORT	NEOCHTRT	T.Downstage	N.Downstage	Relapse2y	Metastasis2y
NEORT	Pearson correlation	1	0.746 **	0.338 **	0.364 **	0.100	0.110
	Sig. (two-tailed)		<0.001	<0.001	<0.001	0.174	0.133
	N	186	186	186	186	186	186
NEOCHTRT	Pearson correlation	0.746 **	1	0.310 **	0.436 **	0.131	0.082
	Sig. (two-tailed)	<0.001		<0.001	<0.001	0.074	0.269
	N	186	186	186	186	186	186
T.downstage	Pearson correlation	0.338 **	0.310 **	1	0.276 **	−0.085	−0.193 **
	Sig. (two-tailed)	<0.001	<0.001		<0.001	0.251	0.008
	N	186	186	186	186	186	186
N.downstage	Pearson correlation	0.364 **	0.436 **	0.276 **	1	−0.021	−0.102
	Sig. (two-tailed)	<0.001	<0.001	<0.001		0.777	0.165
	N	186	186	186	186	186	186
relapse2y	Pearson correlation	0.100	0.131	−0.085	−0.021	1	0.345 **
	Sig. (two-tailed)	0.174	0.074	0.251	0.777		<0.001
	N	186	186	186	186	186	186
metastasis2y	Pearson correlation	0.110	0.082	−0.193 **	−0.102	0.345 **	1
	Sig. (two-tailed)	0.133	0.269	0.008	0.165	<0.001	
	N	186	186	186	186	186	186

**—correlation is significant at the 0.01 level (2-tailed).

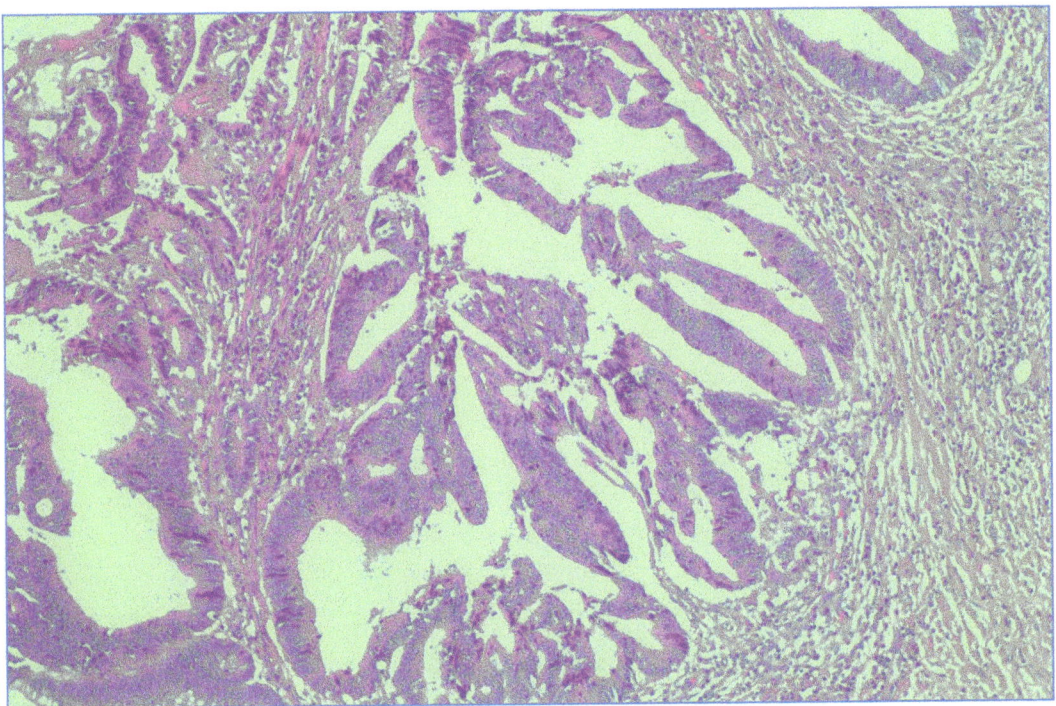

Figure 10. Downstage of rectal adenocarcinoma after neoadjuvant LCRCT radiochemotherapy. Illustrated is a downstaged ypT1 with invasion in submucosa; HE stain × 10 magnification.

The occurrence of distant metastasis and local recurrence within the first 2 years of follow-up was recorded for the patients analyzed. Patients who received neoadjuvant treatment, either radiotherapy alone or long-course radiochemotherapy, had a nonsignificant correlation score with the metastasis rate or local recurrence rate in the first 2 years. However, paradoxically, neoadjuvant treatment was positively correlated with the local recurrence rate at 2 years and with the metastasis rate at 2 years: for neoadjuvant radiochemotherapy, local recurrence was correlated with a Pearson score of 0.131 and metastasis with a Pearson score of 0.082.

Analyzing the downstage rate, we saw that there was an inverse correlation between the tumor downstage rate after neoadjuvant treatment and the 2-year metastasis rate of -0.193, with a statistically significant $p = 0.008$ (Figure 11). Additionally, the nodal downstage rate was negatively correlated with the 2-year metastasis rate, with a Pearson score of -0.102, but this time, there was no statistical significance at $p = 0.165$. The local recurrence rate at 2 years was practically insignificant, with a correlation score close to 0 and a t-test $p > 0.25$ for both tumor downstage and nodal downstage.

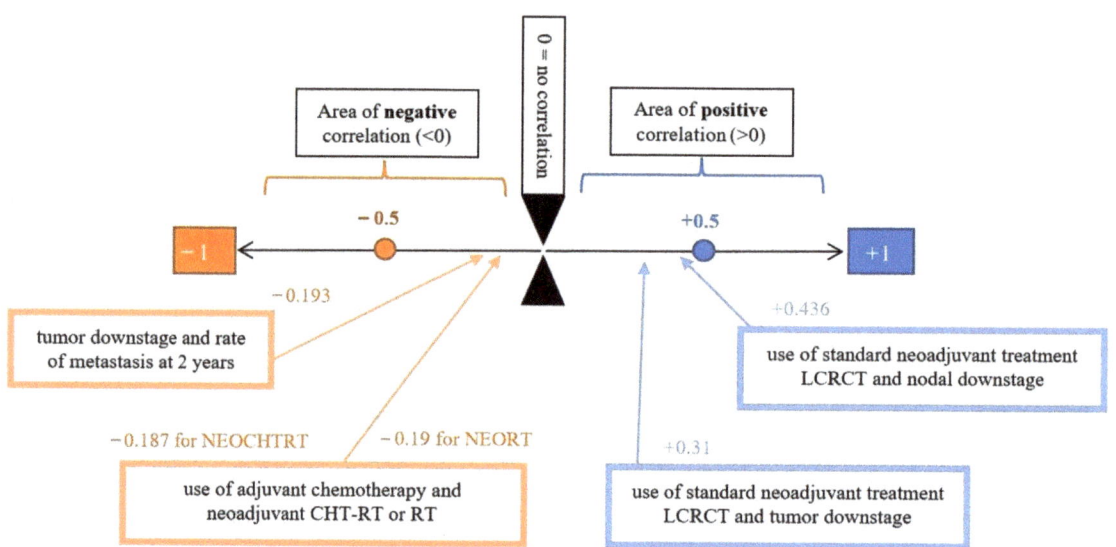

Figure 11. Graphical representation of the correlation between tumor downstage and metastasis rate at 2 years; adjuvant chemotherapy and neoadjuvant treatment; LCRCT and tumor downstage; and LCRCT and nodal downstage.

4. Discussion

The epidemiological data analyzed in the study are similar to other studies conducted on larger cohorts in terms of mean age or sex distribution [28,29]. The present study includes a larger number of patients with upper rectal tumors, as it includes patients with tumors at the rectosigmoid junction. There is currently debate about the optimal treatment modality for high rectal cancer, with suggestions that the peritoneal limit is the key for indicating or omitting neoadjuvant treatment [30]. This principle of choosing the treatment of upper rectal cancers, located at the junction with the sigmoid, poses difficulties for surgeons and oncologists and especially depends on the correct interpretation of preoperative investigations. Sometimes, the multidisciplinary committee may consider that a high rectal cancer does not benefit from neoadjuvant treatment (considering it rather as sigmoid cancer), and then the first intervention would be surgery. In this case, depending on the stage and other postoperative molecular factors, adjuvant chemotherapy may also be omitted, similarly to rectal cancer, which does not preclude the inclusion of patients who did not receive neoadjuvant treatment in this study.

Our main objective was to analyze the association between the use of adjuvant chemotherapy and the postoperative pathological characteristics. The decision to perform adjuvant chemotherapy in patients with stage II-III rectal cancer is mainly based on the presence of a (y)pT > 2 or (y)pN > 0, or a minimum of one out of the following risk factors: a positive resection margin, the presence of lymphovascular invasion, the presence of perineural invasion, or a histopathological grade greater than 1. The only adverse factor encountered on the histopathology report that was uniquely correlated with the use of adjuvant therapy is perineural invasion, despite the fact that the Dutch PROCTOR study [31] showed that PNI+ does not necessarily predict a beneficial effect of adjuvant chemotherapy. This rationale is based more on the association between the presence of perineural invasion and inferior survival [32,33]. According to Swets et al. [32], the presence of extramural invasion, tumor budding, or perineural invasion is associated with much worse overall survival, and the presence of two out of three also decreases disease-free survival and increases the chance of distant metastases. However, none of these features, alone or all together, can predict any benefit of adjuvant chemotherapy.

In pathological stage II, there is inconsistency among oncologists, with most of them choosing to treat these patients with adjuvant chemotherapy according to the NCCN guideline [1]. However, 6.9% of pathologically stage II patients had no risk factors for relapse (n = 13) and did not receive adjuvant treatment, instead following the ESMO [2] or JSCCR [3] guidelines. This rationale is also supported by a retrospective analysis performed in 2022 in Taiwan, which supports omitting adjuvant treatment in ypT0-2N0 patients with good response to neoadjuvant treatment. Kuo et al. [34] conducted a retrospective study of 720 patients with good response after neoadjuvant treatment and found that neither overall survival nor disease-free survival is improved by adjuvant chemotherapy, even for clinically advanced patients.

The findings of other authors show that precisely the lower stages and the presence of downstaging would benefit from adjuvant chemotherapy, thus only fueling the confusion and controversy regarding this subgroup of patients. Breugom et al. [24] consider that adjuvant chemotherapy may be especially useful for patients with tumors located at an upper level, at least 10 cm from the anal margin, in terms of disease-free survival and metastasis. However, these findings do not hold true for overall survival or for tumors located at the lower or middle rectal level.

The high degree of correlation between the administration of adjuvant chemotherapy and the presence of at least one risk factor (Pearson score of +0.633) suggests that if one or more risk factors for relapse are present, a Romanian oncologist would decide to administer adjuvant chemotherapy. The regimen includes at least one antimetabolite (those classically used in Europe and the United States are 5-fluorouracil in combination with leucovorin or orally administered capecitabine, while in Asia, tegafur–gimeracil–oteracil is an option), but most experts' recommendation is to add oxaliplatin. This combination improves disease-free survival, but the addition of oxaliplatin for overall survival is unclear. The phase II ADORE trial [26] of 321 patients with stage II or III rectal cancer treated with neoadjuvant radiochemotherapy, total mesorectal excision, and adjuvant chemotherapy with 5 FU (control arm) or FOLFOX (experimental arm) showed an overall 3-year survival difference of 85.7% versus 95.0% in favor of adjuvant oxaliplatin (HR =.456; 95% CI 0.25–0.97; p = 0.036). The German phase III CAO/ARO/AIO-04 trial [35] found, however, no difference between the two adjuvant groups (with or without oxaliplatin) for 3-year overall survival (88.7% vs. 88%). In our study, the decision to add oxaliplatin to the adjuvant regimen was judged for each individual patient according to biological constants and the risk of relapse. The Japanese national guideline [3] recommends the addition of oxaliplatin only in cases with a higher risk of relapse, concluding that it reduces the risk of relapse or death by about 20% compared with antimetabolite monotherapy.

Another argument for adjuvant treatment often encountered among Romanian physicians, but with less impact according to the Pearson correlation analysis, is the omission of neoadjuvant treatment; thus, there is a higher risk of locoregional or distant relapse. The American guidelines recommend both adjuvant radiochemotherapy and a course of adjuvant chemotherapy after a resection of rectal adenocarcinoma, if not previously offered [36]. Chemotherapy regimens similar to adjuvant treatment in colon cancer are used: fluoropyrimidine monotherapy (possibly administered in an accelerated Gramont-type regimen) with or without oxaliplatin and usually without the addition of irinotecan.

In terms of oncological outcome after treatment, the results obtained in this study are inferior compared to data obtained in other clinical trials [10–14], with a percentage of local relapse or metastasis at 2 years ranging from one quarter to one third of patients. It should be taken into account that more than 50% of the patients included in the study were stage III and not all patients received neoadjuvant treatment. The absence of an organized national population screening program in Romania, both for colorectal cancer and for other common cancers [37], is one of the causes leading to the discovery of cancer in advanced stages.

Our secondary endpoints were to analyze the correlations between the use of neoadjuvant treatment, the rate of tumor or nodal downstage, and the rate of recurrence or metastasis at 2 years. Patients who benefited from tumor downstaging also had lower odds of metastasis, confirming the good prognosis of a response to neoadjuvant treatment, as shown by the analysis in the National Cancer Database performed in the US in 2018 [38]. Local control is not associated with tumor or nodal downstaging, which contradicts a 2018 study [39]. A total of 5 patients out of 77 who received long-course radiochemotherapy had pathological complete response, this percentage of 6.5% being significantly lower than other authors' results of 15–20% [40,41]. This may be explained by the inclusion of a large proportion of patients with pT3 stage in the study, for whom standard neoadjuvant treatment is not aggressive enough in order to obtain complete tumor regression. However, the 3-year survival of patients who had complete pathological response after neoadjuvant radiochemotherapy reported by Tan et al. [41] was 92.4%, only a few percent higher than the survival of the group that did not achieve pathological complete response (88.2%). This difference is statistically significant at $p = 0.002$, but the relatively small gap between the two groups shows that the role of total mesorectal excision performed correctly could be more important than achieving pathological complete response after neoadjuvant treatment. Thus, in patients for whom organ preservation is not established as an objective, fast neoadjuvant treatment, regimens (such as short-course radiotherapy) with immediate surgery and adjuvant chemotherapy may be an option.

Strengths and Limitations of the Study

This study is the first study conducted on a population of patients treated in Romania with locally advanced rectal cancer that analyzes the criteria of choice of adjuvant therapy offered by oncologists. The rationale for the adjuvant treatment of rectal cancer administered in Romania is based on American, European, or Japanese guidelines.

The limitations of the study include the collection of patients from a single hospital unit (as Romania does not yet have a single national registry of cancer patients), which may have led to selection bias. Additionally, some patients were incompletely investigated (lack of CEA dosing) or showed incomplete investigation results (due to a lack of extramural invasion description on preoperative MRI scans). A retrospective analysis cannot provide strong evidence of causality; thus, we recommend future prospective analyses on this topic to confirm our findings. We included in the study patients who received neoadjuvant treatment and patients who did not receive such treatment. The primary endpoint was not influenced by neoadjuvant treatment, and the secondary endpoint analysis on downstaging was only performed on patients who received neoadjuvant treatment.

5. Conclusions

Patients with locally advanced rectal neoplasm treated in Romania will benefit from adjuvant chemotherapy if the patient does not have pathological stage (y)pTNM 0 or I. For pathological stage II patients who have completed neoadjuvant treatment and do not have any risk factor for recurrence, adjuvant treatment may be omitted, but this remains at the oncologist's discretion. The appearance of tumor downstaging decreases the risk of metastases in the first 2 years and is associated with the use of neoadjuvant radiotherapy. The addition of radiosensitizing chemotherapy is associated with a higher chance of nodal downstaging.

Oncology practice in Romania runs the risk of heterogeneity between institutions, and even between physicians in the same institution, due to the lack of standardized national guidelines, large-scale national studies, and a national cancer registry that can centralize this information.

Author Contributions: Conceptualization, H.-D.L. and B.-R.L.; methodology, H.-D.L.; software, H.-D.L.; validation, A.-I.M., R.M. and S.C.; formal analysis, H.-D.L.; investigation, I.-V.A., I.-L.A.-I., A.B. and G.H.; resources, I.-V.A., I.-L.A.-I., A.B. and G.H.; data curation, H.-D.L.; writing—original draft preparation, H.-D.L.; writing—review and editing, A.-I.M., R.M. and S.C.; visualization, R.M.; supervision, B.-R.L.; project administration, H.-D.L., A.-I.M. and G.H. All authors have read and agreed to the published version of the manuscript.

Funding: The publication fees are supported by SNOMR (Romanian National Society of Medical Oncology).

Institutional Review Board Statement: The present study is part of the PhD thesis of the first author, for which he received approval from the Ethics Committee of the Coltea Clinical Hospital, Bucharest, where the study was conducted, according to decision 19090/05.10.2021.

Informed Consent Statement: Informed consent was obtained from all subjects involved in the study.

Data Availability Statement: Data available only on request due to ethical restrictions. The data presented in this study are available on request from the corresponding author and the Coltea Clinical Hospital (secretariat@coltea.ro). The data are not publicly available due to the policy of Coltea Clinical Hospital to have the approval of the Ethics Commitee for each new research study.

Acknowledgments: Special thanks to VERGA I. Nicolae, Head of Department of Radiotherapy, "Coltea" Clinical Hospital, Bucharest, Romania.

Conflicts of Interest: The authors declare no conflict of interest.

References

1. Benson, A.B.; Venook, A.P.; Al-Hawary, M.M.; Azad, N.; Chen, Y.; Ciombor, K.K.; Cohen, S.; Cooper, H.S.; Deming, D.; Garrido-Laguna, I.; et al. NCCN Guidelines Version 4.2022 Rectal Cancer Continue NCCN Guidelines Panel Disclosures. 2023. Available online: https://jnccn.org/view/journals/jnccn/20/10/article-p1139.xml (accessed on 26 March 2023).
2. Glynne-Jones, R.; Wyrwicz, L.; Tiret, E.; Brown, G.; Rödel, C.; Cervantes, A.; Arnold, D. Rectal cancer: ESMO Clinical Practice Guidelines for diagnosis, treatment and follow-up. *Ann. Oncol.* **2017**, *28* (Suppl. 4), iv22–iv40. [CrossRef] [PubMed]
3. Hashiguchi, Y.; Muro, K.; Saito, Y.; Ito, Y.; Ajioka, Y.; Hamaguchi, T.; Hasegawa, K.; Hotta, K.; Ishida, H.; Ishiguro, M.; et al. Japanese Society for Cancer of the Colon and Rectum (JSCCR) guidelines 2019 for the treatment of colorectal cancer. *Int. J. Clin. Oncol.* **2020**, *25*, 1. [CrossRef] [PubMed]
4. Ryan, D.P.; Willett, C.G. Adjuvant Therapy after Neoadjuvant Therapy for Rectal Cancer—UpToDate. *Uptodate.* 2023. Available online: https://www.uptodate.com/contents/adjuvant-therapy-after-neoadjuvant-therapy-for-rectal-cancer?source=mostViewed_widget (accessed on 26 March 2023).
5. Ministerul Sanatatii din Romania. *Traseul Pacientilor cu Cancer Colorectal*; Ministerul Sanatatii din Romania: Bucharest, Romania, 2021. Available online: https://cancer-plan.ro/wp-content/uploads/2022/01/Cancer-colorectal_2021_Traseul-pacientului.pdf (accessed on 26 March 2023).
6. GLOBOCAN 2020. 2020. Available online: https://gco.iarc.fr/today/data/factsheets/cancers/9-Rectum-fact-sheet.pdf (accessed on 24 February 2023).
7. Gobocan Romania 2020. IARC, WHO. 2020. Available online: https://gco.iarc.fr/today/data/factsheets/populations/642-romania-fact-sheets.pdf (accessed on 24 February 2023).
8. Enker, W.E. Total mesorectal excision--the new golden standard of surgery for rectal cancer. *Ann. Med.* **1997**, *29*, 127–133. [CrossRef]
9. Beck, D.E.; Wexner, S.D.; Hull, T.L.; Roberts, P.L.; Saclarides, T.J.; Senagore, A.J.; Stamos, M.J.; Steele, S.R. *The ASCRS Manual of Colon and Rectal Surgery*; Springer: Berlin/Heidelberg, Germany, 2014.
10. Graf, W.; Påhlman, L.; Enblad, P.; Glimelius, B. Anterior versus abdominoperineal resections in the management of mid-rectal tumours. *Acta Chir. Scand.* **1990**, *156*, 231–235.
11. Phillips, R.K.S.; Hittinger, R.; Blesovsky, L.; Fry, J.S.; Fielding, L.P. Local recurrence following 'curative' surgery for large bowel cancer: II. The rectum and rectosigmoid. *Br. J. Surg.* **1984**, *71*, 17–20. [CrossRef]
12. Heald, R. Rectal cancer: The surgical options. *Eur. J. Cancer* **1995**, *31*, 1189–1192. [CrossRef]
13. Gérard, A.; Buyse, M.; Nordlinger, B.; Loygue, J.; Pène, F.; Kempf, P.; Bosset, J.-F.; Gignoux, M.; Arnaud, J.-P.; Desaive, C.; et al. Preoperative Radiotherapy as Adjuvant Treatment in Rectal Cancer. Final results of a randomized study of the European Organization for Research and Treatment of Cancer (EORTC). *Ann. Surg.* **1988**, *208*, 606–614. [CrossRef]
14. Heald, R.; Ryall, R. Recurrence and survival after total mesorectal excision for rectal cancer. *Lancet* **1986**, *327*, 1479–1482. [CrossRef]
15. Erlandsson, J.; Holm, T.; Pettersson, D.; Berglund, A.; Cedermark, B.; Radu, C.; Johansson, H.; Machado, M.; Hjern, F.; Hallböök, O.; et al. Optimal fractionation of preoperative radiotherapy and timing to surgery for rectal cancer (Stockholm III): A multicentre, randomised, non-blinded, phase 3, non-inferiority trial. *Lancet Oncol.* **2017**, *18*, 336–346. [CrossRef] [PubMed]
16. Gastrointestinal Tumor Study Group. Prolongation of the Disease-Free Interval in Surgically Treated Rectal Carcinoma. *N. Engl. J. Med.* **2010**, *312*, 1465–1472. [CrossRef]
17. Liu, S.; Jiang, T.; Xiao, L.; Yang, S.; Liu, Q.; Gao, Y.; Chen, G.; Xiao, W. Total Neoadjuvant Therapy (TNT) versus Standard Neoadjuvant Chemoradiotherapy for Locally Advanced Rectal Cancer: A Systematic Review and Meta-Analysis. *Oncologist* **2021**, *26*, e1555–e1566. [CrossRef] [PubMed]

18. Park, S.E.; Choi, J.H.; Choi, C.H.; Park, S.W.; Kim, B.G.; Cha, S.J.; Hwang, I.G. Additional Chemotherapy with 5-FU plus Leucovorin between Preoperative Chemoradiotherapy and Surgery Improved Treatment Outcomes in Patients with Advanced Rectal Cancer. *J. Cancer* **2019**, *10*, 186. [CrossRef]
19. Bahadoer, R.R.; Dijkstra, E.A.; van Etten, B.; Marijnen, C.A.M.; Putter, H.; Kranenbarg, E.M.-K.; Roodvoets, A.G.H.; Nagtegaal, I.D.; Beets-Tan, R.G.H.; Blomqvist, L.K.; et al. Short-course radiotherapy followed by chemotherapy before total mesorectal excision (TME) versus preoperative chemoradiotherapy, TME, and optional adjuvant chemotherapy in locally advanced rectal cancer (RAPIDO): A randomised, open-label, phase 3 trial. *Lancet Oncol.* **2020**, *22*, 29–42. [CrossRef]
20. Jimenez-Rodriguez, R.M.; Quezada-Diaz, F.; Hameed, I.; Kalabin, A.; Patil, S.; Smith, J.J.; Garcia-Aguilar, J.M. Organ Preservation in Patients with Rectal Cancer Treated with Total Neoadjuvant Therapy. *Dis. Colon Rectum* **2021**, *64*, 1463–1470. [CrossRef]
21. Glynne-Jones, R.; Hollingshead, J. TNT and local recurrence in the RAPIDO trial—untangling the puzzle. *Nat. Rev. Clin. Oncol.* **2023**, *20*, 357–358. [CrossRef]
22. Bosset, J.-F.; Collette, L.; Calais, G.; Mineur, L.; Maingon, P.; Radosevic-Jelic, L.; Daban, A.; Bardet, E.; Beny, A.; Ollier, J.-C. Chemotherapy with Preoperative Radiotherapy in Rectal Cancer. *N. Engl. J. Med.* **2006**, *355*, 1114–1123. [CrossRef]
23. Bosset, J.-F.; Calais, G.; Mineur, L.; Maingon, P.; Stojanovic-Rundic, S.; Bensadoun, R.-J.; Bardet, E.; Beny, A.; Ollier, J.-C.; Bolla, M.; et al. Fluorouracil-based adjuvant chemotherapy after preoperative chemoradiotherapy in rectal cancer: Long-term results of the EORTC 22921 randomised study. *Lancet Oncol.* **2014**, *15*, 184–190. [CrossRef]
24. Sainato, A.; Nunzia, V.C.L.; Valentini, V.; De Paoli, A.; Maurizi, E.R.; Lupattelli, M.; Aristei, C.; Vidali, C.; Conti, M.; Galardi, A.; et al. No benefit of adjuvant Fluorouracil Leucovorin chemotherapy after neoadjuvant chemoradiotherapy in locally advanced cancer of the rectum (LARC): Long term results of a randomized trial (I-CNR-RT). *Radiother. Oncol.* **2014**, *113*, 223–229. [CrossRef]
25. Breugom, A.J.; Swets, M.; Bosset, J.-F.; Collette, L.; Sainato, A.; Cionini, L.; Glynne-Jones, R.; Counsell, N.; Bastiaannet, E.; Broek, C.B.M.V.D.; et al. Adjuvant chemotherapy after preoperative (chemo)radiotherapy and surgery for patients with rectal cancer: A systematic review and meta-analysis of individual patient data. *Lancet Oncol.* **2015**, *16*, 200–207. [CrossRef]
26. Hong, Y.S.; Kim, S.Y.; Lee, J.S.; Nam, B.-H.; Kim, K.-P.; Kim, J.E.; Park, Y.S.; Park, J.O.; Baek, J.Y.; Kim, T.-Y.; et al. Oxaliplatin-Based Adjuvant Chemotherapy for Rectal Cancer After Preoperative Chemoradiotherapy (ADORE): Long-Term Results of a Randomized Controlled Trial. *J. Clin. Oncol.* **2019**, *37*, 3111–3123. [CrossRef]
27. Hong, Y.S.; Nam, B.-H.; Kim, K.-P.; Kim, J.E.; Park, S.J.; Park, Y.S.; Park, J.O.; Kim, S.Y.; Kim, T.-Y.; Kim, J.H.; et al. Oxaliplatin, fluorouracil, and leucovorin versus fluorouracil and leucovorin as adjuvant chemotherapy for locally advanced rectal cancer after preoperative chemoradiotherapy (ADORE): An open-label, multicentre, phase 2, randomised controlled trial. *Lancet Oncol.* **2014**, *15*, 1245–1253. [CrossRef]
28. Høydahl, Ø.; Edna, T.-H.; Xanthoulis, A.; Lydersen, S.; Endreseth, B.H. The impact of age on rectal cancer treatment, complications and survival. *BMC Cancer* **2022**, *22*, 975. [CrossRef]
29. Virostko, J.; Capasso, A.; Yankeelov, T.; Goodgame, B. Recent trends in the age at diagnosis of colorectal cancer in the US National Cancer Data Base, 2004–2015. *Cancer* **2019**, *125*, 3828. [CrossRef]
30. Hui, C.; Baclay, R.; Liu, K.B.; Sandhu, N.B.; Loo, P.; von Eyben, R.M.; Chen, C.; Sheth, V.; Vitzthum, L.; Chang, D.; et al. Rectosigmoid Cancer—Rectal Cancer or Sigmoid Cancer? *Am. J. Clin. Oncol.* **2022**, *45*, 333. [CrossRef]
31. Breugom, A.J.; van Gijn, W.; Muller, E.W.; Berglund, Å.; van den Broek, C.B.M.; Fokstuen, T.; Gelderblom, H.; Kapiteijn, E.; Leer, J.W.H.; Marijnen, C.A.M.; et al. Adjuvant chemotherapy for rectal cancer patients treated with preoperative (chemo)radiotherapy and total mesorectal excision: A Dutch Colorectal Cancer Group (DCCG) randomized phase III trial. *Ann. Oncol.* **2014**, *26*, 696–701. [CrossRef]
32. Swets, M.; Kuppen, P.J.; Blok, E.J.; Gelderblom, H.; van de Velde, C.J.; Nagtegaal, I.D. Are pathological high-risk features in locally advanced rectal cancer a useful selection tool for adjuvant chemotherapy? *Eur. J. Cancer* **2018**, *89*, 1–8. [CrossRef]
33. Song, J.H.; Yu, M.; Kang, K.M.; Lee, J.H.; Kim, S.H.; Nam, T.K.; Jeong, J.U.; Jang, H.S.; Lee, J.W.; Jung, J.-H. Significance of perineural and lymphovascular invasion in locally advanced rectal cancer treated by preoperative chemoradiotherapy and radical surgery: Can perineural invasion be an indication of adjuvant chemotherapy? *Radiother. Oncol.* **2019**, *133*, 125–131. [CrossRef]
34. Kuo, Y.-H.; Lin, Y.-T.; Ho, C.-H.; Chou, C.-L.; Cheng, L.-C.; Tsai, C.-J.; Hong, W.-J.; Chen, Y.-C.; Yang, C.-C. Adjuvant chemotherapy and survival outcomes in rectal cancer patients with good response (ypT0-2N0) after neoadjuvant chemoradiotherapy and surgery: A retrospective nationwide analysis. *Front. Oncol.* **2022**, *12*, 1087778. [CrossRef]
35. Rödel, C.; Graeven, U.; Fietkau, R.; Hohenberger, W.; Hothorn, T.; Arnold, D.; Hofheinz, R.-D.; Ghadimi, M.; Wolff, H.A.; Lang-Welzenbach, M.; et al. Oxaliplatin added to fluorouracil-based preoperative chemoradiotherapy and postoperative chemotherapy of locally advanced rectal cancer (the German CAO/ARO/AIO-04 study): Final results of the multicentre, open-label, randomised, phase 3 trial. *Lancet Oncol.* **2015**, *16*, 979–989. [CrossRef]
36. Ryan, D.P.; Willett, C.G. Adjuvant Therapy for Resected Rectal Adenocarcinoma in Patients not Receiving Neoadjuvant Therapy—UpToDate. *Uptodate*. 2023. Available online: https://www.uptodate.com/contents/adjuvant-therapy-for-resected-rectal-adenocarcinoma-in-patients-not-receiving-neoadjuvant-therapy?source=mostViewed_widget (accessed on 26 March 2023).
37. Scarlat, F.; Scarisoreanu, A.; Verga, N. Absorbed dose distributions using the isodensitometric method for exposures with filter employed for mammographies. *Rom. Rep. Phys.* **2013**, *65*, 168–177.
38. Delitto, D.; George, T.J.; Loftus, T.J.; Qiu, P.; Chang, G.J.; Allegra, C.J.; Hall, W.A.; Hughes, S.J.; Tan, S.A.; Shaw, C.M.; et al. Prognostic Value of Clinical vs Pathologic Stage in Rectal Cancer Patients Receiving Neoadjuvant Therapy. *Gynecol. Oncol.* **2017**, *110*, 460. [CrossRef]

39. Treder, M.; Janssen, S.; Holländer, N.H.; Schild, S.E.; Rades, D. Role of Neoadjuvant Radio-chemotherapy for the Treatment of High Rectal Cancer. *Anticancer. Res.* **2018**, *38*, 5371–5377. [CrossRef]
40. Moore, H.G.; Gittleman, A.E.; Minsky, B.D.; Wong, D.; Paty, P.B.; Weiser, M.; Temple, L.; Saltz, L.; Shia, J.; Guillem, J.G. Rate of Pathologic Complete Response with Increased Interval Between Preoperative Combined Modality Therapy and Rectal Cancer Resection. *Dis. Colon Rectum* **2004**, *47*, 279–286. [CrossRef]
41. Tan, Y.; Fu, D.; Li, D.; Kong, X.; Jiang, K.; Chen, L.; Yuan, Y.; Ding, K. Predictors and Risk Factors of Pathologic Complete Response Following Neoadjuvant Chemoradiotherapy for Rectal Cancer: A Population-Based Analysis. *Front. Oncol.* **2019**, *9*, 497. [CrossRef]

Disclaimer/Publisher's Note: The statements, opinions and data contained in all publications are solely those of the individual author(s) and contributor(s) and not of MDPI and/or the editor(s). MDPI and/or the editor(s) disclaim responsibility for any injury to people or property resulting from any ideas, methods, instructions or products referred to in the content.

Article

Parathyroid Cancer—A Rare Finding during Parathyroidectomy in High Volume Surgery Centre

Petru Radu [1], Dragos Garofil [1,*], Anca Tigora [1], Mihai Zurzu [1], Vlad Paic [1], Mircea Bratucu [1], Mircea Litescu [2], Virgil Prunoiu [3], Valentin Georgescu [1], Florian Popa [1], Valeriu Surlin [4] and Victor Strambu [1]

[1] General Surgery Clinic, Clinical Nephrology Hospital "Dr. Carol Davila", 020021 Bucharest, Romania
[2] Clinical Emergency Hospital "Sfantul Ioan", 042022 Bucharest, Romania
[3] Oncological Institute "Prof. Dr. Alexandru Trestioreanu", 022328 Bucharest, Romania
[4] Sixth Department of Surgery, University of Medicine and Pharmacy of Craiova, Craiova Emergency Clinical Hospital, 200642 Craiova, Romania
* Correspondence: dragosgarofil@gmail.com

Abstract: *Background and Objectives*: Parathyroid cancer is a very rare endocrine tumor, especially in patients with secondary hyperparathyroidism due to end stage renal disease failure. This pathology is difficult to diagnose preoperatively because it has nonspecific clinical manifestations and paraclinical aspects. Our study of the literature identified 34 reported cases of parathyroid carcinoma over the last 40 years in patients undergoing dialysis. We present our experience as illustrative of the features of clinical presentation and histopathological findings of parathyroid carcinoma and assess its management considering the recent relevant literature. *Materials and Methods*: From January 2012 to November 2022, 650 patients with secondary hyperparathyroidism undergoing dialysis were treated at our academic Department of General Surgery and only two cases of parathyroid carcinoma were diagnosed on histopathological examination. *Results*: All patients presented with symptomatic hypercalcemia, with no clinical or imaging suspicion of malignant disease and were surgically treated by total parathyroidectomy. Histopathological examination revealed morphologic aspects of parathyroid carcinoma in two cases and immunostaining of Ki-67 was performed for diagnostic confirmation. Postoperative follow-up showed no signs of recurrence and no oncological adjuvant treatment or surgical reinterventions were needed. *Conclusions*: Parathyroid neoplasia is a particularly rare disease, that remains a challenge when it comes to diagnosis and proper management. Surgical approach is the only valid treatment to remove the malignant tissue and thus improve the patient's prognosis. Medical and oncologic treatment may be beneficial to control hypercalcemia in case of tumor recurrence.

Keywords: parathyroid carcinoma; secondary hyperparathyroidism; hypercalcemia

1. Introduction

Parathyroid carcinoma is a rare endocrine tumor, with an estimated prevalence of 0.005% of all cancers [1] and accounting for less than 1% of parathyroid pathology [2], with the highest incidence of 5% being registered in Japan [3]. Few over 1100 cases of parathyroid malignancy have been reported worldwide [4], the majority (97%) associated with primary hyperparathyroidism (PHPT) [5]. Parathyroid neoplasia is quite uncommon in patients with secondary or tertiary hyperparathyroidism, only 34 cases being reported in the literature associated with end stage renal disease [6], Table 1. Considering gender distribution, both men and women are equally affected, in contrast to benign parathyroid tumors that occur more frequently in women (male:female ratio is 1:4) [7]. It often manifests in individuals during the 4–5th decade of life, being diagnosed approximately 10 years earlier than parathyroid adenomas [8].

Table 1. Parathyroid Carcinoma in patients undergoing dialysis due to chronic renal failure reported in the literature [6].

Case No.	Authors	Year	Age at Diagnosis	Gender	Duration of HD (Years)	Metastasis	Follow-Up (Month)	Status
1	Berland	1982	62	Female	3	No	5	DF
2	Anderson	1983	44	Female		No	17	DFD
3	Ireland	1985	34	Male	5		84	DFD
4	Sherlock	1985	42	Female	7	No	12	DF
5	Krishna	1989	64	Female	9	No	36	DF
6	Kodama	1989	53	Female	7	No	4	DF
7	Iwamoto	1990	46	Male	11	No		
8			55	Female	5	No		
9	Rademaker	1990	46	Female	3	No	84	DF
10			52	Female	2	No	48	DF
11	Tominaga	1995	46	Female	20	Lung		
12	Miki	1996	40	Female	5	Lung	115	
13	Liou	1996	64	Male	0.2	No	12	DF
14	Tseng	1999	20	Female	5	Liver	4	DFD
15	Takami	1999	55	Female	3	No	4	DF
16	Jayawardene	2000	75	Female	3	No		DF
17	Kuji	2000	51	Male	22			
18	Zivaljevic	2002	69	Male	5	No	9	DF
19	Srouji	2004	27	Female	8	No	9	DF
20	Khan	2004	33	Male	10	Lung, Bone	22	AWD
21	Bossola	2005	52	Female	2	No	93	DF
22	Babar-Craig	2005	55	Male				
23	Falvo	2005	61	Male	18	No	18	DF
24	Tzaczyk	2007	55	Male				
25	Diaconescu	2011	48	Male	13	No	54	DF
26	Nasrallah	2014	53	Male	6	No	2	AWD
27	Kim	2016	57	Male	11	No	12	DF
28	Pappa	2017	45	Male	4	No	20	DF
29	Curto	2019	59	Female	40	Lung	6	DF
30	Shen	2019	70	Male	0.5	No	16	DF
31	Won	2019	46		15			
32	Cappellacci	2020	51	Male	15	No	22	DF
33	Malipedda	2020	53	Male	5	No		DF
34	Kada	2021	48	Female	15	No	100	DF

Abbreviations: AWD—alive with disease; DF—disease free; DFD—death from disease.

The etiology and pathogenesis of parathyroid cancer is little understood, for it is usually a sporadic disease [8]. Hereditary cases have also been reported, therefore genetic studies identified several potential genes related to parathyroid cancer such as BRCA2 (breast cancer gene 1), p53, PRAD1 (parathyroid adenomatosis gene 1) or abnormal expression of microRNAs [9]. Moreover, it was diagnosed in association with other hereditary syndromes such as multiple endocrine neoplasia type 1 (MEN 1), type 2A (MEN 2A), Wilm's tumors, breast cancer, retinoblastoma (Rb), polycystic disease, familial isolated hyperparathyroidism (FIHP) and more often with hyperparathyroidism–jaw tumor (HPT–JT) syndrome [8]. HPT–JT syndrome is an autosomal dominant disease caused by mutations in the tumor suppressor gene CDC73, characterized by clinical manifestations of hyperparathyroidism and ossifying fibromas of the maxilla and mandible (5–30%) [10]. Several risk factors have been incriminated in the occurrence of parathyroid cancer, such as previous radiation of the cervical area or chronic stimulation from persistent hypocalcemia. There are no data suggesting that preexisting parathyroid lesions lead to malignant transformation [11].

2. Clinical Presentation

The majority of parathyroid cancers (90%) are hormonally functional tumors, with clinical manifestations of hypercalcemia as a result of excessive PTH serum levels [8]. Initially, the clinical presentation of parathyroid carcinoma is similar to benign hyperplasia and only in advanced stages patients present signs and symptoms of local tumor growth and adjacent tissue invasion [3], Table 2.

Table 2. Clinical and biological features of benign secondary hyperparathyroidism and parathyroid carcinoma [7].

Factor	Benign Secondary Hyperparathyroidism	Parathyroid Carcinoma
Female:Male ratio	4:1	1:1
Average age	55	48
Serum calcium (mg/dL)	≤12	>14
Serum PTH (pg/mL)	10–20× above the upper normal limit	3–10× above the upper normal limit
Palpable cervical mass	Rare	Common
Bone dysfunction	Common	Common

Due to the intensive and constant care services and biochemical routine screening performed by the hemodialysis centers, hyperparathyroidism associated with end stage renal disease is usually detected before the advent of features of hypercalcemia. Therefore, patients usually present mild symptoms such as fatigue, muscle weakness, impaired focus, depression or lethargy [12]. In addition to already existing renal dysfunction, the affliction is accompanied by skeletal impairment (osteopenia, subperiosteal resorption, spontaneous pathological fractures, bone and joint pain, osteitis fibrosa cystica, "salt and pepper" skull) [7,8,12]. None of these clinical aspects are pathognomonic of parathyroid malignancy. Of all parathyroid carcinomas, 10% are nonsecreting tumors and are difficult to diagnose in early stages, thus patients often exhibit palpable neck mass, dysphagia, hoarseness, dyspnea and augmented cervical lymph nodes [4]. Moreover, completely asymptomatic parathyroid neoplasia have been reported in 7 to 46% cases [11,13].

3. Paraclinical Aspects

There is no agreed interval or threshold for PTH and serum calcium levels to define parathyroid cancer. Studies have noted that patients with parathyroid neoplasia present serum calcium levels higher than 3.5 mmol/L and PTH serum levels 3 to 10 times above the normal limit [11]. In addition, Bae et all pointed out that alkaline phosphatase levels higher that 285 IU/L in combination with a tumor size >3 cm can predict the malignant character of a suspicious parathyroid lesion [14].

Imaging investigations are useful and of particular importance for tumor localization but are not able to differentiate adenomas from carcinomas. Ultrasonography is the most used imaging examination for identifying parathyroid abnormalities due to its low cost and noninvasive approach, but its accuracy is questionable when it comes to distinguishing benign form malignant lesions. Parathyroid carcinomas frequently present as hypoechoic, nonhomogeneous tumors, lobulated, with ill-circumscribed margins, thick capsule or intranodular calcification [15]. Moreover, lesions of large size >3 cm, with local tissue invasion and presence of enlarged cervical lymph nodes are aspects that may suggest a positive preoperative diagnosis [16]. Hara et al. also correlated the depth and width of the lesions with the probability of malignancy, concluding that a D/W ratio >1 is suggestive for carcinoma [17].

Scintigraphy with Tc^{99} sestamibi can also be helpful for a precise localization of the parathyroid glands, especially for ectopic sites or hyperactive metastatic parathyroid tissue [18]. Its operating principle is based on the increased and prolonged retention of technetium 99-m within the mitochondria of the abnormal parathyroid gland. This imaging scan also has a high rate of false positive results due to the occasional uptake of the contrast agent within the thyroid gland or cystic degeneration of parathyroid cancer [19]. However, a recent study conducted by Zhang in 2019 demonstrated that parathyroid malignant tumors have a higher uptake level of Tc^{99}-MIBI than benign tumors and the peak of retention index (RI peak, $p < 0.001$) in correlation to serum levels of parathyroid hormone (PTH) may contribute to a preoperative differential diagnosis of parathyroid carcinoma [20].

Both CT and MRI prove their utility in advanced stages of the tumor, providing information related to tumor size, local extension and invasion into adjacent organs (thyroid, trachea, esophagus, cervical muscles, etc.) or presence of metastasis (mediastinal, pulmonary, hepatic or bone) [21]. CT suggestive aspects of parathyroid carcinoma include high short-to-long axis ratio, irregular margins, tumoral calcification, adjacent infiltration and low contrast enhancement [22]. MRI features are similar to CT imaging revealing large parathyroid glands, ill-defined, with increased heterogeneity [16].

PET-CT with 18-FDG (fluorodeoxyglucose positron emission tomography) is a qualitative examination based on emphasizing the increased glucose metabolism of malignant cells. It can provide additional information related to the location and extent of parathyroid carcinoma especially in cases of tumor recurrence, distant spread of the disease or assessment of residual malignant tissue after surgical treatment [16]. However, certain conditions can show a false positive result on PET scans such as postoperative or posttreatment cervical tissue inflammation or infectious lymphadenopathy [19].

In case of suspicion of parathyroid carcinoma, fine needle aspiration cytology (FNAC) is not recommended due to the risk of seeding of malignant cells and high rate of false negative results [8]. On the other hand, FNAC could be performed for the confirmation of parathyroid tissue in aberrant locations, which in association with increased PTH serum levels can suggest a distant metastasis or recurrence of the disease [16].

4. Diagnosis

Parathyroid cancer is difficult to diagnose preoperatively because it has nonspecific clinical manifestations and paraclinical aspects. This pathology can be suspected when patients present with severe hypercalcemia (>14 mg/dL), parathormone elevations and a palpable anterior cervical mass with compressive complications [23].

Intraoperative diagnosis is also doubtful, but certain macroscopic features may raise the suspicion of neoplasia. A parathyroid gland larger than 3 cm, with irregular margins, high consistency, white-gray colored, with cystic or calcified component, enclosed by a dense fibrous capsule is suggestive for carcinoma [8,11]. Cervical lymph node augmentation and local firm adhesion to adjacent structures are additional indicators for malignancy [24].

The diagnosis is usually confirmed postoperatively after the histopathological examination. In 1973, Schantz and Castleman first defined the morphologic aspects of parathyroid carcinoma: cells displayed in a lobular pattern, separated by dense, fibrotic bands, with capsular and vascular invasion and atypical mitosis. Moreover, diffuse nuclear augmentation, macronuclei and a high Ki-67 expression are evocative for neoplastic proliferation [23]. Immunohistochemistry can assist diagnostic accuracy using a highly specific marker (parafibromin) encoded by the CDC73 gene [25,26], which is a test recommended in standardized protocols by the American Association of Endocrine Surgeons Guidelines for Definitive Management of Primary HPT [11].

No pathological staging system for parathyroid carcinoma has been universally adopted considering it is a rare disorder and data collected are mostly retrospective and single institution studies. Nevertheless, the newest edition of the American Joint Committee on Cancer Guidelines introduced a staging system for parathyroid carcinoma in 2017 as presented in Table 3 [23].

Table 3. Parathyroid cancer TNM staging system according to 2017 new edition of AJCC [17].

Stage	Pathological Aspects
Tumor	
Tis	Noninvasive or in situ cancer
T1	Tumor with capsular and surrounding soft tissue invasion
T2	Tumor with invasion of the thyroid gland
T3	Tumor invading the trachea, esophagus or recurrent laryngeal nerve
T4	Tumor invading major blood vessels/spine
Lymph Nodes	
N0	No regional lymph node metastases
N1a	Metastases in central neck lymph nodes
N1b	Metastases in lateral neck lymph nodes
Metastases	
M0	No evidence of distant metastases
M1	Evidence of distant metastases

5. Treatment

5.1. Medical Treatment

Available medical therapy only targets the repercussion of the disease (hypercalcemia) rather than the condition itself and it is recommended for lowering calcium serum levels and management of implicit metabolic disorders. Calcimimetics are the most effective treatment for control of hypercalcemia in patients with secondary hyperparathyroidism awaiting surgery or inoperable parathyroid carcinoma [26]. They are allosteric receptor modulators that increase the receptor's affinity for calcium and reduce PTH secretion. Cinacalcet, a second-generation calcimimetic, approved in 2004 in the United States and European Union, has been successfully used in patients with inoperable parathyroid cancer, correcting hypercalcemia in approximately 66% of cases [16].

Intravenous administration of bisphosphonates can also reduce hypercalcemia by inhibiting osteoclastic activity, but the result is slow to take effect [27]. For a faster result in lowering calcium levels, administration of Calcitonin should be taken into consideration based on its properties to inhibit bone resorption [16].

5.2. Surgical Treatment

Surgical treatment is the only valid therapy to remove the malignant tissue, to control hypercalcemia and thus improve the patient's prognosis. Complete resection with no microscopically invaded margins and averting tearing of the capsule is optimal to achieve the best long-term outcomes [28]. Considering the fact that neoplastic proliferation of parathyroid glands is rarely diagnosed intraoperatively, only local pericapsular excision is performed during the initial operation. In case of macroscopic cancer speculation, most authors concur that an en bloc excision should be executed, consisting of tumor removal, ipsilateral thyroid lobectomy, ipsilateral hemi-thymectomy, paratracheal lymphadenectomy and adjacent cervical muscle resection. On occasion, more invasive tumors may require extensive excisions including tracheal, esophagus, blood vessels or recurrent laryngeal nerve resections [29].

5.3. Adjuvant Treatment

Adjuvant treatments consisting of chemotherapy and radiotherapy have been attempted but the results were discouraging. Parathyroid carcinoma is known to be a radio-resistant tumor, therefore the use of this kind of therapy is controversial [16]. Previous studies presented survival analysis in patients who underwent radiation therapy after surgery and concluded that this treatment did not reduce tumor recurrence, nor improve the prognosis [30]. Sadler et all reported after an analysis performed on 1000 patients with parathyroid carcinoma that radiation therapy was associated with a lower 5-year overall survival [31].

Cytotoxic chemotherapy is even less used than adjuvant radiation because its efficiency has been reported only in isolated cases [19]. The chemotherapy regimen include monotherapy with dacarbazine or combined therapy with dacarbazine-5 fluorouracil-cyclophosphamide or methotrexate-doxorubicin-cyclophosphamide-lomustine [21].

Currently, isolated case reports have shown a response to metastatic disease from parathyroid carcinoma with sorafenib [32]. It is a protein kinase inhibitor which suppresses tumor growth due to its anti-angiogenetic function (blocks VEGF, PDGF receptors and BRAF protein) [19].

Therefore, no other associated therapy has proved highly effective in the management of patients with parathyroid carcinoma and there is no clear protocol to be followed [7].

6. Methods

From January 2012 to November 2022, 650 patients with secondary hyperparathyroidism due to end stage renal disease failure undergoing dialysis were treated at our academic Department of General Surgery as presented in Figure 1. The male:female ratio was approximately 1:1 (333 men and 317 women) with a mean age of 53 (range 20–83). Mean preoperative parathormone (PTH) serum level was 1405 pg/mL (normal range level 17.3–73 pg/mL) with a maximum registered value of 4120 pg/mL. Almost 70% of patients had PTH serum levels over 1000 pg/mL. Mean preoperative calcium level was 12.43 mg/dL, with maximum calcemia level of 17.8 mg/dL.

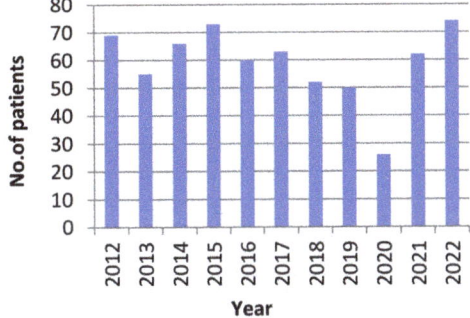

Figure 1. Patients (n = 650) with secondary hyperparathyroidism treated in our clinic in the past 10 years.

All patients were operated under general anesthesia with orotracheal intubation and total parathyroidectomy was performed. There were 29 cases of reintervention for recurrence of secondary hyperparathyroidism due to incomplete resection of the parathyroid glands during initial surgery: three patients with supernumerary parathyroid glands, four patients with ectopic anterior mediastinal localization of one gland, three patients who were scheduled for kidney transplant and thus a subtotal parathyroidectomy was executed and in 19 cases we were not able to intraoperatively identify all four parathyroid glands. The average period of hospitalization was 9 days.

In the past 10 years, among all cases of patients with secondary hyperparathyroidism surgically treated in our clinic, two cases of parathyroid carcinoma were diagnosed using histopathological examination.

Case 1: A 35-year old man with a background of hypertension and family history of autosomal dominant polycystic kidney disease, with chronic renal failure undergoing dialysis for 3 years, was admitted with symptomatic hypercalcemia (calcium serum level −11.6 mg/dL) and elevated PTH serum level (804 pg/mL) accusing muscle weakness, bone pain and fatigue. Ultrasound scan of the anterior cervical region identified three enlarged parathyroid glands with no suspicious imaging aspects. At surgical intervention, four augmented parathyroid glands (1.6 to 2 cm diameter) were macroscopically confirmed, and a total parathyroidectomy was performed. The histological examination revealed predominantly nodular hyperplasia of chief-cells and oxyphilic cells in approximately equal proportions for three of the endocrine glands. The right inferior parathyroid gland presented partially modified histological architecture, nuclei with moderate pleomorphism Figure 2, no mitosis, but evidence of cellular invasion into the capsule and one blood vessel, foci of intralesional necrosis Figure 3, areas of dystrophic calcification processes and moderate chronic inflammatory cell infiltrate Figure 4, aspects suggestive of neoplastic lesion. Immunohistochemical evaluation was performed for Rb (negative), Mdm2-p53 (positive in rare nuclei) and Ki-67 (>5%). In the immediate postoperative period, the patient had low calcium serum levels (7.2 to 8.1 mg/dL) and needed high doses of intravenous calcium gluconate and oral calcium lactate associated with alfacalcidol to maintain safe blood calcium levels. Twenty-four hours after surgery, PTH serum level was detected with a value of 26 pg/mL. The 48-month follow up (ultrasound of the neck and PET-CT) did not show any signs of local recurrence or metastasis.

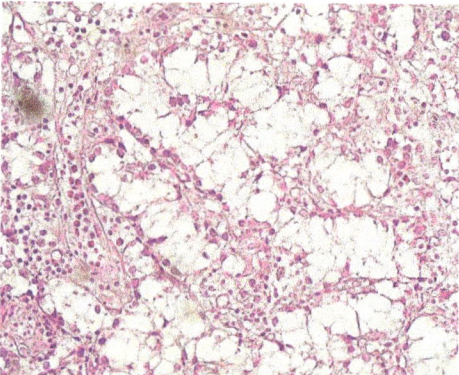

Figure 2. Proliferation of round-oval cells with clear cytoplasm, moderate cytonuclear pleomorphism with centrally located nucleoli or granular chromatin (H and E, ×40).

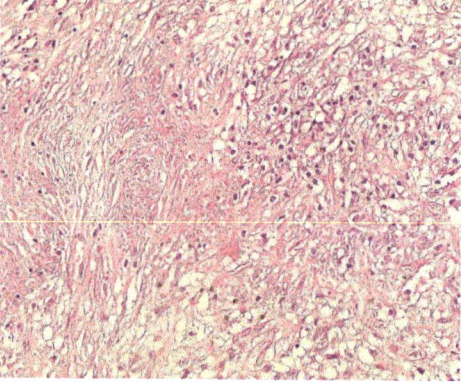

Figure 3. Clear cell proliferation with association of focal areas of intralesional necrosis (H and E, ×40).

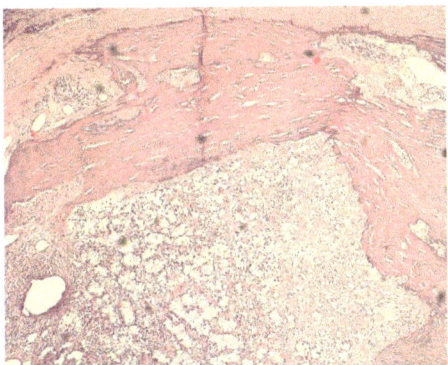

Figure 4. Proliferation of clear cells partially delimited by dystrophic calcification processes and moderate chronic lymphocytic inflammatory cell infiltrate. (H and E, ×10).

Case 2: A 55-year old woman, with background history of hypertension, diabetes mellitus type 2, obesity, general atherosclerosis and chronic renal failure in hemodialysis program for 5 years, was referred for surgical treatment of secondary hyperparathyroidism in late 2015. The patient had signs and symptoms of hypercalcemia (intense bone pain, muscle weakness, osteoporosis, skin lesions of calciphylaxis on the lower limbs, calcification of the main arterial trunks), as shown in Figure 5, with a serum calcium level of 13.2 mg/dL and PTH serum level of 1283 pg/mL. No imaging investigations were performed before surgery. Intraoperatively, all four enlarged parathyroid glands were identified (1.3 to 2 cm diameter) and carefully removed, with no macroscopic suspicion of malignant proliferation. Histological examination uncovered three parathyroid glands with regular nodular hyperplasia and the right inferior gland with cells displayed in a trabecular pattern, outlined by dense, fibrotic bands (intensely desmoplastic stroma), as shown in Figure 6, and surrounding adipose tissue infiltration. Immunostaining of Ki-67 was performed with a tumor cell positivity of 4–5%. Postoperative course was uneventful, with decreasing PTH serum levels (12.3 pg/mL) and normal calcemia (8.3 mg/dL) and no necessary medication for hypocalcemia. At 5 year follow-up patient presented with no signs of tumor recurrence, normal hormone levels and normocalcemia, but further died of acute cardiovascular events.

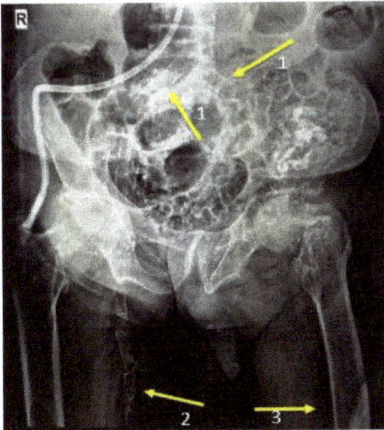

Figure 5. Signs of hypercalcemia in a 55 year old woman with secondary hyperparathyroidism. 1. Calcification of the common iliac arteries; 2. calcification of the right femoral artery; 3. subperiosteal resorption of the left femur.

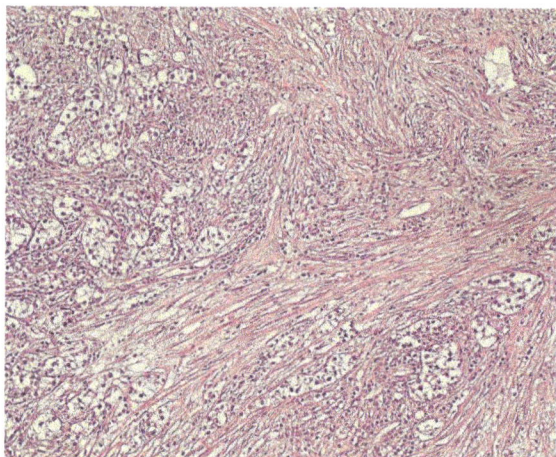

Figure 6. Parathyroid tissue with proliferation of clear cells, with solid–trabecular architecture and intensely desmoplastic stroma. (H and E, ×20).

7. Discussion

Currently, endocrine surgery is a stand-alone sub-specialty of general surgery dedicated to surgical treatment of abdominal and cervical endocrine tumors [33]. Moreover, most studies suggest that surgeons committed to neck surgery performed in high-volume settings are likely to meet better clinical and economic outcomes [34]. Some review studies attempted to define the criteria for high-volume centers/surgeons by analyzing the number of thyroidectomies and parathyroidectomies for primary hyperparathyroidism performed per year in multiple hospitals. Although thyroid and parathyroid interventions have anatomical and surgical similarities, the literature emphasizes that the operative volume is organ specific [34]. Therefore, Iacobone and coll. concluded that >40 parathyroidectomies/year is an appropriate tier to describe an adequate activity and Melfa et all established that 90–100 thyroidectomies/year define a high-volume setting. There are no published reports to suggest any point of reference concerning surgical treatment for secondary hyperparathyroidism. In accordance with recently mentioned aspects, our hospital performs an average of 94 neck surgeries per year (22 for thyroid disease, 7 for primary hyperparathyroidism and 65 for secondary hyperparathyroidism). Given our clinical institution's nephrological field of specialty, the majority of patients admitted have end stage kidney disease and are referred to our surgical department for total parathyroidectomy. Considering the data presented and debated in 2019 at the Conference of the European Society of Endocrine Surgeons, our center meets the criteria for high-volume settings, with a mean of 72 annual surgical interventions for parathyroid disease and is among the few hospitals in the country that address this pathology.

The malignant proliferation of the parathyroid gland is a rare occurrence, the first cases being reported in 1933 by Sainton and 1938 by Armstrong [35]. As yet, few over 1100 cases of parathyroid carcinoma have been described in the literature. Most of the cases are associated with primary hyperparathyroidism, only 3% are related to parathyroid hyperplasia due to end stage renal disease failure. The incidence of this condition varies from 1% in USA to 3% in Italy and 5% in Japan [8]. According to our center's retrospective analysis, the incidence of parathyroid carcinoma in patients undergoing dialysis was 0.3%.

This particular neoplasia appears in sporadic cases and until 2006 it was not recorded by most international organizations such as WHO or SEER Cancer Statistics Review [4]. Its etiology and pathogenesis is unknown and there is little agreement on a systematic oncological surgical approach. Benign parathyroid hyperplasia as a precursor to malignant alteration has not been reported by previous studies [35].

The clinical diagnosis is difficult to state given its similarities to parathyroid adenomas' symptomatology, which comprises renal and skeletal impairment. According to Obara et al. the clinical aspects suggestive for parathyroid malignancy are

- age below 55
- elevated parathormone level (>10 times normal range)
- hypercalcemia
- severe bone symptoms
- renal symptoms
- palpable cervical tumor
- recurrent laryngeal paralysis [36].

The two patients diagnosed in our center presented only 5 of the 7 criteria mentioned. Laboratory parameters to distinguish parathyroid adenoma from carcinoma are also nonspecific.

Imaging investigations (ultrasound, CT, MRI, scintigraphy Tc^{99} sestamibi) are not definitive in the differential diagnosis between the two conditions, unless the patient presents with advanced stage of the disease, with signs of local tumor compression/invasion or metastasis. Therefore, in both listed cases, all four parathyroid glands were identified and removed during surgery with no preoperative imaging studies or inconclusive ones.

Parathyroid glands with malignant proliferation are considered to be large tumors (>3 cm diameter), lobulated, with irregular margins, high consistency and greyish colored [37,38]. None of these aspects were identified intraoperatively in our two case studies (both were <2 cm, smooth outlines, low consistency and normal colored).

The positive diagnosis is set postoperatively on histological examination, which reveals cells displayed in a trabecular pattern, atypical mitosis, fibrous bands and vascular or capsular invasion, aspects that according to some authors are not pathognomonic for neoplasia [38]. According to Erikson et al.'s overview of the 2022 WHO classification of parathyroid tumors, the histological definition of parathyroid carcinoma includes one of the following criteria: (a) cellular invasion of blood vessels, (b) lymphatic invasion, (c) neural invasion, (d) local invasion into proximate anatomic structures or (e) histologically/cytologically registered metastatic disease [39]. Schantz and Castleman's study on 70 patients with parathyroid neoplasia concluded that vascular invasion or the number of mitoses are not reliable predictive indicators of further progression of the disease [40]. The first referred case presented partially modified histological architecture (nuclei with moderate pleomorphism, no mitosis, areas of intralesional necrosis and dystrophic calcification, moderate lymphocytic cell infiltrate and cellular invasion into the capsule and one blood vessel) assessing two of the WHO indicators. The histological analysis in the second case uncovered cells displayed in a trabecular pattern, intensely desmoplastic stroma, capsular invasion and surrounding adipose tissue infiltration, meeting three of the required criteria.

Therefore, additional immunohistochemistry and DNA analysis may be required for further confirmation, but no single marker has proved highly sensitive or specific (Rb, Ki-67, parafibromin). Recent recommendations of WHO (2022) in parathyroid carcinoma include Ki-67 labeling index, a nuclear protein previously identified as a cellular marker for proliferation in breast, prostate and neuroendocrine tumors. Most parathyroid carcinomas show a labeling index that exceeds 5% [39]. Currently, the loss of expression of parafibromin due to CDC73/HRPT2 mutation is considered the most specific indicator of parathyroid carcinoma (77%) [41]. Barazeghi et all (2016) and previous studies from the literature also underlined the implication of TET2 (ten-eleven translocation) gene expression in the pathogenesis of parathyroid cancer. The TET proteins play a regulatory role in cell growth and migration and its deregulated expression lead to reduced levels of 5-hydroxymethylcytosine (5hmC), frequently encountered in various types of neoplasia (breast, prostate, hematological or colorectal tumors) [42]. Unfortunately, sequencing these genes is expensive, difficult to conduct and not available in most pathology laboratories or hospitals without research units. In our center, only immunostaining of Ki-67 is accessible and in both cases presented tumor cell positivity was 4–5%.

The main goal of surgery in patients with secondary end stage kidney disease is to control endocrine function and thus regulate calcium serum levels. In cases of suspicion of parathyroid carcinoma, oncological purpose is taken into consideration. Most studies endorse en bloc resection of the tumor, ipsilateral thyroid lobe and thymus during initial surgery, with avoiding the gland's capsule rupture. This approach improves the patient's prognosis and survival rate with 90% at 5 years and 67% at 10 years [36]. Considering the fact that neoplastic proliferation of parathyroid glands is rarely diagnosed intraoperatively, only local pericapsular excision is performed, with an estimated recurrence at 2–3 years. In our report, the two patients were annually re-evaluated for minimum 4 years after local excision and no relapse was pointed out.

Another issue to be taken into consideration is the risk of neoplastic seeding in subtotal parathyroidectomies or total parathyroidectomies with immediate transplantation of parathyroid tissue in cervical or forearm regions. These type of surgical interventions are recommended to preserve the parathyroid hormone production and to avoid postoperative severe hypocalcemia. Since pathological glands with neoplastic proliferation are difficult to impossible to recognize macroscopically during surgery, there is the possibility of leaving behind malignant tissue in situ. In our center, three young patients with secondary hyperparathyroidism who were scheduled for kidney transplant at the moment of admittance underwent surgery. In these cases, a subtotal parathyroidectomy was performed choosing an alternative surgical approach described by B. Stanescu, which involves mobilization and subcutaneous placement of the remaining inferior parathyroid stump, together with its vascular pedicle above the sternum. Only one of the patients had a kidney transplant, the other two were subsequently admitted to our surgical department at one year for recurrence of the disease and totalization was performed.

Postoperatively, close monitoring of calcemia is mandatory and appropriate administration of calcium medication is necessary to avoid severe hypocalcemia due to "hungry bone syndrome".

Unfortunately, adjuvant oncological treatment with radiotherapy or chemotherapy for this type of cancer has not proved effective.

8. Conclusions

Parathyroid carcinoma is an extremely rare tumor that remains a challenge when it comes to diagnosis and proper treatment. Despite these aspects, in the presence of hyperparathyroidism showing severe hypercalcemia, renal and skeletal impairment, a neoplastic lesion of the parathyroid gland should be suspected. Experienced surgeons and pathologists in high-volume centers have a better chance of diagnosing parathyroid carcinoma and are likely to meet better clinical and economic outcomes. Histopathological examination is the only analysis able to establish the positive diagnosis. Association with immunohistochemistry (Ki-67 labeling index) and sequencing certain tumor suppressing genes (HRPT2, TET2) improves the accuracy of the diagnosis. At present, there are no reliable criteria to predict recurrence risk of the disease, tumor aggressiveness or patient prognosis. Complete surgical resection at the earliest possible time is the ideal treatment to improve patients' survival rate. Parathyroid neoplastic proliferation is difficult to impossible to recognize macroscopically intraoperative; therefore, the risk of seeding malignant tissue in case of subtotal parathyroidectomy or autotransplant has to be considered. Available medical therapy only targets the repercussion of the disease (hypercalcemia) rather than the condition itself.

Author Contributions: Conceptualization, P.R. and D.G.; methodology, P.R. and A.T.; software, M.B.; validation, P.R., F.P. and V.S. (Victor Strambu); formal analysis, M.Z.; investigation, V.P. (Vlad Paic); resources, V.S. (Valeriu Surlin) and V.G.; data curation, V.P. (Virgiliu Prunoiu) and M.L.; writing—original draft preparation, D.G. and V.S. (Victor Strambu); writing—review and editing, all authors; visualization, P.R. and A.T.; supervision V.S. (Victor Strambu); project administration, M.B. All authors have read and agreed to the published version of the manuscript.

Funding: This research received no external funding.

Institutional Review Board Statement: The study was conducted in accordance with the Declaration of Helsinki, and approved by the Research Ethics Committee of Carol Davila University of Medicine and Pharmacy, Bucharest (protocol code 38030/09.12.2022).

Informed Consent Statement: Informed consent was obtained from all subjects involved in the study. Written informed consent has been obtained from the patients to publish this paper.

Data Availability Statement: Data is unavailable due to privacy or ethical restrictions due to GDPR regulations.

Conflicts of Interest: The authors declare no conflict of interest.

References

1. Hundahl, S.A.; Fleming, I.D.; Fremgen, A.M.; Menck, H.R. Two hundred eighty-six cases of parathyroid carcinoma treated in the U.S. between 1985–1995. *Cancer* **1999**, *86*, 538–544. [CrossRef]
2. Bossola, M.; Tazza, L.; Ferrante, A.; Giungi, S.; Carbone, A.; Gui, A.; Luciani, G. Parathyroid carcinoma in a chronic hemodialysis patient: Case report and review of literature. *Tumori* **2005**, *91*, 558–562. [CrossRef] [PubMed]
3. Kirkby-Bott, J.; Lewis, P.; Harmer, C.L.; Smellie, W.J.B. One stage treatment of parathyroid cancer. *Eur. J. Surg. Oncol. EJSO* **2005**, *31*, 78–83. [CrossRef] [PubMed]
4. Talat, N.; Schulte, K.-M. Clinical Presentation, Staging and Long-Term Evolution of Parathyroid Cancer. *Ann. Surg. Oncol.* **2010**, *17*, 2156–2174. [CrossRef] [PubMed]
5. Khan, M. Parathyroid carcinoma in secondary and tertiary hyperparathyroidism1. *J. Am. Coll. Surg.* **2004**, *199*, 312–319. [CrossRef] [PubMed]
6. Kada, S.; Tanaka, M.; Yasoda, A. Parathyroid carcinoma in a patient with secondary hyperparathyroidism and thyroid hemiagenesis: A Case Report and Review of the Literature. *Ear Nose Throat J.* **2021**, *28*, 1455613211036240. [CrossRef] [PubMed]
7. Marcocci, C.; Cetani, F.; Rubin, M.R.; Silverberg, S.J.; Pinchera, A.; Bilezikian, J.P. Parathyroid carcinoma. *J. Bone Miner. Res.* **2008**, *23*, 1869–1880. [CrossRef] [PubMed]
8. Favia, G.; Iacobone, M. Parathyroid Carcinoma. In *Primary, Secondary and Tertiary Hyperparathyroidism*; Springer: Berlin/Heidelberg, Germany, 2016; pp. 183–191.
9. Shane, E. Clinical Review 122: Parathyroid carcinoma. *J. Clin. Endocrinol. Metab.* **2001**, *86*, 485–493. [CrossRef]
10. Woodard, G.E.; Lin, L.; Zhang, J.-H.; Agarwal, S.K.; Marx, S.J.; Simonds, W.F. Parafibromin, product of the hyperparathyroidism–jaw tumor syndrome gene HRPT2, regulates cyclin D1/PRAD1 expression. *Oncogene* **2005**, *24*, 1272–1276. [CrossRef]
11. Ferraro, V.; Sgaramella, L.I.; Di Meo, G.; Prete, F.P.; Logoluso, F.; Minerva, F.; Noviello, M.; Renzulli, G.; Gurrado, A.; Testini, M. Current concepts in parathyroid carcinoma: A single Centre experience. *BMC Endocr. Disord.* **2019**, *19* (Suppl. 1), 46. [CrossRef]
12. Fingeret, A. Contemporary Evaluation and Management of Parathyroid Carcinoma. *JCO Oncol. Pract.* **2022**, *17*, 17. [CrossRef] [PubMed]
13. Sharretts, J.M.; Simonds, W.F. Clinical and molecular genetics of parathyroid neoplasms. *Best Pract. Res. Clin. Endocrinol. Metab.* **2010**, *24*, 491–502. [CrossRef]
14. Bae, J.H.; Choi, H.J.; Lee, Y.; Moon, M.K.; Park, Y.J.; Shin, C.S.; Park, D.J.; Jang, H.C.; Kim, S.T.; Kim, S.W. Preoperative predictive factors for parathyroid carcinoma in patients with primary hyperparathyroidism. *J. Korean Med. Sci.* **2012**, *27*, 890–895. [CrossRef] [PubMed]
15. Tamler, R.; Lewis, M.S.; LiVolsi, V.A.; Genden, E.M. Parathyroid Carcinoma: Ultrasonographic and Histologic Features. *Thyroid* **2005**, *15*, 744–745. [CrossRef] [PubMed]
16. Rodrigo, P.J.; Hernandez-Prera, C.J.; Randolph, W.G.; Zafereo, E.M.; Hartl, M.D.; Silver, E.C.; Suárez, C.; Owen, P.R.; Bradford, R.C.; Mäkitie, A.A.; et al. Parathyroid cancer: An update. *Cancer Treat Rev.* **2020**, *86*, 102012. [CrossRef] [PubMed]
17. Hara, H.; Igarashi, A.; Yano, Y.; Yashiro, T.; Ueno, E.; Aiyoshi, Y.; Ito, K.; Obara, T. Ultrasonographic features of parathyroid carcinoma. *Endocr. J.* **2001**, *48*, 213–217. [CrossRef]
18. Duan, K.; Mete, O. Parathyroid carcinoma: Diagnosis and clinical implications. *Turk. J. Pathol.* **2015**, *31* (Suppl. S1), 80–97. [CrossRef]
19. Machado, N.N.; Wilhelm, M.S. Parathyroid cancer: A review. *Cancers* **2019**, *11*, 1676. [CrossRef]
20. Zhang, M.; Sun, L.; Rui, W.; Guo, R.; He, H.; Miao, Y.; Meng, H.; Liu, J.; Li, B. Semi-quantitative analysis of 99mTc-sestamibi retention level for preoperative differential diagnosis of parathyroid carcinoma. *Quant. Imaging Med. Surg.* **2019**, *9*, 1394–1401. [CrossRef]
21. Wei, C.H.; Harrari, A. Parathyroid carcinoma: Update and guidelines for manangement. *Curr. Treat. Options Oncol.* **2012**, *13*, 11–23. [CrossRef] [PubMed]
22. Takumi, K.; Fukukura, Y.; Hakamada, H.; Nagano, H.; Kumagae, Y.; Arima, H.; Nakajo, A.; Yoshiura, T. CT features of parathyroid carcinomas: Comparison with benign parathyroid lesions. *JPN J. Radiol.* **2019**, *37*, 380–389. [CrossRef] [PubMed]
23. Long, K.; Sippel, R. Current and future treatments for parathyroid carcinoma. *Int. J. Endocr. Oncol.* **2018**, *5*, IJE06. [CrossRef]

24. Holmes, E.C.; Morton, D.L.; Ketcham, A.S. Parathyroid carcinoma: A collective review. *Ann. Surg.* **1969**, *169*, 631–640. [CrossRef] [PubMed]
25. Hu, Y.; Liao, Q.; Cao, S.; Gao, X.; Zhao, Y. Diagnostic performance of parafibromin immunohistochemical staining for sporadic parathyroid carcinoma: A meta-analysis. *Endocrine* **2016**, *54*, 612–619. [CrossRef]
26. Silverberg, S.J.; Rubin, M.R.; Faiman, C.; Peacock, M.; Shoback, D.M.; Smallridge, R.C.; Schwanauer, L.E.; Olson, K.A.; Klassen, P.; Bilezikian, J.P. Cinacalcet hydrochloride reduces the serum calcium concentration in inoperable parathyroid carcinoma. *J. Clin. Endocrinol. Metab.* **2007**, *92*, 3803–3808. [CrossRef]
27. Berenson, J.R. Treatment of hypercalcemia of malignancy with bisphosphonates. *Semin. Oncol.* **2002**, *29*, 12–18. [CrossRef]
28. Villar Del Moral, J.; Jimenez Garcia, A.; Salvador Egea, P.; Martos-Martínez, J.M.; Nuño-Vázquez-Garza, J.M.; Serradilla-Martín, M.; Gómez-Palacio, A.; Moreno-Llorente, P.; Ortega-Serrano, J.; de la Quintana-Basarrate, A. Prognostic factors and staging systems in parathyroid cancer: A multi-center cohort study. *Surgery* **2014**, *156*, 1132–1144. [CrossRef]
29. Sandelin, K.; Auer, G.; Bondeson, L.; Grimelius, L.; Farnebo, L.-O. Prognostic factors in parathyroid cancer: A review of 95 cases. *World J. Surg.* **1992**, *16*, 724–731. [CrossRef]
30. Harari, A.; Waring, A.; Fernandez-Ranvier, G.; Hwang, J.; Suh, I.; Mitmaker, E.; Shen, W.; Gosnell, J.; Duh, Q.-Y.; Clark, O. Parathyroid carcinoma: A 43-year outcome and survival analysis. *J. Clin. Endocrinol. Metab.* **2011**, *96*, 3679–3686. [CrossRef]
31. Sadler, C.; Gow, K.W.; Beierle, E.A.; Doski, J.J.; Langer, M.; Nuchtern, J.G.; Vasudevan, S.A.; Goldfarb, M. Parathyroid carcinoma in more than 1000 patients: A population-level analysis. *Surgery* **2014**, *156*, 1622–1629. [CrossRef]
32. Rozhinskaya, L.; Pigarova, E.; Sabanova, E.; Mamedova, E.; Voronkova, I.; Krupinova, J.; Dzeranova, L.; Tiulpakov, A.; Gorbunova, V.; Orel, N.; et al. Diagnosis and treatment challenges of parathyroid carcinoma in a 27-year-old woman with multiple lung metastases. *Endocrinol. Diab. Metab. Case Rep.* **2017**, *2017*, 16-0113. [CrossRef] [PubMed]
33. Melfa, G. Surgeon volume and hospital volume in endocrine neck surgery: How many procedures are needed for reaching a safety level and acceptable costs? A systematic narrative review. *G. Di Chir.-J. Surg.* **2018**, *39*, 5. [CrossRef] [PubMed]
34. Iacobone, M.; Scerrino, G.; Palazzo, F.F. Parathyroid surgery: An evidence-based volume—Outcomes analysis. *Langenbeck Arch. Surg.* **2019**, *404*, 919–927. [CrossRef] [PubMed]
35. Jayawardene, S.; Owen, W.J.; Goldsmith, D.J.A. Parathyroid carcinoma in a dialysis patient. *Am. J. Kidney Dis.* **2000**, *36*, e26.1–e26.5. [CrossRef]
36. Obara, T.; Fujimoto, Y. Diagnosis and treatment of patients with parathyroid carcinoma: An update and review. *World J. Surg.* **1991**, *15*, 738–744. [CrossRef]
37. Fernandez, J.M.P.; Paiva, C.; Correia, R.; Polonia, J.; da Costa, M.A. Parathyroid carcinoma: From a case report to a review of literature. *Int. J. Surg. Case Rep.* **2018**, *42*, 214–217. [CrossRef]
38. McKeown, P.P.; McGarity, W.C.; Sewell, C.W. Carcinoma of the parathyroid gland: Is it overdiagnosed? A report of three cases. *Am. J. Surg.* **1984**, *147*, 292–298. [CrossRef]
39. Erickson, L.; Mete, O.; Juhlin, C.; Perren, A.; Gill, A. Overview of the 2022 WHO Classification of Parathyroid Tumors. *Endocr. Pathol.* **2022**, *33*, 64–89. [CrossRef]
40. Schantz, A.; Castleman, B. Parathyroid carcinoma. A study of 70 cases. *Cancer* **1973**, *31*, 600–605. [CrossRef]
41. Gill, A.J. Understanding the Genetic Basis of Parathyroid Carcinoma. *Endocr. Pathol.* **2014**, *25*, 30–34. [CrossRef] [PubMed]
42. Barazeghi, E.; Gill, A.J.; Sidhu, S.; Norlén, O.; Dina, R.; Palazzo, F.F.; Hellman, P.; Stålberg, P.; Westin, G. A role for TET2 in parathyroid carcinoma. *Endocr.-Relat. Cancer* **2017**, *24*, 309–318. [CrossRef] [PubMed]

Disclaimer/Publisher's Note: The statements, opinions and data contained in all publications are solely those of the individual author(s) and contributor(s) and not of MDPI and/or the editor(s). MDPI and/or the editor(s) disclaim responsibility for any injury to people or property resulting from any ideas, methods, instructions or products referred to in the content.

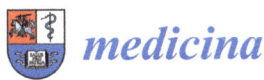

Article

Evaluating the Magnolol Anticancer Potential in MKN-45 Gastric Cancer Cells

Mahsa Naghashpour [1], Dian Dayer [2], Hadi Karami [3], Mahshid Naghashpour [4], Mahin Taheri Moghadam [5], Seyed Mohammad Jafar Haeri [1,*] and Katsuhiko Suzuki [6,*]

1. Department of Anatomical Sciences, Medical School, Arak University of Medical Sciences, Arak 38481-7-6341, Iran
2. Cellular and Molecular Research Center, Medical Basic Sciences Research Institute, Ahvaz Jundishapur University of Medical Sciences, Ahvaz 61357-15794, Iran
3. Department of Molecular Medicine and Biotechnology, Faculty of Medicine, Arak University of Medical Sciences, Arak 38481-7-6341, Iran
4. Department of Basic Medical Sciences, Faculty of Medicine, Abadan University of Medical Sciences, Abadan 6313833177, Iran
5. Department of Anatomical Science, Faculty of Medicine, Ahvaz Jundishapur University of Medical Sciences, Ahvaz 61357-15753, Iran
6. Faculty of Sport Sciences, Waseda University, 2-579-15 Mikajima, Tokorozawa 359-1192, Japan
* Correspondence: smj.haeri@arakmu.ac.ir (S.M.J.H.); katsu.suzu@waseda.jp (K.S.); Tel.: +98-9123276391 (S.M.J.H.)

Abstract: *Background and Objectives:* Combination therapy improves the effect of chemotherapy on tumor cells. Magnolol, used in treating gastrointestinal disorders, has been shown to have anticancer properties. We investigated the synergistic effect of cisplatin and magnolol on the viability and maintenance of MKN-45 gastric cancer cells. *Materials and Methods:* The toxicity of magnolol and/or cisplatin was determined using the MTT technique. The trypan blue method was used to test magnolol and/or cisplatin's effect on MKN-45 cell growth. Crystal violet staining was used to assess the treated cells' tendency for colony formation. The expression of genes linked to apoptosis, cell cycle arrest, and cell migration was examined using the qPCR method. *Results:* According to MTT data, using magnolol and/or cisplatin significantly reduced cell viability. The ability of the treated cells to proliferate and form colonies was also reduced considerably. Magnolol and/or cisplatin treatment resulted in a considerable elevation in *Bax* expression. However, the level of *Bcl2* expression was dramatically reduced. *p21* and *p53* expression levels were significantly increased in the treated cells, while *MMP-9* expression was significantly reduced. *Conclusions:* These findings show that magnolol has a remarkable anti-tumor effect on MKN-45 cells. In combination with cisplatin, magnolol may be utilized to overcome cisplatin resistance in gastric cancer cells.

Keywords: gastric cancer; MKN-45; cisplatin; magnolol

Citation: Naghashpour, M.; Dayer, D.; Karami, H.; Naghashpour, M.; Moghadam, M.T.; Haeri, S.M.J.; Suzuki, K. Evaluating the Magnolol Anticancer Potential in MKN-45 Gastric Cancer Cells. *Medicina* 2023, 59, 286. https://doi.org/10.3390/medicina59020286

Academic Editors: Valentin Titus Grigorean and Daniel Alin Cristian

Received: 31 December 2022
Revised: 20 January 2023
Accepted: 30 January 2023
Published: 1 February 2023

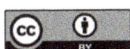

Copyright: © 2023 by the authors. Licensee MDPI, Basel, Switzerland. This article is an open access article distributed under the terms and conditions of the Creative Commons Attribution (CC BY) license (https://creativecommons.org/licenses/by/4.0/).

1. Introduction

Gastric cancer is the most common type of gastrointestinal cancer and the second leading cause of cancer death [1]. Each year, more than 1,000,000 new cases of gastric cancer are recorded [2]. Approximately 70% of these cases are noticed in developed countries, particularly in East Asia [3]. Surgery is the most common treatment for gastric cancer [4]. Chemotherapy is an efficient way to improve the effectiveness of surgery [5]. However, the case response to chemotherapy is predicted to be between 20% and 40%, with a survival time of 6 to 11 months after treatment [6].

Cisplatin is one of the most commonly used medications to treat gastric cancer [6,7]. However, cisplatin does not work for all patients [7]. Furthermore, high-dose chemotherapy has several adverse effects [8]. Chemotherapy resistance is one of the most challenging aspects of treating gastric cancer [9]. DNA/RNA damage repair, drug efflux, apoptosis suppression, and nuclear factor (NF)-κB activation are the four primary methods for preventing cell death after cisplatin treatment [10].

In previous investigations, chemical resistance has been linked to *Bcl-2* overexpression in patients with gastric cancer [11]. Combination therapy addresses critical pathways synergistically or additively and improves treatment efficacy [11]. In South Korea, China, and Japan, the Chinese herb *Magnolia officinalis* is commonly used as a local cure for gastrointestinal issues, coughs, anxiety, and allergic conditions [12]. Magnolol is a hydroxylated biphenyl chemical derived from the stem bark of *Magnolia officinalis* that is frequently used in East Asia to treat acute pain, cough, anxiety, and gastrointestinal issues [13]. Magnolol has been shown to have anti-inflammatory, antioxidant, and tumor-suppressive properties [14]. The inhibitory effect of magnolol on interleukin (IL)-1, tumor necrosis factor (TNF)-α, and IL-6 expression confirms its anti-inflammatory efficacy [15]. Magnolol was shown to have an apparent apoptotic impact in SGC-7901 human gastric cancer cells [16]. Magnolol and its methoxylated derivative, 2-O-methyl magnolol, were recently found to inhibit the proliferation, migration, and invasion of hepatocellular carcinoma cell lines by inducing p21 and p53 activation [17]. The anti-tumor effects of magnolol and 2-O-methyl magnolol in vivo were also established [18]. Magnolol inhibits the cell cycle in human gallbladder cancer cells at the G0/G1 phase [19].

According to several studies, magnolol's metabolic effects are mediated through the NF-κB/MAPK, Nrf2/HO-1, and PI3K/Akt signaling pathways [20]. The two leading causes of cancer cells' resistance to chemotherapy are invasion and metastasis [21]. Magnolol inhibits the invasive capability of MDA-MB cells via downregulating of the NF-κB/MMP-9 signaling pathway [22]. Magnolol's anti-invasive and anti-metastasis properties may also be explained by its anti-angiogenesis activity, which is mediated through vascular endothelial growth factor (VEGF) suppression [23].

Given magnolol's effectiveness in lowering cell growth, invasion, and metastasis, the question of whether magnolol can be utilized to reduce resistance to chemotherapeutic treatments arises [24]. In a recent study, magnolol was shown to be cytotoxic to oral squamous cells [25]. The findings also showed that magnolol therapy makes oral squamous cells more sensitive to cisplatin [25,26]. Chu and colleagues found that magnolol (80 μM) induced cytotoxic effects comparable to cisplatin at a dose of 25 μM in NSCLC cell lines [27]. The current research aims to evaluate the magnolol effects on cisplatin sensitivity in gastric cancer cells.

2. Materials and Methods

This experimental study was approved by the Ethics Committee of Arak University of Medical Sciences, Arak, Iran (Ethical code: IR.ARAKMU.REC.1400.032).

2.1. Reagent Preparation

Magnolol was purchased from Carbosynth Co. (Compton, Berkshire, UK). As a stock reagent, *Magnolol officinalis* alcoholic extract was dissolved in DMSO (dimethyl sulfoxide) at a 100 mM concentration and kept at −20 °C.

2.2. Cell Culture Protocol

The MKN-45 cell line (IBRC C10137) was purchased from the Iranian Biological Resource Center and cultured in RPMI medium containing 20% FBS and 1% penicillin/streptomycin. The cells were incubated at 37 °C with 5% CO_2. The cells were passaged when confluency was reached at 80% [28] (Figure S1).

2.3. MTT Assay

The cells were cultured at 10^4 cells/well density in a 96-well culture plate and incubated at 37 °C with 5% CO_2 for 24 h. Afterward, the culture medium was replaced with 100 μL of 0.5 mg/mL MTT solution, and the plates were incubated for 4 h at 37 °C with 5% CO_2 in the dark. Then each well received 100 μL of DMSO, and the plates were shaken for

15 min. The absorbance of the samples was measured at 570 nm using an ELISA reader (Bio-Rad, Berkeley, CA, USA). The viability of the cells was calculated using the formula: 100 − (absorbance test/absorbance control) × 100 [29]. The IC_{50} values were calculated using Prism software.

2.4. Study Design

The cells were divided into four groups. Group 1 (control group) consisted of MKN-45 cells that received no treatment. Group 2 consisted of MKN-45 cells that received magnolol. Group 3 received cisplatin, and group 4 was treated with a combination of magnolol and cisplatin. All groups were incubated at 37 °C with 5% CO_2 for 24 h and subjected to cell proliferation assay, colony formation analysis, and real-time PCR.

2.5. Cell Proliferation Assay

Cells were plated in 6-well plates at a density of 10^5 cells per well and incubated for 24 h at 37 °C with 5% CO_2. The culture medium was replaced after 48 h of cisplatin and/or magnolol treatment. The cells were cultivated for 24, 48, 72, 96, and 120 h. After that, trypan blue staining was used to determine the number of viable cells. The formula [(number of viable cells in sample/number of viable cells in control) × 100] was used to determine cell proliferation.

2.6. Colony Formation Analysis

To undertake a colony formation analysis, the cells were trypsinized and grown at a density of 20,000 cells/well on a 12-well plate and incubated at 37 °C for 24 h with 5% CO_2. Afterward, the cells were treated in triplicate with cisplatin and/or magnolol for 48 h. The cells were then cultured for seven days with a new culture medium. After incubation, the cells were washed twice with PBS, and a 1:7 mixture of methanol and cold acetic acid was added. The plates were incubated at room temperature for 20 min. The fixative solution was removed in the next step, and the cells were stained with 0.5% crystal violet. The cells were washed four times with distilled water and thoroughly dried at room temperature. The stained colonies were evaluated using an inverted microscope.

2.7. Real-Time PCR

The gene expression of the treated groups was evaluated using real-time PCR. The RNXTM reagent (Sinaclon, Tehran, Iran) was used to extract the RNA according to the manufacturer's instructions. Based on the manufacturer's suggestion, 1 µg of generated RNA was used for cDNA synthesis using a CycleScript cDNA synthesis kit (CycleScript RT PreMix Bioneer, Daejon, Republic of Korea). The real-time PCR reaction was performed using an Ampliqon RealQ Plus Master kit for SYBR Green I® (Ampliqon, Copenhagen, Denmark) on a Lightcycler® Detection System (Roche, New York, NY, USA). The genes and primers used in real-time PCR are listed in Table 1. The relative expression of the genes was compared using β-actin as the housekeeping gene. The reactions were prepared in a 20 µL mixture containing 10 µL Master Mix kit, 0.5 µL of each primer (200 nM), 3 µL cDNA (300 ng), and 7 µL nuclease-free water. The PCR protocol consisted of a 10 min denaturation at 95 °C followed by 45 cycles at 94 °C for 15 s and 60 °C for 30 s. Two separate reactions without cDNA or RNA served as negative calibrators. The gene expression of different groups was compared using the $2^{-\Delta\Delta Ct}$ technique. The MIQE (the minimum information for publication of quantitative real-time PCR experiments) guideline was followed for all qPCR studies.

Table 1. Characteristics of primers used in qPCR test.

Gene Name	Primer Sequence
β-actin-hum-F	CAGCCTCAAGATCATCAGCAATG
β-actin-hum-R	CATGAGTCCTTCCACGATACCA
Bax-hum-F	AAGAAGCTGAGCGAGTGTCT
Bax-hum-R	TGCCGTCAGAAAACATGTCAG
MMP-9-hum-F	TAAGGAGTACTCGACCTGTACCA
MMP-9-hum-R	GAGGAACAAACTGTATCCTTGGTC
Bcl-2-hum-F	GGATGCCTTTGTGGAACTG
Bcl-2-hum-R	CAGCCAGGAGAAATCAAACAG
P53-hum-F	CAGACCTATGGAAACTACTTCCTG
P53-hum-R	ATTCTGGGAGCTTCATCTGGA
P21-hum-F	ATGTGGACCTGTCACTGTCTT
P21-hum-R	CGTTTGGAGTGGTAGAAATCTGTC

2.8. Statistical Analysis

Statistical analysis was performed by GraphPad Prism 6.0 software. All analyses were done in triplicate. One-way ANOVA followed by Tukey post hoc analysis was used to assess the differences between various means. The difference between the two independent groups was determined using the t-test. All experimental data were presented as the mean $\pm$ SEM. The level of significance for all tests was set at $p < 0.05$.

3. Results

3.1. The Effects of Magnolol and/or Cisplatin on MKN-45 Cells' Viability

According to MTT data, magnolol treatment reduced cell viability dose-dependently (Figure 1). The algorithm of cisplatin's effect on MKN-45 cells was similar to that of magnolol (Figure 1). However, the combination of magnolol and cisplatin resulted in a substantially more significant reduction in cell viability (Figure 1). IC_{50} values of magnolol, cisplatin, and their combination were 6.53, 7, and 3.25 µM, respectively.

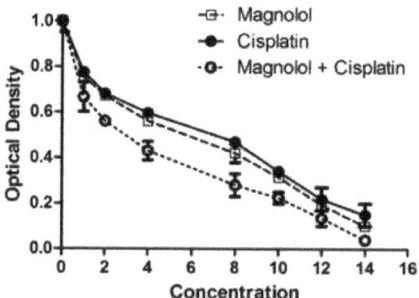

Figure 1. Changes in MKN Cells' viability following magnolol and/or cisplatin therapy. The results of the MTT assay showed diminished optical density after treating of MKN-45 cell line with magnolol and/or cisplatin.

3.2. The Effects of Magnolol and/or Cisplatin on MKN-45 Cells' Proliferation

According to the results of proliferation analysis, the cell growth rate was reduced to 62% and 59% of the control group after 24 h of treatment with magnolol and cisplatin, respectively ($p < 0.05$). However, the combination of the two medications decreased cellular proliferation by 55.5% compared to the control ($p < 0.05$). The tendency of lower cell proliferation in all treatment groups relative to the control group persisted until the fifth day of therapy. In the groups treated with magnolol, cisplatin, and magnolol plus cisplatin for five days, the proliferation amount reduced to 38.0%, 36.5%, and 36.7% of the control, respectively ($p < 0.05$) (Figure 2).

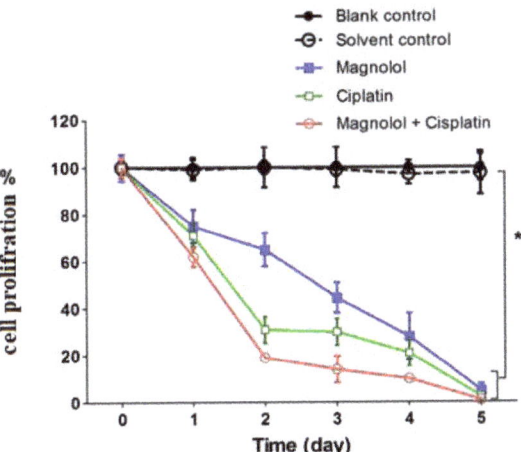

Figure 2. Proliferation assay following treatment of MKN-45 cells with magnolol and/or cisplatin. MKN-45 cells were treated with magnolol and/or cisplatin for 24 h. Then, the proliferation rate was calculated by counting the number of viable cells during five days compared to the control group (*: A significant difference between the cell proliferation % of the control group and other groups.)

3.3. The Effects of Magnolol and/or Cisplatin on the Ability of MKN-45 Cells to Form Colonies

Following magnolol injection, the ability of MKN-45 cells to form colonies was significantly reduced. The cells that received cisplatin therapy showed a more significant decrease in colony formation. The cells that were given a combination of magnolol and cisplatin had the least ability to form colonies (Figure 3A–E).

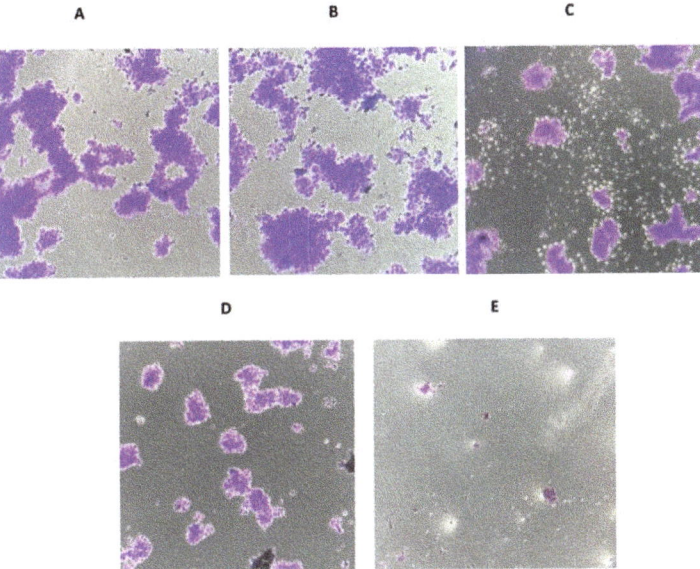

Figure 3. The effect of magnolol and/or cisplatin on colony formation in MKN-45 cells. (**A**) control group 1 (no treatment), (**B**) control group 2 (treated with PBS), (**C**) treated with magnolol, (**D**) treated with cisplatin, (**E**) treated with magnolol and cisplatin.

3.4. The Effects of Magnolol and/or Cisplatin on the Expression of Apoptosis-Dependent Genes

Real-time PCR data revealed increased *Bax* expression following magnolol and/or cisplatin treatment. The group treated with magnolol showed the maximum increased level of *Bax* expression compared to the control group. In addition, a substantial increase in *Bax* expression in the groups treated with cisplatin or cisplatin + magnolol was noted ($p < 0.001$). The result showed no significant increase in *Bax* expression in the magnolol-treated group compared to the magnolol + cisplatin-treated group ($p > 0.05$). However, a substantial increase in *Bax* expression was noted in the magnolol + cisplatin-treated group compared to the cisplatin-treated group ($p < 0.001$) (Figure 4a). In all treated groups, *Bcl2* expression was significantly reduced compared to the control group ($p < 0.001$). The group that received cisplatin with magnolol had the lowest level of *Bcl2* expression. The group that received magnolol + cisplatin showed a considerable reduction in *Bcl2* expression compared to those that received magnolol or cisplatin alone ($p < 0.001$) (Figure 4b).

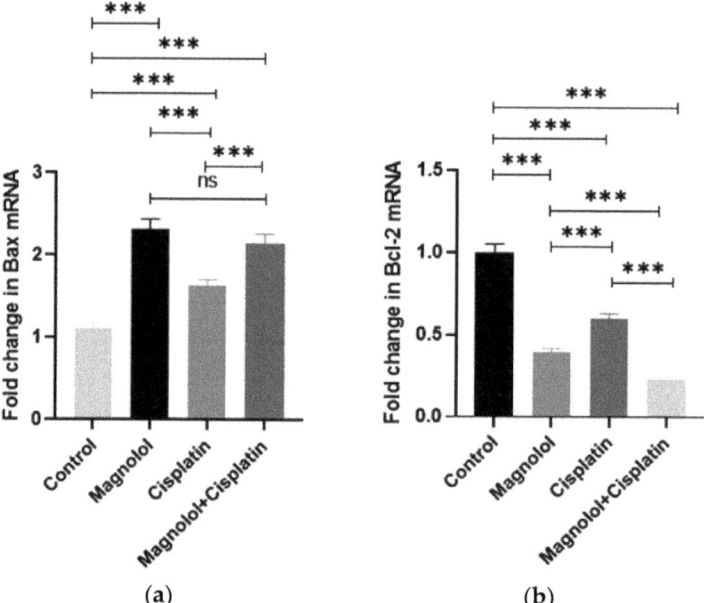

Figure 4. Changes in apoptotic-related genes following magnolol and/or cisplatin therapy. (**a**) A substantial increase in *Bax* expression after magnolol and/or cisplatin application. (**b**) A significantly decreased level of *Bcl2* expression after magnolol and/or cisplatin application. β-actin was used as the reference gene for normalizing the relative quantitative expression of target genes. All experiments were performed in triplicate. *** $p < 0.001$, ns: not significant.

3.5. The Effects of Magnolol and/or Cisplatin on the Expression of Cell Cycle Regulator Genes

Magnolol and/or cisplatin treatment induced a significant increase in *p53* expression in comparison with the control group ($p < 0.001$) (Figure 5a). The group treated with magnolol + cisplatin showed the most significantly increased level of *P53*. There was no significant difference in P53 expression between the group that received magnolol alone and those treated with magnolol + cisplatin ($p > 0.05$). However, the combination therapy induced a significant elevation in *P53* expression compared with the group treated with cisplatin alone ($p < 0.001$) (Figure 5a). *p21* expression changes followed the same pattern as *p53* expression changes after magnolol and/or cisplatin treatment (Figure 5b).

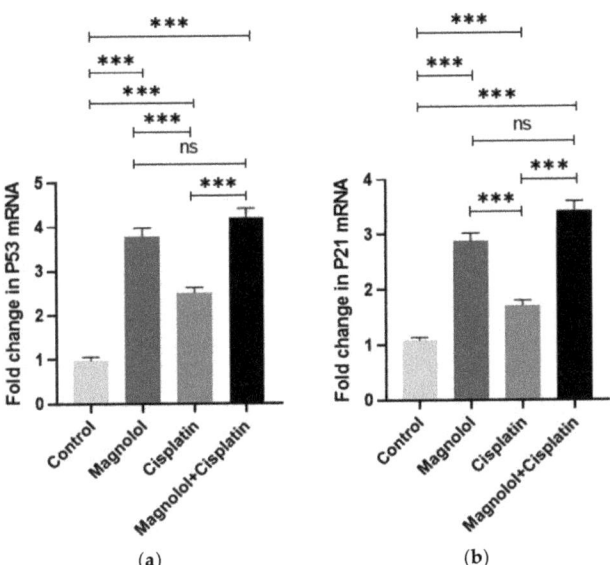

(a)   (b)

Figure 5. Changes in cell cycle regulator genes following magnolol and/or cisplatin therapy. (**a**) All treated groups showed significantly elevated levels of *p53* compared to the control group. The group that received a combination of magnolol and cisplatin had the maximum expression of *p53*. (**b**) All treated groups showed significantly elevated levels of *p21* compared to the control group. The group that received a combination of magnolol and cisplatin had the maximum expression of *p21*. β-actin was used as the reference gene for normalizing the relative quantitative expression of target genes. All experiments were performed in triplicate. ns: not significant. *** $p < 0.001$.

3.6. The Effects of Magnolol and/or Cisplatin on the Expression of Extracellular Matrix Remodeling Gene Expression

MMP-9 showed significantly reduced expression in the groups who received magnolol and/ or cisplatin ($p < 0.001$) (Figure 6). The group that received cisplatin presented the lowest expression of *MMP-9*. There was a significant difference between the treated groups in *MMP9* expression ($p < 0.001$) (Figure 6).

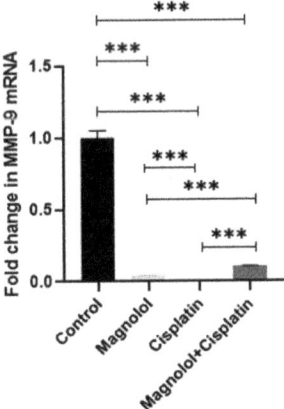

Figure 6. Changes in *MMP-9* wxpression following magnolol and/or cisplatin therapy treatment of MKN-45 cells with magnolol and/or cisplatin resulted in a substantial decrease in *MMP9* expression compared to the control group. β-actin was used as the reference gene for normalizing the relative quantitative expression of target genes. All experiments were performed in triplicate. *** $p < 0.001$.

4. Discussion

This study aimed to see if magnolol could improve cisplatin cytotoxicity in gastric cancer cells. Cisplatin is commonly used to treat progressive gastric cancer [30]. However, cisplatin therapy has some unfavorable and harmful effects on normal cells [31]. Cisplatin induces unwanted apoptosis in blood, nerve, stomach, and kidney cells. Cisplatin binds to purine residues, causes DNA damage, and inhibits the cell cycle [27]. Cisplatin induces reactive oxygen species production and lipid peroxidation, resulting in unwanted ototoxicity. Another significant issue in gastric cancer treatment is cancer cells' resistance to cisplatin [32]. Some evidence suggests that chemotherapy treatments without cisplatin considerably enhance survival time, progression-free survival, and response rate in gastric cancer patients [33]. In this regard, scientists worldwide are looking for natural compounds with anti-tumor properties. Some studies propose cisplatin and natural compound combination therapy to avoid the harmful effects of cisplatin [34]. Magnolol's anti-cancer activity has been proven in several earlier investigations of various cancers [35]. Rasul et al. showed magnolol-induced apoptosis in SGC-7901 human gastric cancer cells.

This study investigated the effect of magnolol with or without cisplatin on MKN-45 gastric cancer cells in vitro. According to our findings, magnolol and cisplatin inhibited MKN-45 cell survival, proliferation, and colony formation ability in a dose-dependent way. Futhermore, the combination of magnolol and cisplatin had a substantially more significant death effect on cells [36]. According to Hyun et al. study, magnolia extract suppressed the survival of cervical cancer cells [37]. Regarding Ong et al.'s study results, magnolol inhibited the growth, colony formation, and proliferative capacity of non-small cell lung cancer cells [38]. Jian et al. found that treating human A549-bearing nude mice with honokiol, a bioactive component derived from magnolia, suppressed tumor growth considerably. When honokiol was combined with cisplatin, its anti-tumor efficacy was significantly increased [39]. In the next step, we investigated the mechanism by which magnolol lowers the viability of MKN-45 cells. In this regard, changes in apoptosis-related genes were studied.

The data demonstrated a noticeable increase in *Bax* expression and a significant decrease in *Bcl2* expression following magnolol and/or cisplatin treatment. The data from Park et al.'s study showed an increase in *Bax* expression and a reduction of *Bcl2* expression following the treatment of colon cancer cells with magnolol. According to their findings, magnolol causes cytochrome c movement from the mitochondria to the cytoplasm, leading to caspase-3 activation and cell death [40]. According to Rasul et al., magnolol has an apparent apoptotic effect mediated by an increase in *Bax/Bcl2* and caspase-3 expressions. The researchers reported that magnolol-induced apoptosis in gastric cancer cells could be related to increased mitochondrial membrane permeability and caspase pathway activation or decreased PI3K/Akt [41]. The exact mechanism by which magnolol reduces the viability of cancer cells is unclear [42]. Tsai et al.'s study revealed that magnolol inhibits apoptosis in non-small cell lung cancer cells via caspase-independent mechanisms. According to the observations, magnolol enhances the release of *Bid*, *Bax*, and cytochrome c from mitochondria. However, magnolol does not affect the expression of caspase-3, -8, or -9. The researchers concluded that magnolol inhibits non-small cell lung cancer cell proliferation by suppressing the PI3K/AKT and ERK1/2 pathways [43].

The next step of our study was to see how magnolol treatment affected the expression of cell cycle-regulating genes. In the groups treated with magnolol and/or cisplatin, we found a significant increase in *p53* and *p21* expression. The *p53* tumor suppressor gene is a critical transcription factor that controls angiogenesis, cell cycle, and DNA repair gene expression [44]. *p53* stops the cell cycle at stage G1 in response to DNA damage. *p53* is critical for genome preservation and is required for maintaining the shape and number of genomes [45]. Alterations in the *p53* gene were found in 77% of gastric cancer patients [46]. *p21* is defined as a downstream target of the tumor suppressor *p53*. *p53* binds to the *p21* promoter and stimulates its transcription [47]. *p21* is a cyclin-dependent kinase inhibitor that controls the activity of several cyclins and cyclin-dependent kinases involved in cell cycle regulation [48]. *p53* and *p21* have been suggested as critical biomarkers in cancer diagnosis. The findings of a clinical investigation showed that *p53* overexpression was associated with an improved response to chemotherapy in individuals with gastric cancer [49]. The increased levels of *p53* and *p21* expression identified in our study revealed that magnolol or magnolol plus cisplatin treatment could activate cell cycle arrest.

These results indicate that magnolol increases cellular sensitivity to cisplatin in MKN-45 cells. Hsu et al. discovered that magnolol treatment of colon cancer cells results in a significant increase in *p21* expression via the Ras/Raf-1-mediated activation of ERK [50]. According to a study by Shen et al., magnolol decreases the mitotic phase and the progress of G2/M in a dose-dependent manner [51]. According to the findings of a study on the effect of magnolol on rat xenograft cells, magnolol inhibits and dramatically suppresses β-catenin nuclear transfer and attaches the TGF β-catenin complexes to the DNA-bound axis in the nucleus [51]. In SW480 and HCT116 human colon cancer cells, these processes result in decreased regulation of target β-catenin/TCF genes such as c-myc, MMP-7, and plasminogen activator urokinase. In HCT116 nude mouse xenograft cells, magnolol also slows invasion and demonstrates anticancer efficacy [51]. In human umbilical vein endothelial cells, magnolol also suppresses the proliferation of basal fibroblast growth factor and the creation of capillary tubules [52]. The findings of the Zhou et al. investigation showed that magnolol increased cell cycle arrest at the G2/M phase by elevating *p21* and *p53* expression and reducing cyclin-B1 and CDK-1 expression [53].

The final phase of our research examined the effects of magnolol/cisplatin treatment on MKN-45 cell migration and invasion. The findings revealed that magnolol and cisplatin dramatically reduced gastric cancer cell migration, which correlated to a reduction in *MMP-9* expression. This finding is similar to earlier cellular studies that showed magnolol promotes cancer cell migration and invasion by reducing the NF-κB signaling pathway and MMP activity in breast cell lines and cholangiocarcinoma, respectively [54]. According to previous research, *MMP-9* is overexpressed in cancer cells [55]. It has been demonstrated that *p53* inactivation induces *MMP-9* production via enhancing glycolysis [56]. Hypoxia generally causes cell necrosis, leukocyte infiltration, and the release of TNF-α and IL-6 in tumor cells [57]. This condition causes *MMP-9* overexpression by activating the PI3k/AKT and MAPK pathways [58]. Furthermore, tumor hypoxia stimulates HIF-1 expression, increasing *MMP-9* activity [59]. The increase in *MMP-9* expression in tumor tissues plays a vital role in realizing the metastatic process's sequential phases [60]. Our study's considerable reduction in *MMP-9* suggested that magnolol and/or cisplatin treatment might have an anti-invasive and anti-metastatic effect. According to Liu et al.'s report, magnolol inhibited breast cancer cell invasion by down-regulating NF-κB and MMP-9 [22]. According to Nagas et al., magnolol substantially lowers malignancy in the human fibrosarcoma cell line HT-1080 by reducing *MMP-9* activity [61]. Finally, our findings, which are comparable with evidence from previous in vitro and in vivo investigations, confirm magnolol's anti-tumor activities in MKN-45 gastric cancer cells. Our results also indicate that magnolol improves cisplatin's anti-tumor efficacy.

5. Conclusions

Using magnolol as a single drug or combined with cisplatin may be a novel treatment for gastric cancer patients. However, more in vivo and clinical research is needed to determine the precise effects of magnolol on normal and malignant cells. More investigation is recommended to determine the exact molecular mechanisms of magnolol on normal and cancer cells.

Supplementary Materials: The following supporting information can be downloaded at https://www.mdpi.com/article/10.3390/medicina59020286/s1, Figure S1: The changes in morphological characteristics of MKN-45 cells during magnolol and/or cisplatin treatment. A. MKN-45 gastric cancer cells without treatment (control group). B. Magnolol therapy induced a significantly reduced number of viable cells. C. Cisplatin therapy resulted in a reduced number of viable cells and colonies. D. Cisplatin and magnolol combination therapy had the maximum inhibitory effect on MKN-45 cell viability. Figure S2: The results of electrophoresis. The real-time PCR products were loaded on 1% agarose gel and detected using a transilluminator (Jal Doc, Iran).

Author Contributions: Conceptualization, S.M.J.H. and H.K.; methodology, M.N. (Mahsa Naghashpour), D.D. and H.K.; software, M.N. (Mahsa Naghashpour); validation, M.T.M.; formal analysis, M.N. (Mahsa Naghashpour); investigation, project administration, funding acquisition, resources, and supervision, S.M.J.H.; data curation, D.D.; writing—original draft preparation, M.N. (Mahsa Naghashpour) and M.N. (Mahshid Naghashpour); writing—review and editing, K.S. All authors have read and agreed to the published version of the manuscript.

Funding: This research was funded by the Voice Chancellor for Research, Arak University of Medical Sciences, Arak, Iran, grant number 6345.

Institutional Review Board Statement: Not applicable.

Informed Consent Statement: Not applicable.

Data Availability Statement: The data presented in this study are available upon request from the corresponding author.

Acknowledgments: The authors would like to thank the staff of Cellular and Molecular Research Center, Medical Basic Sciences Research Institute, Ahvaz Jundishapur University of Medical Sciences, Ahvaz, Iran, for their assistance in molecular and cellular analysis.

Conflicts of Interest: The authors declared no conflict of interest.

References

1. Xie, Y.; Shi, L.; He, X.; Luo, Y. Gastrointestinal cancers in China, the USA, and Europe. *Gastroenterol. Rep.* **2021**, *9*, 91–104. [CrossRef] [PubMed]
2. Ilic, M.; Ilic, I. Epidemiology of stomach cancer. *World J. Gastroenterol.* **2022**, *28*, 1187. [CrossRef] [PubMed]
3. Lu, B.; Li, N.; Luo, C.-Y.; Cai, J.; Lu, M.; Zhang, Y.-H.; Chen, H.-D.; Dai, M. Colorectal cancer incidence and mortality: The current status, temporal trends and their attributable risk factors in 60 countries in 2000–2019. *Chin. Med. J.* **2021**, *134*, 1941–1951. [CrossRef]
4. Joshi, S.S.; Badgwell, B.D. Current treatment and recent progress in gastric cancer. *CA Cancer J. Clin.* **2021**, *71*, 264–279. [CrossRef]
5. Lin, Z.; Cai, M.; Zhang, P.; Li, G.; Liu, T.; Li, X.; Cai, K.; Nie, X.; Wang, J.; Liu, J. Phase II, single-arm trial of preoperative short-course radiotherapy followed by chemotherapy and camrelizumab in locally advanced rectal cancer. *J. Immunother. Cancer* **2021**, *9*. [CrossRef]
6. Lehtomäki, K.; Mustonen, H.; Kellokumpu-Lehtinen, P.-L.; Joensuu, H.; Hermunen, K.; Soveri, L.-M.; Boisen, M.K.; Dehlendorff, C.; Johansen, J.S.; Haglund, C. Lead time and prognostic role of serum CEA, CA19-9, IL-6, CRP, and YKL-40 after adjuvant chemotherapy in colorectal cancer. *Cancers* **2021**, *13*, 3892. [CrossRef]
7. Wu, L.; Cai, S.; Deng, Y.; Zhang, Z.; Zhou, X.; Su, Y.; Xu, D. PD-1/PD-L1 enhanced cisplatin resistance in gastric cancer through PI3K/AKT mediated P-gp expression. *Int. Immunopharmacol.* **2021**, *94*, 107443. [CrossRef]
8. Araújo, D.; Cabral, I.; Vale, N.; Amorim, I. Canine Gastric Cancer: Current Treatment Approaches. *Vet. Sci.* **2022**, *9*, 383. [CrossRef] [PubMed]
9. Shetty, N.P.; Prabhakaran, M.; Srivastava, A.K. Pleiotropic nature of curcumin in targeting multiple apoptotic-mediated factors and related strategies to treat gastric cancer: A review. *Phytother. Res.* **2021**, *35*, 5397–5416. [CrossRef]
10. Kanno, Y.; Chen, C.-Y.; Lee, H.-L.; Chiou, J.-F.; Chen, Y.-J. Molecular mechanisms of chemotherapy resistance in head and neck cancers. *Front. Oncol.* **2021**, *11*, 640392. [CrossRef]
11. Liu, J.; Li, J.; Sun, Z.; Duan, Y.; Wang, F.; Wei, G.; Yang, J.-H. Bcl-2-associated transcription factor 1 Ser290 phosphorylation mediates DNA damage response and regulates radiosensitivity in gastric cancer. *J. Transl. Med.* **2021**, *19*, 339. [CrossRef] [PubMed]
12. Ahmad, R.S. A systematic review on multi-nutritional and phytopharmacological importance of *Perilla* frutescens. *Int. J. Green Pharm.* **2022**, *16*. [CrossRef]
13. She, J.; Gu, T.; Pang, X.; Liu, Y.; Tang, L.; Zhou, X. Natural Products Targeting Liver X Receptors or Farnesoid X Receptor. *Front. Pharmacol.* **2021**, *12*. [CrossRef]
14. Mukherjee, S.; Dutta, A.; Chakraborty, A. External modulators and redox homeostasis: Scenario in radiation-induced bystander cells. *Mutat. Res. Rev. Mutat. Res.* **2021**, *787*, 108368. [CrossRef] [PubMed]
15. Wang, H.; He, Y.; Sun, Z.; Ren, S.; Liu, M.; Wang, G.; Yang, J. Microglia in depression: An overview of microglia in the pathogenesis and treatment of depression. *J. Neuroinflamm.* **2022**, *19*, 132. [CrossRef]
16. Yang, W.; Huang, G. Extraction methods and activities of natural glucans. *Trends Food Sci. Technol.* **2021**, *112*, 50–57. [CrossRef]
17. Zheng, Z.; Zhang, L.; Hou, X. Potential roles and molecular mechanisms of phytochemicals against cancer. *Food Funct.* **2022**, *13*, 9208–9225. [CrossRef] [PubMed]

18. Yang, J.; Wang, L.; Guan, X.; Qin, J.-J. Inhibiting STAT3 Signaling Pathway by Natural Products for Cancer Prevention and Therapy: In Vitro and In Vivo Activity and Mechanisms of Action. *Pharmacol. Res.* **2022**, 106357. [CrossRef]
19. Zhu, D.; Gu, X.; Lin, Z.; Yu, D.; Wang, J. High expression of PSMC2 promotes gallbladder cancer through regulation of GNG4 and predicts poor prognosis. *Oncogenesis* **2021**, *10*, 43. [CrossRef]
20. Liu, X.; Wang, Y.; Wu, D.; Li, S.; Wang, J.; Han, Z.; Wang, K.; Yang, Z.; Wei, Z. Magnolol prevents acute alcoholic liver damage by activating PI3K/Nrf2/PPARγ and inhibiting NLRP3 signaling pathway. *Front. Pharmacol.* **2019**, *10*, 1459. [CrossRef]
21. Asif, P.J.; Longobardi, C.; Hahne, M.; Medema, J.P. The role of cancer-associated fibroblasts in cancer invasion and metastasis. *Cancers* **2021**, *13*, 4720. [CrossRef] [PubMed]
22. Liu, Y.; Cao, W.; Zhang, B.; Liu, Y.; Wang, Z.; Wu, Y.; Yu, X.; Zhang, X.; Ming, P.; Zhou, G. The natural compound magnolol inhibits invasion and exhibits potential in human breast cancer therapy. *Sci. Rep.* **2013**, *3*, 3098. [CrossRef] [PubMed]
23. Chen, C.-H.; Hsu, F.-T.; Chen, W.-L.; Chen, J.-H. Induction of apoptosis, inhibition of MCL-1, and VEGF-A expression are associated with the anti-cancer efficacy of magnolol combined with regorafenib in hepatocellular carcinoma. *Cancers* **2021**, *13*, 2066. [CrossRef] [PubMed]
24. Ranaware, A.M.; Banik, K.; Deshpande, V.; Padmavathi, G.; Roy, N.K.; Sethi, G.; Fan, L.; Kumar, A.P.; Kunnumakkara, A.B. Magnolol: A neolignan from the magnolia family for the prevention and treatment of cancer. *Int. J. Mol. Sci.* **2018**, *19*, 2362. [CrossRef] [PubMed]
25. Peng, C.-Y.; Yu, C.-C.; Huang, C.-C.; Liao, Y.-W.; Hsieh, P.-L.; Chu, P.-M.; Yu, C.-H.; Lin, S.-S. Magnolol inhibits cancer stemness and IL-6/Stat3 signaling in oral carcinomas. *J. Formos. Med. Assoc.* **2022**, *121*, 51–57. [CrossRef]
26. Bijani, F.; Zabihi, E.; Bijani, A.; Nouri, H.R.; Nafarzadeh, S.; Seyedmajidi, M. Evaluation of apoptotic effect of crocin, cisplatin, and their combination in human oral squamous cell carcinoma cell line HN5. *Dent. Res. J.* **2021**, *18*, 70.
27. Baharuddin, P.; Satar, N.; Fakiruddin, K.S.; Zakaria, N.; Lim, M.N.; Yusoff, N.M.; Zakaria, Z.; Yahaya, B.H. Curcumin improves the efficacy of cisplatin by targeting cancer stem-like cells through p21 and cyclin D1-mediated tumour cell inhibition in non-small cell lung cancer cell lines. *Oncol. Rep.* **2016**, *35*, 13–25. [CrossRef]
28. Samie, K.A.; Dayer, D.; Eshkiki, Z.S. Human Colon Cancer HT29 Cell Line Treatment with High-Dose LAscorbic Acid Results to Reduced Angiogenic Proteins Expression and Elevated Pro-apoptotic Proteins Expression. In *Current Molecular Medicine*; Bentham Science Publishers: Bussum, The Netherlands, 2023.
29. Dayer, D.; Tabandeh, M.R.; Kazemi, M. The radio-sensitizing effect of pharmacological concentration of ascorbic acid on human pancreatic Cancer cells. *Anti-Cancer Agents Med. Chem.* **2020**, *20*, 1927–1932. [CrossRef]
30. Lee, K.-W.; Chung, I.-J.; Ryu, M.-H.; Park, Y.I.; Nam, B.-H.; Oh, H.-S.; Lee, K.H.; Han, H.S.; Seo, B.-G.; Jo, J.-C. Multicenter phase III trial of S-1 and cisplatin versus S-1 and oxaliplatin combination chemotherapy for first-line treatment of advanced gastric cancer (SOPP trial). *Gastric Cancer* **2021**, *24*, 156–167. [CrossRef]
31. Ongnok, B.; Chattipakorn, N.; Chattipakorn, S.C. Doxorubicin and cisplatin induced cognitive impairment: The possible mechanisms and interventions. *Exp. Neurol.* **2020**, *324*, 113118. [CrossRef]
32. Spirina, L.V.; Avgustinovich, A.V.; Afanas' ev, S.G.; Cheremisina, O.V.; Volkov, M.Y.; Choynzonov, E.L.; Gorbunov, A.K.; Usynin, E.A. Molecular mechanism of resistance to chemotherapy in gastric cancers, the role of autophagy. *Curr. Drug Targets* **2020**, *21*, 713–721. [CrossRef]
33. Peng, W.; Zhang, F.; Wang, Z.; Li, D.; He, Y.; Ning, Z.; Sheng, L.; Wang, J.; Xia, X.; Yu, C. Large scale, multicenter, prospective study of apatinib in advanced gastric cancer: A real-world study from China. *Cancer Manag. Res.* **2020**, *12*, 6977. [CrossRef] [PubMed]
34. Bai, Z.; Yao, C.; Zhu, J.; Xie, Y.; Ye, X.-Y.; Bai, R.; Xie, T. Anti-tumor drug discovery based on natural product β-elemene: Anti-tumor mechanisms and structural modification. *Molecules* **2021**, *26*, 1499. [CrossRef]
35. Chen, Y.; Huang, K.; Ding, X.; Tang, H.; Xu, Z. Magnolol inhibits growth and induces apoptosis in esophagus cancer KYSE-150 cell lines via the MAP kinase pathway. *J. Thorac. Dis.* **2019**, *11*, 3030. [CrossRef] [PubMed]
36. Rasul, A.; Yu, B.; Khan, M.; Zhang, K.; Iqbal, F.; Ma, T.; Yang, H. Magnolol, a natural compound, induces apoptosis of SGC-7901 human gastric adenocarcinoma cells via the mitochondrial and PI3K/Akt signaling pathways. *Int. J. Oncol.* **2012**, *40*, 1153–1161. [CrossRef] [PubMed]
37. Hyun, S.; Kim, M.S.; Song, Y.S.; Bak, Y.; Ham, S.Y.; Lee, D.H.; Hong, J.; Yoon, D.Y. Peroxisome proliferator-activated receptor-gamma agonist 4-O-methylhonokiol induces apoptosis by triggering the intrinsic apoptosis pathway and inhibiting the PI3K/Akt survival pathway in SiHa human cervical cancer cells. *J. Microbiol. Biotechnol.* **2015**, *25*, 334–342. [CrossRef]
38. Ong, C.P.; Lee, W.L.; Tang, Y.Q.; Yap, W.H. Honokiol: A review of its anticancer potential and mechanisms. *Cancers* **2019**, *12*, 48. [CrossRef] [PubMed]
39. Jiang, Q.-q.; Fan, L.-y.; Yang, G.-l.; Guo, W.-H.; Hou, W.-l.; Chen, L.-j.; Wei, Y.-q. Improved therapeutic effectiveness by combining liposomal honokiol with cisplatin in lung cancer model. *BMC Cancer* **2008**, *8*, 242. [CrossRef]
40. Park, J.B.; Lee, M.S.; Cha, E.Y.; Lee, J.S.; Sul, J.Y.; Song, I.S.; Kim, J.Y. Magnolol-induced apoptosis in HCT-116 colon cancer cells is associated with the AMP-activated protein kinase signaling pathway. *Biol. Pharm. Bull.* **2012**, *35*, 1614–1620. [CrossRef]
41. Rasul, A.; Ding, C.; Li, X.; Khan, M.; Yi, F.; Ali, M.; Ma, T. Dracorhodin perchlorate inhibits PI3K/Akt and NF-κB activation, up-regulates the expression of p53, and enhances apoptosis. *Apoptosis* **2012**, *17*, 1104–1119. [CrossRef]

42. Tang, Y.; Wang, L.; Yi, T.; Xu, J.; Wang, J.; Qin, J.-J.; Chen, Q.; Yip, K.-M.; Pan, Y.; Hong, P. Synergistic effects of autophagy/mitophagy inhibitors and magnolol promote apoptosis and antitumor efficacy. *Acta Pharm. Sin. B* **2021**, *11*, 3966–3982. [CrossRef] [PubMed]
43. Tsai, J.-R.; Chong, I.-W.; Chen, Y.-H.; Hwang, J.-J.; Yin, W.-H.; Chen, H.-L.; Chou, S.-H.; Chiu, C.-C.; Liu, P.-L. Magnolol induces apoptosis via caspase-independent pathways in non-small cell lung cancer cells. *Arch. Pharmacal Res.* **2014**, *37*, 548–557. [CrossRef] [PubMed]
44. Smith, N.D.; Rubenstein, J.N.; Eggener, S.E.; Kozlowski, J.M. The p53 tumor suppressor gene and nuclear protein: Basic science review and relevance in the management of bladder cancer. *J. Urol.* **2003**, *169*, 1219–1228. [CrossRef] [PubMed]
45. Shaltiel, I.A.; Aprelia, M.; Saurin, A.T.; Chowdhury, D.; Kops, G.J.; Voest, E.E.; Medema, R.H. Distinct phosphatases antagonize the p53 response in different phases of the cell cycle. *Proc. Natl. Acad. Sci. USA* **2014**, *111*, 7313–7318. [CrossRef]
46. Tamura, G. Alterations of tumor suppressor and tumor-related genes in the development and progression of gastric cancer. *World J. Gastroenterol. WJG* **2006**, *12*, 192. [CrossRef]
47. Lagger, G.; Doetzlhofer, A.; Schuettengruber, B.; Haidweger, E.; Simboeck, E.; Tischler, J.; Chiocca, S.; Suske, G.; Rotheneder, H.; Wintersberger, E. The tumor suppressor p53 and histone deacetylase 1 are antagonistic regulators of the cyclin-dependent kinase inhibitor p21/WAF1/CIP1 gene. *Mol. Cell. Biol.* **2003**, *23*, 2669–2679. [CrossRef]
48. Nagaki, M.; Sugiyama, A.; Naiki, T.; Ohsawa, Y.; Moriwaki, H. Control of cyclins, cyclin-dependent kinase inhibitors, p21 and p27, and cell cycle progression in rat hepatocytes by extracellular matrix. *J. Hepatol.* **2000**, *32*, 488–496. [CrossRef]
49. Zeestraten, E.C.; Benard, A.; Reimers, M.S.; Schouten, P.C.; Liefers, G.J.; Van de Velde, C.J.; Kuppen, P.J. The prognostic value of the apoptosis pathway in colorectal cancer: A review of the literature on biomarkers identified by immunohistochemistry. *Biomark. Cancer* **2013**, *5*, BIC-S11475. [CrossRef]
50. Hsu, Y.F.; Lee, T.S.; Lin, S.Y.; Hsu, S.P.; Juan, S.H.; Hsu, Y.H.; Zhong, W.B.; Lee, W.S. Involvement of Ras/Raf-1/ERK actions in the magnolol-induced upregulation of p21 and cell-cycle arrest in colon cancer cells. *Mol. Carcinog. Publ. Coop. Univ. Tex. MD Cancer Cent.* **2007**, *46*, 275–283. [CrossRef]
51. Shen, J.; Ma, H.; Zhang, T.; Liu, H.; Yu, L.; Li, G.; Li, H.; Hu, M. Magnolol inhibits the growth of non-small cell lung cancer via inhibiting microtubule polymerization. *Cell. Physiol. Biochem.* **2017**, *42*, 1789–1801. [CrossRef]
52. He, Q.; Liu, Q.; Chen, Y.; Meng, J.; Zou, L. Long-zhi decoction medicated serum promotes angiogenesis in human umbilical vein endothelial cells based on autophagy. *Evid.-Based Complement. Altern. Med.* **2018**, *2018*, 6857398. [CrossRef] [PubMed]
53. Zhou, Y.; Bi, Y.; Yang, C.; Yang, J.; Jiang, Y.; Meng, F.; Yu, B.; Khan, M.; Ma, T.; Yang, H. Magnolol induces apoptosis in MCF-7 human breast cancer cells through G2/M phase arrest and caspase-independent pathway. *Die Pharm.-Int. J. Pharm. Sci.* **2013**, *68*, 755–762.
54. Jiao, L.; Bi, L.; Lu, Y.; Wang, Q.; Gong, Y.; Shi, J.; Xu, L. Cancer chemoprevention and therapy using chinese herbal medicine. *Biol. Proced. Online* **2018**, *20*, 1. [CrossRef] [PubMed]
55. Choi, J.Y.; Jang, Y.S.; Min, S.Y.; Song, J.Y. Overexpression of MMP-9 and HIF-1α in breast cancer cells under hypoxic conditions. *J. Breast Cancer* **2011**, *14*, 88–95. [CrossRef] [PubMed]
56. Jia, L.; Huang, S.; Yin, X.; Zan, Y.; Guo, Y.; Han, L. Quercetin suppresses the mobility of breast cancer by suppressing glycolysis through Akt-mTOR pathway mediated autophagy induction. *Life Sci.* **2018**, *208*, 123–130. [CrossRef] [PubMed]
57. Sun, X.; Xue, Z.; Yasin, A.; He, Y.; Chai, Y.; Li, J.; Zhang, K. Colorectal Cancer and Adjacent Normal Mucosa Differ in Apoptotic and Inflammatory Protein Expression. *Eng. Regen.* **2022**, *2*, 279–287. [CrossRef]
58. Jin, T.; Li, D.; Yang, T.; Liu, F.; Kong, J.; Zhou, Y. PTPN1 promotes the progression of glioma by activating the MAPK/ERK and PI3K/AKT pathways and is associated with poor patient survival. *Oncol. Rep.* **2019**, *42*, 717–725. [CrossRef]
59. Pezzuto, A.; Carico, E. Role of HIF-1 in cancer progression: Novel insights. A review. *Curr. Mol. Med.* **2018**, *18*, 343–351. [CrossRef]
60. Patra, K.; Jana, S.; Sarkar, A.; Mandal, D.P.; Bhattacharjee, S. The inhibition of hypoxia-induced angiogenesis and metastasis by cinnamaldehyde is mediated by decreasing HIF-1α protein synthesis via PI3K/Akt pathway. *Biofactors* **2019**, *45*, 401–415. [CrossRef]
61. Nagase, H.; Ikeda, K.; Sakai, Y. Inhibitory effect of magnolol and honokiol from Magnolia obovata on human fibrosarcoma HT-1080 invasiveness in vitro. *Planta Med.* **2001**, *67*, 705–708. [CrossRef]

Disclaimer/Publisher's Note: The statements, opinions and data contained in all publications are solely those of the individual author(s) and contributor(s) and not of MDPI and/or the editor(s). MDPI and/or the editor(s) disclaim responsibility for any injury to people or property resulting from any ideas, methods, instructions or products referred to in the content.

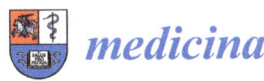

Article

Validation of a New Prognostic Score in Patients with Ovarian Adenocarcinoma

Oana Gabriela Trifanescu [1,2,†], Radu Iulian Mitrica [1,2], Laurentia Nicoleta Gales [1,3,*], Serban Andrei Marinescu [4,†], Natalia Motas [5,6], Raluca Alexandra Trifanescu [7,8,†], Laura Rebegea [9], Mirela Gherghe [10], Dragos Eugen Georgescu [11,*], Georgia Luiza Serbanescu [1,2], Haj Hamoud Bashar [12,†], Serban Dragosloveanu [13], Daniel Alin Cristian [14] and Rodica Maricela Anghel [1,2]

1. Discipline of Oncology, "Carol Davila" University of Medicine and Pharmacy, 022328 Bucharest, Romania
2. Department of Radiotherapy, "Prof. Dr. Al. Trestioreanu" Institute of Oncology, 022328 Bucharest, Romania
3. Department of Oncology, "Prof. Dr. Al. Trestioreanu" Institute of Oncology, 022328 Bucharest, Romania
4. Department of Surgery, "Prof. Dr. Al. Trestioreanu" Institute of Oncology, 022328 Bucharest, Romania
5. Department of Thoracic Surgery, "Prof. Dr. Al. Trestioreanu" Institute of Oncology, 022328 Bucharest, Romania
6. Discipline of Thoracic Surgery, "Carol Davila" University of Medicine and Pharmacy, 022328 Bucharest, Romania
7. Discipline of Endocrinology, "Carol Davila" University of Medicine and Pharmacy, 011863 Bucharest, Romania
8. "C.I. Parhon" Institute of Endocrinology, 011863 Bucharest, Romania
9. Discipline of Oncology, Faculty of Medicine and Pharmacy, "Dunarea de Jos" University, 800010 Galati, Romania
10. Department of Nuclear Medicine, "Prof. Dr. Al. Trestioreanu" Institute of Oncology, 022328 Bucharest, Romania
11. "Dr. Ion Cantacuzino" Department of Surgery, "Carol Davila" University of Medicine and Pharmacy, 030167 Bucharest, Romania
12. Department for Gynecology, Obstetrics and Reproductive Medicine, Saarland University Hospital, 66421 Homburg, Germany
13. Discipline of Orthopedics, "Foisor" Orthopedics Hospital, "Carol Davila" University of Medicine and Pharmacy, 022328 Bucharest, Romania
14. Discipline of Surgery, Coltea Clinical Hospital, "Carol Davila" University of Medicine and Pharmacy, 022328 Bucharest, Romania
* Correspondence: laurentia.gales@umfcd.ro (L.N.G.); gfdragos@yahoo.com (D.E.G.)
† These authors contributed equally to this work.

Abstract: *Background and Objectives:* This study aimed to assess the impact of clinical prognostic factors and propose a prognostic score that aids the clinician's decision in estimating the risk for patients in clinical practice. *Materials and Methods:* The study included 195 patients diagnosed with ovarian adenocarcinoma. The therapeutic strategy involved multidisciplinary decisions: surgery followed by adjuvant chemotherapy (80%), neoadjuvant chemotherapy followed by surgery (16.4%), and only chemotherapy in selected cases (3.6%). *Results:* After a median follow-up of 68 months, in terms of progression-free survival (PFS) and overall survival (OS), Eastern Cooperative Oncology Group (ECOG) performance status of 1 and 2 vs. 0 (hazard ratio—HR = 2.71, 95% confidence interval—CI, 1.96–3.73, $p < 0.001$ for PFS and HR = 3.19, 95%CI, 2.20–4.64, $p < 0.001$ for OS), menopausal vs. premenopausal status (HR = 2.02, 95%CI, 1.35–3,0 $p < 0.001$ and HR = 2.25, 95%CI = 1.41–3.59, $p < 0.001$), ascites (HR = 1.95, 95%CI 1.35–2.80, $p = 0.03$, HR = 2.31, 95%CI = 1.52–3.5, $p < 0.007$), residual disease (HR = 5.12, 95%CI 3.43–7.65, $p < 0.0001$ and HR = 4.07, 95%CI = 2.59–6.39, $p < 0.0001$), and thrombocytosis (HR = 2.48 95%CI = 1.72–3.58, $p < 0.0001$, HR = 3.33, 95%CI = 2.16–5.13, $p < 0.0001$) were associated with a poor prognosis. An original prognostic score including these characteristics was validated using receiver operating characteristic (ROC) curves (area under the curve—AUC = 0.799 for PFS and AUC = 0.726 for OS, $p < 0.001$). The median PFS for patients with none, one, two, three, or four (or more) prognostic factors was not reached, 70, 36, 20, and 12 months, respectively. The corresponding median overall survival (OS) was not reached, 108, 77, 60, and 34 months, respectively. *Conclusions:* Several negative prognostic factors were identified: ECOG performance status ≥ 1, the

Citation: Trifanescu, O.G.; Mitrica, R.I.; Gales, L.N.; Marinescu, S.A.; Motas, N.; Trifanescu, R.A.; Rebegea, L.; Gherghe, M.; Georgescu, D.E.; Serbanescu, G.L.; et al. Validation of a New Prognostic Score in Patients with Ovarian Adenocarcinoma. *Medicina* 2023, 59, 229. https://doi.org/10.3390/medicina59020229

Academic Editor: Vasilios Pergialiotis

Received: 15 December 2022
Revised: 8 January 2023
Accepted: 19 January 2023
Published: 26 January 2023

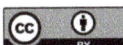

Copyright: © 2023 by the authors. Licensee MDPI, Basel, Switzerland. This article is an open access article distributed under the terms and conditions of the Creative Commons Attribution (CC BY) license (https://creativecommons.org/licenses/by/4.0/).

presence of ascites and residual disease after surgery, thrombocytosis, and menopausal status. These led to the development of an original prognostic score that can be helpful in clinical practice.

Keywords: prognostic factors; prognostic score; ovarian carcinoma; adenocarcinoma

1. Introduction

Worldwide, ovarian cancer represents a significant health burden, representing the second cause of gynecological-tumor-associated mortality, according to the latest estimates of GLOBOCAN 2020 [1]. More than two-thirds of patients are diagnosed in the advanced stages of the disease because of unspecific symptoms and a lack of efficient screening and detection methods [2]. Despite adopting new treatment techniques and developing new therapeutic agents, the outcome for patients with gynecological tumors remains poor, especially in developing countries [1,3,4].

The clinician must be guided in choosing a personalized therapeutic strategy by thoroughly exploring the patients' prognostic factors. Identifying these risk factors is vital to classify the patient in a specific risk group and estimate the risk of progression and death. These results must be correlated and interpreted in a multidisciplinary tumor board regarding selecting the correct treatment sequence between chemotherapy, targeted therapy, surgery, or radiotherapy [5,6].

A variety of adverse prognostic factors have been proposed for ovarian cancer. These include low-performance status, menopause, late-stage disease, mucinous histology and poor histologic differentiation, residual disease post-surgery, hypoalbuminemia, and thrombocytosis [7–17].

The most established prognostic factor in ovarian cancer is the presence of remaining cancer cells after a radical surgery aimed to remove as much of the tumor as possible. Based on the amount of residual disease, the risk can be stratified as follows: complete resection (R0): no cancer cells detectable, with best prognosis; microscopic residual disease (R1): cancer cells detectable only under the microscope, with intermediate prognosis; and macroscopic residual disease (R2): visible evidence of cancer remaining in the body post-surgery, with the worst prognosis [18]. Complete cytoreduction is associated with improved outcomes in all patients with ovarian cancer. As such, the residual disease status is a significant predictor of poor survival [10,19–23].

Thrombocytosis, defined as an elevated platelet count, has also been identified as a prognostic factor in patients with ovarian cancer. It is associated with advanced stages of the disease and decreased survival, as it may be caused by paracrine circuits involving thrombopoietic cytokines that stimulate tumor growth [15,16].

Another relevant marker of poor prognosis is hypoalbuminemia, defined as decreased levels of serum albumin (typically below 3.5 g/dL), and has been correlated with worse outcomes in advanced stages and may be a potential predictor of post-surgical survival [17]. A clinical surrogate for hypoalbuminemia is the presence of ascites, as low levels of albumin can cause an imbalance in oncotic and hydrostatic forces, leading to the leakage of fluids out of blood vessels into the abdominal cavity and has been associated with decreased survival and an increased risk of postoperative complications [24].

The study's primary objectives were to assess the impact of clinical and pathological prognostic factors and establish a simple prognostic score that can help clinicians estimate patients' risk and personalize the treatment in current medical practice. Identifying such a risk-factor-based prognostic score with predictive value in everyday routine can be helpful for clinicians and provide a meaningful benefit in treatment outcomes for ovarian cancer patients.

2. Materials and Methods

2.1. Patients

The ambispective study included 195 patients diagnosed with ovarian adenocarcinoma between 2007–2019. The study was approved by "Prof. Dr. Al. Trestioreanu" Bucharest Institute of Oncology Ethical Committee No. 22333/2022. No specific informed consent form (ICF) was used because all patients signed the institutional ICF giving consent to full use of their medical records for research purposes. The study was conducted in harmonization with the Declaration of Helsinki.

Patient's medical records were analyzed retrospectively between 2007–2010 and prospectively between 2011–2019. Histopathological confirmation of ovarian carcinoma, stage IC-IV, good performance status (ECOG 0-2), acceptable hematologic, liver, and renal function tests to allow the treatment administration, and consent of patients were among the inclusion criteria. The exclusion criteria included ECOG $\geq$ 3, lack of informed consent of patients, the impossibility of delivering chemotherapy, abnormal hematologic, liver, and renal function tests, and losing contact with the patients during the follow-up period.

2.2. Treatment

The therapeutic strategy involved multidisciplinary decisions, including surgery followed by adjuvant chemotherapy, neoadjuvant chemotherapy followed by surgery, or only chemotherapy in selected cases (multiple comorbidities, poor general health status). Bilateral salpingo-oophorectomy, hysterectomy, and omentectomy, with or without para-aortic lymphadenectomy, were among the surgical interventions required to obtain no macroscopic residual disease, along with the possible resection of any other involved segment (bowel, diaphragm, hepatic resection, appendectomy, partial cystectomy, metastasectomy). First-line chemotherapy included at least four cycles of platinum salts doublets, and the protocols included paclitaxel 175 mg/m^2 and carboplatin (AUC = 5) or cisplatin (75 mg/m^2).

2.3. Statistical Analysis

The statistical analysis was realized with IBM SPSS, version 23.0 (Chicago, IL, USA) for Windows and Excel, and included all eligible patients. Progression-free survival (PFS) and overall survival (OS) represented the endpoints of the analysis. The Kaplan–Meier method was used for generating survival curves. The univariate analysis using the log-rank test was used for studying the influence of relevant parameters on survival and time to disease progression, and multivariate analysis was used according to the stepwise Cox proportional hazards model to identify independent prognostic factors and estimate their effect on the time to disease progression and overall survival. The confidence interval (CI) considered for the calculated quantitative variables was 95%, and the p-value considered statistically significant was <0.05. ROC curves were used to measure the model's efficacy and estimate the method's sensibility and specificity. An AUC closer to 1 is considered efficient, and AUC values > 0.6 validate the model.

3. Results

3.1. Baseline Characteristics

The median age of patients was 54 $\pm$ 10.63 years (range between 18 and 82 years).

A complete physical examination was required to assess patients' clinical status, and the performance status was evaluated according to the ECOG scale. Most patients (61.7%) presented good performance status (ECOG 0), 35.6% with ECOG 1, and 0.7% with ECOG 2.

Most patients were postmenopausal at the time of diagnosis (63.6%). Known as a risk factor for ovarian cancer, the prevalence of nulliparity was 15.4% in our study's cohort.

In our cohort, the stage distribution included: 9.7% in stage IC, 11.8% in location IIA, 1% in stage IIB, 9.8% in stage IIC, 4.1% in stage IIIA, 3.1% in stage IIIB, 43.6% in stage IIIC, and 16.9% in stage IV. Therefore, two-thirds of the patients (66.7%) were diagnosed with an advanced stage of the disease and metastasis. Most patients presented with large ovarian tumors, with a mean size of 87.6 ± 47.8 mm (range between 10–250 mm) (Figure 1). The CA125 level at diagnosis was elevated in 76% of patients, with a mean value of 616 ± 922 U/mL (range 4–4892 U/mL). Additionally, significant ascites (>500 mL) was observed at the diagnosis in 35.8% of patients.

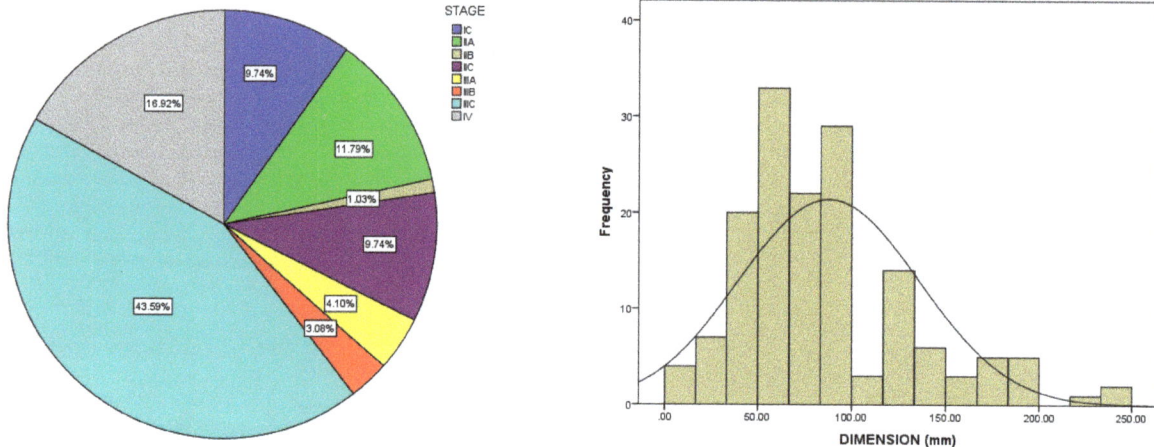

Figure 1. Tumor characteristics according to International Federation of Gynecology and Obstetrics (FIGO) staging and tumor dimension.

The histopathological report confirmed the diagnosis of ovarian epithelial adenocarcinoma in all patients. Most tumors were included in the serous subtype (72.9%), 12.8% in the endometrioid subtype, 13.3% mucinous, and 1% were included in the clear cell carcinoma subtype. Moreover, 62.9% were poorly differentiated tumors (G3), 27.4% were moderately differentiated (G2), and 9.7% were well differentiated (G1).

A multidisciplinary team decided on the therapeutic strategy. It included surgery followed by adjuvant chemotherapy in 156 patients (80%), neoadjuvant chemotherapy followed by surgery in 30 patients (16.4%), and only chemotherapy in 3.6% of patients (poor performance status, comorbidities).

Oncologic Outcome and Prognostic Factors

After a median follow-up of 68 months (range 7–191), the median PFS for all stages was 32 months, and the median OS was 84 months. For stage IIIC, the median PFS was 20 months, and the median OS was 51 months, whereas for stage IV, the median PFS was 14 months, and the median OS was 40 months.

Some important risk factors were identified (Tables 1 and 2).

ECOG performance status 1 or 2 (combined) compared to 0 was associated with poor prognostic outcome, a median PFS of 15 months vs. 60 months, and an OS of 38 vs. 112 months.

The presence of ascites represented a poor prognostic factor. PFS for patients with ascites was 22 months compared to 48 months for patients without ascites ($p = 0.027$). Moreover, OS was 44 months versus 120 months in favor of patients without ascites at the time of diagnosis ($p = 0.005$). The presence of ascites was associated with a 1.95 times higher risk of disease progression and a 2.31 times higher risk of death.

There was also a statistically significant difference regarding PFS for patients with thrombocytosis (defined as more than 450,000 platelets/mm^3) at the time of diagnosis versus patients with a standard value of platelets. Therefore, the median PFS and OS for patients with normal values of platelets were 60 and 150 months, and for patients with thrombocytosis, median PFS and OS were only 20 and 36 months ($p = 0.0001$). The presence of thrombocytosis at the time of diagnosis was associated with a 2.48 times higher risk of disease progression and a 3.33 times higher risk of death.

The most important prognostic factor was the presence of residual disease after surgery evaluated according to the surgeon's description and through imaging techniques (84.6% had a CT or MRI post-surgery before starting chemotherapy). In our series of patients, 49.23% of patients presented with residual disease after surgery. The presence of residual disease after surgery was associated with a shorter PFS (15 vs. 156 months, $p = 0.0001$) and statistically significant reduced OS (38 months vs. median not reached, $p = 0.0003$). Patients with residual disease after surgery had a five times higher risk of disease progression than patients without residual disease and a four times higher risk of death.

Additionally, the quantity of residual disease after surgery represents a prognostic factor. For patients without the residual disease, PFS was 156 months; for patients with residual disease less than 1 cm, PFS was 20 months; for patients with residual disease more than 1 cm, PFS was only 12 months ($p < 0.0001$). Median OS for patients without residual disease was not reached; for patients with residual disease less than 1 cm, OS was 60 months; for patients with the residual disease more than 1 cm, OS was only 34 months ($p = 0.0002$).

Table 1. Progression-free survival (PFS) and overall survival (OS) according to prognostic factors.

Characteristics	PFS		OS	
	Median PFS (Months)	p	Median OS (Months)	p
Eastern Cooperative Oncology Group (ECOG)				
ECOG 0	60		112	
ECOG 1	20	0.002	40	0.0001
ECOG 2	10	0.001	30	0.0001
Menopause				
No	60		150	
Yes	24	0.001	60	0.005
Residual disease				
Yes	15		38	
No	156	<0.0001	NR	0.0003
R1 cm				
0	156		NR	
0–1 cm	20	<0.0001	60	0.0002
More 1 cm	12	<0.0001	34	0.0001
G				
G2	72		150	
G3	21	<0.0001	50	0.0001
Histopathology (HP)				
Serous	24	0.002	62	NS
Mucinous	60	NS	72	
Endometrioid	70	NS	110	
Clear Cell	30	NS	NR	
Ascites				
Yes	22		44	
No	48	0.027	120	0.005
Thrombocytosis				
Yes	60		36	
No	20	0.0001	152	0.0001

Table 2. Multivariate analysis of the prognostic factors for PFS and OS.

Characteristics	HR	PFS PFS 95%CI	p	HR	OS OS 95%CI	p
ECOG						
ECOG 0	1			1		
ECOG 1, 2	2.71	1.96–3.73	0.001	3.19	2.20–4.64	0.001
Thrombocytosis						
No	1			1		
Yes	2.48	1.72–3.58	0.0001	3.33	2.16–5.13	0.0001
Menopause						
No	1			1		
Yes	2.02	1.35–3.01	0.001	2.25	1.41–3.59	0001
R0						
Yes	1			1		
No	5.12	3.43–7.65	0.0001	4.07	2.59–6.39	0.0001
G						
G2	1			1		
G3	2.50	1.77–3.53	0.001	2.24	1.65–3.24	0.001
HP						
Serous	1			1		
Non-serous	0.68	0.61–0.90	0.008	0.56	0.5–1	NS
Ascites						
No	1			1		
Yes	1.95	1.35–2.80	0.03	2.31	1.52–3.5	0.007

The most frequent histopathological subtype for postmenopausal women was high-grade serous carcinoma, whereas the incidence of the two histopathological subtypes was similar for premenopausal women. PFS was statistically significantly higher in premenopausal patients (60 vs. 24 months, $p = 0.001$), and the OS was 150 months vs. 60 months ($p = 0.005$).

3.2. Prognostic Score

After carefully analyzing the risk factors, the following variables were considered for establishing a prognostic score that could estimate the patient's outcome, the necessary therapeutic strategy, and follow-up intensity:

- performance status ECOG $\geq$ 1,
- presence of ascites,
- menopausal status,
- residual disease after surgery,
- presence of thrombocytosis.

In our series of patients, 28 (14.4%) patients had no risk factors, 43 (22.1%) patients had one risk factor, 42 (21.5%) patients had two risk factors, 36 (18.5%) had three risk factors, 40 (20.6%) had four risk factors, and 6 (3%) had five risk factors at diagnosis.

Each additional risk factor contributed to a statistically significant reduction in PFS ($p = 0.0001$) and OS ($p = 0.001$). Patients with no risk factors and a score of 0 had not reached median PFS and OS (Figure 2a for PFS and Figure 2b for OS). Patients with one risk factor had a median PFS of 70 months and an estimated median OS of 108 months. Patients with two risk factors had a median PFS of 36 months and a median OS of 77 months. Patients with three risk factors had a median PFS of 20 months and a median OS of 60 months. Patients with four or more poor prognostic factors had a median PFS of 12 months and an estimated OS of 34 months. These data sustain the use of the clinical prognostic score in the patient's initial evaluation.

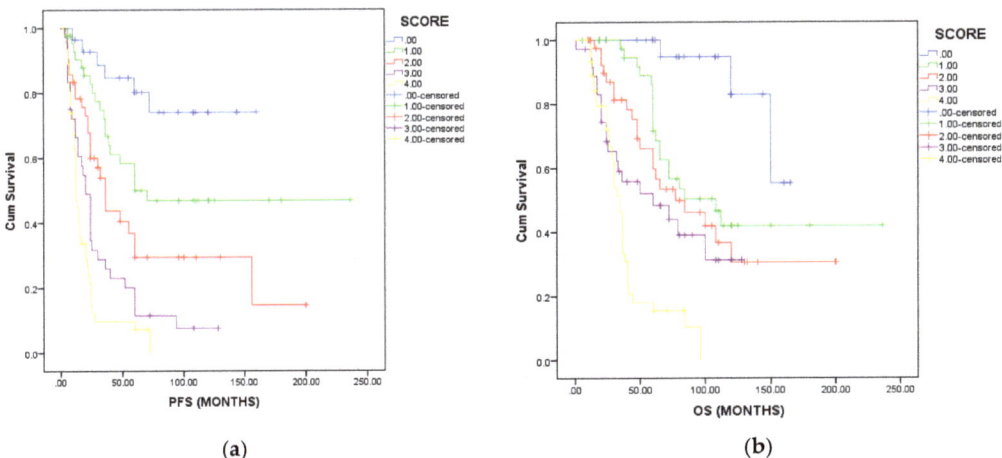

Figure 2. Progression-free survival (**a**) and overall survival (**b**) according to the number of risk factors.

ROC curves were used to validate the prognostic score and to characterize its sensibility and specificity. The prognostic score has an area under the curve of 0.799 ($p = 0.0001$, 95%CI 0.721–0.86) for PFS and an area under the curve of 0.726 ($p = 0.0001$, 95%CI 0.710–0.850) for OS. Therefore, these results demonstrate that this prognostic score could be helpful in medical practice due to its good sensibility and specificity (Figure 3a for PFS and Figure 3b for OS).

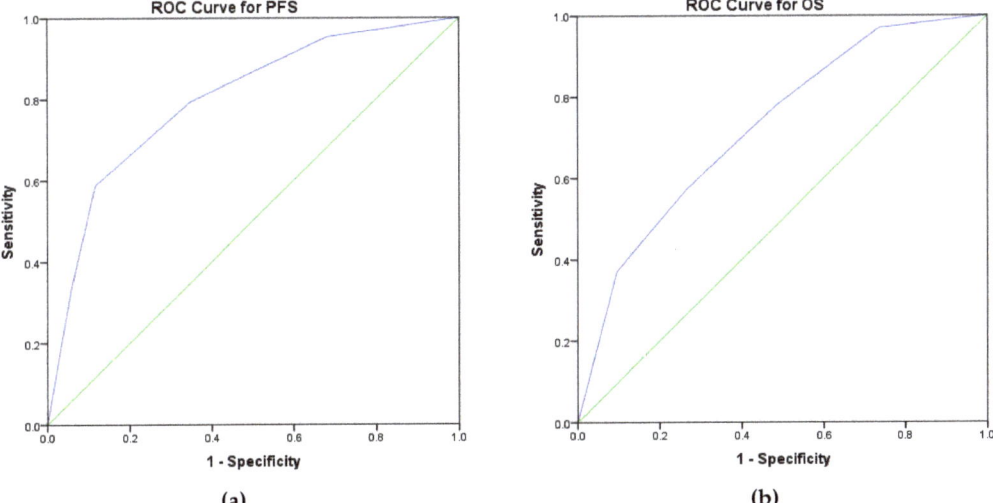

Figure 3. ROC curves estimating the specificity and sensitivity of the prognostic score ((**a**)-PFS and (**b**)-OS).

4. Discussion

Despite using new therapeutic agents and developing new treatment techniques, the outcome for patients with gynecological tumors remains poor, especially in developing countries [1,3]. Correctly identifying prognostic factors in ovarian cancer is vital, supporting the clinician in classifying the patient in a specific risk group and estimating the risk of disease progression and death. Furthermore, correctly identifying all prognostic factors leads to the right choice of therapeutic strategies and can help choose a personalized treatment. This can be achieved by associating standard treatment with additional therapeutic options such as antiangiogenic agents, PARP inhibitors, targeted therapy, immunotherapy, or radiotherapy. Identifying risk factor sets with predictive value in everyday practice can be a helpful tool.

The 195 patients with ovarian carcinoma included in this study had an extended median follow-up (68 months, range 7–191 months), allowing the identification of several adverse prognostic factors. Thus, the main prognostic factors were the stage of the disease, ECOG performance status 1 or 2 compared to 0, the presence of ascites, the degree of tumor differentiation, serous histopathological subtype compared to non-serous tumors, and menopausal status. The most important prognostic factor in our study was the presence and the amount of residual disease after surgery.

To our knowledge, an integrated prognostic score correlating these factors is yet to be developed. As such, we consider that this comprehensive method of calculating a predictive clinical marker is a novelty that the clinician needs.

The most robust data regarding the identification of prognostic factors in ovarian carcinoma originate from the analysis of three prospective studies (AGO-OVAR 3, 5, 7) conducted in Europe. The studies' initial purpose was to evaluate the role of a third chemotherapeutic agent (epirubicin or topotecan) added to the classic combination of paclitaxel and carboplatin/cisplatin [7–9].

Considering the negative result of the study, researchers proposed a prospective analysis of several prognostic factors for patients with ovarian carcinoma. The study included 3126 patients and proved through a univariate and a multivariate analysis that age, FIGO stage IIIC and IV compared to stage IIIB tumors or earlier stages, grade G2 and G3 compared to G1, mucinous histopathological subtype versus serous, ECOG 2 performance status versus ECOG 0, and the presence of ascites over 500 mL are independent prognostic factors.

The study showed that only a third of the included patients met the criteria for complete resection. The minimum residual disease was defined as a tumor between 1 and 10 mm, and macroscopic residual disease was defined as a tumor over 1 cm. The complete resection of the tumor was associated with a reduction in disease progression and death of 66% and 68%, respectively. The benefit of radical surgery was maintained for all stages of the disease.

Similar results were reported by a study including 1895 patients with stage III disease [10]. Following R0 resection as a comparison standard, the study observed that the presence of residual disease between 0–10 mm or over 10 mm was associated with a rise in the risk of disease progression HR = 1.96 (95%CI, 1.70–2.26; $p = 0.001$) and HR = 2.36 (95%CI 2.04–2.73; $p = 0.001$). Moreover, the risk of death was also increased by the presence of residual disease less than 1 cm (HR = 2.11; $p = 0.001$) or over 1 cm (HR = 2.47; $p = 0.001$) compared to those without residual disease or those with macroscopic residual disease. The study concluded that age, performance status, histopathology (mucinous vs. serous and endometrioid), and residual disease after surgery were poor prognostic factors.

Another study was published in Gynecologic Oncology Journal, and the objective was to evaluate the impact of cytoreduction and residual disease in 326 patients with stage IV ovarian adenocarcinoma. Optimal surgical resection was obtained in 54.9% of patients, 30.8% presented residual disease between 1–10 mm, and 14.3% showed residual disease over 10 mm after cytoreduction. The median OS was statistically significantly better for patients who underwent optimal cytoreduction without the residual disease (50 months) compared to patients with the residual disease between 1–10 mm when OS was 25 months or patients with the residual disease over 1 cm when OS was only 16 months.

The multivariate analysis confirmed the inferiority regarding the lack of surgical intervention (HR = 2.51, $p = 0.0001$), of residual disease between 1 and 10 mm (HR =1.5, $p = 0.046$), and residual disease over 1 cm (HR = 2.17, $p = 0.002$) compared to optimal cytoreduction, without the macroscopic residual disease. The study identified other prognostic factors, such as performance status, presence of ascites over 500 mL, and extension of the disease to the abdominal wall or liver metastasis, which are associated with a reserved prognosis [19].

Even more recent studies have elaborated a predictive model of response after neoadjuvant chemotherapy and discovered that patients with complete or near complete response (CRS3) (28%) after platinum salts doublet had a better PFS and OS compared to patients with partial CRS2 or no/minimal response CRS1 (HR = 0. 55, 95%CI, p = 0.001 for PFS and 0.65, p = 0.002 for OS) [20]. A similar study found that these data are valid for residual ovarian tumors and omental metastasis [21]. A recent systematic review identified that the Peritoneal Cancer Index (PCI) with an AUC of 0.69–0.92 [22] and Predictive Index Value (PIV) with an AUC of 0.66–0.98 were the most critical scores for complete resection [23].

Menopausal status is a known factor associated with ovarian adenocarcinoma, with over 65% of patients being postmenopausal at diagnosis [11]. Limited data are mentioned in the literature regarding ovarian adenocarcinoma in premenopausal patients; thus, the diagnosis is delayed in most cases. The proportion of young patients in our study is similar to the data mentioned in the literature [12,13].

A study that included 496 patients with malignant epithelial tumors reported an increased incidence of ovarian carcinoma with aging. Similar to our results, the percentage of patients with endometrioid carcinoma was higher in young patients compared to postmenopausal patients [14]. Although most patients are diagnosed during menopause, the reproductive characteristics of the patients, such as nulliparity or reduced number of pregnancies and the use of contraceptive pills, represent the most important risk factors [25]. Nulliparous patients had a higher risk of ovarian cancer than patients who gave birth (HR = 0.69, p = 0.001) and a significantly higher risk of clear cell carcinoma (RR = 0.35). In contrast, patients with serous carcinoma had the lowest risk reduction (RR = 0.81) [26].

Another important prognostic factor identified in our patients was the presence of thrombocytosis at diagnosis. In a study including 619 ovarian carcinoma patients, the aim was to establish the relationship between the number of thrombocytes in the peripheral blood smear, time to disease progression, and overall survival of patients. The study demonstrated that thrombocytosis is associated with advanced stages of the disease and decreased survival. Moreover, a rise in thrombopoietin values and IL-6 was observed, which explains the existence of a paracrine circuit where the increase in thrombopoietic cytokines leads to paraneoplastic thrombocytosis, which stimulates tumor growth [15].

A study that included more than 100 patients with ovarian cancer considered the value of pretreatment platelet count and tumor markers such as CA125 and proposed a reliable and straightforward to use in clinical practice score for patients with stage IV disease. A combined platelet and CA125 score of 0, 1, and 2 were determined based on the presence of thrombocytosis defined as more than 400,000/μL, elevated CA125 level defined as more than 1200 U/mL, or both. Median PFS was significantly lower in patients with a Platelet-CA125 score of 2 (19.6 months) compared with patients with a score of 0 (32.0 months; p = 0.011). Multivariate analysis identified both Platelet-CA125 scores of 2 and 1 as independent poor prognostic factors both for overall survival (p = 0.004, p < 0.001) and progression (p = 0.033, p = 0.017) in comparison with a score of 0 [16].

Another study aimed to validate a nomogram that predicts the 3-year recurrence risk of ovarian carcinoma. The items included in the nomogram were FIGO stage, histological grade, histological type, lymph node metastasis status, and serum CA125 level at diagnosis. The ROC curve of the nomogram showed that the AUC was 0.828 and identified a threshold value with reasonable specificity and sensitivity [27]. The study also showed that patients with thrombocytosis (53%) had a statistically significant lower PFS than those with a normal platelet count. OS was 2.62 years for patients with thrombocytosis and 4.65 years for patients with a normal thrombocyte count. The multivariate analysis showed that by analyzing according to age, stage of disease, grading, histopathological subtype, and residual disease after surgery, thrombocytosis remains an adverse prognostic factor for survival (p < 0.001).

Hypoalbuminemia at diagnosis was identified as a poor prognostic factor in advanced stages. More than that, after neoadjuvant treatment, if albumin levels return to normal, this may be a potential predictor of survival after surgery [17].

Markers of angiogenesis such as vascular endothelial growth factors VEGF and oxidative stress markers such as malondialdehyde may be used as prognostic markers, but their use on a large scale is limited [6,28–31].

In recurrent ovarian cancer, too, such a risk score that included patient's characteristics (ECOG performance status, age, quality of life, and nausea/vomiting) and treatment characteristics, such as platinum-free interval, showed a good predictive value with an AUC of 0.81 [32].

The future will belong to risk scores that include gene signatures. Such a score will be developed and validated based on the expression and augmentation of ovarian-cancer-related genes used to predict the outcome and chemoresistance in ovarian cancer patients [33].

New data are expected from the OTTA-SPOT (Ovarian Tumor Tissue Analysis consortium—Stratified Prognosis of Ovarian Tumors). They developed 276 gene expression signatures, identifying patients likely to achieve 5-year survival [34].

5. Conclusions

Several negative prognostic factors were identified: ECOG performance status ≥ 1, ascites, the presence and quantity of residual disease after surgery, thrombocytosis, and menopausal status. These results led to the development of an original prognostic score, which can be useful in clinical practice. Therefore, the clinical prognostic score could allow medical oncologists and surgeons to identify patients with adverse prognostic factors, for which treatment should be individualized through the escalation of therapeutic strategies.

Author Contributions: Conceptualization, O.G.T., R.M.A., L.N.G.; S.A.M. and D.E.G.; methodology, O.G.T., R.A.T. and H.H.B.; software, S.A.M. and H.H.B.; validation, L.R.; formal analysis, M.G. and N.M.; investigation, O.G.T., G.L.S., R.I.M. and L.N.G.; resources, O.G.T., R.M.A., L.N.G. and G.L.S.; data curation, S.D., D.A.C., S.A.M. and D.E.G.; writing—original draft preparation, O.G.T. and R.A.T.; writing—review and editing, L.N.G., S.A.M., H.H.B. and R.M.A.; visualization, D.E.G., L.R. and M.G.; supervision, D.E.G.; project administration, R.M.A.; All authors have read and agreed to the published version of the manuscript.

Funding: This research received no external funding.

Institutional Review Board Statement: The study was conducted in accordance with the Declaration of Helsinki and approved by the Institutional Review Board (or Ethics Committee) of Institute of Oncology "Prof. Dr Alexandru Trestioreanu" Bucharest Nr 22333/2022 for studies involving humans.

Informed Consent Statement: Informed consent was obtained from all subjects involved in the study.

Data Availability Statement: All data generated and analyzed are included within this research article.

Acknowledgments: Publication of this paper was supported by the University of Medicine and Pharmacy Carol Davila, through the institutional program Publish not Peris.

Conflicts of Interest: The authors declare no conflict of interest.

References

1. Sung, H.; Ferlay, J.; Siegel, R.L.; Laversanne, M.; Soerjomataram, I.; Jemal, A.; Bray, F. Global Cancer Statistics 2020: GLOBOCAN Estimates of Incidence and Mortality Worldwide for 36 Cancers in 185 Countries. *CA Cancer J. Clin.* **2021**, *71*, 209–249. [CrossRef]
2. Cannistra, S.A. Cancer of the Ovary. *N. Engl. J. Med.* **2004**, *351*, 2519–2529. [CrossRef]
3. Trifanescu, O.G.; Gales, L.N.; Serbanescu, G.L.; Zgura, A.F.; Iliescu, L.; Mehedintu, C.; Anghel, R.M. Long-Term Oncological Outcome in Patients with Cervical Cancer after 3 Trimodality Treatment (Radiotherapy, Platinum-Based Chemotherapy, and Robotic Surgery). *Medicine* **2021**, *100*, e25271. [CrossRef]
4. Siegel, R.L.; Miller, K.D.; Fuchs, H.E.; Jemal, A. Cancer Statistics, 2022. *CA Cancer J. Clin.* **2022**, *72*, 7–33. [CrossRef] [PubMed]

5. Bristow, R.E.; Tomacruz, R.S.; Armstrong, D.K.; Trimble, E.L.; Montz, F.J. *Survival Effect of Maximal Cytoreductive Surgery for Advanced Ovarian Carcinoma during the Platinum Era: A Meta-Analysis*; Centre for Reviews and Dissemination: York, UK, 2002.
6. Trifanescu, O.G.; Gales, L.N.; Tanase, B.C.; Marinescu, S.A.; Trifanescu, R.A.; Gruia, I.M.; Paun, M.A.; Rebegea, L.; Mitrica, R.; Serbanescu, L.; et al. Prognostic Role of Vascular Endothelial Growth Factor and Correlation with Oxidative Stress Markers in Locally Advanced and Metastatic Ovarian Cancer Patients. *Diagnostics* **2023**, *13*, 166. [CrossRef] [PubMed]
7. du Bois, A. A Randomized Clinical Trial of Cisplatin/Paclitaxel Versus Carboplatin/Paclitaxel as First-Line Treatment of Ovarian Cancer. *Cancer Spectrum Knowl. Environ.* **2003**, *95*, 1320–1329. [CrossRef] [PubMed]
8. Pfisterer, J.; Weber, B.; Reuss, A.; Kimmig, R.; du Bois, A.; Wagner, U.; Bourgeois, H.; Meier, W.; Costa, S.; Blohmer, J.-U.; et al. Randomized Phase III Trial of Topotecan Following Carboplatin and Paclitaxel in First-Line Treatment of Advanced Ovarian Cancer: A Gynecologic Cancer Intergroup Trial of the AGO-OVAR and GINECO. *JNCI J. Natl. Cancer Inst.* **2006**, *98*, 1036–1045. [CrossRef] [PubMed]
9. du Bois, A.; Weber, B.; Rochon, J.; Meier, W.; Goupil, A.; Olbricht, S.; Barats, J.-C.; Kuhn, W.; Orfeuvre, H.; Wagner, U.; et al. Addition of Epirubicin As a Third Drug to Carboplatin-Paclitaxel in First-Line Treatment of Advanced Ovarian Cancer: A Prospectively Randomized Gynecologic Cancer Intergroup Trial by the Arbeitsgemeinschaft Gynaekologische Onkologie Ovarian Cancer Study Group and the Groupe d'Investigateurs Nationaux Pour l'Etude Des Cancers Ovariens. *J. Clin. Oncol.* **2016**, *24*, 1127–1135. [CrossRef]
10. Winter, W.E., III; Maxwell, G.L.; Tian, C.; Carlson, J.W.; Ozols, R.F.; Rose, P.G.; Markman, M.; Armstrong, D.K.; Muggia, F.; McGuire, W.P. Prognostic Factors for Stage III Epithelial Ovarian Cancer: A Gynecologic Oncology Group Study. *J. Clin. Oncol.* **2007**, *25*, 3621–3627. [CrossRef]
11. Rampersad, A.C.; Wang, Y.; Smith, E.R.; Xu, X.-X. Menopause and Ovarian Cancer Risk: Mechanisms and Experimental Support. *Am. J. Clin. Exp. Obstet. Gynecol.* **2015**, *2*, 14–23.
12. Riman, T.; Nilsson, S.; Persson, I.R. Review of Epidemiological Evidence for Reproductive and Hormonal Factors in Relation to the Risk of Epithelial Ovarian Malignancies. *Acta Obstet. Gynecol. Scand.* **2004**, *83*, 783–795. [CrossRef] [PubMed]
13. Trifanescu, O.G.; Gales, L.N.; Trifanescu, R.A.; Anghel, R.M. Clinical Prognostic Factors in pre- and Post-Menopausal Women with Ovarian Carcinoma. *Acta Endocrinol.* **2018**, *14*, 353–359. [CrossRef]
14. Jung, E.J.; Eom, H.M.; Byun, J.M.; Kim, Y.N.; Lee, K.B.; Sung, M.S.; Kim, K.T.; Jeong, D.H. Different Features of the Histopathological Subtypes of Ovarian Tumors in Pre- and Postmenopausal Women. *Menopause* **2017**, *24*, 1028. [CrossRef] [PubMed]
15. Stone, R.L.; Nick, A.M.; McNeish, I.A.; Balkwill, F.; Han, H.D.; Bottsford-Miller, J.; Rupaimoole, R.; Armaiz-Pena, G.N.; Pecot, C.V.; Coward, J.; et al. Paraneoplastic Thrombocytosis in Ovarian Cancer. *N. Engl. J. Med.* **2012**, *366*, 610–618. [CrossRef] [PubMed]
16. Chen, J.-P.; Huang, Q.-D.; Wan, T.; Tu, H.; Gu, H.-F.; Cao, J.-Y.; Liu, J.-H. Combined Score of Pretreatment Platelet Count and CA125 Level (PLT-CA125) Stratified Prognosis in Patients with FIGO Stage IV Epithelial Ovarian Cancer. *J. Ovarian Res.* **2019**, *12*, 72. [CrossRef] [PubMed]
17. Dai, D.; Balega, J.; Sundar, S.; Kehoe, S.; Elattar, A.; Phillips, A.; Singh, K. Serum Albumin as a Predictor of Survival after Interval Debulking Surgery for Advanced Ovarian Cancer (AOC): A Retrospective Study. *J. Investig. Surg.* **2022**, *35*, 426–431. [CrossRef]
18. Sørensen, S.M.; Schnack, T.H.; Høgdall, C. Impact of Residual Disease on Overall Survival in Women with Federation of Gynecology and Obstetrics Stage IIIB-IIIC vs Stage IV Epithelial Ovarian Cancer after Primary Surgery. *Acta Obstet. Gynecol. Scand.* **2019**, *98*, 34–43. [CrossRef]
19. Ataseven, B.; Grimm, C.; Harter, P.; Heitz, F.; Traut, A.; Prader, S.; du Bois, A. Prognostic Impact of Debulking Surgery and Residual Tumor in Patients with Epithelial Ovarian Cancer FIGO Stage IV. *Gynecol. Oncol.* **2016**, *140*, 215–220. [CrossRef]
20. Cohen, P.A.; Powell, A.; Böhm, S.; Gilks, C.B.; Stewart, C.J.R.; Meniawy, T.M.; Bulsara, M.; Avril, S.; Brockbank, E.C.; Bosse, T.; et al. Pathological Chemotherapy Response Score Is Prognostic in Tubo-Ovarian High-Grade Serous Carcinoma: A Systematic Review and Meta-Analysis of Individual Patient Data. *Gynecol. Oncol.* **2019**, *154*, 441–448. [CrossRef]
21. Santoro, A.; Angelico, G.; Piermattei, A.; Inzani, F.; Valente, M.; Arciuolo, D.; Spadola, S.; Mulè, A.; Zorzato, P.; Fagotti, A.; et al. Pathological Chemotherapy Response Score in Patients Affected by High Grade Serous Ovarian Carcinoma: The Prognostic Role of Omental and Ovarian Residual Disease. *Front. Oncol.* **2019**, *9*, 778. [CrossRef]
22. Jónsdóttir, B.; Lomnytska, M.; Poromaa, I.S.; Silins, I.; Stålberg, K. The Peritoneal Cancer Index Is a Strong Predictor of Incomplete Cytoreductive Surgery in Ovarian Cancer. *Ann. Surg. Oncol.* **2021**, *28*, 244–251. [CrossRef] [PubMed]
23. Engbersen, M.P.; Lahaye, M.J.; Lok, C.A.R.; Koole, S.N.; Sonke, G.S.; Beets-Tan, R.G.H.; Van Driel, W.J. Peroperative Scoring Systems for Predicting the Outcome of Cytoreductive Surgery in Advanced-Stage Ovarian Cancer—A Systematic Review. *Eur. J. Surg. Oncol.* **2021**, *47*, 1856–1861. [CrossRef] [PubMed]
24. Ge, L.-N.; Wang, F. Prognostic Significance of Preoperative Serum Albumin in Epithelial Ovarian Cancer Patients: A Systematic Review and Dose–Response Meta-Analysis of Observational Studies. *Cancer Manag. Res.* **2018**, *10*, 815–825. [CrossRef] [PubMed]
25. Moorman, P.G.; Calingaert, B.; Palmieri, R.T.; Iversen, E.S.; Bentley, R.C.; Halabi, S.; Berchuck, A.; Schildkraut, J.M. Hormonal Risk Factors for Ovarian Cancer in Premenopausal and Postmenopausal Women. *Am. J. Epidemiol.* **2008**, *167*, 1059–1069. [CrossRef]
26. Wentzensen, N.; Poole, E.M.; Trabert, B.; White, E.; Arslan, A.A.; Patel, A.V.; Setiawan, V.W.; Visvanathan, K.; Weiderpass, E.; Adami, H.-O.; et al. Ovarian Cancer Risk Factors by Histologic Subtype: An Analysis from the Ovarian Cancer Cohort Consortium. *J. Clin. Oncol.* **2016**, *34*, 2888–2898. [CrossRef]
27. Hu, J.; Jiao, X.; Zhu, L.; Guo, H.; Wu, Y. Establishment and Verification of the Nomogram That Predicts the 3-Year Recurrence Risk of Epithelial Ovarian Carcinoma. *BMC Cancer* **2020**, *20*, 938. [CrossRef]

28. Yu, L.; Deng, L.; Li, J.; Zhang, Y.; Hu, L. The Prognostic Value of Vascular Endothelial Growth Factor in Ovarian Cancer: A Systematic Review and Meta-Analysis. *Gynecol. Oncol.* **2013**, *128*, 391–396. [CrossRef]
29. Didžiapetrienė, J.; Bublevič, J.; Smailytė, G.; Kazbarienė, B.; Stukas, R. Significance of Blood Serum Catalase Activity and Malondialdehyde Level for Survival Prognosis of Ovarian Cancer Patients. *Medicina* **2014**, *50*, 204–208. [CrossRef]
30. Komatsu, H.; Oishi, T.; Itamochi, H.; Shimada, M.; Sato, S.; Chikumi, J.; Sato, S.; Nonaka, M.; Sawada, M.; Wakahara, M.; et al. Serum Vascular Endothelial Growth Factor-A as a Prognostic Biomarker for Epithelial Ovarian Cancer. *Int. J. Gynecol. Cancer* **2017**, *27*, 1325–1332. [CrossRef]
31. Trifanescu, O.; Gruia, M.I.; Gales, L.; Trifanescu, R.; Pascu, A.M.; Poroch, V.; Toma, S.; Poiana, C.; Anghel, R. Malondialdehyde as a Prognostic Marker in Patients with Ovarian Adenocarcinoma. *Rev. Chim.* **2019**, *70*, 2561–2565. [CrossRef]
32. Armbrust, R.; Richter, R.; Woopen, H.; Hilpert, F.; Harter, P.; Sehouli, J. Impact of Health-Related Quality of Life (HRQoL) on Short-Term Mortality in Patients with Recurrent Ovarian, Fallopian or Peritoneal Carcinoma (the NOGGO-AGO QoL Prognosis-Score-Study): Results of a Meta-Analysis in 2209 Patients. *ESMO Open* **2021**, *6*, 100081. [CrossRef] [PubMed]
33. Lu, H.-Y.; Tai, Y.-J.; Chen, Y.-L.; Chiang, Y.-C.; Hsu, H.-C.; Cheng, W.-F. Ovarian Cancer Risk Score Predicts Chemo-Response and Outcome in Epithelial Ovarian Carcinoma Patients. *J. Gynecol. Oncol.* **2020**, *32*, e18. [CrossRef] [PubMed]
34. Millstein, J.; Budden, T.; Goode, E.L.; Anglesio, M.S.; Talhouk, A.; Intermaggio, M.P.; Leong, H.S.; Chen, S.; Elatre, W.; Gilks, B.; et al. Prognostic Gene Expression Signature for High-Grade Serous Ovarian Cancer. *Ann. Oncol.* **2020**, *31*, 1240–1250. [CrossRef] [PubMed]

Disclaimer/Publisher's Note: The statements, opinions and data contained in all publications are solely those of the individual author(s) and contributor(s) and not of MDPI and/or the editor(s). MDPI and/or the editor(s) disclaim responsibility for any injury to people or property resulting from any ideas, methods, instructions or products referred to in the content.

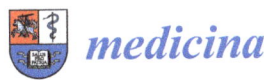

Article

Cancer-Oriented Comprehensive Nursing Services in Republic of Korea: Lessons from an Oncologist's Perspective

Suk Hun Ha [1], Moonho Kim [1], Hyojin Kim [2], Boram No [2], Ara Go [2], Miso Choi [2], Seol Lee [2] and Yongchel Ahn [1,*]

1. Department of Hematology and Oncology, Gangneung Asan Hospital, University of Ulsan College of Medicine, 38 Bangdong-gil, Sacheon-myeon, Gangneung-si 25440, Gangwon-do, Republic of Korea
2. Department of Nursing, Gangneung Asan Hospital, University of Ulsan College of Medicine, 38 Bangdong-gil, Sacheon-myeon, Gangneung-si 25440, Gangwon-do, Republic of Korea
* Correspondence: lephenixmed@gmail.com; Tel.: +82-33-610-3149

Abstract: *Background and objectives:* As is well known, cancer patients require extensive medical attention as they undergo surgery, chemotherapy, radiotherapy, and supportive care. The importance of high-quality cancer-directed nursing, combined with precision medicine, to maximize their survival outcomes and help them achieve a better quality of life cannot be overemphasized. In this context, we offered a new cancer-oriented comprehensive nursing system to our inpatients and reviewed its clinical outcomes in comparison with those from the preexisting general cancer ward. *Materials and Methods*: From March 2019 to February 2020, a total of 102 cancer patients and 42 nurses were enrolled in this pilot study. We aimed to analyze their performance in three main categories: structure, process, and patient/nurse outcomes. *Results*: First, structural (nurse staffing and environment) upgrades were installed in the cancer-oriented comprehensive nursing ward, including an improved nurse-patient ratio (1:8 in the comprehensive ward as compared with 1:14 in the general ward), wider space between beds (1.5 m versus 1.0 m), fully automatic beds with fall prevention sensors, etc. Second, the nursing process was improved (missed care 0.1 event/month vs. 1.3 event/month). Third, both patient and nurse outcomes showed preferable results in the comprehensive ward. The patient satisfaction level was higher in the comprehensive nursing ward than in the general ward (willing to revisit: 91.7% and 78.4%, respectively; willing to recommend to others: 95.0% and 76.8%, respectively). Pressure ulcers, as a patient safety indicator, were also decreased (0.3 events/month vs. 0.8 events/month). However, the fall incidence was similar in both groups (1.6 events/month vs. 1.5 events/month). In terms of nurse outcomes, turnover intention was stabilized and nurses' job satisfaction in the comprehensive ward was superior to that of their counterparts. *Conclusions*: Our study was a pilot study to demonstrate that cancer patient-oriented comprehensive nursing services can be helpful in improving the quality of cancer treatment and nurses' job satisfaction. Continued interest in and efforts to improve nursing care delivery are also crucial in achieving and maintaining the best possible cancer patient care.

Keywords: cancer; comprehensive nursing service; outcome

1. Introduction

In the Republic of Korea, unlike in other developed countries, inpatient nursing care has been shared by the patient's family members or paid caregivers. For example, family members are allowed to stay in hospital rooms to help with the daily medical care of patients, which enables a relatively small number of medical staff to manage a larger number of patients. We have maintained this individual-patient nursing care system for more than 70 years [1,2]. However, medical problems such as increased opportunistic infections or unexpected falls are more frequently observed when non-medical personnel take part in nursing than in nurse-centered caregiving [3]. In addition, about 40% of inpatients are now cared for by patient-paid caregivers because of the rapid progress of industrialization/urbanization, the increase in the aging population, and the subsequent expansion of the nuclear family. Securing a private caregiver inevitably brings about increased medical expenses for the patients, and it has now become a public healthcare issue.

In an effort to solve this healthcare problem, our government kicked off a pilot project called the "Patient-Sitter Program" in 2006 [4]. The current model of comprehensive nursing care was built to extend beyond the simple concept of co-nursing and was officially initiated with a national insurance subsidy in 2016 [5,6]. This inpatient nursing service features nursing staff reinforcement, along with hospital facility improvements. Registered nurses (RNs) and nursing assistants (NAs) are sufficiently assigned to the comprehensive nursing ward, while patients only need to pay a quarter of the caregiving fee instead of hiring a private caregiver [1]. As of December 2019, this comprehensive nursing system was successfully implemented, with 49,000 beds in 534 institutions [6]. Reports on the performance of this service mainly focused on patient and nurse satisfaction from the nurses' perspectives. Studies generally showed that the risk of infection and accidents was reduced in this service, while achieving patient satisfaction [1–3,7,8]. However, the levels of job satisfaction for the nurses revealed inconsistent results for each study [9–11].

In measuring quality of health care, Donabedian's three components (structure, process, and outcomes) approach is widely used [12]. He believed that structure measures have an effect on process measures, which in turn, affect outcome measures, but he also mentioned that cause and effect are more complex in the real world. On the basis of the Donabedian model, we postulated that our desired impact of 'high-quality nursing care for cancer patients' was determined by three different types of measures, namely structure, process, and outcome.

To date, academic research on the comprehensive nursing ward is mainly focused only on nursing-related fields. There are few studies currently available regarding the influence of comprehensive nursing applied to patients suffering from malignancies. As is well known, cancer patients require complex medical attention as they undergo surgery, chemotherapy, radiotherapy, and concurrent supportive care. The importance of offering sophisticated cancer patient-directed nursing, combined with anticancer treatments, to maximize patient survival outcomes and achieve a better quality of life, cannot be overemphasized. In this context, we adopted this new nursing system in one of the hematology-oncology wards (called cancer-oriented comprehensive nursing wards) to review its operational outcomes in comparison with those in the preexisting general cancer ward.

2. Materials and Methods

2.1. Study Setting

A tertiary hospital (827 beds) staffed with 246 doctors and 703 RNs is located on the east coast of the Republic of Korea. In 2018, 11,946 patients diagnosed with cancer were admitted to the hospital (average 32.4 patients/day, bed turnover rate 85.7%) and 5682 inpatients received chemotherapy in cancer care wards. Besides a preexisting general cancer ward (58 beds with 25 RNs only), we started to run a new cancer-oriented comprehensive nursing ward (46 beds with 25 RNs and 12 NAs) in December 2017. These two wards mainly cared for medical hematology-oncology patients. A total of 11,946 inpatients (average 32.4 patients/day, bed turnover rate 85.7%) were admitted, and 5682 patients received chemotherapy in 2018.

2.2. Participant Selection and Data Collection

Respondents (patients and nurses) who had consented to participate were enrolled in this preliminary study. First, patients who met the following criteria were eligible: (a) diagnosed with cancer, (b) community-dwelling, and (c) without any missing data. We determined the patient sample size using G*Power version 3.1.9.2. The sample size was calculated based on the effect size of 0.5, a significance level of 0.05, and a power of 0.80, and the minimum sample size was 52 in each group. From March 2019 to February 2020, data were collected for 104 patients (52 patients in the comprehensive ward and 52 in the general ward, respectively). A total of 102 patients were ultimately analyzed (two patients in the general ward submitted incomplete questionnaire form). Second, 42 nurses volunteered to participate in this study (23 nurses out of 25 in comprehensive ward and 19 out of 25 in general ward, respectively). Each questionnaire form (either for patients or for nurses) informed respondents about the confidentiality of their answers and the voluntary nature of their participation. Additionally, the purpose and method of the study were clearly specified and consent for participation was obtained. Participants could always stop the survey at by their own choice, without any penalty.

2.3. Measurements

In order to assess the quality of nursing services with simple but consistent variables, we adopted the Donabedian model for examining the quality of care to analyze our clinical outcomes regarding the cancer-focused comprehensive nursing service in three main categories: structure, process, and patient/nurse outcomes (Figure 1) [1,12].

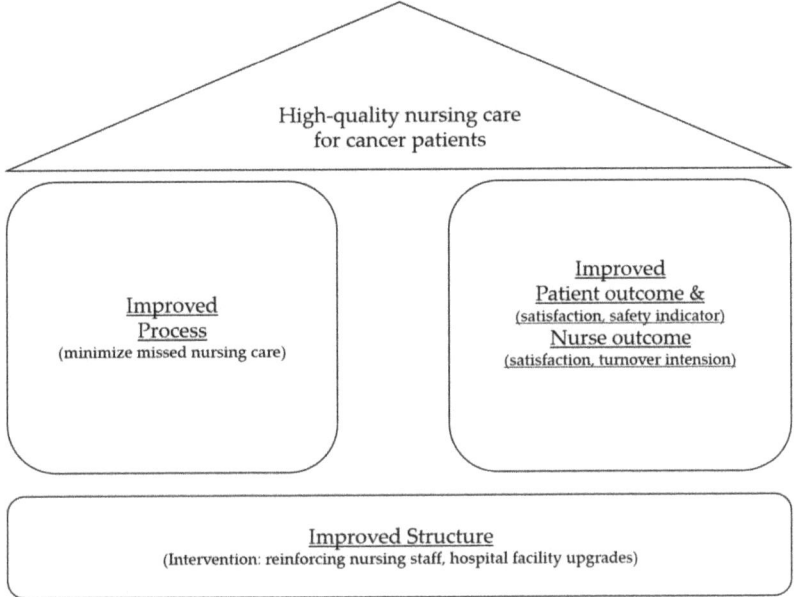

Figure 1. Conceptual framework of our study.

2.3.1. Structure

At first, we looked into structural improvements made in the cancer-oriented comprehensive nursing ward. Changes in the number of nursing staff, the nurse-patient ratio, and any hospital facility upgrades were documented.

2.3.2. Process

The indicator of the process category included any item of missed nursing care (or care left undone) in our study. Nursing care indicates (a) communication and information sharing; (b) education, including care planning, discharge planning, and decisions; (c) fundamental physical care; and (d) emotional and psychological care. Missed nursing care encompasses any unfinished or delayed clinical, administrative, or emotional care that was not completed or was postponed during a nurse's given duty time [13]. The reporting and tracking of missed nursing care in the study population was performed by a nurse in charge, under the supervision of head nurse, on a monthly basis.

2.3.3. Patient/Nurse Outcome

Patient satisfaction and safety indicators, such as falls and infections, were assessed as patient outcomes. Using the patient satisfaction index [2], a questionnaire comprised of 35 questions (on a 5-point Likert scale) was utilized to compare patient satisfaction between the comprehensive nursing ward and the general ward. The patient satisfaction in physical, therapeutic, environmental, emotional, and informative nursing was included. A higher score in the survey indicated a higher level of patient satisfaction. Moreover, we additionally asked patients whether they wanted to re-visit the comprehensive ward based on the followings: "If there is a need to admit to the hospital, would you want to use comprehensive nursing ward again?" and "Are you willing to encourage other patients to try this ward?" [14,15]

In terms of nurse outcome, job satisfaction and turnover intention (or will to resign) were evaluated. First, a well-designed tool to measure nurses' job satisfaction was adopted in our study, which was composed of 20 questions (assessed on the 5-point Likert scale) [16–18]. The higher the score, the higher the job satisfaction. Questionnaire items included satisfaction with the professional position, payment level, interaction, autonomy, job requirements, administrative affairs, and the relationship between nurses and other healthcare professionals. Second, turnover intention was measured using 6 questions (on a 5-point Likert scale) [19,20]. A higher score indicated a nurse's higher will to resign. In order to guarantee anonymity and to obtain accurate answers, we decided not to ask nurses for personal data, such as age, education level, and service period.

2.4. Statistical Analysis

When comparing the characteristics of patients in two different groups, the Chi-square test and the Fisher exact test were used for categorical variables, and the Student's t-test and the Mann–Whitney U test were used for continuous variables. For the analysis of the study's main outcome (comparison of satisfaction between the two wards), we used the Student's t-test with the score results from each group. The statistical significance referred to a value of $p < 0.05$. Data were analyzed using IBM SPSS version 24.0 for Windows (SPSS Inc., Chicago, IL, USA).

3. Results

3.1. Structure

Structural (nursing staffing and environment) upgrades were made in the cancer-oriented comprehensive nursing ward. The nursing staff was reinforced in this special ward (46 beds with 25 RNs and 12 NAs) when compared with the general ward (58 beds with only 25 RNs). This finally resulted in the improved nurse-patient ratio (1:8 in the comprehensive ward as compared with 1:14 in the general ward).

Environmental upgrades were made to promote patient safety, including a wider space between beds (1.5 m vs. 1.0 m), fully automatic beds with fall prevention sensors, etc. Mobile toilets, shampoo aids, a sink, and room shower equipment are available for patients to perform activities of daily living, with the help of circulating NAs. Furthermore, auxiliary nurse stations were arranged by the corridor to further support nurses' work, and closed-circuit televisions were also installed to monitor any safety risks, such as falls (Table 1).

3.2. Process

We examined missed nursing care as an indicator of the process category. From March to November 2019, the incidence of missed delivery nursing care was only one in the comprehensive ward, as opposed to twelve in the general ward (an average 0.1 and 1.3 events per month, respectively) (Figure 2).

Table 1. The environmental improvements in the comprehensive nursing ward.

Category	Facilities and Equipment	General Ward	Comprehensive Ward	Purpose
Ward	Auxiliary nurse station per team	None	A table with one PC * per team	Proximity nursing
	Patient lounge	Shared and small	More spacious	Providing comfortable space
	Corridor surveillance cameras	Same		Incident/accident monitoring
	Corridor guard rail	In compliance with government regulations	Twice as protective as required per the regulations	Fall prevention
Patient room	Interval between beds	1.5 m	2 m	Infection prevention
	Emergency call bell per bed	Same		Fall prevention
	Mat with fall prevention sensor	None	Yes	
	Electric bed with remote control	Beds in private rooms only	All of the beds	Patient convenience
	Air mattress	None	Yes	Bedsore prevention
	Sink per room	Same		Infection prevention
	Alcohol-rub dispenser per bed	Same		
	Toilet in room	Beds in OB/GYN ** ward and private rooms	About 30% of beds	Patient convenience
	Shower room	Beds in private rooms only	About 30% of beds	
Medical equipment	Wheelchair, walker	In compliance with the government regulations	More than 1.5 times as many as required per the regulations	Fall prevention
	Mobile toilet	None	Yes	Sanitary nursing
	Shampoo aid	None	Yes	
	Bath bed	None	Yes	
	Oxygen monitor	In compliance with the government regulations	Twice as many as required per the regulations	Vital sign measurement
	Non-invasive sphygmomanometer	In compliance with the government regulations	Twice as many as required per the regulations	
	Bladder scan	Same		Residual urine check
	Various and detailed patient information	Handout only	Handout and video guide	Educating patients and visiting guardians

* PC, personal computer; ** OB/GYN, obstetrics and gynecology.

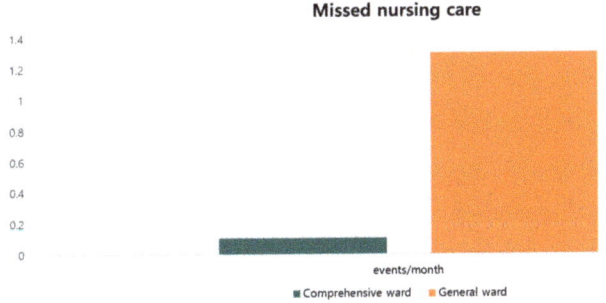

Figure 2. Missed nursing care (events/month).

3.3. Outcomes

3.3.1. Patient Outcome

A survey regarding the patient outcome in both groups was performed by the time the patient was discharged. The mean age of patients was similar in between groups (62.38 ± 17.67 years and 62.62 ± 10.22 years in the comprehensive ward and the general ward, respectively). More than 60% were male (61.5% and 60%, respectively) and the Eastern Cooperative Oncology Group performance status was either 0 or 1 in most of the patients in both wards (82.7% and 76%, respectively). Colorectal cancer patients accounted for the largest proportion (28.9% and 32.0%, respectively) in our study. The differences in the nursing requirement severity between the two wards were not statistically significant

(p = 0.06). The detailed baseline characteristics of inpatients with solid or hematologic malignancies are summarized in Table 2.

Table 2. Baseline characteristics of patients (n = 102).

Characteristic	Comprehensive Nursing Ward (n = 52)	General Ward (n = 50)	p
	n (%) or M ± SD *	n (%) or M ± SD	
Age (years, range)	62.38 ± 11.17 (19–86)	62.62 ± 10.22 (38–84)	0.84
Sex			0.87
Male	32 (61.5%)	30 (60%)	
Female	20 (38.5%)	20 (40%)	
Living status			0.39
Living with family	27 (75%)	34 (82.9%)	
Living alone	9 (25%)	7 (17.1%)	
ECOG PS **			0.32
0–1	43 (82.7%)	38 (76%)	
2	5 (9.6%)	6 (12%)	
3	3 (5.8%)	2 (4%)	
4	1 (1.9%)	4 (8%)	
Length of stay (days, range)	9.98 ± 4.51 (2–29)	10.50 ± 6.40 (3–33)	0.56
Reason for admission			0.33
Elective	44 (88%)	39 (78%)	
Emergency	8 (12%)	11 (22%)	
Cancer stage (solid tumor)			0.22
I-II	10 (25.0%)	7 (14.6%)	
III-IV	30 (75.0%)	41 (85.4%)	
Cancer type			0.78
Breast	12 (23.1%)	9 (18.0%)	
Colorectal	15 (28.9%)	16 (32.0%)	
Hepatobiliary/Pancreatic	3 (5.8%)	4 (8.0%)	
Lung	6 (11.5%)	6 (12.0%)	
Stomach	2 (3.9%)	5 (10.0%)	
Hematologic malignancies	13 (25.0%)	7 (14.0%)	
Others	1 (1.8%)	3 (6.0%)	
Nursing requirement severity			0.06
I-II	51 (98.1%)	44 (88%)	
III-IV	1 (1.9%)	6 (12%)	

* M ± SD, mean ± standard deviation; ** ECOG PS, Eastern Cooperative Oncology Group performance status.

Patient satisfaction was measured by the patient satisfaction index. The scores of all five items (i.e., physical, therapeutic, environmental, emotional, and informational nursing satisfaction) were statistically higher in the comprehensive ward than those in the general ward (Table 3). We also conducted an additional survey on patients' willingness to revisit and willingness to recommend to others (willing to revisit: 91.7% vs. 78.4%, willing to recommend to others: 95.0% vs. 76.8%) (Figure 3A). In terms of patient safety, the incidence of pressure ulcers was improved in the comprehensive ward (0.3 event/month in the comprehensive ward and 0.8 events/month in the general ward). However, there was no difference in the incidence of falls between the two wards (1.6 event/month vs. 1.5 event/month) (Figure 3B).

Table 3. Scores using the patient satisfaction index ($n = 102$).

Characteristic	Comprehensive Nursing Ward ($n = 52$)	General Ward ($n = 50$)	p
	Score *, M ± SD **	Score, M ± SD	
Physical satisfaction	4.32 ± 0.66	4.02 ± 0.71	<0.01
Therapeutic satisfaction	4.33 ± 0.69	4.09 ± 0.66	<0.01
Environmental satisfaction	4.41 ± 0.70	3.95 ± 0.77	<0.01
Emotional satisfaction	4.39 ± 0.66	3.99 ± 0.75	<0.01
Informational satisfaction	4.29 ± 0.69	3.97 ± 0.88	<0.01

* The scores range from 1 to 5; ** M ± SD, mean ± standard deviation.

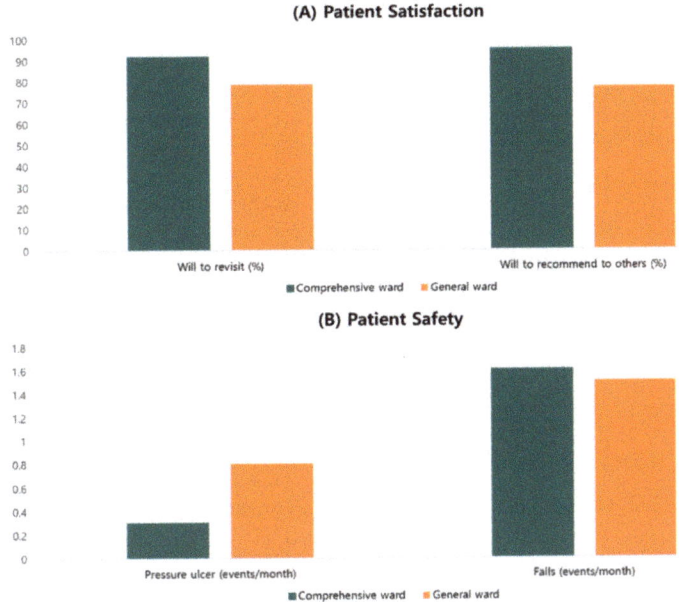

Figure 3. (**A**) Patient satisfaction (willing to re-visit and recommend to others, %); (**B**) patient safety (pressure ulcers and falls, events/month).

3.3.2. Nurse Outcome

The nurse outcome survey was conducted simultaneously three months after the start of the study in both groups. The overall job satisfaction of nurses was found to be better in the comprehensive ward (M ± SD; 3.54 ± 0.33) than that in the general ward (M ± SD; 3.09 ± 0.55). We also found that a nurse's intention to resign (or reposition) was more stable in the comprehensive ward than that in the general ward (M ± SD; 3.10 ± 0.51 vs. 3.87 ± 0.49, $p < 0.01$) (Table 4).

Table 4. Comparison of nurses' job satisfaction and turnover intention ($n = 42$).

Characteristic	Comprehensive Nursing Ward ($n = 23$)	General Ward ($n = 19$)	p
	Score *, M ± SD **	Score, M ± SD	
Job satisfaction	3.54 ± 0.33	3.09 ± 0.55	<0.01
Turnover intention	3.10 ± 0.51	3.87 ± 0.49	<0.01

* The score ranges from 1 to 5; ** M ± SD, mean ± standard deviation.

4. Discussion

In this study, we evaluated new comprehensive nursing care services in view of the structure, process, and patient/nurse outcomes. We compared not only subjective items (patient and nurse satisfaction) but also objective items, such as falls, pressure ulcers, and missed nursing care errors. Innovative changes were identifiable in all the subjective and objective variables (except for the incidence of falls), which are essential to maintain the high standard of cancer treatment.

In Western countries, the nursing care delivery system has evolved to a nurse-centered scheme which strictly restricts non-medical personnel from staying with patients to help with medical care. On the other hand, due to a lack of medical staff (mainly doctors and nurses) and equipment, some of the healthcare provider's duties are still passed on to the family members or paid caregivers in our country. This outdated nursing system really can be potentially harmful to cancer patients because anticancer treatment requires the multidisciplinary collaboration of healthcare workers, as well as an enormous amount of medical resources [21]. We aimed to estimate the performance outcomes of a cancer-centered comprehensive nursing ward (which features nursing staff reinforcement and hospital environment upgrades), in comparison with the current general cancer ward as a new way of hematology-oncology patient nursing care.

The nursing staff is crucial in delivering the best available medical care for cancer patients [22]. To improve their quality of life, it is very important to simultaneously provide high-quality nursing services and anticancer treatment. In this respect, we postulated that a comprehensive nursing system could provide us with good insight into ideal inpatient services for cancer patients. It can also relieve the financial burden on cancer patients and their family members. Patients with malignancy, especially advanced or metastatic, often have difficulty performing routine daily activities, so their need for caregiving services is relatively higher than those of non-cancer patients. Under this new system, with the help of a national insurance subsidy, cancer patients only need to pay a quarter of the caregiving fee instead of hiring a private caregiver when they use the comprehensive nursing services [1].

In this study, we conducted a pilot study, for the first time in a literature review, on the operational performance of a cancer-focused comprehensive ward. With reference to previous studies [1,2], we chose simple but clinically useful parameters from each category (structure, process, and outcome) in regards to an oncologist's perspective. In the structure, the most significant changes were made in the software aspect (the number of RNs and NAs was increased to achieve a nurse-patient ratio of 1:8) in addition to hardware aspects (facility upgrades). In the general ward, one duty nurse takes charge of fourteen patients, i.e., cancer patients were put at great risk of exposure to poorer quality medical care, even if this was not the intention of the system. We further reinforced the system with seven NAs to provide the patients with meal, bathing, personal hygiene, and toileting assistance. Thus, the RNs were able to invest more time in their profession-related tasks, such as patient education, occupational training, etc. We determined that a comprehensive nursing system can help to maintain a desirable nurse-patient ratio so as to create a healthier work environment for both patients and medical staff [23]. As stated above, we performed many renovations to hospital environments to ensure patient safety and comfort during the hospital stay. In the near future, we hope that environmental improvement in the general ward can also be ensured through the use of government support programs.

A previous study proposed nursing time, missed nursing care, and service quality as process outcomes [1]. We selected missed care because it is the single most important representative of process outcomes, as it is easy to monitor and share among doctors, RNs, NAs, and other healthcare providers. We observed that care left undone is dramatically reduced in the comprehensive nursing ward.

Many studies demonstrated that patient satisfaction and hospital reuse intention are consistently higher in comprehensive nursing wards [1,24]. We also observed the same result, with statistical differences, in the cancer patients using the comprehensive service. We also evaluated whether the cancer-focused comprehensive ward could be helpful in securing patient safety because cancer patients are vulnerable to pressure ulcers and pathologic fractures from falls. Interestingly, we observed that the incidence of falls was similarly low between the two groups. This might be partly explained by our baseline characteristics of relatively young age and good performance status in our study.

When the nursing staff is satisfied with their jobs, we can expect that a higher quality of nursing services can be ensured. This is why it is vital to take a close look at nursing outcomes when evaluating a cancer-directed comprehensive nursing care. In the literature review, studies have thus far shown mixed results concerning this topic. Some studies reported higher nurse satisfaction [25]; others showed a lack of statistical difference [23]; while another revealed lower nurse satisfaction [26]. In our study, job satisfaction was higher in the comprehensive ward than in the general ward. However, there were a few things to consider: although the differences in nursing severity were not statistically significant, nursing severity in the general ward patients was somewhat higher. Moreover, experienced nurses were assigned in the early stages of the comprehensive ward operation. Therefore, care must be taken in interpreting our job satisfaction results. Based on these findings, we must closely monitor the nursing staff and equipment to maintain a higher level of patient/nurse outcomes [27,28], which secures professional care for cancer patients.

There are some limitations in our study. First, our findings originated from a preliminary, non-randomized study with a small sample size that was not representative of the larger population. Second, the purpose and method of the research were clearly communicated to the participants, and the non-blinded nature of study design could definitely result in inevitable statistical bias; there was evident superiority and inferiority in our variables between the two groups, including clear differences in manpower and resources. Third, the self-reporting form of the questionnaire was the main source of information to evaluate the quality of nursing care. Fourth, among the various nurse-related outcomes, only job satisfaction and turnover intention were included. In patient-related outcomes, only patient satisfaction, ulcer sores, and incidental falls were analyzed. Further studies are needed to encompass other important aspects of medical care, such as opportunistic infection rates, length of hospital stay, thromboembolic events, and survival outcomes.

5. Conclusions

Our study was a pilot study to demonstrate that a cancer-oriented comprehensive nursing service would be successful both in improving the quality of cancer care and the nursing staff's job satisfaction. We believe that our experiences are not confined only to medical hematology-oncologists or cancer nurses in the Republic of Korea. In other words, to achieve and maintain high-quality cancer patient care, continued interest and efforts to improve the nursing care delivery system are also crucial.

Author Contributions: Conceptualization, Y.A.; methodology, M.K.; software, H.K.; validation, B.N.; formal analysis, A.G.; investigation, M.C.; resources, S.L.; data curation, S.H.H.; writing—original draft preparation, M.K. and S.H.H.; writing—review and editing, Y.A.; visualization, M.K.; supervision, Y.A. All authors have read and agreed to the published version of the manuscript.

Funding: This research received no external funding.

Institutional Review Board Statement: This study was conducted in accordance with Declaration of Helsinki, and we obtained the approval of the Gangneung Asan Hospital Institutional Review Board (IRB No. 2019-01-029-003; Approval Date: 1 February 2019).

Informed Consent Statement: All the participants were fully informed about study's aim and purpose and provided written informed consent.

Data Availability Statement: Our data are readily available upon reasonable request.

Conflicts of Interest: The authors declare no conflict of interest.

References

1. Kim, J.; Kim, S.; Park, E.; Jeong, S.; Lee, E. Policy Issues and New Direction for Comprehensive Nursing Service in the National Health Insurance. *J. Korean Acad. Nurs. Adm.* **2017**, *23*, 312–322. [CrossRef]
2. Lee, S.; Yu, S.; Kim, M.; Kim, H. Impact of South Korea's Comprehensive Nursing Service Policy on Nurse and Patient Outcomes. *Healthcare* **2020**, *8*, 223. [CrossRef] [PubMed]
3. Park, K.-O.; Yu, M.; Kim, J.-K. Experience of Nurses Participating in Comprehensive Nursing Care. *J. Korean Acad. Nurs. Adm.* **2017**, *23*, 76–89. [CrossRef]
4. You, S.-J.; Choi, Y.-K. Institutionalization of a Patient-Sitter Program in Acute Care Hospitals. *J. Korea Contents Assoc.* **2013**, *13*, 370–379. [CrossRef]
5. Kim, J.; Choi, H.S. Research Trends in Korea on Integrated Nursing Care Service: A Scoping Review. *Korean J. Adult Nurs.* **2020**, *32*, 455–471. [CrossRef]
6. Policy Direction of Comprehensive Nursing Care. Available online: http://www.nhis.or.kr/bbs7/boards/B0040/21012 (accessed on 2 December 2022).
7. Shin, S.-R.; Park, K.-Y. Comparing Satisfaction with Nursing Care and Factors Relevant to Hospital Revisit Intent among Hospitalized Patients in Comprehensive Nursing Care Units and General Care Units. *J. Korean Acad. Nurs. Adm.* **2015**, *21*, 469–479. [CrossRef]
8. Park, J.H.; Lee, M.H. Effects of Nursing and Care = Giving Integrated Service on nursing work performance, nurses' job satisfaction and patient safety. *J. Korean Acad. Soc. Home Care Nurs.* **2017**, *24*, 14–22.
9. Bang, M.R.; Sim, S.S.; Lee, D.-S. Comparison of Patient-Sitter Ward Nurses and General Ward Nurses on Work-Related Musculoskeletal Symptoms, Occupational Stress and Nursing Work Environments. *J. Korean Biol. Nurs. Sci.* **2015**, *17*, 169–178. [CrossRef]
10. Lim, H.-S.; Song, E.J. Influences of Emotional Labor, Hardiness on Job Satisfaction of Nurses in Comprehensive Nursing Care Service Units. *J. Korea Acad. Ind. Coop. Soc.* **2020**, *21*, 65–72.
11. Kim, S.-E.; Han, J.-Y. Clinical Nurses' Job Stress, Emotional labor, Nursing Performance, and Burnout in Comprehensive Nursing Care Service Wards and General Wards. *J. Korean Acad. Nurs. Adm.* **2017**, *23*, 336–345. [CrossRef]
12. Donabedian, A. *An Introduction to Quality Assurance in Health Care*; Oxford University Press: Oxford, UK, 2002.
13. Recio-Saucedo, A.; Dall'Ora, C.; Maruotti, A.; Ball, J.; Briggs, J.; Meredith, P.; Redfern, O.C.; Kovacs, C.; Prytherch, D.; Smith, G.B.; et al. What impact does nursing care left undone have on patient outcomes? Review of the literature. *J. Clin. Nurs.* **2018**, *27*, 2248–2259. [CrossRef]
14. Lee, M.-A.; Gong, S.-W.; Cho, S.-J. Relationship among Nursing Service Quality, Medical Service Satisfaction, and Hospital Revisit Intent. *J. Korean Acad. Nurs. Adm.* **2012**, *18*, 96–105. [CrossRef]
15. Parasuraman, A.; Zeithaml, V.A.; Berry, L.L. Reassessment of Expectations as a Comparison Standard in Measuring Service Quality: Implications for Further Research. *J. Mark.* **1994**, *58*, 111–124. [CrossRef]
16. Weiss, D.J.; Dawis, R.V.; England, G.W.; Lofquist, L.H. Manual for the Minnesota Satisfaction Questionnaire. In *Minnesota Studies in Vocational Rehabilitation*; University of Minnesota, Industrial Relations Center: Minneapolis, MN, USA, 1967.
17. Park, I.J. A Validation Study of the Minnesota Satisfaction Questionnaire (MSQ). Unpublished. Master's Thesis, University of Minnesota, Minneapolis, MN, USA, 2005.
18. Stamps, P.L.; Piedmont, E.B.; Slavitt, D.B.; Haase, A.M. Measurement of Work Satisfaction among Health Professionals. *Med. Care* **1978**, *16*, 337–352. [CrossRef] [PubMed]
19. Kim, M.R. *Influential Factors on Turnover Intention of Nurses: The Effect of Nurse's Organizational Commitment and Career Commitment to Turnover Intention*; Ewha Woman's University: Seoul, Republic of Korea, 2007.
20. Mobley, W.H. *Employee Turnover: Causes, Consequences, and Control*; Addison-Wesley Publishing Co.: Reading, UK, 1982.
21. Deribe, B.; Ayalew, M.; Geleta, D.; Gemechu, L.; Bogale, N.; Mengistu, K.; Gadissa, A.; Dula, D.; Ababi, G.; Gebretsadik, A. Perceived Quality of Nursing Care Among Cancer Patients Attending Hawassa University Comprehensive Specialized Hospital Cancer Treatment Center; Hawassa Southern Ethiopia: Cross-Sectional Study. *Cancer Manag. Res.* **2021**, *13*, 1225–1231. [CrossRef]
22. The Lancet Oncology. The importance of nurses in cancer care. *Lancet Oncol.* **2015**, *16*, 737. [CrossRef] [PubMed]
23. Kim, B.H.; Kang, H.Y. Job satisfaction, job stress, burnout, and turnover intention of comprehensive nursing care service ward nurses and general ward nurses. *J. Korea Acad. Ind. Coop. Soc.* **2018**, *19*, 459–469.
24. Jung, Y.A.; Sung, K.M. A Comparison of Patients' Nursing Service Satisfaction, Hospital Commitment and Revisit Intention between General Care Unit and Comprehensive Nursing Care Unit. *J. Korean Acad. Nurs. Adm.* **2018**, *24*, 30–39. [CrossRef]
25. Yeun, Y.-R. Effects of Comprehensive Nursing Service on the Nursing Performance, Job Satisfaction and Customer Orientation among Nurses. *J. Korea Acad. Ind. Coop. Soc.* **2015**, *16*, 317–323. [CrossRef]
26. Shim, O.S.; Lee, H.J. A comparative study on the job satisfaction, nursing professionalism and nursing work environment of nurses in comparative nursing care service wards and nurses in general wards. *J. Converg. Inform. Technol.* **2017**, *7*, 25–33.

27. Aiken, L.H.; Sloane, D.M.; Bruyneel, L.; Van den Heede, K.; Griffiths, P.; Busse, R.; Diomidous, M.; Kinnunen, J.; Kózka, M.; Lesaffre, E.; et al. Nurse staffing and education and hospital mortality in nine European countries: A retrospective observational study. *Lancet* **2014**, *383*, 1824–1830. [CrossRef] [PubMed]
28. Kim, B.; Lee, K.-S.; Park, Y.-K.; Choi, Y.-A.; Cho, S.-M.; Kim, S.-Y.; Han, G.-Y.; Shim, M. A Study of Nurses' Perception of the Comprehensive Nursing Service. *Korean J. Fam. Pract.* **2017**, *7*, 99–104. [CrossRef]

Disclaimer/Publisher's Note: The statements, opinions and data contained in all publications are solely those of the individual author(s) and contributor(s) and not of MDPI and/or the editor(s). MDPI and/or the editor(s) disclaim responsibility for any injury to people or property resulting from any ideas, methods, instructions or products referred to in the content.

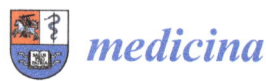 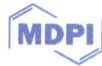

Review

Exploring Biomarkers in Breast Cancer: Hallmarks of Diagnosis, Treatment, and Follow-Up in Clinical Practice

Laura Lopez-Gonzalez [1,2,†], Alicia Sanchez Cendra [3,†], Cristina Sanchez Cendra [3], Eduardo David Roberts Cervantes [3], Javier Cassinello Espinosa [3], Tatiana Pekarek [4], Oscar Fraile-Martinez [2,4], Cielo García-Montero [2,4], Ana María Rodriguez-Slocker [1], Laura Jiménez-Álvarez [4,5], Luis G. Guijarro [2,6], Soledad Aguado-Henche [1,2], Jorge Monserrat [2,4,*], Melchor Alvarez-Mon [2,4,7], Leonel Pekarek [2,3,4], Miguel A. Ortega [2,4,8,‡] and Raul Diaz-Pedrero [1,2,5,‡]

1. Department of Surgery, Medical and Social Sciences, Faculty of Medicine and Health Sciences, University of Alcalá, 28801 Alcala de Henares, Spain; laura.lgonzalez@uah.es (L.L.-G.); anarodriguezslocker@gmail.com (A.M.R.-S.); soledad.aguado@uah.es (S.A.-H.); raul.diazp@uah.es (R.D.-P.)
2. Ramón y Cajal Institute of Sanitary Research (IRYCIS), 28034 Madrid, Spain; oscarfra.7@hotmail.com (O.F.-M.); cielo.gmontero@gmail.com (C.G.-M.); luis.gonzalez@uah.es (L.G.G.); mademons@gmail.com (M.A.-M.); leonel.pekarek@gmail.com (L.P.); miguel.angel.ortega92@gmail.com (M.A.O.)
3. Oncology Service, Guadalajara University Hospital, 19002 Guadalajara, Spain; ali.96sc@gmail.com (A.S.C.); csc.orbis@gmail.com (C.S.C.); edy_roberts@hotmail.com (E.D.R.C.); jcassinelloespinosa@gmail.com (J.C.E.)
4. Department of Medicine and Medical Specialities, Faculty of Medicine and Health Sciences, University of Alcalá, 28801 Alcala de Henares, Spain; tatianapekarek@gmail.com (T.P.); laura.jimenezal@gmail.com (L.J.-Á.)
5. Department of General and Digestive Surgery, General and Digestive Surgery, Príncipe de Asturias Universitary Hospital, 28805 Alcala de Henares, Spain
6. Unit of Biochemistry and Molecular Biology, Department of System Biology (CIBEREHD), University of Alcalá, 28801 Alcala de Henares, Spain
7. Immune System Diseases-Rheumatology, Oncology Service an Internal Medicine (CIBEREHD), University Hospital Príncipe de Asturias, 28806 Alcala de Henares, Spain
8. Cancer Registry and Pathology Department, Principe de Asturias University Hospital, 28806 Alcala de Henares, Spain
* Correspondence: jorge.monserrat@uah.es
† These authors contributed equally to this work.
‡ These authors also contributed equally to this work.

Abstract: Breast cancer is a prevalent malignancy in the present day, particularly affecting women as one of the most common forms of cancer. A significant portion of patients initially present with localized disease, for which curative treatments are pursued. Conversely, another substantial segment is diagnosed with metastatic disease, which has a worse prognosis. Recent years have witnessed a profound transformation in the prognosis for this latter group, primarily due to the discovery of various biomarkers and the emergence of targeted therapies. These biomarkers, encompassing serological, histological, and genetic indicators, have demonstrated their value across multiple aspects of breast cancer management. They play crucial roles in initial diagnosis, aiding in the detection of relapses during follow-up, guiding the application of targeted treatments, and offering valuable insights for prognostic stratification, especially for highly aggressive tumor types. Molecular markers have now become the keystone of metastatic breast cancer diagnosis, given the diverse array of chemotherapy options and treatment modalities available. These markers signify a transformative shift in the arsenal of therapeutic options against breast cancer. Their diagnostic precision enables the categorization of tumors with elevated risks of recurrence, increased aggressiveness, and heightened mortality. Furthermore, the existence of therapies tailored to target specific molecular anomalies triggers a cascade of changes in tumor behavior. Therefore, the primary objective of this article is to offer a comprehensive review of the clinical, diagnostic, prognostic, and therapeutic utility of the principal biomarkers currently in use, as well as of their clinical impact on metastatic breast cancer. In doing so, our goal is to contribute to a more profound comprehension of this complex disease and, ultimately, to enhance patient outcomes through more precise and effective treatment strategies.

Citation: Lopez-Gonzalez, L.; Sanchez Cendra, A.; Sanchez Cendra, C.; Roberts Cervantes, E.D.; Espinosa, J.C.; Pekarek, T.; Fraile-Martinez, O.; García-Montero, C.; Rodriguez-Slocker, A.M.; Jiménez-Álvarez, L.; et al. Exploring Biomarkers in Breast Cancer: Hallmarks of Diagnosis, Treatment, and Follow-Up in Clinical Practice. *Medicina* **2024**, *60*, 168. https://doi.org/10.3390/medicina60010168

Academic Editor: Valentin Titus Grigorean

Received: 12 December 2023
Revised: 2 January 2024
Accepted: 9 January 2024
Published: 17 January 2024

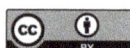

Copyright: © 2024 by the authors. Licensee MDPI, Basel, Switzerland. This article is an open access article distributed under the terms and conditions of the Creative Commons Attribution (CC BY) license (https://creativecommons.org/licenses/by/4.0/).

Keywords: breast cancer; biomarkers; serological; histological; translational medicine

1. Introduction

Breast cancer, recognized as the most prevalent cancer worldwide, is also the leading cause of cancer-related mortality among women in both developed and developing nations. As of 2022, this disease accounted for approximately 3 million new cases globally, which constituted roughly 13% of all cancer diagnoses. During the same period, it led to more than 600,000 deaths [1]. Specifically, breast cancer represents 25% of all neoplasms in women, with an overall incidence rate of 50 per 100,000. However, this incidence rate varies, as evidenced by Belgium's notably higher rate of 113 cases per 100,000 women [2,3].

Over recent decades, there has been a significant 30–40% rise in the incidence of breast cancer. This increase can primarily be attributed to the widespread adoption of mammography screening programs, especially targeting women in higher-risk age groups. Consequently, these initiatives have enabled an earlier detection of the disease, undeniably improving patient prognosis [4].

Regarding risk factors, several have been identified as particularly significant. Age, for instance, emerges as a crucial factor, with women over 50 facing a greater risk. Furthermore, a family history of breast cancer, as well as a previous diagnosis in males, increases this risk. Genetic factors also play a role, with mutations in genes such as BRCA1, BRCA2, TP53, CDH1, PTEN, and STK11 significantly raising the risk [5,6]. Additionally, lifestyle factors such as obesity, long-term use of hormone replacement therapies (including birth control pills and HRT), and excessive alcohol consumption, particularly among women aged 55 and older, have been linked to an increased risk of developing metastatic breast cancer [7–9].

In terms of screening and early detection, the U.S. Preventive Services Task Force (USPSTF) plays a pivotal role. As per their 2021 guidelines, they recommend that women of average risk begin biennial mammography screening at age 50 and continue until age 74 [10]. The diagnostic process typically starts with a thorough physical examination and breast imaging tests like mammography or ultrasound to identify any suspicious lumps or areas of thickening. If a lump is detected, the next step usually involves a needle biopsy to confirm the presence of cancer cells. Additional diagnostic tools, such as MRI for high-risk patients and CT or PET scans, help to further understand the extent of the cancer and its potential spread [11,12].

Regarding the stage at diagnosis, about 64% of women are found to have localized cancer, 27% have regional involvement, and 6% are diagnosed at an advanced stage. Identifying the specific type of cancer is heavily reliant on histological and pathological markers [13,14]. Moreover, molecular classification, which involves evaluating hormone receptors and HER2/neu expression, is critical for determining both therapeutic approaches and prognostic outcomes [15,16].

The treatment of metastatic breast cancer is intricately tailored based on these molecular markers. For example, in HER2-negative metastatic tumors with positive hormone receptors, the first-line treatment involves hormone blockade combined with aromatase inhibitors or antiestrogens, often paired with a CDK 4/6 inhibitor like palbociclib. In contrast, for triple-negative tumors, assessing PDL1 status is essential to decide on the use of atezolizumab; otherwise, chemotherapy is considered, though it offers limited benefits [17]. The role of BRCA1 and BRCA2 expression in these patients cannot be overstated, as it greatly influences the choice of targeted therapy, such as poly ADP-ribose polymerase inhibitors. In the case of HER2-positive metastatic tumors, the first-line treatment typically includes trastuzumab-, pertuzumab-, and taxane-based chemotherapy [18]. It is important to note that the treatment landscape for metastatic breast cancer is continually evolving, with ongoing clinical trials showing the effectiveness of new therapies, like the combination of conjugated antibodies with chemotherapy [19].

Finally, during the course of metastatic disease, follow-up imaging tests and the monitoring of serological tumor markers are crucial for detecting any signs of recurrence. This allows for timely adjustments in systemic treatment based on peripheral blood samples [20]. The emergence of new biomarkers, including circulating tumor cells and genetic markers, is increasingly playing a vital role in the diagnosis and prognosis of breast cancer, further enhancing the management of and treatment outcomes for patients with advanced stages of the disease.

2. Luminal A

The designation "luminal" for certain breast cancer subtypes arises from their gene expression profiles, which bear a resemblance to the luminal epithelium of the breast. These cancers typically express luminal cytokeratins 8 and 18. Among these subtypes, the most prevalent and the one associated with the best prognosis is Luminal A breast cancer. This subtype accounts for approximately 40% of all breast cancer cases [21]. Luminal A breast cancer is characterized by high expression levels of genes associated with hormonal receptors and low expression of the HER2 gene group, coupled with a low proliferation gene signature.

2.1. Histological Biomarkers

Hormone receptors play a pivotal role as primary biomarkers in luminal breast cancer. There are two primary forms of the estrogen receptor (ER), namely ERα and ERβ. However, only ERα holds a validated clinical role, being expressed in 70–75% of breast cancers [22]. Similarly, the progesterone receptor (PR) exists in two forms, PRA and PRB. These receptors (ERα, PRA, and PRB) are typically identified using immunohistochemical techniques on biopsy tissue samples. A critical threshold for the positive identification of these receptors is their expression greater than or equal to 1% of tumor cells. Notably, the expression of PR often increases as a result of ER signaling; hence, cells expressing ER are likely to express PR as well. It is rare for tumors that are ER-negative to be PR-positive [23,24].

The primary clinical significance of hormone receptors lies in selecting patients for adjuvant therapy with hormonal drugs. These treatments include selective ER modulators (such as tamoxifen), third-generation aromatase inhibitors (like anastrozole, letrozole, or exemestane), LH-RH agonists (including leuprolide and goserelin), pure ER antagonists (such as fulvestrant), oophorectomy, or other endocrine therapies [25]. Consequently, these receptors have predictive utility. Additionally, they offer prognostic utility; hormone receptor-positive tumors have been linked to improved survival and a lower annual recurrence rate within the first five years post treatment [26].

Conversely, HER2, another critical biomarker, belongs to the epidermal growth factor receptor (EGFR) family and plays a role in numerous tumor signaling pathways. Its analysis is generally conducted on biopsy tissue samples, utilizing immunohistochemistry or in situ hybridization techniques. Luminal-type breast cancers, characterized by low HER2 receptor expression, are typically not considered for anti-HER2 treatments like trastuzumab or pertuzumab [27].

Additionally, the Ki-67 protein serves as an important biomarker for assessing tumor proliferative activity, given its involvement in cell division. Although there is no universally established cutoff point, major guidelines suggest that high proliferative activity is indicated by values above 30%, while low activity is below 10% [28,29]. For instance, a Ki-67 level of 20% indicates that 20% of the tumor cells are actively dividing. Generally, luminal tumors exhibit low Ki-67 levels. In research conducted by Viale et al., the prognostic and predictive value of Ki-67 was explored, revealing that higher values correlate with a poorer prognosis [30].

2.2. Serological Biomarkers

Serological markers are of significant importance in both the diagnosis and prognosis of breast cancer, with Ki67, CA 15-3, BAX, and Bcl-2 being notably characteristic in luminal subtype tumors [31,32]. Although Ki-67 is typically assessed in tumor tissue, its potential as a serological biomarker for estimating cell proliferation has been explored. For instance, a study by Cheang et al. revealed that Luminal B tumors exhibited a higher Ki67 index and were associated with poorer recurrence-free survival compared to Luminal A tumors [33].

Focusing on the role of BAX and Bcl-2, these proteins are intricately linked to apoptosis and their expression carries prognostic implications in breast cancer. BAX is crucial in inducing apoptosis, whereas Bcl-2 prevents programmed cell death. This balance is key to cell survival. A specific study examining the expression of Bcl-2 and BAX as prognostic markers in breast cancer found that Bcl-2 expression correlated with a better prognosis across all molecular subtypes, including Luminal A breast cancer [34,35].

Another important serological marker is CA 15-3, a protein component of MUC 1 found in epithelial cells. It is frequently utilized as a tumor marker for detecting and monitoring breast cancer [36]. However, it is noteworthy that CA 15-3 levels can also rise in other conditions, such as gastrointestinal and lung neoplasms. The specificity of CA 15-3 as a prognostic marker for Luminal A breast cancer requires further study. Additionally, carcinoembryonic antigen (CEA) and CA 27.29 are other tumor markers relevant in breast cancer, especially for monitoring patients in advanced stages. Elevated CEA levels may signal tumor activity but can also increase due to non-cancerous conditions like inflammatory gastrointestinal diseases. CA 27.29 may be particularly valuable in metastatic breast cancer [37].

Moreover, chronic inflammation, with cytokines acting as mediators, is recognized as a risk factor for tumor development. Research involving the detection of cytokines in the blood for tumor diagnosis has shown preliminary utility. Cytokines such as CXCL12, CXCL1, CXCL8, and CXCR4, when combined with the CA 15-3 antigen panel, may serve as early biomarkers in the diagnosis of breast cancer, particularly for luminal-type cancers [38].

2.3. Genetic Biomarkers

It is crucial to acknowledge that the identification of genetic alterations in breast cancer is essential not only for determining prognosis and guiding treatment decisions but also for genetic counseling and screening of individuals at risk. Gene expression analysis platforms, such as Oncotype DX and MammaPrint, analyze multiple genes from tumor tissue samples. These analyses provide insights into the tumor's specific characteristics, including its aggressiveness, recurrence risk, and the necessity for therapy initiation [39]. Within this framework, genetic alterations in breast cancer can be broadly categorized into two types: somatic mutations and germline mutations.

Somatic mutations, which are unique to tumor cells and not passed down through generations, play a significant role in breast cancer. In Luminal A breast cancer, a primary somatic mutation is found in the PIK3CA gene in approximately 49% of cases [40]. This gene is instrumental in cell signaling regulation and is a part of the PI3K/AKT/mTOR pathway, often leading to enhanced cell growth and survival [41]. Another noteworthy gene is GATA3, which is involved in cellular differentiation and is present in 14% of Luminal A tumors. GATA3 expression is associated with higher hormonal receptor expression and a more favorable prognosis [42]. Additionally, the TP53 gene, known for its critical role in maintaining DNA integrity, is altered in about 12% of cases, often indicating increased tumor aggressiveness and a poorer prognosis [43]. The MAP3K1 gene, with a mutation rate of 14% in this tumor subtype, highlights the genetic heterogeneity of luminal tumors. However, its exact role remains to be fully understood. It has been observed that specific genes, like MCM4, correlate with survival in the Luminal A subtype but not in Luminal B, HER2-positive, or triple-negative subtypes [44].

In contrast, germline mutations are inherited from one's parents and are present in all body cells, including germ cells. A well-studied genetic alteration in breast cancer is the BRCA1 gene mutation. Individuals with this mutation have an elevated risk of developing breast cancer, particularly at a younger age [45]. These mutations are more prevalent in hereditary breast cancer cases and are linked to a higher likelihood of developing bilateral breast cancer and luminal-type tumors. Awareness of BRCA1 mutations can significantly influence treatment choices, such as the consideration of prophylactic mastectomy [46]. However, it is important to note that while germline mutations increase the risk of breast cancer, they do not definitively determine whether an individual will develop the disease [47].

2.4. Circulating Tumor Cells and MicroRNAs

MicroRNAs (miRNAs) are small RNA molecules playing a crucial role in gene expression regulation. Acting as either oncogenes or tumor suppressors, their impact is determined by their specific functions and the genes they regulate. The exploration of miRNA expression abnormalities in breast cancer, including the Luminal A subtype, represents a significant area of contemporary research. This research is key to understanding the molecular architecture of these tumor types [48].

A prominent miRNA in Luminal A breast cancer is miR-21. Research, including a study by Kalinina et al., indicates that miR-21 overexpression may foster tumor cell proliferation and hinder apoptosis. Furthermore, there is evidence suggesting that miR-21 might influence the response to hormonal therapy, a cornerstone in the treatment of Luminal A breast cancer [49]. Additional miRNAs associated with Luminal A breast cancer include miR-34a, miR-126, miR-206, and the miR-221/222 cluster [50]. These miRNAs are being closely studied for their roles in the progression and treatment response of this cancer subtype.

The investigation of circulating tumor cells (CTCs) in the peripheral blood of patients with non-metastatic breast cancer is increasingly being recognized as crucial in both research and clinical practice. CTCs, which are tumor cells that break away from the primary tumor and enter the bloodstream, possess the ability to migrate to distant sites and potentially initiate metastases. Their detection is typically conducted using methods like flow cytometry, polymerase chain reaction (PCR), and various cell capture techniques. A notable correlation has been established between the presence of CTCs and poorer clinical outcomes, including reduced progression-free and overall survival. This association underscores the potential of CTCs as valuable prognostic indicators in early-stage breast cancer [51].

Recent advancements in research suggest that the identification and analysis of CTCs could significantly enhance risk stratification and the personalization of treatment for breast cancer patients. Particularly in non-metastatic cases, analyzing CTCs can offer insights into minimal residual disease—the presence of cancer cells remaining in the body post initial treatment. This information is vital for assessing the efficacy of adjuvant therapies, thereby aiding in customizing treatment plans to optimize outcomes and monitoring [52]. Pierga et al.'s research indicated that the detection of CTCs can predict early metastatic recurrence following neoadjuvant chemotherapy in operable and locally advanced breast cancer patients [53]. Furthermore, a study examining the expression of epidermal growth factor receptor (EGFR) and the cell surface protein CD133 in CTCs of breast cancer patients found a significant link between positive EGFR expression in CTCs and luminal-type tumors [54].

In conclusion, understanding various biomarkers is crucial for personalized medicine in Luminal A breast cancer. Histological biomarkers, including hormone receptors (ERα, PRA, PRB), HER2, and Ki-67, are key in diagnosis, prognosis, and treatment. Serological markers like Ki-67, CA 15-3, BAX, and Bcl-2 are important for prognosis and monitoring. Genetic biomarkers, both somatic (e.g., PIK3CA, GATA3, TP53, MAP3K1 mutations) and germline (like BRCA1 mutations), provide insights into the disease's origins and treatments. MicroRNAs, especially miR-21, play a role in tumor biology and response to therapy. Circulating tumor cells (CTCs) have emerged as a novel biomarker for understanding metastasis and prognosis in non-metastatic breast cancer, helping in assessing residual disease and treatment planning.

3. Luminal B

Luminal breast cancer accounts for approximately two-thirds of all breast carcinomas globally. Presently, there is an emphasis on individualized therapies tailored to the biological characteristics unique to each luminal subtype. Within these subtypes, Luminal B breast cancer is comparatively less common. Similar to Luminal A, Luminal B is characterized by positive hormone receptors. However, in contrast to Luminal A, which is typically HER2-negative, Luminal B can be either HER2-positive or -negative. Notably, Luminal B is associated with a higher rate of cell proliferation than Luminal A, which correlates with a less favorable prognosis due to its increased aggressiveness. In the context of early-stage breast cancer, Luminal B demonstrates poorer outcomes in terms of 5- and 10-year event-free survival (EFS), irrespective of adjuvant systemic therapy, when compared to Luminal A [55].

3.1. Histological Biomarkers

As previously mentioned in the context of Luminal A breast cancer, Luminal B tumors are also characterized by a high expression of ERs and PRs. This characteristic renders these tumors responsive to endocrine therapy targeting these receptors, often leading to a better prognosis due to the availability of an effective therapeutic target. However, despite the general effectiveness of hormonal therapy, some patients with Luminal B breast cancer may develop resistance over time. This resistance can manifest as cancer recurrence or continued tumor growth despite ongoing hormonal therapy [56]. The mechanisms behind hormone resistance are varied, encompassing alterations in hormone receptor expression, engagement of alternative signaling pathways, and genetic modifications.

A critical aspect of Luminal B breast cancer is the expression of the HER2 receptor, which significantly influences both treatment and prognosis. Contrary to Luminal A, which is usually HER2-negative, Luminal B can exhibit HER2 positivity. Recent updates in the classification of intrinsic subtypes now include Luminal B with HER2 overexpression [57]. This distinction is crucial for treatment considerations; while HER2 positivity may worsen the prognosis, it also opens the possibility for targeted therapies against HER2, such as trastuzumab. In cases where HER2 is not overexpressed, the treatment strategy primarily revolves around hormonal therapy and chemotherapy, tailored to the individual patient's characteristics [58].

The Ki-67 index, a key marker for Luminal B breast cancer, can be evaluated using immunohistochemical techniques on tissue samples. Luminal B is distinguished by a higher Ki-67 percentage than Luminal A, correlating with a less favorable prognosis, an increased risk of recurrence, and faster disease progression [59]. Ki-67 levels also play a significant role in determining treatment approaches. Patients with Luminal B breast cancer exhibiting high Ki-67 levels are often considered for adjuvant chemotherapy or a combination of a cell cycle inhibitor with hormonal therapy [60]. Cheang et al. developed an immunohistochemical assay to differentiate Luminal B tumors from Luminal A based on the Ki-67 index and explored its utility in predicting breast cancer recurrence-free survival and overall disease survival [61].

3.2. Serological Biomarkers

Numerous serological markers have been identified as crucial in determining prognosis, aiding in treatment selection, and understanding the behavior of Luminal B breast cancer. Beyond the Ki-67 index, which shows elevated expression in both tissue and blood in Luminal B tumors, indicating a poorer prognosis compared to Luminal A, there are other cell proliferation markers of interest. These include the proliferating cell nuclear antigen (PCNA) and topoisomerase II, which may play significant roles in the pathology of Luminal B breast cancer [62].

Additionally, the expression of specific genes and proteins such as p62, also known as sequestosome-1 (SQSTM1), has been identified. p62 is instrumental in the regulation of autophagy and selective protein degradation in cells. Another notable marker is aldehyde dehydrogenase 1 family member A3 (ALDH1A3), involved in aldehyde oxidation, potentially influencing chemotherapy resistance. The presence of these markers is associated with a poorer prognosis in Luminal B breast cancer [63].

Furthermore, components of the MCM complex, including MCM2, MCM4, and MCM6, are essential proteins involved in DNA replication. These proteins are vital in the preparation and initiation of DNA replication, a key process for cell proliferation. In differentiating between breast cancer subtypes, MCM2, MCM4, and MCM6 gain relevance due to their association with cell proliferation. Given that Luminal B breast cancer is characterized by a higher rate of cell proliferation compared to Luminal A, the expression levels of these markers may be elevated in Luminal B, thus aiding in the distinction between these subtypes [64].

3.3. Genetic Biomarkers

Luminal B breast cancer is characterized by several significant genetic alterations with varying frequencies. Beyond the expression of hormonal receptors, this subtype may also exhibit an overexpression of HER-2 in some cases, which is linked to a poorer prognosis [65–67]. Research has indicated that certain genetic polymorphisms are associated with the Luminal B subtype, suggesting their potential in predicting subtypes and guiding personalized treatment strategies [68,69].

Mutations in the PIK3CA gene, present in about 32% of Luminal B cases, can activate the PI3K/AKT/mTOR signaling pathway, contributing to breast cancer development and progression. Additionally, TP53 gene mutations are relatively common in this subtype, occurring in approximately 31% of cases, which is a higher frequency than in Luminal A breast cancer [70]. These mutations are considered possible predictors of resistance to endocrine therapy. Both TP53 and PIK3CA mutations are associated with increased tumor aggressiveness and an unfavorable prognosis [71].

In response to these genetic alterations, targeted therapies have been developed, such as PI3K inhibitors like alpelisib and idelalisib, and mTOR inhibitors like everolimus. These therapies are selected based on tumor characteristics and patient response to treatment [72]. These genes are instrumental in the proliferation and prognosis of Luminal B breast cancer, providing potential targets for diagnosis, prognosis, and treatment strategies. Additionally, in the metastatic setting, other less common biomarkers for targeted therapy options (MSI/MMR, TMB, NTRK) and comprehensive profiling of genomic profiles are utilized to identify uncommon targets and determine additional treatment options.

Moreover, research into non-coding cis-regulatory elements, DNA regions that do not encode proteins but are crucial in gene expression regulation, has highlighted their potential impact on gene activity. These elements contribute to the molecular and biological characteristics of Luminal B breast cancer, offering insights into the subtype's distinct nature [73].

3.4. Circulating Tumor Cells and MicroRNAs

In Luminal B breast cancer, the influence of microRNAs on disease progression and treatment response has been a subject of considerable research. One microRNA that has been extensively studied in this context, similar to its role in Luminal A, is miR-21. This microRNA is linked with tumor proliferation and resistance to chemotherapy in breast cancer. Song et al.'s research revealed that 25 out of 32 histological breast tissue samples from cancer patients showed miR-21 overexpression compared to the normal mammary epithelium. Furthermore, a close correlation was observed between the incidence of lymph node metastasis and miR-21 expression, suggesting its significant role in metastasis and, therefore, in prognostication. The study also found that four different breast cancer cell lines exhibited varying levels of miR-21 overexpression, hinting at its potential as a classifier for these tumors [74].

Another microRNA, miR-145, has been recognized as a potential tumor suppressor in breast cancer. Research indicates that miR-145 can inhibit angiogenesis and tumor growth by suppressing N-RAS and VEGF [75]. It is also known to hinder breast cancer cell migration by regulating TGF-β1 expression, either directly or indirectly, further underscoring its tumor-suppressive capabilities [76]. Additionally, microRNAs like miR-221 and miR-222 have been associated with a decreased expression of hormonal receptors and a diminished response to hormonal treatments, highlighting their importance in the context of Luminal B breast cancer [77].

In Luminal B breast cancer, circulating tumor cells (CTCs) can express specific markers such as hormone receptors (ERs/PRs) and HER2, which are distinctive features of this breast cancer subtype. The expression of these markers in CTCs can vary, providing insights into tumor heterogeneity and its evolution during disease progression [78]. Although detecting CTCs poses challenges due to their low concentration in blood, their prognostic significance has been established by various studies. However, as of now, there is no definitive evidence supporting the use of any biomarker for stratifying patients based on individual prognosis or for guiding personalized treatment in this context [79].

A study by Galardi et al. explored the prognostic role of CTC count and its utility in monitoring treatment with palbociclib, a kinase inhibitor, as well as in predicting treatment response. This study concluded that initial CTC count did not provide a clear predictive value in patients treated with palbociclib. However, CTCs proved useful as indicators for identifying patients who were developing early resistance to the treatment. Additionally, CTC counts at the time of disease progression were shown to offer valuable prognostic information regarding subsequent responses to palbociclib [80].

The quantity of detected CTCs has been linked with the prognosis of breast cancer patients. These cells can also offer information about treatment response and the effectiveness of therapies. The field of CTC research in breast cancer is dynamic and continually evolving, with new technologies and methodologies being developed to improve the sensitivity and specificity of CTC detection.

In summary, Luminal B breast cancer, distinguished by its aggressiveness, shares some markers with Luminal A but crucially differs in HER2 positivity and a higher Ki-67 index, signaling a more challenging prognosis. These markers not only guide but also necessitate targeted therapies and often more aggressive treatment like chemotherapy. Furthermore, serological markers and CTC analysis provide deeper insights into tumor characteristics, crucially aiding in the selection of targeted therapies, particularly against the PI3K/AKT/mTOR pathway. Additionally, microRNAs such as miR-21 and miR-145 are instrumental in understanding disease progression. Overall, the integration of various biomarkers is essential for tailoring effective treatments and improving patient outcomes in Luminal B breast cancer. The most relevant histological, serological, and genetic markers, as well as microRNAs of luminal-type metastatic breast cancer, are concisely summarized in Figure 1.

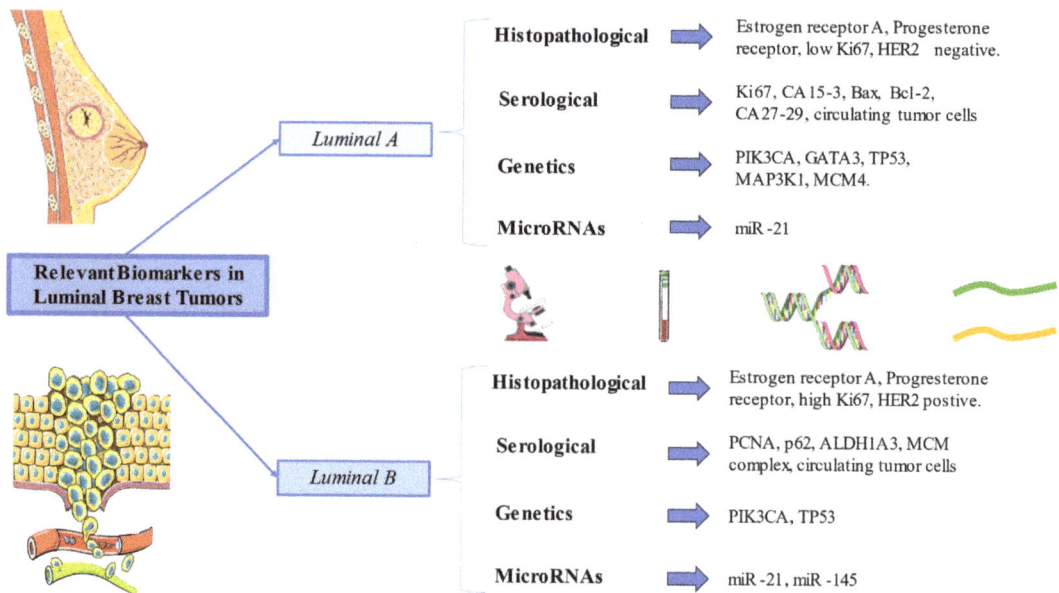

Figure 1. Summary of the most relevant biomarkers in metastatic Luminal A and B tumors.

4. HER2

4.1. Histological Biomarkers

Approximately 30% of breast cancers test positive for human epidermal growth factor receptor 2 (HER2), previously known as HER2/neu or ERBB-2. HER2, a transmembrane receptor with tyrosine kinase activity, belongs to the epidermal growth factor receptor (EGFR) family and plays a crucial role in cell signaling, differentiation, and angiogenesis [81].

Typically, HER2-positive breast cancer does not express hormone receptors like ER or PR and is characterized by a high proliferative index (KI-67). Initially, the overexpression or amplification of HER2 is assessed using immunohistochemistry (IHC), rated on a scale from 0 to 3 based on staining intensity. In ambiguous cases, such as IHC grade 2, in situ hybridization techniques like fluorescence in situ hybridization (FISH) and chromogenic in situ hybridization (CISH) are employed. These methods determine the amplification of specific genes, including HER2, by identifying and quantifying extra gene copies, which are indicative of increased cancer risk and aggressiveness [82]. FISH utilizes fluorescent probes, while CISH employs chromogenic enzyme-marked probes, resulting in a visible color change under the microscope. Both techniques are essential in determining HER2 status and guiding treatment decisions.

The clinical value of HER2 testing lies in its predictive power, identifying women who could benefit from targeted treatments. Therefore, assessing HER2 status in new cases of invasive and metastatic breast cancer is recommended according to various guidelines. The main treatments targeting HER2 include drugs like trastuzumab, pertuzumab, and lapatinib [83]. Conversely, HER2 overexpression has been linked to drug resistance, such as to paclitaxel, and increased tumor aggressiveness [84]. Although HER2 detection has prognostic value, indicating higher recurrence and mortality rates without adjuvant therapy, the clinical significance of this information is debatable, particularly with early use of HER2-directed agents in treatment.

HER2-positive breast cancer displays intertumoral heterogeneity, with up to 45% of cases expressing hormone receptors and exhibiting various molecular subtypes [85]. While hormone receptor status does not define the overall genetic profile, specific genetic aberrations characterize HER2-positive cancer subgroups. HER2-enriched tumors respond well to anti-HER2 therapy, potentially reducing chemotherapy requirements. However, "HER2 low" tumors, with fewer HER2 receptors, respond poorly to HER2-targeted treatments, prompting the exploration of alternatives like immunotherapy [86].

The presence of tumor-infiltrating lymphocytes (TILs) in tissue samples signals the immune response against cancer cells. TIL assessment is a growing research area with implications for prognosis and treatment. Higher TIL quantities often correlate with better outcomes in certain breast cancer subtypes, suggesting that an active immune response can limit tumor growth and progression. Studies indicate that TIL presence, particularly in triple-negative and HER2-positive tumors, may enhance responsiveness to chemotherapy and anti-HER2 treatments [87].

4.2. Serological Biomarkers

In HER2-positive breast cancer, monitoring biomarkers in the blood can offer valuable insights into treatment response and disease progression. While HER2 overexpression is commonly analyzed in tissue samples, HER2/neu can also be detected in circulating DNA, which is released by tumor cells into the bloodstream. This detection of HER2 amplification in circulating DNA serves as an indicator of tumor burden and response to treatment [88].

Similarly to other molecular subtypes of breast cancer, tumor markers like CA 15.3, CEA, and CA 27.29 are also useful. These markers aid in diagnosis and help monitor the effectiveness of specific treatments.

4.3. Genetic Biomarkers

HER2-positive breast cancer patients often exhibit intratumoral genetic variability, a phenomenon widely observed in various human cancers, including breast cancer. In these cancers, HER2 overexpression and amplification can display a heterogeneous pattern [89]. Three types of cellular distributions have been identified based on HER2 status heterogeneity: "clustered", featuring two distinct tumor clones (one with HER2 amplification and another with a normal status); "mosaic", where a diffused mix of cells with different HER2 states exists; and "dispersed", characterized by isolated HER2-amplified cells amidst a majority of HER2-negative tumor cells.

Genomic analysis, including gene copy number profiling and massive parallel sequencing, has been conducted on heterogeneous HER2 breast cancers. This analysis has identified driver genetic alterations restricted to HER2-negative cells. In vitro models have shown that the overexpression/amplification of BRF2 and DSN1, along with the HER2 I767M mutation, compensate for the lack of HER2 amplification in the HER2-negative components of these breast carcinomas [90].

Studies have linked the increased frequency of chromosome 17 polysomy with HER2 heterogeneity in breast cancer. While rare, chromosome 17 polysomy often appears as a gain or amplification of the centromere of chromosome 17 (CEP17). In these cases, it is crucial to refer to it as "abnormal CEP17 copy number", particularly when evaluated using FISH in interphase nuclei. The independent increase in CEP17 copy numbers in heterogeneous HER2 carcinomas suggests a possible link to chromosomal instability [91].

The response to neoadjuvant chemotherapy in HER2-positive breast cancer can also vary based on PIK3CA mutations and hormone receptor status. In HER2-positive/ER-positive patients, a better prognosis and reduced benefit from trastuzumab have been reported, along with lower rates of TP53 mutations and reduced HER2 expression [92]. Other mutations in genes like p53, PTEN, PIK2CA, or TOP2A may contribute to the progression and treatment resistance of HER2-positive breast cancer.

Furthermore, mutations in BRCA1 and BRCA2 are more commonly associated with HER2-positive breast cancer. Research suggests that HER2-positive patients with BRCA mutations might be more sensitive to certain treatments, including PARP inhibitors like olaparib [93].

4.4. Circulating Tumor Cells and MicroRNAs

The role of microRNAs in HER2-positive breast cancer has garnered significant interest in recent research. Various studies have explored how microRNAs regulate HER-2 and impact the progression of this breast cancer subtype. For instance, microRNAs such as microRNA-125a, microRNA-125b, and microRNA-148a have been identified for their role in regulating HER-2, showing an inhibitory effect on its expression under certain conditions [94].

Similar to its role in luminal tumors, microRNA-21 in HER2-positive breast cancer has been linked to the activation of the HER-2 pathway. It functions by suppressing tumor suppressor genes and promoting cell proliferation, a role paralleled by microRNA-205. Conversely, research suggests that microRNA-26a may inhibit cell proliferation and invasion in HER2-positive breast cancer by modulating the expression of genes associated with these processes [95].

In HER2-positive breast cancer, research has focused on the expression of specific molecules in circulating tumor cells (CTCs). One key area of study is the detection of HER2/Neu mRNA in the blood, which helps assess the presence of the HER2 protein in CTCs. High levels of HER2/Neu mRNA are linked to increased risks of recurrence and mortality [96].

Cytokeratin 19 (CK19), found in epithelial cells, is a common immunohistochemical marker in breast cancer diagnosis. Its presence in cancer cells confirms the epithelial origin of the tumor and aids in identifying specific breast cancer subtypes. CK19's role extends to evaluating tumor aggressiveness and response to treatments, including HER2-targeted therapies. The presence of CK19 mRNA in CTCs is associated with a worse prognosis, particularly in patients with triple-negative and HER2/Neu-negative tumors, indicating potential aggressiveness and treatment resistance [97,98].

Additionally, the breast-specific protein mammaglobin and its expression in CTCs are being studied in HER2-positive breast cancer. Mammaglobin mRNA in the blood correlates with shorter survival times and lower overall survival rates in these patients [99].

In summary, HER2-positive breast cancer, notable for its HER2 receptor overexpression and lack of hormone receptors, makes up about 30% of breast cancers. HER2 status, key for treatment decisions, is assessed using immunohistochemistry and, if necessary, in situ hybridization techniques like FISH and CISH. The presence of HER2 overexpression in CTCs directs the use of targeted therapies such as trastuzumab or lapatinib. Serological biomarkers like CA 15.3 and CEA are important for monitoring disease progression. This cancer subtype also shows genetic variability, including HER2 heterogeneity and mutations in genes like PIK3CA, which affect treatment response and prognosis. MicroRNAs such as microRNA-125a and -21 also play roles in regulating HER-2 expression and cancer progression. The analysis of molecules in CTCs, like HER2/Neu mRNA, provides insights into recurrence risk and treatment response. Overall, the combination of histological, serological, genetic biomarkers, microRNAs, and CTCs is crucial in understanding HER2-positive breast cancer and developing personalized treatment plans.

5. Therapeutic Implication of Specific Biomarkers in Luminal A, Luminal B, and HER-2 Breast Cancer

5.1. CDK4/6 Inhibitors

The CCND1 gene is amplified in approximately 15% of breast cancer cells, and cyclin D1 is overexpressed in up to 67%. Overexpression of cyclin D1 increases cyclin-dependent kinases 4 and 6 (CDK4/6) and stimulates cell division, making this pathway an attractive target in cancer therapy [100–104]. Abemaciclib is a small-molecule inhibitor of CDK4, CDK6, and CDK9. Amplification of CCND1 and overexpression of cyclin D1 are common in hormone receptor-positive breast cancers, implying greater sensitivity to CDK4/6 inhibition.

The clinical trial MONARCH 2 [100], which evaluated abemaciclib for advanced HR+/HER2- breast cancer that progressed during or after endocrine therapy, significantly reduced the risk of disease progression or death. The median progression-free survival was 16.4 months with abemaciclib compared to 9.3 months with a placebo. In MONARCH 3 [101], abemaciclib improved progression-free survival in first-line treatment for advanced HR+/HER2- breast cancer in postmenopausal women, in combination with aromatase inhibitors. Abemaciclib was also approved as a second-line treatment based on the results of the MONARCH 1 trial [102]. The monarchE trial [103] demonstrated a clinically significant benefit by reducing invasive disease events when abemaciclib was added to endocrine therapy in high-risk early-stage HR+/HER2- breast cancer.

Palbociclib is another potent CDK4/6 inhibitor, and the PALOMA-2 trial [104] demonstrated its effectiveness in first-line treatment for advanced HR+/HER2- breast cancer in postmenopausal women. The combination of palbociclib and letrozole significantly increased progression-free survival compared to the placebo. The PALOMA-3 trial [105] with palbociclib evaluated its effectiveness in combination with fulvestrant as second-line treatment for advanced HR+/HER2- breast cancer. Palbociclib doubled the median progression-free survival compared to the placebo.

The MONALEESA-2 trial [106] evaluated ribociclib as a first-line treatment for advanced HR+/HER2- breast cancer in postmenopausal women, showing a significant improvement in progression-free survival and overall survival. The MONALEESA-3 trial [107] compared ribociclib as a first- and second-line treatment for advanced HR+/HER2- breast cancer, demonstrating a significant improvement in progression-free survival and overall survival in both settings. MONALEESA-7 [108] investigated ribociclib in combination with endocrine therapy for early-stage HR+/HER2- breast cancer in premenopausal and perimenopausal women, showing a substantial increase in progression-free survival and overall survival.

Despite the clinical success of CDK4/6 inhibitors, they have side effects such as diarrhea, thromboembolism, hematological toxicity, and interstitial lung disease. Resistance to these inhibitors is an ongoing challenge, and studies like neoMONARCH [109] explore molecular signatures associated with sensitivity or resistance to guide treatment decisions.

In conclusion, amplification of CCND1 and overexpression of cyclin D1 are key in many breast cancers, making CDK4/6 inhibitors like abemaciclib, palbociclib, and ribociclib effective treatments. Clinical trials have confirmed their benefits in various stages of breast cancer, though challenges remain with side effects and resistance. Ongoing research is crucial to enhance treatment efficacy and patient response.

5.2. mTOR Inhibitors

The mammalian target of rapamycin (mTOR) is a protein kinase that plays a role in cellular proliferation and survival. Rapamycin, also known as sirolimus, inhibits mTOR signaling by binding to the FK-binding protein 12 (FKBP12), disrupting the mTOR Complex 1 (mTORC1). Rapamycin analogs (rapalogs) were developed to enhance solubility and pharmacokinetic properties.

Everolimus, an mTOR inhibitor, was evaluated in the BOLERO-1 trial [110] as a first-line treatment for advanced HER2+ breast cancer. When combined with trastuzumab and paclitaxel, everolimus did not show improvements in key outcomes in the overall population but did benefit HR-/HER2+ patients. The interaction between the HR, HER2, and PI3K pathways could contribute to resistance in HR+/HER2+ patients.

The combination of everolimus with letrozole synergistically inhibited cell proliferation and induced apoptosis in ER+ breast cancer cells. The BOLERO-2 trial [111] studied everolimus with exemestane in non-steroidal aromatase inhibitor refractory breast cancer, showing an increase in progression-free survival. Everolimus, in combination with exemestane, was approved in 2012 for advanced HR+/HER2- breast cancer. mTOR inhibitors, such as everolimus, have various adverse effects, including neutropenia, stomatitis, diarrhea, and alopecia. Ongoing research explores their potential in triple-negative breast cancer (TNBC), where preclinical studies suggest a cytostatic effect [112].

To summarize, mTOR inhibitors like everolimus have shown promise in treating advanced breast cancer. While results in HER2+ cases were mixed, they have been effective in HR+ breast cancer, especially when combined with drugs like letrozole and exemestane. Approved for advanced HR+/HER2- breast cancer in 2012, these inhibitors, despite their side effects, are now being explored for potential use in triple-negative breast cancer.

5.3. PI3K Inhibitors

Approximately 40% of HR+/HER2- breast cancers have activating mutations in the PIK3CA gene, leading to the hyperactivation of the catalytic subunit p110α of phosphatidylinositol 3-kinase (PI3K). Mutations in PI3K p110α promote tumor-like behavior in mammary epithelial cells and confer resistance to endocrine therapy and conventional chemotherapy, correlating with unfavorable clinical outcomes.

The clinical trial SOLAR-1 [113] enrolled postmenopausal patients with advanced HR+/HER2- breast cancer who experienced disease progression during or after aromatase inhibitor therapy. Participants were administered alpelisib, a PI3K inhibitor, or a placebo in combination with the estrogen receptor antagonist fulvestrant. A modest clinical benefit was observed in the non-mutated PIK3CA subgroup, with alpelisib increasing progression-free survival by 1.8 months, although the effect was not statistically significant. However, for patients with PIK3CA mutations, the median progression-free survival almost doubled, from 5.7 months with placebo to 11.0 months with alpelisib. Based on the positive results of SOLAR-1, the FDA approved alpelisib in combination with fulvestrant for advanced HR+/HER2- breast cancer with PIK3CA mutations in postmenopausal women.

The most common grade 3 or higher adverse events with alpelisib are hyperglycemia and maculopapular rash. Both are considered specific effects of PI3Kα inhibition, owing to the role of this pathway in glucose metabolism and the differentiation and survival of keratinocytes. Indeed, there have been several case reports of alpelisib-induced diabetic ketoacidosis, even in non-diabetic patients.

The utility of alpelisib as a second-line agent is complicated by the recent availability of CDK 4/6 inhibitors and their introduction into the standard first-line treatment for HR+/HER2- breast cancer. In the SOLAR-1 trial, only nine patients (5%) who received alpelisib had previously been treated with a CDK 4/6 inhibitor. BYLieve is a non-comparative Phase II trial of alpelisib plus endocrine therapy [114]. However, larger comparative studies are needed to better define the role of alpelisib in breast cancer therapy. Ongoing Phase III clinical trials explore the use of alpelisib with other agents, including its combination with trastuzumab and pertuzumab for HER2+ breast cancer with PI3KCA mutations (EPIK-B2) [115] and with nab-paclitaxel for triple-negative breast cancer (EPIK-B3) [116]. The results of these and other trials are expected to better delineate the utility of alpelisib and possibly define new roles for its application in the therapy of metastatic disease.

In brief, alpelisib, a PI3K inhibitor, has proven effective for HR+/HER2- breast cancer with PIK3CA mutations, as shown in the SOLAR-1 trial. It notably increases progression-free survival and is FDA-approved in combination with fulvestrant. Despite its efficacy, alpelisib's role in treatment regimens is evolving, particularly due to side effects like hyperglycemia, and ongoing research is comparing it with other therapies.

5.4. Anti-HER2 Antibodies

HER2 is a transmembrane receptor tyrosine kinase involved in various cellular processes. The amplification of the HER2 gene is linked to poor outcomes in breast cancer, leading to the development of agents targeting HER2. Trastuzumab, an anti-HER2 monoclonal antibody, was the first drug developed and approved for clinical use. It demonstrated efficacy in metastatic and early-stage HER2-positive breast cancer, showing benefits in terms of progression-free survival and overall survival. There are clinical trials, such as H0648g, M77001, BCIRG-006, and HERA, which assess the efficacy of trastuzumab in different settings, including metastatic and adjuvant treatment [117]. Although these drugs have significantly improved outcomes, they can also cause adverse effects, such as cardiotoxicity and pulmonary toxicity.

Pertuzumab, an anti-HER2 drug that acts on a different domain of the receptor than trastuzumab, showed synergy when combined with trastuzumab and chemotherapy. Clinical trials such as CLEOPATRA [118] and APHINITY [119] demonstrated the benefits of dual HER2 blockade in both metastatic breast cancer and early-stage high-risk settings. Its effectiveness has been demonstrated in patients with affected lymph nodes and small tumors. Although there are therapeutic issues that still need clarification, such as early recurrence in HER2+ breast cancer, anti-HER2 monoclonal antibodies are also essential in advanced disease. The combination of trastuzumab–pertuzumab with chemotherapy is standard in first-line treatment, and subsequent lines of treatment largely depend on these antibodies, often in combination with other HER2-targeted drugs, such as tyrosine kinase inhibitors. One advantage is that subcutaneous formulations of anti-HER2 antibodies with hyaluronidase have been developed and have been approved by the Food and Drug Administration, providing an alternative to the intravenous route [120].

Margetuximab is a monoclonal antibody against HER2 that, compared to trastuzumab, features a modified Fc domain, increasing affinity for CD16A and reducing affinity for CD32B. This modification enhances antibody-dependent cellular cytotoxicity (ADCC) of the innate immune system. In the SOPHIA trial [121], which compared margetuximab with trastuzumab in the treatment of advanced breast cancer following progression after HER2-targeted therapies, margetuximab demonstrated an increase in progression-free survival by approximately 1 month in the intention-to-treat population. The benefit of margetuximab was selective for patients with the CD16A-158F allele, while it did not provide clinical benefit in V/V homozygotes CD16A-158 compared to trastuzumab. Based on these findings, the Food and Drug Administration approved margetuximab in combination with chemotherapy as a third-line treatment for metastatic HER2+ breast cancer. Common adverse events were similar to those of trastuzumab, although infusion-related reactions were more frequent with margetuximab.

Several studies have also been conducted on the use of these therapies in neoadjuvant treatment. The Phase II clinical trial, NeoSphere [122], evaluated various combinations of pertuzumab, trastuzumab, and docetaxel in the neoadjuvant setting for HER2+ breast cancer treatment. Although the combination of all three agents showed the highest rate of pathological complete responses (46%), it did not demonstrate superiority in progression-free survival, possibly due to the small size of the study. Another trial, WSG-ADAPT HR-/HER2+ [123], tested the combination of pertuzumab–trastuzumab with or without paclitaxel in the same setting, showing a high rate of pathological complete responses (91%) with the addition of paclitaxel. At 5 years of follow-up, disease-free survival was 98% with paclitaxel and 89% without paclitaxel, although it did not reach statistical significance. Larger trials are needed to assess the significance of survival outcomes, but the high rate of pathological complete responses justifies reconsidering the use of this combination in neoadjuvant treatment.

Therefore, despite lingering therapeutic questions, these anti-HER2 monoclonal antibodies play a crucial role in various stages of HER2+ breast cancer treatment. They are essential tools, demonstrating effectiveness in both adjuvant therapy and advanced disease.

5.5. PARP Inhibitors

Mutations in the BRCA1 and BRCA2 genes increase the risk of breast cancer, with cumulative risks of 72% for BRCA1 and 69% for BRCA2 mutation carriers. The use of PARP inhibitors, such as olaparib and talazoparib, has shown effectiveness in treating breast cancer with BRCA1 or BRCA2 mutations. These inhibitors target Poly (ADP-ribose) polymerase (PARP) 1 and 2, crucial in DNA repair. Studies in 2005 demonstrated that tumors with BRCA mutations are particularly sensitive to PARP inhibition, leading to chromosomal instability and apoptosis [124].

The OlympiAD trial [124] compared the efficacy of olaparib with the physician's choice of single-agent chemotherapy in patients with HER2-negative metastatic breast cancer and germline mutations in BRCA1 or BRCA2 (gBRCAm). Olaparib demonstrated a significant extension in progression-free survival compared to TPC, reducing the risk of disease progression or death by 42% in the intention-to-treat population. Although there was no significant improvement in overall survival in the total population, subgroup analysis revealed a clinically significant benefit in patients without prior treatment. In 2018, the FDA approved olaparib for the treatment of HER2-negative metastatic breast cancer with gBRCAm.

Talazoparib, another PARP inhibitor, was approved by the Food and Drug Administration for use in gBRCAm HER2-negative locally advanced or metastatic breast cancer based on the outcomes of the EMBRACA trial [125], a Phase III trial that compared the efficacy of talazoparib with standard chemotherapy in this subgroup of patients.

To summarize, mutations in BRCA1 and BRCA2 significantly increase breast cancer risk, and PARP inhibitors like olaparib and talazoparib have been effective in targeting these mutations. These inhibitors work by disrupting DNA repair processes, particularly in tumors with BRCA mutations. The OlympiAD trial showed that olaparib notably extended progression-free survival in patients with HER2-negative metastatic breast cancer and BRCA mutations, leading to its FDA approval in 2018. Similarly, talazoparib, proven effective in the EMBRACA trial, was also FDA-approved for treating advanced breast cancer in patients with BRCA mutations. These developments mark significant advancements in personalized breast cancer therapy.

The complexities, clinical trial outcomes, side effects, and ongoing challenges associated with each of these therapeutic agents are summarized in Table 1.

Table 1. This table summarizes the therapeutic implications of specific biomarkers in breast cancer, including clinical trial outcomes, side effects, challenges, and the corresponding references for each therapeutic agent.

Biomarker/Therapeutic Agent	Description	Clinical Trials and Outcomes	Side Effects/Challenges	References
"DK4/6 Inhibitors"				
Abemaciclib	Targets CDK4/6, effective in hormone receptor-positive breast cancer	MONARCH 2 [100], 3 [101], 1 [102], and E [103] trials showed improved progression-free survival	Diarrhea, thromboembolism, hematological toxicity, interstitial lung disease	[100–103]
Palbociclib	A potent CDK4/6 inhibitor	PALOMA-2 [104] and 3 [105] trials demonstrated effectiveness	Similar side effects as abemaciclib	[104,105]
Ribociclib	Another CDK4/6 inhibitor	MONALEESA-2 [106], 3 [107], and 7 [108] trials showed improvements	Comparable side effects to other CDK4/6 inhibitors	[106–108]
"mTOR Inhibitors"				
Everolimus	Inhibits mTOR signaling, effective in ER+ breast cancer	BOLERO-1 [110] and 2 [111] trials, mixed results in HER2+ cases	Neutropenia, stomatitis, diarrhea, alopecia	[110,111]
"PI3K Inhibitors"				
Alpelisib	Targets PI3K, effective in HR+/HER2- breast cancer with PIK3CA mutations	SOLAR-1 [113] trial showed improved progression-free survival	Hyperglycemia, maculopapular rash	[113]

Table 1. Cont.

Biomarker/Therapeutic Agent	Description	Clinical Trials and Outcomes	Side Effects/Challenges	References
"Anti-HER2 Antibodies"				
Trastuzumab	Targets HER2 receptor	Various trials (H0648g, M77001, BCIRG-006, HERA) [117]	Cardiotoxicity, pulmonary toxicity	[117]
Pertuzumab	Acts on a different domain of HER2	CLEOPATRA [118] and APHINITY [119] trials showed benefits	Similar side effects to trastuzumab	[118,119]
Margetuximab	Modified anti-HER2 antibody	SOPHIA trial [121] showed increased progression-free survival	Infusion-related reactions	[121]
"PARP Inhibitors"				
Olaparib	Targets PARP, effective in BRCA1/2 mutation breast cancer	OlympiAD [124] trial showed extended progression-free survival	Similar side effects to other PARP inhibitors	[124]
Talazoparib	Another PARP inhibitor	EMBRACA [125] trial, effective in gBRCAm HER2-negative advanced breast cancer	Comparable side effects to olaparib	[125]

6. Triple-Negative

Triple-negative breast cancer (TNBC), characterized by the absence of estrogen receptor (ER), progesterone receptor (PR), and human epidermal growth factor receptor 2 (HER2), accounts for 10–15% of all breast cancers. TNBC's epidemiologic profile is complex, with notable implications. Epidemiologically, it predominantly affects younger women, making age a significant risk factor. Women under 40 years of age are more likely to be diagnosed with TNBC compared to other breast cancer subtypes.

Beyond age, TNBC shows racial disparities in incidence, disproportionately affecting Hispanic and African American women. These ethnic groups often present with more advanced stages of the disease at diagnosis. Genetics also play a crucial role in TNBC, with a significant number of cases linked to BRCA1 mutations, many of which are hereditary. Understanding the genetic basis of TNBC is essential for effective risk assessment and personalized treatment strategies.

Given TNBC's aggressive nature and the scarcity of targeted treatments, developing clinical biomarkers for this cancer type is crucial. These biomarkers aim to provide comprehensive information about prognosis, predict treatment response, analyze unique genetic and molecular characteristics for personalized medicine, and identify potential therapeutic targets. Consequently, several serologic, histologic, and genetic biomarkers for TNBC are currently being developed.

6.1. Histological Biomarkers: PD-L1 and Novel Histological Biomarkers

Identifying biomarkers that can predict prognosis and guide treatment decisions is critical for improving outcomes in triple-negative breast cancer (TNBC) patients. Recent research has emphasized the clinical importance of programmed death-ligand 1 (PD-L1) in TNBC. PD-L1 has become a significant biomarker in metastatic TNBC, with studies exploring its expression and clinical implications.

One notable finding is PD-L1's role as a negative prognostic factor in TNBC. Muenst et al. [126] demonstrated that patients with PD-L1-positive tumors had poorer overall and disease-free survival compared to those with PD-L1-negative tumors, suggesting its potential as a prognostic marker. Furthermore, PD-L1 expression in TNBC is crucial, particularly regarding immunotherapy. PD-L1 on tumor cells helps evade immune detection by interacting with the PD-1 receptor on immune cells. Blocking this interaction with immune checkpoint inhibitors, like anti-PD-1 or anti-PD-L1 antibodies, can reactivate antitumor immune responses. The IMpassion130 trial [127] showed that adding the PD-L1 inhibitor atezolizumab to nab-paclitaxel improved survival in patients with newly diagnosed metastatic or locally advanced PD-L1-positive TNBC. The FDA has approved atezolizumab combined with nab-paclitaxel for treating unresectable locally advanced or metastatic PD-L1-positive TNBC [128], representing a new approach in TNBC treatment.

However, challenges remain, including variable PD-L1 testing concordance among pathologists and the dynamic expression of PD-L1. Standardizing PD-L1 testing is essential for accurate clinical decision-making [129]. Immunotherapy targeting PD-L1 shows promise in managing metastatic TNBC, with PD-L1 expression emerging as a predictive indicator for immunotherapy response. While combination treatments have shown enhanced results, further research is needed to understand the response and resistance mechanisms better.

Additionally, tumor-infiltrating lymphocytes (TILs) have gained attention as innovative histological biomarkers in TNBC. Studies, including those by Loi et al. [130] and Adams et al. [131], indicate that a higher quantity of TILs, particularly CD8+ TILs, correlates with improved clinical outcomes in TNBC. This suggests TILs' potential as a positive prognostic factor. However, caution is needed when assessing TILs using machine learning algorithms, as challenges and limitations exist in this approach [132].

In summary, both PD-L1 and TILs have emerged as important biomarkers in TNBC, offering insights into prognosis and guiding treatment decisions. While PD-L1-targeted immunotherapy has shown promising results, TILs provide a valuable prognostic perspective. Continued research and standardization of assessments are necessary to optimize these biomarkers' clinical utility in TNBC.

6.2. Serological Biomarkers: The Importance of Follow-Up

Serological biomarkers are essential in diagnosing, prognosticating, and managing triple-negative breast cancer (TNBC), a subtype of breast cancer characterized by the absence of estrogen receptor (ER), progesterone receptor (PR), and human epidermal growth factor receptor 2 (HER2) expression. Understanding these biomarkers can provide insights into TNBC and inform personalized treatment approaches.

CA15-3 has emerged as a significant biomarker in TNBC, linked to disease progression and prognosis. Li et al.'s meta-analysis of 36 studies indicated that CA15-3 levels differ among breast cancer subtypes, suggesting its utility in differentiating TNBC from other forms [133]. Fu and Li emphasized the importance of combining CA15-3 with other tumor markers for more accurate clinical assessments [134], while Zhu et al. highlighted its role in monitoring therapy outcomes and disease progression in metastatic breast cancer [135]. Additionally, Wang et al. identified CA15-3 as a key biomarker in nipple discharge, aiding in diagnosis and prognosis [136], and Oliveira et al.'s development of a microfluidic device for CA15-3 detection underscores its practical application in clinical settings [137].

Carcinoembryonic antigen (CEA) is another crucial serological biomarker for monitoring TNBC. Anoop et al. found that elevated serum CEA levels in metastatic breast cancer patients were significantly associated with poorer survival outcomes, indicating its prognostic value in metastatic TNBC [138]. Li et al.'s meta-analysis further supported CEA's association with larger tumor size, lymph node involvement, and advanced tumor stage [139]. Yang et al.'s study demonstrated that increased CEA levels during therapy could predict a poor therapeutic response [140]. However, CEA is not exclusive to breast cancer and can be elevated in other conditions, necessitating its interpretation alongside other clinical factors.

In conclusion, serological biomarkers like CA15-3 and CEA are promising tools in TNBC management. They offer non-invasive methods for early diagnosis and tailoring treatments. Despite challenges such as validation and standardization, these biomarkers hold the potential to revolutionize the approach and management of this aggressive cancer subtype.

6.3. Genetic Biomarkers

Genetic biomarkers are pivotal in understanding the biology of triple-negative breast cancer (TNBC), guiding treatment strategies, and improving patient outcomes. Identifying these biomarkers can aid in diagnosing and prognosing TNBC.

TP53, also known as tumor protein p53, is a tumor suppressor gene crucial for genomic stability. In TNBC, TP53 mutations occur more frequently than in other breast cancer subtypes, associated with a more aggressive phenotype, higher tumor grade, and poorer prognosis [141]. Studies have demonstrated the link between TP53 mutations and higher risks of distant recurrence and reduced overall survival in TNBC patients [142], indicating its prognostic potential. For example, Petrovic et al. found that TP53 mutations were more common in TNBC than other breast cancer subtypes [143]. Moreover, TP53 mutations have been linked to a higher risk of developing TNBC, larger tumor size, and lymph node involvement [144,145]. These mutations also correlate with resistance to common chemotherapeutic agents like anthracyclines and taxanes [146], highlighting their role in guiding treatment decisions.

BRCA1 and BRCA2 mutations are also crucial in TNBC. These tumor suppressor genes are involved in DNA repair, and mutations in them increase breast cancer risk, including TNBC. BRCA mutations are more prevalent in TNBC patients and may offer benefits from targeted therapies like PARP inhibitors. The presence of BRCA mutations necessitates risk assessment and genetic counseling for patients and their families [147]. A study found that testing for BRCA mutations in TNBC patients under 50 could be a cost-effective strategy, reducing the incidence of future breast and ovarian cancers [148]. Noh et al. reported associations between BRCA mutations and younger onset age, higher nuclear grade, and poorer histological grade in TNBC patients [149]. Additionally, these mutations have been linked to increased risks of distant metastasis and decreased survival [150].

TNBC patients with BRCA mutations can benefit from PARP inhibitors, which exploit DNA repair deficiencies caused by these mutations. Clinical trials have shown promising results in terms of response rates and progression-free survival with PARP inhibitor treatments in TNBC patients with BRCA mutations [151,152].

In conclusion, TP53 and BRCA mutations significantly impact the development, progression, and treatment of TNBC. These mutations are associated with increased TNBC risks, specific clinicopathological characteristics, and responsiveness to targeted therapies.

6.4. Circulating Tumor Cells and MicroRNAs: New Findings

MicroRNAs (miRNAs) are emerging as key regulators in the pathogenesis of TNBC with their dysregulation implicated in the disease's progression, diagnosis, and prognosis [153]. Studies have identified specific miRNAs, including miR-145, miR-296, and miR-93, as potential diagnostic and prognostic tools in TNBC [154]. Additionally, circulating miRNAs have been proposed as non-invasive biomarkers for TNBC, aiding in disease monitoring [155]. These miRNAs offer potential for early-stage diagnosis, prognosis, and prediction of therapeutic response.

Their role in TNBC extends to influencing cancer progression, metastasis, and drug resistance [156]. MiRNAs are also involved in regulating the epithelial–mesenchymal transition (EMT) and cancer stem cell properties, impacting the disease's phenotype [157]. MiRNA expression profiling is instrumental in identifying specific miRNA signatures for TNBC, with bioinformatic analysis revealing miR-934 as a potential EMT regulator [158]. Integrated analysis of data related to circulating miRNAs can unveil drug resistance mechanisms in TNBC [52], highlighting their therapeutic potential.

Circulating tumor cells (CTCs) also play a crucial role in TNBC. Their presence has been linked to early metastatic relapse after neoadjuvant chemotherapy [159] and disease-free survival in breast cancer, marking them as a prognostic marker [160]. CTCs offer insights into disease progression and treatment response in TNBC. Their association with residual cancer burden is an independent prognostic factor in patients with residual TNBC [161]. Case studies, like one utilizing a tumor-informed CTC test in an advanced TNBC patient, demonstrate CTCs' utility in identifying therapeutic targets and monitoring treatment response [162]. Additionally, the role of CTCs in metastasis and chemotherapy effectiveness is under investigation, suggesting their therapeutic target potential [163].

In this sense, miRNAs and CTCs hold significant promise as prognostic and diagnostic tools in TNBC. Their association with survival, treatment response, and residual disease burden underscores their clinical importance in managing TNBC. The most relevant histological, serological, and genetic markers, as well as microRNAs of HER2+ and triple negative metastatic breast cancer, are concisely summarized in Figure 2.

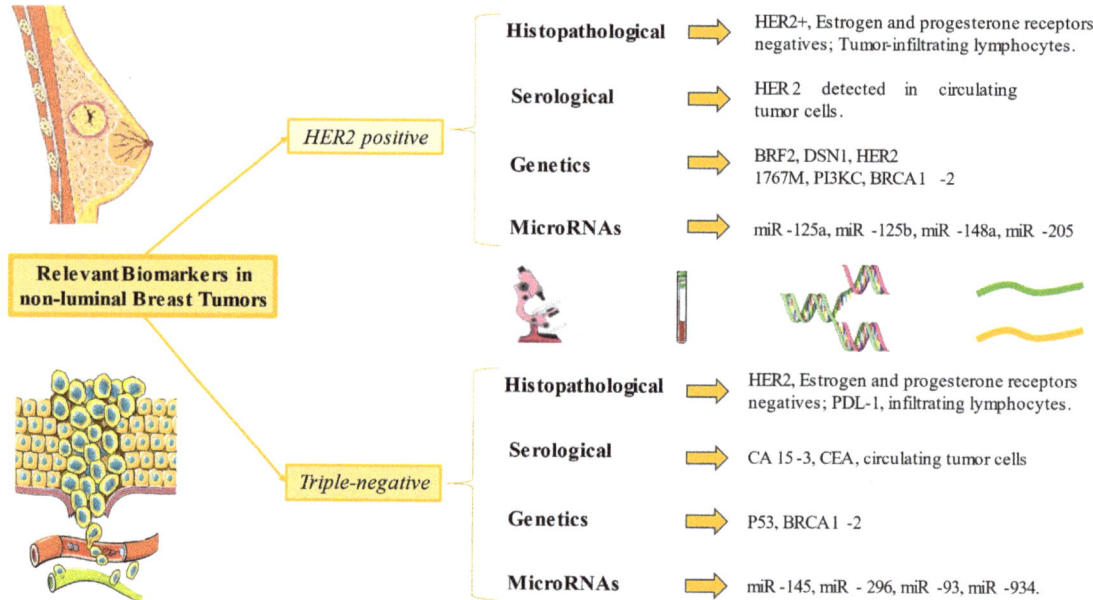

Figure 2. Summary of the most relevant biomarkers in metastatic HER2+ and triple-negative tumors.

7. Limitations

The integration of biomarkers in breast cancer treatment faces multifaceted challenges. Economically, the implementation of advanced detection technologies and targeted therapies based on biomarkers is costly, posing a significant barrier in resource-limited settings and developing countries. It should be noted that the interpretation of these biomarkers requires specialized training, a resource often lacking in less developed healthcare systems. Standardized methodologies are critical for the reliability of biomarker data, emphasizing the importance of uniform practices in sample collection and analysis to ensure data quality [164]. Furthermore, disparities in access to cutting-edge technologies for biomarker analysis lead to inequalities in breast cancer treatment across different regions or even in different parts of the same country [165]. Lastly, the use of genetic data in patient treatment raises ethical concerns, highlighting the need for comprehensive consent processes and robust data protection strategies to safeguard patient privacy and ensure the ethical handling of sensitive information [166].

In summary, while biomarkers offer a promising approach to breast cancer treatment, their integration is hindered by several technical and practical challenges. These include the high cost of advanced detection technologies, the need for specialized training in biomarker analysis, uneven access to necessary technology, and ethical concerns related to genetic data. Addressing these issues is crucial for leveraging biomarkers effectively in breast cancer care, requiring both technical advancements and policy considerations.

8. Conclusions

In conclusion, this article emphasizes the necessity of a multidisciplinary approach in managing metastatic breast cancer. It advocates for the integration of serological, histological, and genetic analyses, coupled with the examination of circulating tumor cells and microRNAs, thereby enhancing diagnostic accuracy. Moreover, this comprehensive strategy not only tailors treatments to individual patient profiles but also significantly improves the monitoring of disease progression. Consequently, these advancements herald a promising shift towards more precise and effective breast cancer care, signifying a pivotal moment in oncology.

Author Contributions: Conceptualization, L.P., M.A.O. and R.D.-P.; methodology, L.P. and M.A.O.; validation, R.D.-P.; investigation, L.L.-G., A.S.C., C.S.C., E.D.R.C., J.C.E., T.P., M.A.O., O.F.-M., C.G.-M., A.M.R.-S., L.J.-Á., S.A.-H., L.P., M.A.-M., L.G.G. and R.D.-P.; data curation, L.P.; writing—original draft preparation, L.L.-G., A.S.C., C.S.C., E.D.R.C., J.C.E., T.P. and L.P. writing—review and editing, O.F.-M., C.G.-M., A.M.R.-S., L.J.-Á., L.G.G., S.A.-H., J.M., L.P. and M.A.O.; visualization, L.P. and M.A.O.; supervision, M.A.O. and L.G.G.; project administration, M.A.O. and M.A.-M.; funding acquisition, M.A.-M. All authors have read and agreed to the published version of the manuscript.

Funding: The study was supported by the Comunidad de Madrid (P2022/BMD-7321), ProACapital, and HALE KULANI, S.L. and MJR.

Institutional Review Board Statement: Not applicable.

Informed Consent Statement: Not applicable.

Conflicts of Interest: The authors declare no conflicts of interest.

References

1. Giaquinto, A.N.; Sung, H.; Miller, K.D.; Kramer, J.L.; Newman, L.A.; Minihan, A.; Jemal, A.; Siegel, R.L. Breast Cancer Statistics, 2022. *CA Cancer J. Clin.* **2022**, *6*, 524–541. [CrossRef] [PubMed]
2. Arnold, M.; Morgan, E.; Rumgay, H.; Mafra, A.; Singh, D.; Laversanne, M.; Vignat, J.; Gralow, J.R.; Cardoso, F.; Siesling, S.; et al. Current and future burden of breast cancer: Global statistics for 2020 and 2040. *Breast* **2022**, *66*, 15–23. [CrossRef] [PubMed]
3. Gorasso, V.; Silversmit, G.; Arbyn, M.; Cornez, A.; De Pauw, R.; De Smedt, D.; Grant, I.; Wyper, G.M.A.; Devleesschauwer, B.; Speybroeck, N. The non-fatal burden of cancer in Belgium, 2004–2019: A nationwide registry-based study. *BMC Cancer* **2022**, *22*, 58. [CrossRef] [PubMed]
4. Zaheer, S.; Shah, N.; Maqbool, S.A.; Soomro, N.M. Estimates of past and future time trends in age-specific breast cancer incidence among women in Karachi, Pakistan: 2004–2025. *BMC Public Health* **2019**, *19*, 1001. [CrossRef] [PubMed]
5. Kamińska, M.; Ciszewski, T.; Łopacka-Szatan, K.; Miotła, P.; Starosławska, E. Breast cancer risk factors. *Menopausal Rev.* **2015**, *14*, 196–202. [CrossRef]
6. Collins, A. The genetics of breast cancer: Risk factors for disease. *Appl. Clin. Genet.* **2011**, *4*, 11–19. [CrossRef] [PubMed]
7. Criscitiello, C.; Corti, C. Breast Cancer Genetics: Diagnostics and Treatment. *Genes* **2022**, *9*, 1593. [CrossRef]
8. Freudenheim, J.L. Alcohol's Effects on Breast Cancer in Women. *Alcohol Res. Curr. Rev.* **2020**, *40*, 11. [CrossRef]
9. Vinogradova, Y.; Coupland, C.; Hippisley-Cox, J. Use of hormone replacement therapy and risk of breast cancer: Nested case-control studies using the QResearch and CPRD databases. *BMJ* **2020**, *371*, m3873. [CrossRef]
10. Soori, M.; Platz, E.A.; Brawley, O.W.; Lawrence, R.S.; Kanarek, N.F. Inclusion of the US Preventive Services Task Force Recommendation for Mammography in State Comprehensive Cancer Control Plans in the US. *JAMA Netw. Open* **2022**, *5*, e229706. [CrossRef]
11. He, Z.; Chen, Z.; Tan, M.; Elingarami, S.; Liu, Y.; Li, T.; Deng, Y.; He, N.; Li, S.; Fu, J.; et al. A review on methods for diagnosis of breast cancer cells and tissues. *Cell Prolif.* **2020**, *53*, e12822. [CrossRef] [PubMed]
12. Wang, L. Early Diagnosis of Breast Cancer. *Sensors* **2017**, *17*, 1572. [CrossRef] [PubMed]
13. Smolarz, B.; Nowak, A.Z.; Romanowicz, H. Breast Cancer—Epidemiology, Classification, Pathogenesis and Treatment (Review of Literature). *Cancers* **2022**, *10*, 2569. [CrossRef] [PubMed]
14. Vondeling, G.T.; Menezes, G.L.; Dvortsin, E.P.; Jansman, F.G.A.; Konings, I.R.; Postma, M.J.; Rozenbaum, M.H. Burden of early, advanced and metastatic breast cancer in The Netherlands. *BMC Cancer* **2018**, *18*, 262. [CrossRef]
15. Kapp, A.V.; Jeffrey, S.S.; Langerød, A.; Børresen-Dale, A.L.; Han, W.; Noh, D.Y.; Bukholm, I.R.; Nicolau, M.; Brown, P.O.; Tibshirani, R. Discovery and validation of breast cancer subtypes. *BMC Genom.* **2006**, *7*, 231. [CrossRef] [PubMed]

16. Yersal, O. Biological subtypes of breast cancer: Prognostic and therapeutic implications. *World J. Clin. Oncol.* **2014**, *5*, 412–424. [CrossRef] [PubMed]
17. Miglietta, F.; Bottosso, M.; Griguolo, G.; Dieci, M.V.; Guarneri, V. Major advancements in metastatic breast cancer treatment: When expanding options means prolonging survival. *ESMO Open* **2022**, *7*, 100409. [CrossRef] [PubMed]
18. Waks, A.G.; Winer, E.P. Breast Cancer Treatment. *JAMA* **2019**, *321*, 288–300. [CrossRef]
19. Harbeck, N.; Gnant, M. Breast cancer. *Lancet* **2017**, *389*, 1134–1150. [CrossRef]
20. Duffy, M.J. Serum Tumor Markers in Breast Cancer: Are They of Clinical Value? *Clin. Chem.* **2006**, *52*, 345–351. [CrossRef]
21. Gao, J.J.; Swain, S.M. Luminal A Breast Cancer and Molecular Assays: A Review. *Oncologist* **2018**, *23*, 556–565. [CrossRef]
22. Li, Z.; Wei, H.; Li, S.; Wu, P.; Mao, X. The Role of Progesterone Receptors in Breast Cancer. *Drug Des. Dev. Ther.* **2022**, *16*, 305–314. [CrossRef] [PubMed]
23. Prat, A.; Pineda, E.; Adamo, B.; Galván, P.; Fernández, A.; Gaba, L.; Díez, M.; Viladot, M.; Arance, A.; Muñoz, M. Clinical implications of the intrinsic molecular subtypes of breast cancer. *Breast* **2015**, *24*, S26–S35. [CrossRef] [PubMed]
24. Kennecke, H.; Yerushalmi, R.; Woods, R.; Cheang, M.C.; Voduc, D.; Speers, C.H.; Nielsen, T.O.; Gelmon, K. Metastatic Behavior of Breast Cancer Subtypes. *J. Clin. Oncol.* **2010**, *28*, 3271–3277. [CrossRef] [PubMed]
25. Hou, Y.; Peng, Y.; Li, Z. Update on prognostic and predictive biomarkers of breast cancer. *Semin. Diagn. Pathol.* **2022**, *39*, 322–332. [CrossRef] [PubMed]
26. Mueller, C.; Haymond, A.; Davis, J.B.; Williams, A.; Espina, V. Protein biomarkers for subtyping breast cancer and implications for future research. *Expert Rev. Proteom.* **2018**, *15*, 131–152. [CrossRef] [PubMed]
27. Slamon, D.J.; Clark, G.M.; Wong, S.G.; Levin, W.J.; Ullrich, A.; McGuire, W.L. Human Breast Cancer: Correlation of Relapse and Survival with Amplification of the HER-2/neu Oncogene. *Science* **1987**, *235*, 177–182. [CrossRef] [PubMed]
28. Marchiò, C.; Annaratone, L.; Marques, A.; Casorzo, L.; Berrino, E.; Sapino, A. Evolving concepts in HER2 evaluation in breast cancer: Heterogeneity, HER2-low carcinomas and beyond. *Semin. Cancer Biol.* **2021**, *72*, 123–135. [CrossRef]
29. Roulot, A.; Héquet, D.; Guinebretière, J.-M.; Vincent-Salomon, A.; Lerebours, F.; Dubot, C.; Rouzier, R. Tumoral heterogeneity of breast cancer. *Ann. Biol. Clin.* **2016**, *74*, 653–660. [CrossRef]
30. Panal Cusati, M.; Herrera de la Muela, M.; Hardisson Hernaez, D.; Choqueneira Dionisio, M.; Román Guindo, A.; de Santiago Garcia, F.J. Correlación entre la expresión de Ki67 con factores clásicos pronósticos y predictivos en el cáncer de mama precoz. *Rev. Senol. Y Patol. Mamar.* **2014**, *27*, 163–169. [CrossRef]
31. Chachaima-Mar, J.; Pineda-Reyes, J.; Marín, R.; Lozano-Miranda, Z.; Chian, C. Perfil inmunofenotípico de cáncer de mama de pacientes atendidas en un hospital general de lima, perú. *Rev. Medica Hered.* **2021**, *31*, 235–241. [CrossRef]
32. Tarighati, E.; Keivan, H.; Mahani, H. A review of prognostic and predictive biomarkers in breast cancer. *Clin. Exp. Med.* **2022**, *23*, 1–16. [CrossRef] [PubMed]
33. Weigelt, B.; Peterse, J.L.; van't Veer, L.J. Breast cancer metastasis: Markers and models. *Nat. Rev. Cancer* **2005**, *5*, 591–602. [CrossRef] [PubMed]
34. Suero, L.; Carrero, Y.; Jara, G.; Valencia, S.; Tayupanta, J.; Tapia, S. Marcadores tumorales pronósticos en cáncer de mama: Bax y bcl-2. *Enfermería Investig.* **2022**, *7*, 24–31. [CrossRef]
35. Castillo, L.; Bonilla, F.; Reigosa, A.; Fernández, Á. Expresión de p53 y Bcl-2 en carcinoma ductal infiltrante de mama localmente avanzado. Su relación con el subtipo intrínseco molecular como factor pronóstico. *Investig. Clínica* **2018**, *59*, 325–338. [CrossRef]
36. Arenillas Medina, M.P.; Ortiz Tejedor, J.G. Marcador tumoral CA 15-3 en carcinoma invasivo de mama de tipo no especial (ductal). *Anatomía Digit.* **2022**, *5*, 58–75. [CrossRef]
37. Heylen, J.; Punie, K.; Smeets, A.; Neven, P.; Weltens, C.; Laenen, A.; Wildiers, H. Elevated CA 15.3 in Newly Diagnosed Breast Cancer: A Retrospective Study. *Clin. Breast Cancer* **2022**, *22*, 579–587. [CrossRef]
38. de los Miranda, M.Á. Expresión y Significación Clínica de las Citoquinas en el Cáncer de Mama—Dialnet. Dialnet. Available online: http://hdl.handle.net/10651/30131 (accessed on 8 November 2023).
39. Garcia-Martinez, L.; Zhang, Y.; Nakata, Y.; Chan, H.L.; Morey, L. Epigenetic mechanisms in breast cancer therapy and resistance. *Nat. Commun.* **2021**, *12*, 1786. [CrossRef]
40. Alzahrani, A.S. PI3K/Akt/mTOR inhibitors in cancer: At the bench and bedside. *Semin. Cancer Biol.* **2019**, *59*, 125–132. [CrossRef]
41. Low, S.; Zembutsu, H.; Nakamura, Y. Breast cancer: The translation of big genomic data to cancer precision medicine. *Cancer Sci.* **2017**, *109*, 497–506. [CrossRef]
42. Husni Cangara, M.; Miskad, U.A.; Masadah, R.; Nelwan, B.J.; Wahid, S. Gata-3 and KI-67 expression in correlation with molecular subtypes of breast cancer. *Breast Dis.* **2021**, *40*, S27–S31. [CrossRef]
43. Dumitrescu, R.G. Interplay Between Genetic and Epigenetic Changes in Breast Cancer Subtypes. In *Methods in Molecular Biology*; Springer: New York, NY, USA, 2018; pp. 19–34. [CrossRef]
44. Morales, D.A.; Echeverría, I.C. Biomarcadores mamarios en procesos metastásicos en mujeres ecuatorianas. *Rev. Fac. Cienc. Médicas* **2019**, *44*, 24–33. [CrossRef]
45. Sanabria, M.C.; Muñoz, G.; Vargas, C.I. Análisis de las mutaciones más frecuentes del gen BRCA1 (185delAG y 5382insC) en mujeres con cáncer de mama en Bucaramanga, Colombia. *Biomédica* **2009**, *29*, 61. [CrossRef]
46. Franceschini, G.; Di Leone, A.; Terribile, D.; Sanchez, M.A.; Masetti, R. Bilateral prophylactic mastectomy in BRCA mutation carriers: What surgeons need to know. *Ann. Ital. Chir.* **2019**, *90*, 1–2. [CrossRef] [PubMed]

47. Goldhirsch, A.; Winer, E.P.; Coates, A.S.; Gelber, R.D.; Piccart-Gebhart, M.; Thürlimann, B.; Senn, H.J.; Albain, K.S.; André, F.; Bergh, J.; et al. Personalizing the treatment of women with early breast cancer: Highlights of the St Gallen International Expert Consensus on the Primary Therapy of Early Breast Cancer 2013. *Ann. Oncol.* **2013**, *24*, 2206–2223. [CrossRef]
48. The Cancer Genome Atlas (TCGA) Research Network. Comprehensive molecular portraits of human breast tumours. *Nature* **2012**, *490*, 61–70. [CrossRef]
49. Kalinina, T.S.; Kononchuk, V.V.; Yakovleva, A.K.; Alekseenok, E.Y.; Sidorov, S.V.; Gulyaeva, L.F. Association between Lymph Node Status and Expression Levels of Androgen Receptor, miR-185, miR-205, and miR-21 in Breast Cancer Subtypes. *Int. J. Breast Cancer* **2020**, *2020*, 3259393. [CrossRef] [PubMed]
50. Souza, K.C.; Evangelista, A.F.; Leal, L.F.; Souza, C.P.; Vieira, R.A.; Causin, R.L.; Neuber, A.C.; Pessoa, D.P.; Passos, G.A.; Reis, R.; et al. Identification of Cell-Free Circulating MicroRNAs for the Detection of Early Breast Cancer and Molecular Subtyping. *J. Oncol.* **2019**, *2019*, 8393769. [CrossRef]
51. Sieuwerts, A.M.; Kraan, J.; Bolt, J.; van der Spoel, P.; Elstrodt, F.; Schutte, M.; Martens, J.W.; Gratama, J.W.; Sleijfer, S.; Foekens, J.A. Anti-Epithelial Cell Adhesion Molecule Antibodies and the Detection of Circulating Normal-Like Breast Tumor Cells. *J. Natl. Cancer Inst.* **2009**, *101*, 61–66. [CrossRef]
52. Piñeiro, R.; Martínez-Pena, I.; López-López, R. Relevance of CTC Clusters in Breast Cancer Metastasis. *Adv. Exp. Med. Biol.* **2020**, *1220*, 93–115. [CrossRef]
53. Valdivia-Silva, J.; Pérez-Tulich, L.; Flores-Olazo, L.; Málaga-Julca, M.; Ubidia, A.; Fleschman, A.; Guio, H. Desarrollo de un sistema microfluidico (lab-on-achip) accesible y de bajo costo para detección de células tumorales circulantes de cáncer de mama. *Acta Medica Peru.* **2020**, *37*, 40–47. [CrossRef]
54. Pierga, J.; Bidard, F.; Mathiot, C.; Brain, É.; Delaloge, S.; Giachetti, S.; Marty, M. Circulating tumor cell detection predicts early metastatic relapse after neoadjuvant chemotherapy in large operable and locally advanced breast cancer in a phase ii randomized trial. *Clin. Cancer Res.* **2008**, *14*, 7004–7010. [CrossRef]
55. Mittal, A.; Mani, N. Molecular classification of breast cancer. *Indian J. Pathol. Oncol.* **2021**, *8*, 241–247. [CrossRef]
56. Lamb, C.A.; Vanzulli, S.I.; Lanari, C. Hormone receptors in breast cancer: More than estrogen receptors. *Medicina* **2019**, *79*, 540–545. [PubMed]
57. Łukasiewicz, S.; Czeczelewski, M.; Forma, A.; Baj, J.; Sitarz, R.; Stanisławek, A. Breast Cancer-Epidemiology, Risk Factors, Classification, Prognostic Markers, and Current Treatment Strategies-An Updated Review. *Cancers* **2021**, *13*, 4287. [CrossRef]
58. Aktas, A.; Gunay-Gurleyik, M.; Aker, F.; Kaan-Akgok, Y.; Atag, E. Does neoadjuvant chemotherapy provide any benefit for surgical de-escalation in luminal B, HER2(-) breast cancers? *Cirugía Cir.* **2023**, *91*, 186–194. [CrossRef]
59. Orrantia-Borunda, E.; Anchondo-Nuñez, P.; Acuña-Aguilar, L.E.; Gómez-Valles, F.O.; Ramírez-Valdespino, C.A. Subtypes of Breast Cancer. In *Breast Cancer*; Mayrovitz, H.N., Ed.; Exon Publications: Brisbane, Australia, 2022.
60. Viale, G.; Hanlon Newell, A.E.; Walker, E.; Harlow, G.; Bai, I.; Russo, L.; Dell'Orto, P.; Maisonneuve, P. Ki-67 (30-9) scoring and differentiation of Luminal A- and Luminal B-like breast cancer subtypes. *Breast Cancer Res. Treat.* **2019**, *178*, 451–458. [CrossRef]
61. Cheang, M.; Chia, S.; David, V.; Gao, D.; Leung, S.; Snider, J.; Nielsen, T. Ki67 index, her2 status, and prognosis of patients with luminal b breast cancer. *JNCI J. Natl. Cancer Inst.* **2009**, *101*, 736–750. [CrossRef]
62. Terkelsen, T.; Pernemalm, M.; Gromov, P.; Børresen-Dale, A.L.; Krogh, A.; Haakensen, V.D.; Lethiö, J.; Papaleo, E.; Gromova, I. Proteómica de alto rendimiento del líquido intersticial del cáncer de mama: Identificación de biomarcadores serológicamente relevantes específicos de subtipos tumorales. *Mol. Oncol.* **2021**, *15*, 429–461. [CrossRef]
63. Ozaki, A.; Motomura, H.; Tamori, S.; Onaga, C.; Nagashima, Y.; Kotori, M.; Akimoto, K. High expression of p62 and aldh1a3 is associated with poor prognosis in luminal b breast cancer. *Anticancer Res.* **2022**, *42*, 3299–3312. [CrossRef]
64. Issac, M.; Yousef, E.; Tahir, M.; Gaboury, L. Mcm2, mcm4, and mcm6 in breast cancer: Clinical utility in diagnosis and prognosis. *Neoplasia* **2019**, *21*, 1015–1035. [CrossRef] [PubMed]
65. Cancello, G.; Maisonneuve, P.; Rotmensz, N.; Viale, G.; Mastropasqua, M.; Pruneri, G.; Colleoni, M. Prognosis in women with small node-negative operable breast cancer by immunohistochemically selected subtypes. *Breast Cancer Res. Treat.* **2011**, *127*, 713–720. [CrossRef]
66. Shimoda, M.; Hori, A.; Wands, J.; Tsunashima, R.; Naoi, Y.; Miyake, T.; Noguchi, S. Endocrine sensitivity of estrogen receptor-positive breast cancer is negatively correlated with aspartate-β-hydroxylase expression. *Cancer Sci.* **2017**, *108*, 2454–2461. [CrossRef] [PubMed]
67. Haque, R.; Ahmed, S.; Inzhakova, G.; Shi, J.; Avila, C.; Polikoff, J.; Press, M. Impact of breast cancer subtypes and treatment on survival: An analysis spanning two decades. *Cancer Epidemiol. Biomark. Prev.* **2012**, *21*, 1848–1855. [CrossRef]
68. Xu, X.; Lu, L.; Zhu, L.; Tan, Y.; Li, Y.; Bao, L. Predicting the molecular subtypes of breast cancer using nomograms based on three-dimensional ultrasonography characteristics. *Front. Oncol.* **2022**, *12*, 838787. [CrossRef] [PubMed]
69. Kuol, N.; Yan, X.; Barriga, V.; Karakkat, J.; Vassilaros, S.; Fyssas, I.; Apostolopoulos, V. Pilot study: Immune checkpoints polymorphisms in greek primary breast cancer patients. *Biomedicines* **2022**, *10*, 1827. [CrossRef]
70. Ragu, M.; Lim, J.; Ng, P.; Yip, C.; Rajadurai, P.; Teo, S.; Pan, J. Tp53 somatic mutations in asian breast cancer are associated with subtype-specific effects. *Breast Cancer Res.* **2023**, *25*, 48. [CrossRef] [PubMed]
71. Halim, F.; Azhar, Y.; Suwarman, S.; Hernowo, B. P53 mutation as plausible predictor for endocrine resistance therapy in luminal breast cancer. *F1000research* **2022**, *11*, 330. [CrossRef]

72. Zhu, K.; Wu, Y.; He, P.; Fan, Y.; Zhong, X.; Zheng, H.; Luo, T. PI3K/AKT/mTOR-Targeted Therapy for Breast Cancer. *Cells* **2022**, *11*, 2508. [CrossRef]
73. Barzaman, K.; Karami, J.; Zarei, Z.; Hosseinzadeh, A.; Kazemi, M.H.; Moradi-Kalbolandi, S.; Safari, E.; Farahmand, L. Breast cancer: Biology, biomarkers, and treatments. *Int. Immunopharmacol.* **2020**, *84*, 106535. [CrossRef]
74. Song, B.; Wang, C.; Liu, J.; Wang, X.; Lv, L.; Wei, L.; Song, X. Microrna-21 regulates breast cancer invasion partly by targeting tissue inhibitor of metalloproteinase 3 expression. *J. Exp. Clin. Cancer Res.* **2010**, *29*, 29. [CrossRef] [PubMed]
75. Ding, Y.; Zhang, C.; Zhang, J.; Zhang, N.; Li, T.; Fang, J.; Sun, X. Mir-145 inhibits proliferation and migration of breast cancer cells by directly or indirectly regulating tgf-β1 expression. *Int. J. Oncol.* **2017**, *50*, 1701–1710. [CrossRef] [PubMed]
76. Lv, P.; Zhang, Z.; Hou, L.; Zhang, Y.; Lu, L.; Wang, C.; Shi, F. Meta-analysis of the clinicopathological significance of mirna-145 in breast cancer. *Biosci. Rep.* **2020**, *40*, BSR20193974. [CrossRef] [PubMed]
77. Davey, M.G.; Lowery, A.J.; Miller, N.; Kerin, M.J. MicroRNA Expression Profiles and Breast Cancer Chemotherapy. *Int. J. Mol. Sci.* **2021**, *22*, 10812. [CrossRef]
78. Zubair, M.; Wang, S.; Ali, N. Advanced Approaches to Breast Cancer Classification and Diagnosis. *Front. Pharmacol.* **2021**, *11*, 632079. [CrossRef] [PubMed]
79. Galardi, F.; De Luca, F.; Biagioni, C.; Migliaccio, I.; Curigliano, G.; Minisini, A.M.; Bonechi, M.; Moretti, E.; Risi, E.; McCartney, A.; et al. Circulating tumor cells and palbociclib treatment in patients with ER-positive, HER2-negative advanced breast cancer: Results from a translational sub-study of the TREnd trial. *Breast Cancer Res.* **2021**, *23*, 38. [CrossRef] [PubMed]
80. Alimirzaie, S.; Bagherzadeh, M.; Akbari, M.R. Liquid biopsy in breast cancer: A comprehensive review. *Clin. Genet.* **2019**, *95*, 643–660. [CrossRef]
81. Zhang, H.; Karakas, C.; Tyburski, H.; Turner, B.M.; Peng, Y.; Wang, X.; Katerji, H.; Schiffhauer, L.; Hicks, D.G. HER2-low breast cancers: Current insights and future directions. *Semin. Diagn Pathol.* **2022**, *39*, 305–312. [CrossRef]
82. Goud, K.I.; Dayakar, S.; Vijayalaxmi, K.; Babu, S.J.; Reddy, P.V. Evaluation of HER-2/neu status in breast cancer specimens using immunohistochemistry (IHC) & fluorescence in-situ hybridization (FISH) assay. *Indian J. Med. Res.* **2012**, *135*, 312–317.
83. Wynn, C.S.; Tang, S.C. Anti-HER2 therapy in metastatic breast cancer: Many choices and future directions. *Cancer Metastasis Rev.* **2022**, *41*, 193–209. [CrossRef]
84. Haghnavaz, N.; Asghari, F.; Komi DE, A.; Shanehbandi, D.; Baradaran, B.; Kazemi, T. La positividad para Her2 puede conferir resistencia a la terapia con paclitaxel en líneas celulares de cáncer de mama. *Células Artif. Nanomedicina Biotecnol.* **2017**, *46*, 518–523. [CrossRef] [PubMed]
85. Tarantino, P.; Hamilton, E.; Tolaney, S.M.; Cortes, J.; Morganti, S.; Ferraro, E.; Marra, A.; Viale, G.; Trapani, D.; Cardoso, F.; et al. HER2-Low Breast Cancer: Pathological and Clinical Landscape. *J. Clin. Oncol.* **2020**, *38*, 1951–1962. [CrossRef] [PubMed]
86. Vranić, S.; Bešlija, S.; Gatalica, Z. Targeting HER2 expression in cancer: New drugs and new indications. *Bosn. J. Basic. Med. Sci.* **2021**, *21*, 1–4. [CrossRef] [PubMed]
87. Denkert, C.; von Minckwitz, G.; Darb-Esfahani, S.; Lederer, B.; Heppner, B.I.; Weber, K.E.; Budczies, J.; Huober, J.; Klauschen, F.; Furlanetto, J.; et al. Tumour-infiltrating lymphocytes and prognosis in different subtypes of breast cancer: A pooled analysis of 3771 patients treated with neoadjuvant therapy. *Lancet Oncol.* **2018**, *19*, 40–50. [CrossRef] [PubMed]
88. Litton, J.K.; Burstein, H.J.; Turner, N.C. Molecular Testing in Breast Cancer. *Am. Soc. Clin. Oncol. Educ. Book.* **2019**, *39*, e1–e7. [CrossRef] [PubMed]
89. Liang, Y.; Zhang, H.; Song, X.; Yang, Q. Metastatic heterogeneity of breast cancer: Molecular mechanism and potential therapeutic targets. *Semin. Cancer Biol.* **2020**, *60*, 14–27. [CrossRef]
90. Ng, C.K.; Martelotto, L.G.; Gauthier, A.; Wen, H.C.; Piscuoglio, S.; Lim, R.S.; Cowell, C.F.; Wilkerson, P.M.; Wai, P.; Rodrigues, D.N.; et al. Intra-tumor genetic heterogeneity and alternative driver genetic alterations in breast cancers with heterogeneous HER2 gene amplification. *Genome Biol.* **2015**, *16*, 107. [CrossRef] [PubMed]
91. Schettini, F.; Prat, A. Dissecting the biological heterogeneity of HER2-positive breast cancer. *Breast* **2021**, *59*, 339–350. [CrossRef]
92. Martínez-Sáez, O.; Chic, N.; Pascual, T.; Adamo, B.; Vidal, M.; González-Farré, B.; Sanfeliu, E.; Schettini, F.; Conte, B.; Brasó-Maristany, F.; et al. Frequency and spectrum of PIK3CA somatic mutations in breast cancer. *Breast Cancer Res.* **2020**, *22*, 45. [CrossRef]
93. Cortesi, L.; Rugo, H.S.; Jackisch, C. An Overview of PARP Inhibitors for the Treatment of Breast Cancer. *Target. Oncol.* **2021**, *16*, 255–282. [CrossRef]
94. Zhang, M.; Bai, X.; Zeng, X.; Liu, J.; Liu, F.; Zhang, Z. circRNA-miRNA-mRNA in breast cancer. *Clin. Chim. Acta* **2021**, *523*, 120–130. [CrossRef] [PubMed]
95. Wang, H.; Tan, Z.; Hu, H.; Liu, H.; Wu, T.; Zheng, C.; Wang, X.; Luo, Z.; Wang, J.; Liu, S.; et al. microRNA-21 promotes breast cancer proliferation and metastasis by targeting LZTFL1. *BMC Cancer* **2019**, *19*, 738. [CrossRef] [PubMed]
96. Yu, M.; Bardia, A.; Wittner, B.S.; Stott, S.L.; Smas, M.E.; Ting, D.T.; Isakoff, S.J.; Ciciliano, J.C.; Wells, M.N.; Shah, A.M.; et al. Circulating breast tumor cells exhibit dynamic changes in epithelial and mesenchymal composition. *Science* **2013**, *339*, 580–584. [CrossRef] [PubMed]
97. Liang, D.H.; Hall, C.; Lucci, A. Circulating Tumor Cells in Breast Cancer. *Recent Results Cancer Res.* **2020**, *215*, 127–145. [CrossRef] [PubMed]

98. Aceto, N.; Bardia, A.; Miyamoto, D.T.; Donaldson, M.C.; Wittner, B.S.; Spencer, J.A.; Yu, M.; Pely, A.; Engstrom, A.; Zhu, H.; et al. Circulating tumor cell clusters are oligoclonal precursors of breast cancer metastasis. *Cell* 2014, *158*, 1110–1122. [CrossRef] [PubMed]
99. Bidard, F.C.; Proudhon, C.; Pierga, J.Y. Circulating tumor cells in breast cancer. *Mol. Oncol.* 2016, *10*, 418–430. [CrossRef] [PubMed]
100. Sledge, G.W.; Toi, M., Jr.; Neven, P.; Sohn, J.; Inoue, K.; Pivot, X.; Burdaeva, O.; Okera, M.; Masuda, N.; Kaufman, P.A.; et al. MONARCH 2: Abemaciclib in Combination With Fulvestrant in Women With HR+/HER2- Advanced Breast Cancer Who Had Progressed While Receiving Endocrine Therapy. *J. Clin. Oncol.* 2017, *35*, 2875–2884. [CrossRef]
101. Goetz, M.P.; Toi, M.; Campone, M.; Sohn, J.; Paluch-Shimon, S.; Huober, J.; Park, I.H.; Trédan, O.; Chen, S.C.; Manso, L.; et al. MONARCH 3: Abemaciclib As Initial Therapy for Advanced Breast Cancer. *J. Clin. Oncol.* 2017, *35*, 3638–3646. [CrossRef]
102. Dickler, M.N.; Tolaney, S.M.; Rugo, H.S.; Cortés, J.; Diéras, V.; Patt, D.; Wildiers, H.; Hudis, C.A.; O'Shaughnessy, J.; Zamora, E.; et al. MONARCH 1, A Phase II Study of Abemaciclib, a CDK4 and CDK6 Inhibitor, as a Single Agent, in Patients with Refractory HR+/HER2- Metastatic Breast Cancer. *Clin. Cancer Res.* 2017, *23*, 5218–5224. [CrossRef]
103. Johnston, S.R.D.; Harbeck, N.; Hegg, R.; Toi, M.; Martin, M.; Shao, Z.M.; Zhang, Q.Y.; Martinez Rodriguez, J.L.; Campone, M.; Hamilton, E.; et al. Abemaciclib Combined With Endocrine Therapy for the Adjuvant Treatment of HR+, HER2-, Node-Positive, High-Risk, Early Breast Cancer (monarchE). *J. Clin. Oncol.* 2020, *38*, 3987–3998. [CrossRef]
104. Finn, R.S.; Martin, M.; Rugo, H.S.; Jones, S.; Im, S.A.; Gelmon, K.; Harbeck, N.; Lipatov, O.N.; Walshe, J.M.; Moulder, S.; et al. Palbociclib and Letrozole in Advanced Breast Cancer. *N. Engl. J. Med.* 2016, *20*, 1925–1936. [CrossRef] [PubMed]
105. Cristofanilli, M.; Rugo, H.S.; Im, S.A.; Slamon, D.J.; Harbeck, N.; Bondarenko, I.; Masuda, N.; Colleoni, M.; DeMichele, A.; Loi, S.; et al. Overall Survival with Palbociclib and Fulvestrant in Women with HR+/HER2- ABC: Updated Exploratory Analyses of PALOMA-3, a Double-blind, Phase III Randomized Study. *Clin. Cancer Res.* 2022, *28*, 3433–3442. [CrossRef] [PubMed]
106. Hortobagyi, G.N.; Stemmer, S.M.; Burris, H.A.; Yap, Y.S.; Sonke, G.S.; Hart, L.; Campone, M.; Petrakova, K.; Winer, E.P.; Janni, W.; et al. Overall Survival with Ribociclib plus Letrozole in Advanced Breast Cancer. *N. Engl. J. Med.* 2022, *386*, 942–950. [CrossRef] [PubMed]
107. Slamon, D.J.; Neven, P.; Chia, S.; Fasching, P.A.; De Laurentiis, M.; Im, S.A.; Petrakova, K.; Bianchi, G.V.; Esteva, F.J.; Martín, M.; et al. Phase III Randomized Study of Ribociclib and Fulvestrant in Hormone Receptor-Positive, Human Epidermal Growth Factor Receptor 2-Negative Advanced Breast Cancer: MONALEESA-3. *J. Clin. Oncol.* 2018, *36*, 2465–2472. [CrossRef] [PubMed]
108. Lu, Y.S.; Im, S.A.; Colleoni, M.; Franke, F.; Bardia, A.; Cardoso, F.; Harbeck, N.; Hurvitz, S.; Chow, L.; Sohn, J.; et al. Updated Overall Survival of Ribociclib plus Endocrine Therapy versus Endocrine Therapy Alone in Pre- and Perimenopausal Patients with HR+/HER2- Advanced Breast Cancer in MONALEESA-7: A Phase III Randomized Clinical Trial. *Clin. Cancer Res.* 2022, *28*, 851–859. [CrossRef]
109. Hurvitz, S.A.; Martin, M.; Press, M.F.; Chan, D.; Fernandez-Abad, M.; Petru, E.; Rostorfer, R.; Guarneri, V.; Huang, C.S.; Barriga, S.; et al. Potent Cell-Cycle Inhibition and Upregulation of Immune Response with Abemaciclib and Anastrozole in neoMONARCH, Phase II Neoadjuvant Study in HR+/HER2- Breast Cancer. *Clin. Cancer Res.* 2020, *26*, 566–580. [CrossRef]
110. Hurvitz, S.A.; Andre, F.; Jiang, Z.; Shao, Z.; Mano, M.S.; Neciosup, S.P.; Tseng, L.M.; Zhang, Q.; Shen, K.; Liu, D.; et al. Combination of everolimus with trastuzumab plus paclitaxel as first-line treatment for patients with HER2-positive advanced breast cancer (BOLERO-1): A phase 3, randomised, double-blind, multicentre trial. *Lancet Oncol.* 2015, *16*, 816–829. [CrossRef] [PubMed]
111. Beaver, J.A.; Park, B.H. The BOLERO-2 trial: The addition of everolimus to exemestane in the treatment of postmenopausal hormone receptor-positive advanced breast cancer. *Future Oncol.* 2012, *8*, 651–657. [CrossRef]
112. Hatem, R.; El Botty, R.; Chateau-Joubert, S.; Servely, J.L.; Labiod, D.; de Plater, L.; Assayag, F.; Coussy, F.; Callens, C.; Vacher, S.; et al. Targeting mTOR pathway inhibits tumor growth in different molecular subtypes of triple-negative breast cancers. *Oncotarget* 2016, *7*, 48206–48219. [CrossRef]
113. André, F.; Ciruelos, E.M.; Juric, D.; Loibl, S.; Campone, M.; Mayer, I.A.; Rubovszky, G.; Yamashita, T.; Kaufman, B.; Lu, Y.S.; et al. Alpelisib plus fulvestrant for PIK3CA-mutated, hormone receptor-positive, human epidermal growth factor receptor-2-negative advanced breast cancer: Final overall survival results from SOLAR-1. *Ann. Oncol.* 2021, *32*, 208–217. [CrossRef]
114. Rugo, H.S.; Lerebours, F.; Ciruelos, E.; Drullinsky, P.; Ruiz-Borrego, M.; Neven, P.; Park, Y.H.; Prat, A.; Bachelot, T.; Juric, D.; et al. Alpelisib plus fulvestrant in PIK3CA-mutated, hormone receptor-positive advanced breast cancer after a CDK4/6 inhibitor (BYLieve): One cohort of a phase 2, multicentre, open-label, non-comparative study. *Lancet Oncol.* 2021, *22*, 489–498. [CrossRef] [PubMed]
115. Hurvitz, S.A.; Chia, S.K.L.; Ciruelos, E.M.; Hu, X.; Im, S.-A.; Janni, W.; Jerusalem, G.; Lacouture, M.; O'Regan, R.; Rugo, H.S.; et al. 352TiP EPIK-B2: A phase III study of alpelisib (ALP) as maintenance therapy with trastuzumab (T) and pertuzumab (P) in patients (pts) with PIK3CA-mutated (mut) human epidermal growth factor receptor-2–positive (HER2+) advanced breast cancer (ABC). *Ann. Oncol.* 2020, *31*, S389–S390. [CrossRef]
116. Sharma, P.; Farooki, A.; Fasching, P.A.; Loi, S.; Peterson, K.; Prat, A.; Tripathy, D.; Xu, B.; Yardley, D.A.; Mills, D.; et al. 349TiP EPIK-B3: A phase III, randomised, double-blind (DB) placebo (PBO)-controlled study of alpelisib (ALP) + nab-paclitaxel (nab-PTX) in advanced triple-negative breast cancer (TNBC) with either PIK3CA mutation or phosphatase and tensin homolog (PTEN) loss without PIK3CA mutation. *Ann. Oncol.* 2020, *31*, S387–S388. [CrossRef]
117. Jacobs, A.T.; Martinez Castaneda-Cruz, D.; Rose, M.M.; Connelly, L. Targeted therapy for breast cancer: An overview of drug classes and outcomes. *Biochem. Pharmacol.* 2022, *204*, 115209. [CrossRef] [PubMed]

118. Swain, S.M.; Miles, D.; Kim, S.B.; Im, Y.H.; Im, S.A.; Semiglazov, V.; Ciruelos, E.; Schneeweiss, A.; Loi, S.; Monturus, E.; et al. Pertuzumab, trastuzumab, and docetaxel for HER2-positive metastatic breast cancer (CLEOPATRA): End-of-study results from a double-blind, randomised, placebo-controlled, phase 3 study. *Lancet Oncol.* **2020**, *21*, 519–530. [CrossRef]
119. Piccart, M.; Procter, M.; Fumagalli, D.; de Azambuja, E.; Clark, E.; Ewer, M.S.; Restuccia, E.; Jerusalem, G.; Dent, S.; Reaby, L.; et al. Adjuvant Pertuzumab and Trastuzumab in Early HER2-Positive Breast Cancer in the APHINITY Trial: 6 Years' Follow-Up. *J. Clin. Oncol.* **2021**, *39*, 1448–1457. [CrossRef]
120. Heo, Y.A.; Syed, Y.Y. Subcutaneous Trastuzumab: A Review in HER2-Positive Breast Cancer. *Target. Oncol.* **2019**, *14*, 749–758. [CrossRef] [PubMed]
121. Rugo, H.S.; Im, S.A.; Cardoso, F.; Cortes, J.; Curigliano, G.; Musolino, A.; Pegram, M.D.; Bachelot, T.; Wright, G.S.; Saura, C.; et al. Margetuximab Versus Trastuzumab in Patients With Previously Treated HER2-Positive Advanced Breast Cancer (SOPHIA): Final Overall Survival Results From a Randomized Phase 3 Trial. *J. Clin. Oncol.* **2023**, *41*, 198–205. [CrossRef]
122. Gianni, L.; Pienkowski, T.; Im, Y.H.; Tseng, L.M.; Liu, M.C.; Lluch, A.; Starosławska, E.; de la Haba-Rodriguez, J.; Im, S.A.; Pedrini, J.L.; et al. 5-year analysis of neoadjuvant pertuzumab and trastuzumab in patients with locally advanced, inflammatory, or early-stage HER2-positive breast cancer (NeoSphere): A multicentre, open-label, phase 2 randomised trial. *Lancet Oncol.* **2016**, *17*, 791–800. [CrossRef]
123. Nitz, U.A.; Gluz, O.; Christgen, M.; Grischke, E.M.; Augustin, D.; Kuemmel, S.; Braun, M.; Potenberg, J.; Kohls, A.; Krauss, K.; et al. De-escalation strategies in HER2-positive early breast cancer (EBC): Final analysis of the WSG-ADAPT HER2+/HR- phase II trial: Efficacy, safety, and predictive markers for 12 weeks of neoadjuvant dual blockade with trastuzumab and pertuzumab ± weekly paclitaxel. *Ann. Oncol.* **2017**, *28*, 2768–2772. [CrossRef]
124. Robson, M.E.; Tung, N.; Conte, P.; Im, S.A.; Senkus, E.; Xu, B.; Masuda, N.; Delaloge, S.; Li, W.; Armstrong, A.; et al. OlympiAD final overall survival and tolerability results: Olaparib versus chemotherapy treatment of physician's choice in patients with a germline BRCA mutation and HER2-negative metastatic breast cancer. *Ann. Oncol.* **2019**, *30*, 558–566. [CrossRef] [PubMed]
125. Litton, J.K.; Hurvitz, S.A.; Mina, L.A.; Rugo, H.S.; Lee, K.H.; Gonçalves, A.; Diab, S.; Woodward, N.; Goodwin, A.; Yerushalmi, R.; et al. Talazoparib versus chemotherapy in patients with germline BRCA1/2-mutated HER2-negative advanced breast cancer: Final overall survival results from the EMBRACA trial. *Ann. Oncol.* **2020**, *31*, 1526–1535. [CrossRef] [PubMed]
126. Muenst, S.; Schaerli, A.R.; Gao, F.; Däster, S.; Trella, E.; Droeser, R.A.; Muraro, M.G.; Zajac, P.; Zanetti, R.; Gillanders, W.E.; et al. Expression of programmed death ligand 1 (PD-L1) is associated with poor prognosis in human breast cancer. *Breast Cancer Res. Treat.* **2014**, *146*, 15–24. [CrossRef] [PubMed]
127. Gonzalez-Ericsson, P.I.; Stovgaard, E.S.; Sua, L.F.; Reisenbichler, E.; Kos, Z.; Carter, J.M.; Michiels, S.; Le Quesne, J.; Nielsen, T.O.; Laenkholm, A.V.; et al. The path to a better biomarker: Application of a risk management framework for the implementation of PD-L1 and TILs as immuno-oncology biomarkers in breast cancer clinical trials and daily practice. *J. Pathol.* **2020**, *250*, 667–684. [CrossRef] [PubMed]
128. 128. Planes-Laine, G.; Rochigneux, P.; Bertucci, F.; Chrétien, A.S.; Viens, P.; Sabatier, R.; Gonçalves, A. PD-1/PD-L1 Targeting in Breast Cancer: The First Clinical Evidences Are Emerging. A Literature Review. *Cancers* **2019**, *11*, 1033. [CrossRef]
129. Franzoi, M.A.; Romano, E.; Piccart, M. Immunotherapy for early breast cancer: Too soon, too superficial, or just right? *Ann. Oncol.* **2021**, *32*, 323–336. [CrossRef] [PubMed]
130. Loi, S.; Drubay, D.; Adams, S.; Pruneri, G.; Francis, P.A.; Lacroix-Triki, M.; Joensuu, H.; Dieci, M.V.; Badve, S.; Demaria, S.; et al. Tumor-Infiltrating Lymphocytes and Prognosis: A Pooled Individual Patient Analysis of Early-Stage Triple-Negative Breast Cancers. *J. Clin. Oncol.* **2019**, *37*, 559–569. [CrossRef]
131. Adams, S.; Gray, R.J.; Demaria, S.; Goldstein, L.; Perez, E.A.; Shulman, L.N.; Martino, S.; Wang, M.; Jones, V.E.; Saphner, T.J.; et al. Prognostic Value of Tumor-Infiltrating Lymphocytes in Triple-Negative Breast Cancers From Two Phase III Randomized Adjuvant Breast Cancer Trials: ECOG 2197 and ECOG 1199. *J. Clin. Oncol.* **2014**, *32*, 2959–2966. [CrossRef]
132. Meng, S.; Li, L.; Zhou, M.; Jiang, W.; Niu, H.; Yang, K. Distribution and prognostic value of tumor-infiltrating T cells in breast cancer. *Mol. Med. Rep.* **2018**, *18*, 4247–4258. [CrossRef]
133. Liu, S.; Lachapelle, J.; Leung, S.; Gao, D.; Foulkes, W.D.; Nielsen, T.O. CD8+ lymphocyte infiltration is an independent favorable prognostic indicator in basal-like breast cancer. *Breast Cancer Res.* **2012**, *14*, R48. [CrossRef]
134. Thagaard, J.; Broeckx, G.; Page, D.B.; Jahangir, C.A.; Verbandt, S.; Kos, Z.; Gupta, R.; Khiroya, R.; Abduljabbar, K.; Acosta Haab, G.; et al. Pitfalls in machine learning-based assessment of tumor-infiltrating lymphocytes in breast cancer: A report of the International Immuno-Oncology Biomarker Working Group on Breast Cancer. *J. Pathol.* **2023**, *260*, 498–513. [CrossRef] [PubMed]
135. Hing, J.X.; Mok, C.W.; Tan, P.T.; Sudhakar, S.S.; Seah, C.M.; Lee, W.P.; Tan, S.M. Clinical utility of tumour marker velocity of cancer antigen 15-3 (CA 15-3) and carcinoembryonic antigen (CEA) in breast cancer surveillance. *Breast* **2020**, *52*, 95–101. [CrossRef] [PubMed]
136. Fu, Y.; Li, H. Assessing Clinical Significance of Serum CA15-3 and Carcinoembryonic Antigen (CEA) Levels in Breast Cancer Patients: A Meta-Analysis. *Med. Sci. Monit.* **2016**, *22*, 3154–3162. [CrossRef] [PubMed]
137. Chu, W.G.; Ryu, D.W. Clinical significance of serum CA15-3 as a prognostic parameter during follow-up periods in patients with breast cancer. *Ann. Surg. Treat. Res.* **2016**, *90*, 57–63. [CrossRef] [PubMed]
138. Wang, G.; Qin, Y.; Zhang, J.; Zhao, J.; Liang, Y.; Zhang, Z.; Qin, M.; Sun, Y. Nipple Discharge of CA15-3, CA125, CEA and TSGF as a New Biomarker Panel for Breast Cancer. *Int. J. Mol. Sci.* **2014**, *15*, 9546–9565. [CrossRef] [PubMed]

139. Hasan, D. Diagnostic impact of CEA and CA 15-3 on monitoring chemotherapy of breast cancer patients. *J. Circ. Biomark.* **2022**, *11*, 57–63. [CrossRef]
140. Anoop, T.M.; Joseph, P.R.; Soman, S.; Chacko, S.; Mathew, M. Significance of serum carcinoembryonic antigen in metastatic breast cancer patients: A prospective study. *World J. Clin. Oncol.* **2022**, *13*, 529–539. [CrossRef] [PubMed]
141. Li, X.; Dai, D.; Chen, B.; Tang, H.; Xie, X.; Wei, W. Clinicopathological and Prognostic Significance of Cancer Antigen 15-3 and Carcinoembryonic Antigen in Breast Cancer: A Meta-Analysis including 12,993 Patients. *Dis. Markers* **2018**, *2018*, 9863092. [CrossRef]
142. Yang, Y.; Zhang, H.; Zhang, M.; Meng, Q.; Cai, L.; Zhang, Q. Elevation of serum CEA and CA15-3 levels during antitumor therapy predicts poor therapeutic response in advanced breast cancer patients. *Oncol. Lett.* **2017**, *14*, 7549–7556. [CrossRef]
143. Huszno, J.; Grzybowska, E. TP53 mutations and SNPs as prognostic and predictive factors in patients with breast cancer (Review). *Oncol. Lett.* **2018**, *16*, 34–40. [CrossRef]
144. Kim, J.Y.; Park, K.; Jung, H.H.; Lee, E.; Cho, E.Y.; Lee, K.H.; Bae, S.Y.; Lee, S.K.; Kim, S.W.; Lee, J.E.; et al. Association between Mutation and Expression of TP53 as a Potential Prognostic Marker of Triple-Negative Breast Cancer. *Cancer Res. Treat.* **2016**, *48*, 1338–1350. [CrossRef] [PubMed]
145. Uscanga-Perales, G.I.; Santuario-Facio, S.K.; Sanchez-Dominguez, C.N.; Cardona-Huerta, S.; Muñoz-Maldonado, G.E.; Ruiz-Flores, P.; Barcenas-Walls, J.R.; Osuna-Rosales, L.E.; Rojas-Martinez, A.; Gonzalez-Guerrero, J.F.; et al. Genetic alterations of triple negative breast cancer (TNBC) in women from Northeastern Mexico. *Oncol. Lett.* **2019**, *17*, 3581–3588. [CrossRef]
146. Wang, S.; Zhang, K.; Tang, L.; Yang, Y.; Wang, H.; Zhou, Z.; Pang, J.; Chen, F. Association Between Single-Nucleotide Polymorphisms in Breast Cancer Susceptibility Genes and Clinicopathological Characteristics. *Clin. Epidemiol.* **2021**, *13*, 103–112. [CrossRef] [PubMed]
147. Walerych, D.; Napoli, M.; Collavin, L.; Del Sal, G. The rebel angel: Mutant p53 as the driving oncogene in breast cancer. *Carcinogenesis* **2012**, *33*, 2007–2017. [CrossRef] [PubMed]
148. Mitri, Z.I.; Abuhadra, N.; Goodyear, S.M.; Hobbs, E.A.; Kaempf, A.; Thompson, A.M.; Moulder, S.L. Impact of TP53 mutations in Triple Negative Breast Cancer. *NPJ Precis. Oncol.* **2022**, *6*, 64. [CrossRef]
149. Atchley, D.P.; Albarracin, C.T.; Lopez, A.; Valero, V.; Amos, C.I.; Gonzalez-Angulo, A.M.; Hortobagyi, G.N.; Arun, B. KClinical and Pathologic Characteristics of Patients With *BRCA*-Positive and *BRCA*-Negative Breast Cancer. *J. Clin. Oncol.* **2008**, *26*, 4282–4288. [CrossRef] [PubMed]
150. Gonzalez-Angulo, A.M.; Timms, K.M.; Liu, S.; Chen, H.; Litton, J.K.; Potter, J.; Lanchbury, J.S.; Stemke-Hale, K.; Hennessy, B.T.; Arun, B.K.; et al. Incidence and Outcome of BRCA Mutations in Unselected Patients with Triple Receptor-Negative Breast Cancer. *Clin. Cancer Res.* **2011**, *17*, 1082–1089. [CrossRef]
151. Lee, A.; Moon, B.-I.; Kim, T.H. BRCA1/BRCA2 Pathogenic Variant Breast Cancer: Treatment and Prevention Strategies. *Ann. Lab. Med.* **2020**, *40*, 114–121. [CrossRef]
152. Plascak, J.J.; Rundle, A.G.; Xu, X.; Mooney, S.J.; Schootman, M.; Lu, B.; Roy, J.; Stroup, A.M.; Llanos, A.A.M. Associations between neighborhood disinvestment and breast cancer outcomes within a populous state registry. *Cancer* **2021**, *128*, 131–138. [CrossRef]
153. Cheng, T.; Wu, Y.; Liu, Z.; Yu, Y.; Sun, S.; Guo, M.; Sun, B.; Huang, C. CDKN2A-mediated molecular subtypes characterize the hallmarks of tumor microenvironment and guide precision medicine in triple-negative breast cancer. *Front. Immunol.* **2022**, *13*, 970950. [CrossRef]
154. Sharma, P.; Klemp, J.R.; Kimler, B.F.; Mahnken, J.D.; Geier, L.J.; Khan, Q.J.; Elia, M.; Connor, C.S.; McGinness, M.K.; Mammen, J.M.; et al. Germline BRCA mutation evaluation in a prospective triple-negative breast cancer registry: Implications for hereditary breast and/or ovarian cancer syndrome testing. *Breast Cancer Res. Treat.* **2014**, *145*, 707–714. [CrossRef] [PubMed]
155. Tang, Q.; Ouyang, H.; He, D.; Yu, C.; Tang, G. Microrna-based potential diagnostic, prognostic and therapeutic applications in triple-negative breast cancer. *Artif. Cells Nanomedicine Biotechnol.* **2019**, *47*, 2800–2809. [CrossRef] [PubMed]
156. Piña-Sánchez, P.; Valdez-Salazar, H.; Ruiz-Tachiquín, M. Circulating micrornas and their role in the immune response in triple-negative breast cancer (review). *Oncol. Lett.* **2020**, *20*, 224. [CrossRef] [PubMed]
157. Malla, R.R.; Kumari, S.; Gavara, M.M.; Badana, A.K.; Gugalavath, S.; Kumar, D.K.G.; Rokkam, P. A perspective on the diagnostics, prognostics, and therapeutics of micrornas of triple-negative breast cancer. *Biophys. Rev.* **2019**, *11*, 227–234. [CrossRef] [PubMed]
158. Qattan, A.; Al-Tweigeri, T.; Alkhayal, W.; Suleman, K.; Tulbah, A.; Amer, S. Clinical identification of dysregulated circulating micrornas and their implication in drug response in triple negative breast cancer (tnbc) by target gene network and meta-analysis. *Genes* **2021**, *12*, 549. [CrossRef] [PubMed]
159. Cullinane, C.; Fleming, C.; O'Leary, D.; Hassan, F.; Kelly, L.; O'Sullivan, M.J.; Corrigan, M.A.; Redmond, H.P. Association of circulating tumor dna with disease-free survival in breast cancer. *JAMA Netw. Open* **2020**, *3*, e2026921. [CrossRef] [PubMed]
160. Mao, S.; Chang, C.; Pei, Y.; Guo, Y.; Chang, J.; Li, H. Potential management of circulating tumor dna as a biomarker in triple-negative breast cancer. *J. Cancer* **2018**, *9*, 4627–4634. [CrossRef]
161. Stecklein, S.R.; Kimler, B.F.; Yoder, R.; Schwensen, K.; Staley, J.M.; Khan, Q.J.; O'Dea, A.P.; Nye, L.E.; Elia, M.; Heldstab, J.; et al. Ctdna and residual cancer burden are prognostic in triple-negative breast cancer patients with residual disease. *NPJ Breast Cancer* **2023**, *9*, 10. [CrossRef]
162. Azzi, G.; Krinshpun, S.; Tin, A.; Maninder, M.; Malashevich, A.K.; Malhotra, M.; Vega, R.R.; Billings, P.R.; Rodriguez, A.; Aleshin, A. Treatment response monitoring using a tumor-informed circulating tumor dna test in an advanced triple-negative breast cancer patient: A case report. *Case Rep. Oncol.* **2022**, *15*, 473–479. [CrossRef]

163. Xiang, J.; Hurchla, M.A.; Fontana, F.; Su, X.; Amend, S.R.; Esser, A.K.; Douglas, G.J.; Mudalagiriyappa, C.; Luker, K.E.; Pluard, T. Cxcr4 protein epitope mimetic antagonist pol5551 disrupts metastasis and enhances chemotherapy effect in triple-negative breast cancer. *Mol. Cancer Ther.* **2015**, *14*, 2473–2485. [CrossRef]
164. Neves Rebello Alves, L.; Dummer Meira, D.; Poppe Merigueti, L.; Correia Casotti, M.; do Prado Ventorim, D.; Ferreira Figueiredo Almeida, J.; Pereira de Sousa, V.; Cindra Sant'Ana, M.; Gonçalves Coutinho da Cruz, R.; Santos Louro, L.; et al. Biomarkers in Breast Cancer: An Old Story with a New End. *Genes* **2023**, *14*, 1364. [CrossRef] [PubMed]
165. Unger-Saldaña, K. Challenges to the early diagnosis and treatment of breast cancer in developing countries. *World J. Clin. Oncol.* **2014**, *5*, 465–477. [CrossRef] [PubMed]
166. Roux, A.; Cholerton, R.; Sicsic, J.; Moumjid, N.; French, D.P.; Giorgi Rossi, P.; Balleyguier, C.; Guindy, M.; Gilbert, F.J.; Burrion, J.B.; et al. Study protocol comparing the ethical, psychological and socio-economic impact of personalised breast cancer screening to that of standard screening in the "My Personal Breast Screening" (MyPeBS) randomised clinical trial. *BMC Cancer* **2022**, *22*, 507. [CrossRef] [PubMed]

Disclaimer/Publisher's Note: The statements, opinions and data contained in all publications are solely those of the individual author(s) and contributor(s) and not of MDPI and/or the editor(s). MDPI and/or the editor(s) disclaim responsibility for any injury to people or property resulting from any ideas, methods, instructions or products referred to in the content.

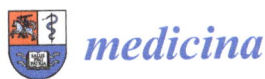 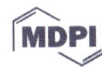

Review

Cancer Pain and Non-Invasive Brain Stimulation—A Narrative Review

Valentina-Fineta Chiriac [1,2], Daniel Ciurescu [2,*] and Daniela-Viorica Moșoiu [2,3]

1. Departament of Medical Oncology, "Dr Pompei Samarian" County Emergency Hospital, 910071 Călărași, Romania
2. Faculty of Medicine, Transilvania University, 500036 Brașov, Romania
3. HOSPICE Casa Speranței, 500074 Brașov, Romania
* Correspondence: daniel.ciurescu@unitbv.ro; Tel.: +40-722-559-551

Abstract: *Background and Objectives*: Pain is the most prevalent symptom in cancer patients. There is a paucity of data regarding non-invasive brain stimulation (NIBS) for the treatment of chronic pain in patients with cancer. The purpose of this article is to review the techniques of NIBS and present the published experiences of the oncological population. *Materials and Methods*: Databases including MEDLINE, Scopus, Web of Science, and the Cochrane Library were searched for articles on cancer patients with pain that was managed with non-invasive brain stimulation techniques. We included articles in English that were published from inception to January 2023. As studies were limited in number and had different designs and methodologies, a narrative review was considered as the best option to integrate data. *Results*: Four studies focusing on transcranial magnetic stimulation, six articles on transcranial direct current stimulation, and three articles regarding cranial electric stimulation were found and reviewed. *Conclusions*: Data are limited and not robust. Further studies in this field are required. Guidelines on NIBS for non-malignant chronic pain conditions provide good premises for cancer-related chronic pain.

Keywords: pain; neoplasm; non-invasive brain stimulation; repetitive transcranial magnetic stimulation (rTMS); transcranial direct current stimulation (tDCS); cranial electric stimulation (CES)

Citation: Chiriac, V.-F.; Ciurescu, D.; Moșoiu, D.-V. Cancer Pain and Non-Invasive Brain Stimulation—A Narrative Review. *Medicina* 2023, 59, 1957. https://doi.org/10.3390/medicina59111957

Academic Editors: Valentin Titus Grigorean and Daniel Alin Cristian

Received: 18 September 2023
Revised: 22 October 2023
Accepted: 31 October 2023
Published: 6 November 2023

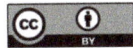

Copyright: © 2023 by the authors. Licensee MDPI, Basel, Switzerland. This article is an open access article distributed under the terms and conditions of the Creative Commons Attribution (CC BY) license (https://creativecommons.org/licenses/by/4.0/).

1. Introduction

Cancer is one of the leading causes of death, but its major social impact regards morbidity [1]. Pain affects half of patients receiving treatment and more than two-thirds of patients with metastatic or terminal cancer [1,2]. Cancer-related pain is the most frequent and feared symptom [3].

Jan Stjernsward, one of the pioneers and author of WHO analgesic ladder, had the vision in the 1980's 'to achieve world freedom from cancer pain by the year 2000' [4]. Twenty-three years after that deadline, not much has changed in the management of pain.

In the light of recent advances in cancer therapy with improved disease-free survival and overall survival, pain has become even more challenging in daily practice [5,6].

Drugs are the main treatment for pain, with opioids being the most effective pharmacological treatment. The reality shows that these are insufficient in terms of efficacy. Up to 20% of patients will not obtain relief of pain, despite a constant update of pain treatment [7,8]. Moreover, pharmacological interventions have side effects that can influence patients' awareness and self-control and all in all, can decrease quality of life [9].

The nervous system has the ability to adapt to environmental changes. This process is called neuroplasticity. Even pain is considered a "learned concept" by the International Association for the Study of Pain [10]. The implication of neural networks and neuroplasticity have been proposed as mechanisms in the search for the pathophysiology of cancer-related pain [11]. This idea provides a new possible intervention in the field of neuromodulation of cancer pain [12].

Neuromodulation relates to "the alteration of nerve activity through targeted delivery of a stimulus, such as electrical stimulation or chemical agents, to specific neurological sites in the body" [13]. Neuromodulation can be considered as a method to restore neural activity, similar to a cardiac pacemaker re-establishing cardiac rhythm. It includes spinal cord stimulation, peripheral nerve stimulation and deep brain stimulation, as well as a vast category of non-invasive brain stimulation (NIBS).

NIBS primarily includes repetitive transcranial magnetic stimulation (rTMS), transcranial electric stimulation using direct current (tDCS), and cranial electrotherapy stimulation (CES). Other new but not very well established methods are transcranial electric stimulation using alternating current (tACS), transcranial random noise stimulation (tRNS), reduced impedance non-invasive cortical electrostimulation (RINCE), and transcranial ultrasound stimulation (TUS).

The efficiency of non-invasive brain neuromodulation techniques for chronic pain has been recently investigated using an updated Cochrane database review [14]. They provide low quality evidence for single-dose high-frequency rTMS of the motor cortex as well as for tDCS. The effect on pain appears to be of short duration. However the results are not conclusive, as studies were conducted on a small number of patients with different chronic conditions [14].

Several guidelines exists and are providing rTMS and tDCS with good levels of evidence for chronic pain such as fibromyalgia, neuropathic pain, or migraine [15–17].

Not much is known regarding these methods in the management of cancer pain. With the exception of two articles [15,18] that each included one study, the main database reviews on NIBS in chronic pain [14,16,17] have excluded studies on cancer patients. Even though these new techniques are mentioned in articles presenting advances in cancer pain management [19,20], no comprehensive review of the existing data exists. Recently, a systematic review and meta-analysis was performed on just four trials involving non-invasive brain stimulation in patients with cancer [21].

With an understanding of the knowledge gap in this category of patients and the urgent need to improve pain management, our primary goal was to perform a systematic review on this topic. Some disadvantages were soon noted. Studies were numerically poorly represented and diverse regarding study design and methodology. We decided to remain faithful to our main idea to provide a comprehensive review of the existing data on NIBS for the management of cancer pain. Therefore, a change in study design was made. A narrative review was considered best to fit the data found.

2. Materials and Methods

A wide literature search was conducted at the beginning of January 2023 using the following databases: MEDLINE (via PubMed), Scopus, Web of Science (via Clarivate), Cochrane Library, LILACS, BBO (Brazilian Library of Dentistry) and other Latin American databases (via VHL Regional Portal), and multiple databases from more than 70 countries using WorldWideScience.org and the Grey Literature Database (via DANS easy).

Keywords such as 'transcranial direct current stimulation', 'transcranial magnetic stimulation', 'cranial electrical stimulation', 'noninvasive brain stimulation', 'pain', and 'cancer' were used. The search strategy combined MeSH (Medical Subject Headings) terms and synonyms with significant occurrences in major databases. The search was individualized according to the specificity of each database. The Boolean operators "AND" and "OR" were used to combine the searches. The main database search strategies are presented in Supplementary Table S1.

The inclusion criteria were as follows:

1. Articles involving adult patients with histological confirmed cancer and cancer-related pain (both tumour- or treatment-related pain)
2. Articles describing studies that used non-invasive brain stimulation, including the following:

- transcranial direct current stimulation (tDCS) or
- transcranial magnetic stimulation (rTMS) or
- cranial electric stimulation (CES)

as a method of treating cancer-related pain.

The exclusion criteria were letters to the editor, reviews, and case reports.

An English language filter was applied. No time span was imposed. All articles from database inception to the time of research—January 2023—were included.

The titles and abstracts found in the search were evaluated if they met the inclusion criteria. Duplicate records were automatically removed. Relevant articles were retrieved in the full text and read. A manual search was also performed on the reference lists of articles included in this study. The flow diagram is shown in Figure 1. This narrative review followed the recommendations proposed by Green on how to write narrative reviews for peer-review journals [22].

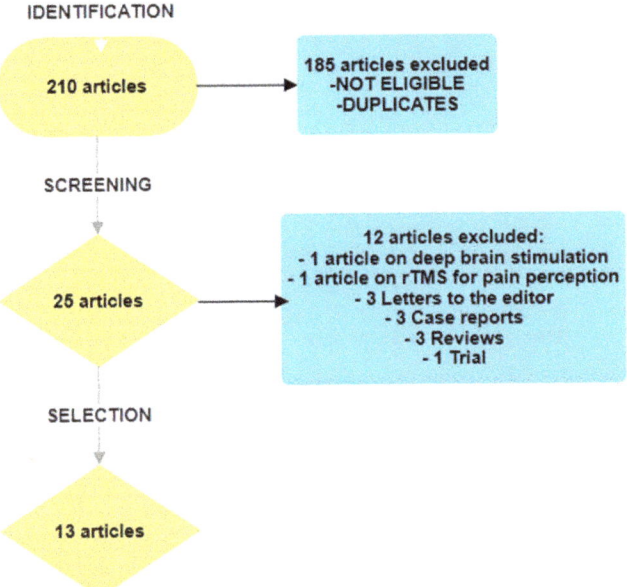

Figure 1. Flow chart of article selection.

Articles that presented clinical trials were examined through the lens of the IMMPACT recommendations [23]. The domains of interest were as follows: (1) pain scoring on an 11-point scale, (2) physical functioning using the Brief Pain Inventory, (3) emotional functioning using Beck Depression Inventory or equal, (4) participant ratings of improvement and satisfaction with treatment, (5) reporting of adverse events, and (6) participant disposition (e.g., adherence to the treatment regimen and reasons for premature withdrawal from the trial). These six items were searched for in each article and if found, each was given one point. A maximum of six points was possible. The scores that each paper received can be found in Tables 1–3.

Table 1. Studies of rTMS in the management of cancer-related pain.

First author Country of origin Year of publication	Khedr [24] Egipt 2015	Khedr [25] Egipt 2015	Goto [26] Japan 2020	Tang [27] China 2022
Type of study	Randomized clinical trial.	Preliminary randomized trial.	Pilot randomized controlled, single-blind, four-way crossover study.	Randomized double-blind, parallel-group, sham-controlled, clinical trial.
IMMPACT Recommendations Score	4/6	4/6	3/6	4/6
Type of pain	Neuropathic pain with a score ≥ 4 on the Douleur Neuropathique 4 questionnaire.	Visceral pain.	Neuropathic pain with a minimum grade 2 severity based on the National Cancer Institute Common Terminology Criteria for Adverse Events (NCI-CTCAE, version 4.0) scale.	Lung cancer pain.
Inclusion criteria	• Age: 18–65 years; • Malignant neuropathic pain resistant to medical treatments for at least 2 months.	• Age: 18–65 years; • Malignant visceral pain resistant to medical treatment for at least 2 months or associated with significant adverse effect from medication.	• Age: >20 years; • Any stage of cancer; • Patients with a confirmed treatment plan consisting of taxane-based or oxaliplatin based chemotherapy; • Neuropathic pain and/or peripheral sensory neuropathy; • A performance status of Karnofsky 80%; • 30 mm score in VAS of pain or dysesthesia intensity.	• Age: 18–70 years; • Confirmed diagnosis of advanced NSCLC by pathology or cytology; • Pain symptoms and confirmed as cancer pain by oncologist; • Experienced worst pain score ≥ 4 on NRS at the site of pain; • Clear awareness and could cooperate to evaluate pain severity; • Estimated that the survival time is more than 3 months; • Completion of signed informed consents and voluntary participation in this study.
Exclusion criteria	• Intracranial metallic devices, pacemakers, or other devices; • Recent myocardial ischaemia, unstable angina; • History of epilepsy.	• Intracranial metallic devices, pacemakers, or other devices; • Extensive myocardial ischaemia, unstable angina; • Epilepsy.	• Implanted devices; • History of seizures; • Metal implants in the head; • Higher brain dysfunction; • Severe depression (>41 scores of the Beck Depression Inventory).	• Brain tumour patients; • History of seizure; • Implanted pacemaker, stent, and other metal substances; • Acute pain anywhere in the body due to other diseases; • Serious psychiatric diagnoses (e.g., psychosis).
Period of study	January 2010–May 2013	January 2010–January 2012	April 2015–October 2016	January 2020–March 2021
Study patients	Intervention group Control group	Intervention group Control group	Pilot study, no control group	Intervention group Control group

200

Table 1. *Cont.*

Initial number of patients	17	17	17	11	21	21
Final number of patients	15	15	15	11	20	19
Losses (no/%)	2 (11.7%)	2 (11.7%)	2 (11.7%)	0	1 (4.7%)	2 (9.5%)
Age (years) mean ± SD	47 ± 9.2	48 ± 9.7	51 ± 9.7	57.8 ± 3.9	64.8 ± 7.8	58.5 ± 8.9	59.6 ± 7.7
Gender Male Female	1 16	2 15	10 7	8 9	0 11	12 8	10 9
Duration of disease (months)	15.4 ± 15.9	16.8 ± 16.3	15 ± 19.6	12.3 ± 14.9	Unknown	Unknown
Oncologic Pathology/Cancer (no patients)	Post mastectomy 14 Soft tissue sarcoma 1 Giant cell glioma 1 Femoral mass 1	Post mastectomy 15 Soft tissue sarcoma 2	Pancreas 4 Hepatic 7 Gall bladder 2 Stomach 1 NH lymphoma 1 Peritoneal mesothelioma 1	Pancreas 5 Hepatic 6 Gall Bladder 2 Stomach 2 Oesophagus 1 NH lymphoma 1	Breast 9 Gynecologic 2	Lung cancer 42
Treatment analgesic	Tramadol 100 mg bid Pregabalin 75 mg bid Gabapentin 400 mg bid Amitriptyline 25 mg bid	Tramadol 100 mg bid Pregabalin 75 mg bid Gabapentin 400 mg bid Amitriptyline 25 mg bid	Tramadol 100 mg bid Scopolamina 20 mg tid Amitriptilina 25 mg bid	Tramadol 100 mg bid Scopolamina 20 mg tid Amitriptilina 25 mg bid	Unknown	Morphine sulfate controlled-release tablets or oxycodone hydrochloride sustained-release tablets

Table 1. Cont.

STIMULATION DETAILS	Target/Coil type/Orientation/Stimulation Frequency/Intensity/Time	Contralateral to pain M1 hand; F8 coil/AP; 20 Hz (10 s, 10 trains, with intertrain interval 30 s); 80% RMT; 10 min.	Contralateral side of pain M1 hand or dominant hemisphere for epigastric pain; F8 coil/AP; 20 Hz (10 s, 10 trains, with intertrain of 30 s); 80% RMT; 10 min.	5 Hz, 10 s, 10 trains, with intertrain of 50 s, F8 coil; Stimulation types: 1. PA 90%: PA coil direction with 90% RMT target M1 stimulation, 2. PA 100%: PA coil direction with 100% RMT target M1 stimulation, 3. Ipsilateral PA 90%: PA coil direction with 90% RMT stimulation ipsilateral to the target M1 (if the target M1 was "the right-hand area", then ipsilateral target M1 was "the right leg area"), 4. LM 90%: LM coil direction with 90% RMT target M1 stimulation.	DLPFC left side; F8 coil; 10 Hz (15 pulse trains (1.5 s), with intertrain of 3 s); 80% RMT.
	No of pulses/sessions No of sessions	2000 pulses; 10 sessions; daily; 2 weeks.	2000 pulses; 10 session; daily; 2 weeks.	500 pulses; 4 sessions in 2 months.	1500 pulses; 15 sessions; daily; 3 weeks.
	Endpoints	Primary VAS after 10th session and 1 month later; Secondary VDS, LANSS, and HAM-D after 10th session and 1 month later.	Primary VAS after 10th session and 1 month later; Secondary VDS and HAM-D after 10th session and 1 month later; Serum Dynorphin.	P-VAS; SF-MPQ2; D-VAS.	NRS; OME, Quality of life; HAM-A; HAM-D.
	Adverse events	No	No	No	two patients with transient scalp numbness or facial muscle twitching

Table 1. *Cont.*

Results	• Reduction in pain score at the end of rTMS protocol (49% on VRS and 36.7% on VAS).
	• Effect maintained for 2 weeks with reduction (45.6% on VRS and 35.5% on VAS) but not at 1 month.
	• Reduction in LANNS score at the end of rTMS protocol—21.9% and at 2 weeks—20.9%.
	• Reduction in HAM-D at the end of rTMS protocol—24.4% and at 2 weeks—23.6%.
	• Percentage of pain relief in the VAS scale; the number of responders (30% or more pain relief) were 13 (86.6%), 12 (80%), and 4 (26.6%) at the three time points of assessment in the real group.
		• Pain relief in malignant visceral pain for at least 15 days, with reduction in pain score at the end of rTMS protocol (35.6% on VRS and 30% on VAS) and at 2 weeks after the last session (39.7% on VRS and 26% on VAS). The effect is not maintained at one month.
		• No significant differences in HAM-D.
		• Serum human Dyn level shows no significant difference between patients with visceral pain treated with real rTMS and sham rTMS.
			• Amelioration in pain or disesthesia mainly in the targeted extremity. At the target extremity:
			  – P-VAS scores significantly decreased after LM 90% ($p = 0.03$).
			  – D-VAS scores significantly decreased after PA 90% ($p = 0.03$) and LM 90% ($p = 0.04$).
			  – SF-MPQ2 score decreased significantly after PA 90% ($p = 0.01$).
			• At the three non target extremities:
			  – only D-VAS scores significantly decreased after PA 90% ($p = 0.047$).
				• Decrease in NRS in the treatment group starting from the 3rd day to the 3rd week (decrease of 41.09% in the rTMS group and 23.23% in the sham group).
				• On week 3, the OME in the rTMS group was similar to that of baseline ($p = 0.02$), while the sham group was significantly higher than that of baseline ($p = 0.02$). The physiology and psychology domains of WHOQOL-BREF scores showed significant improvements with rTMS group versus sham group ($p = 0.02$). HAM-A and HAMD scores in the rTMS group showed significant improvements after 3 weeks of treatment when compared with baseline ($p = 0.005$ and $p = 0.011$).

Abbreviations: rTMS, repetitive transcranial magnetic stimulation; NRS, numeric rating scale; VAS, visual analogue scale; VDS, verbal descriptor scale; SD, standard deviation; NSCLC, Non-Small Cell Lung Cancer; NHL, Non-Hodgkin Lymphoma; AP, antero-posterior; LM, lateral-medial; M1, motor cortex cortical area; RMT, resting motor threshold; DLPFC, dorsolateral prefrontal cortex; HAM-A, Hamilton anxiety rating scale; HAM-D, Hamilton depression rating scale; P-VAS, pain visual analogue scale; LANSS, Leeds assessment of neuropathic symptoms and signs; OME, oral morphine equivalent; SF-MPQ2, Short-form McGill Pain Questionnaire 2; D-VAS, Dysesthesia visual analogue scale; WHOQOL-BREF, World Health Organization Quality of Life-BREF.

Table 2. Randomized studies of tDCS in the management of cancer-related pain.

First author Country of origin Year of publication	Ibrahim [28] Egipt 2018	Stamenkovic [29] Serbia 2020	Hanna [30] Egipt 2022
Type of study	Prospective, randomized, double-blind sham-controlled.	Prospective, randomized, double-blind sham-controlled.	Prospective, randomized, sham-controlled.
IMMPACT Recommendations Score	4/6	4/6	3/6
Type of pain	HCC; Chronic abdominal/visceral pain.	Lung cancer; Acute pain post thoracotomy.	Post mastectomy pain syndrome scored ≥ 4 in DN4.
Inclusion criteria	• Age: >18 years; • Chronic abdominal pain due to primary liver cancer or on top of cirrhosis that was resistant to medical treatment for at least 2 months or associated with significant adverse effects from medication.	• Age: 18–80 years; • Willingness to participate; • Ability to understand the protocol and provide written informed consent; • Scheduled thoracotomy for confirmed primary malignant lung disease and planned tracheal extubation in the operating room immediately after surgery.	• Age: 25–69 years; • Females with unilateral/single mastectomy, total mastectomy (with sentinel lymph node dissection), modified radical mastectomy (with axillary lymph node dissection), nipple-sparing mastectomy (with either sentinel or axillary lymph node dissection), and skin-sparing mastectomy; • No or mild lymphedema; • Female patients with PMPS; • Presence of neuropathic pain post mastectomy surgery by DN4 questionnaire; • Patients with neuropathic pain that lasted for 6 months or more.

Table 2. Cont.

Exclusion criteria	• History of chronic pain syndrome; • Intracranial metallic devices or with cardiac pacemakers; • Extensive myocardial ischemia; • History of epilepsy.		• Pregnancy; • Treatment for neurological or psychiatric diseases; • Any chronic pain condition; • History of alcohol or drug abuse; • Chemotherapy; • History of previous thoracic or cardiac surgery; • Allergy to medications used in the study; • Presence of pacemaker, automatic implantable cardioverter/defibrillator, or any other implanted device in the head, spinal cord, or peripheral nerves; • Confirmed brain lesion, including tumour or metastasis.		• Epilepsy or a history of epilepsy or epileptic drugs; • Intake; • Medical diagnoses of psychological or neurological disorders; • History of migraines; • Scalp or skin condition (e.g., psoriasis or eczema); • Metalic implants, including intracranial electrodes, surgical clips, shrapnel, or a pacemaker, or any metallic accessories or cloth; • Head injury resulting in a loss of consciousness that has required further investigation (e.g., a brain scan); • Seizure; • Chance of pregnancy and patients on contraceptive pills; • Moderate or severe lymphedema.	
Period of study	April 2015 to February 2016		15 June 2016 to 27 March 2018.		Unknown	
Study patients	Intervention group	Control group	Intervention group	Control group	Intervention grpup	Control group
Initial number of patients	24	24	30	31	20	18
Final number of patients	20	20	27	28	15	15
Losses (no/%)	4 (16%)	4 (16%)	3 (10%)	3 (9.6%)	5 (20%)	3 (6%)
Age (years) mean ± SD	58.9 ± 5.6	56.85 ± 9.16	61.44 ± 7.98	61.89 ± 5.79	40.5 ± 2.8	40.2 ± 3.1
Gender						
Male	14	13	16	23	0	0
Female	6	7	11	5	15	15
Oncologic pathology	HCC		Lung cancer		Breast cancer	
Treatment analgesic	Tramadol hydrochloride 50 mg twice daily.		Unknown		Unknown	

Table 2. Cont.

Endpoints		VAS; VDS; HAM-D.	Morphine dose; VAS—pain rest, movement, and couch; VAS—anxiety; Beck depression inventory; PRO.	VAS; Beck depression inventory; ROM.
Stimulation details	Anode location	Primary motor cortex of the contralateral most painful abdominal area.	Left primary motor cortex.	Bilateral M1.
	Cathode location	Contralateral supraorbital region.	Contralateral supraorbital region.	Supraorbital region.
	Stimulation details	Duration: 10 sessions/2 weeks; Intensity: 2 mA; Duration of a session: 30 min; Device: neuroConn Germany.	Duration: 5 daily sessions; Intensity: 1.2 mA; Duration of a session: 20 min; Device: neuroelectrics.	Duration: 5 daily sessions; Intensity: 2 mA; Duration of a session: 20 min × 2 (20 min each side); Device: unknown.
Side effects		Slight burning sensation in three patients; Skin redness under the active electrode in two patients.	None declared.	None declared.
Outcome		• For the active stimulation group—reduction in VDS ($p = 0.001$) and VAS ($p = 0.001$) and HAM-D ($p = 0.012$); • The effect started from the 5th session and continued to 1 month after stimulation, while in the sham group, the effect persisted for 5 days only.	• Cumulative morphine dose in the first 120 h after surgery was significantly lower in the tDCS compared to sham group $p = 0.043$; • On postoperative day 5, VAS pain score with cough was significantly lower in the tDCS group ($p = 0.018$) and pain interference with cough was 80% lower ($p = 0.013$).	• In the stimulation group, there was a significant difference between pre- and post treatment mean values of: – Pain ($p = 0.001$). Pain decreased by 32% post treatment; – Depression index ($p = 0.003$): depression decreased by 3.7% post treatment; – Shoulder extension ($p = 0.002$): shoulder extension increased by 5.5% post treatment; – Shoulder flexion ($p = 0.001$): shoulder flexion increased by 4.8% post treatment.

Abbreviations: tDCS, transcranial direct current stimulation; HCC, hepatocellular carcinoma; VAS, visual analogue scale; VDS, verbal descriptor scale; PRO, patient-reported outcomes; HAM-D, Hamilton Depression Scale; Beck, Beck Depression Inventory; ROM, range of motion; PMPS, post mastectomy pain syndrome; DN4, Douleur Neuropathique 4 questionnaire; SD, standard deviation; M1, primary motor cortex area.

Table 3. Studies of CES in the management of cancer-related pain.

	Lyon [31]	Lyon [32]	Yennurajalingam [33]
First author	Lyon [31]	Lyon [32]	Yennurajalingam [33]
Country of origin	USA	USA	USA
Year of publication	2010	2015	2018
Type of study	Pilot feasibility study.	Randomized, sham-controlled trial.	Preliminary study, one group, open label.
IMMPACT Recommendation Score	4/6	4/6	4/6
Inclusion criteria	• Stage I-IIIA breast cancer; • Female; • Age 18 years or older; • Able to read and speak English; • Scheduled to receive at least four cycles of an anthracycline-containing chemotherapy regimen.	• Stage I-IIIA breast cancer; • Performance score ECOG < 2; • Scheduled to receive at least four cycles of adjuvant or neoadjuvant chemotherapy.	• Advanced cancer; • One or more of the four symptoms (depression, anxiety, sleep disturbance, and pain) with average intensity of ≥3/10 on the Edmonton Symptom Assessment Scale.
Exclusion criteria	• Major psychiatric conditions; • Treatment with antidepressants or anxiolytics; • Implanted devices (cardiac pacemakers).	• Previous chemotherapy; • Dementia; • Active psychosis; • History of seizure disorder; • Any implanted electrical device; • Began or changed a medication regimen for depression or other psychiatric condition within 30 days prior to study enrolment.	• Systemic anti-inflammatory medications; • Mental illness (schizophrenia, bipolar disorder); • Delirium (Memorial Delirium Assessment Scale (MDAS) score ≥ 7); • Participating in other structured behavioural intervention(s); • Pregnancy; • Presence of an implantable device (pacemaker); • Cancer of the head and/or neck or brain tumour or brain metastasis; • A history of seizure.
Stimulation details	Alpha-Stim Stress Control System Intensity: 100 µA; Frequency: 0.5 Hz; Duration: 60 min;	Alpha-Stim Stress Control System Intensity: 100 µA; Frequency: 0.5 Hz; Duration: 60 min;	Alpha-Stim M Intensity: 100 µA; Frequency: 0.5 Hz; Duration: 60 min;
Period of stimulation	Daily for 6–8 weeks depending on chemotherapy schedule.	Daily for the chemotherapy period and 2 weeks after; (6–32 weeks).	Daily for 4 weeks.

Table 3. Cont.

Outcomes	Feasability; HADS; BPI; BFI; GSDS.				ESAS; HADS; PSQI; BPI; MDAS; NCCN Distress Thermometer Safety.	
Groups	Active	Sham	Standard	Active	Sham	Not sham-controlled
Number of patients initially	13	36	36	84	83	36
Number of patients analyzed	10	10	12	77	75	33
Losses number (%)	0%	0%	0%	7 (8.33%)	8 (10.6%)	3 (8.33%)
Age (years) ± SD	47.54 ± 9.1	46.6 ± 5.64	50.5 ± 18.28	51.04 ± 1.21	51.91 ± 0.97	59
Results	<ul><li>Feasability of CES;</li><li>No significant data regarding symptom relief.</li></ul>			<ul><li>No benefit of CES on depression, anxiety, pain, fatigue, and sleep disturbances.</li></ul>		<ul><li>Feasible and safe;</li><li>Improvement in pain BPI pain ($p = 0.013$);</li><li>Improvement in PSQI daytime dysfunction ($p = 0.002$);</li><li>Improvment in ESAS anxiety ($p = 0.001$); ESAS depression ($p = 0.025$);</li><li>Improvement in HADS depression ($p = 0.024$).</li></ul>

Abbreviations: CES, cranial electric stimulation; HADS, Hospital Anxiety and Depression Scale; ECOG, Eastern Cooperative Oncology Group Performance Status; BPI, Brief Pain Inventory; BFI, Brief Fatigue Inventory; GSDS, General Sleep Disturbance Scale; ESAS, Edmonton Symptom Assessment Scale; PSQI, Pittsburgh Sleep Quality Index; MDAS, Memorial Delirium Assessment Scale.

3. Results and Discussions

In total, 210 articles were identified. After excluding duplicates and screening for eligibility based on the title and abstract, 25 articles were selected for full-text reading. Twelve articles were excluded; one treated deep brain stimulation [34] and one discussed rTMS as a method used to study pain perception [35]. Furthermore, the following articles were excluded: three letters to the editor, three case records, three reviews, and one trial that did not consider pain as a major endpoint. The flow diagram is presented in Figure 1.

The 13 articles included were divided according to the non-invasive brain stimulation method used in cancer patients.

- Transcranial magnetic stimulation (rTMS)—four articles
- Transcranial direct current stimulation (tDCS)—six articles
- Cranial electric stimulation (CES)—three articles

After a short overview of each technique, articles on the topic will be discussed.

3.1. Transcranial Magnetic Stimulation

3.1.1. Brief Technique Overview

Transcranial magnetic stimulation (TMS) was the first non-invasive brain stimulation used for research and therapeutic purposes. It uses the electric current produced by a dynamic magnetic field through electromagnetic induction. Single-pulse TMS was initially designed and used as a non-invasive method to study human pain perception [35], but its potential therapeutic role has rapidly surfaced. Repetitive TMS (rTMS) can induce long-lasting changes in brain activity. Based on this mechanism, it has been proven to be safe and well tolerated, as well as effective in numerous psychiatric and neurological conditions [17].

By enhancing neuroplasticity, rTMS has the ability to indirectly modulate central structures such as the cingulate, orbitofrontal, and prefrontal cortical regions that are implicated in pain processing [36], as well as in the pain–emotion connection [37]. It can also potentiate descending inhibitory pathways [19,38]. Another proposed mechanism is based on the effect of increasing endogenous opioids in the nervous system [39]. The implications of BDNF brain-derived neurotrophic factor (BDNF) have also been hypothesized [40].

Different sessions regarding intensity and length of time or type of impulses have been investigated from that period, and many trials have shown some benefits in chronic pain suppression [14]. The Cochrane review from 2018 indicates low and very low quality evidence for prefrontal rTMS, whereas motor cortex stimulation has been accepted as a potential method to reduce pain for short periods of time [14].

In neuropathic pain, it is considered that the damage to the peripheral nervous system implies a dysfunction in the somatosensory processing in the central nervous system [41]. rTMS has been shown to have a beneficial effect on neuropathic pain by modulating neural activity in the brain [14,42,43]. The main area of stimulation was considered the primary motor area, not the dorsolateral prefrontal cortex (DLPFC) [44]. The Cochrane systematic review and French recommendations concluded that only high-frequency stimulation (>5 Hz), with >500 stimuli and only multiple sessions, have beneficial results [14,45]. rTMS of the M1 (primary motor cortex area) contralateral to the pain side in neuropathic pain has been considered to be effective through stimulation with high frequency (>5 Hz), with level of evidence A, at a constant over the years [17,46]. A small response of rTMS to chronic pain was identified in the Cochrane review [14] with a 7% reduction in pain and quality of life. Moreover, the Latin American [15] consensus recommend level A for rTMS over M1 for fibromyalgia and neuropathic pain and level B for myofascial or musculoskeletal pain, complex regional pain, and migraine.

3.1.2. Begining of rTMS in Cancer Pain

The first cases of rTMS in cancer patients were described by a French team from Nantes. In each case [37,47] good response to rTMS for refractory cancer pain was recorded.

The effect was observed after a few days, with a reduction in pain, as well as a drastic reduction in analgesic drugs needed [47]. This technique has potential benefits for pain, mood, anxiety, and depression and is considered by the authors as a possible adjuvant method in the context of multidisciplinary management of palliative care [37].

3.1.3. Studies Using rTMS for Cancer Pain Treatment

Four studies focusing on rTMS and cancer pain were identified (Table 1), three clinical trials [24,25,27], and one pilot study [26]. All trials received a score of four based on the IMMPACT recommendations, whereas the pilot study gathered three points.

Two studies investigated neuropathic pain [24,26], and one focused on visceral pain [25]. All four studies used the visual analogue scale (VAS) or numerical rating scale (NRS) to evaluate pain intensity. The population analyzed in this study was diverse. The first Egyptian study [24] mostly included women with neuropathic pain after mastectomy. All patients were undergoing active oncologic treatment, either chemotherapy or radiotherapy. A Japanese study [26] also investigated neuropathic pain in women, but they included patients with neuropathic pain and/or peripheral sensory neuropathy who received a chemotherapy regimen based on taxane or oxaliplatin. It is worth mentioning the different inclusion criteria for pain evaluation. The first study [24] used the DN4 score (Douleur Neuropathique 4) and included patients with a questionnaire score equal to or greater than four who were resistant to treatment for at least two months. Goto [26] defined neuropathic pain as a minimum grade 2 severity based on the National Cancer Institute Common Terminology Criteria for Adverse Events (NCI-CTCAE, version 4.0) scale. In their study, they used a combination of patient-reported symptoms and clinical assessment to select participants with chemotherapy-induced peripheral neuropathy (CIPN). One year after their previous study, the same Egyptian team published a new study [25] using the same procedure but focusing on malignant visceral pain. They included diverse oncologic localizations. The pain investigated in all cases was localized in the upper abdomen (either the right or left hypochondrium or epigastrium) and was resistant to medical treatment for at least two months or associated with significant adverse effects from medication. The latest study [27] coming from China included only lung cancer patients, with cancer pain evaluated as equal to or greater than four on the NRS. The type of pain, whether neuropathic or nociceptive, was not mentioned.

Patients with intracranial metallic devices, other metallic implanted devices (e.g., pacemakers), a history of seizures, and severe cardiac or psychiatric conditions were not permitted to participate. The number of participants was modest, with Tang [27] having the maximum (39) number of patients, whereas Khedr included 30 patients in both his studies [24,25], and Goto analyzed only 11 patients [26]. The randomized sham-controlled studies had all well-balanced groups in terms of age, duration of illness, and initial pain evaluation score. Interestingly, all patients in the two Egyptian studies [24,25] were on the same analgesic medication.

The stimulation received was also different. Khedr [24,25] used in both of his studies 10 daily sessions of rTMS at 20 Hz, applied to the motor cortical area corresponding to the hand area in the painful side or the dominant hemisphere in the case of epigastric pain. Tang [27] used a different approach, positioning the F8 coil in the dorsolateral prefrontal cortex (DLPFC), providing 1500 pulses for 15 sessions in three weeks. Goto's pilot study [26] used four different types of stimulation, with differences in coil direction, intensity, and position, which they applied in random order to 11 patients, with one stimulation per week. A summary of the details regarding the stimulation is presented in Table 1.

The benefit was evaluated using the VAS or NRS as the principal endpoint. Moreover, the studies used the verbal descriptor scale (VDS), Hamilton scale for depression (HAD), Leeds assessment of neuropathic symptoms and signs (LANSS) [24], oral morphine equivalent (OME), quality of life [27], and McGill Pain Questionnaire 2 (SF-MPQ2) [26]. One study used blood samples to test for the level of serum human dynorphine [25].

The results of all four studies were positive. The first randomized clinical trial [24] reported the benefit of rTMS based on the VAS score but also on the decrease in medication in the treated group compared to the control group. As shown in other studies on non-cancer pain, the effect on pain appeared after several sessions and maintained some effect after the end of stimulation but was not present at the one month follow up. Interestingly, at one month, the reduction in the HAD and LANSS scores was still significant. It should be noted that participants reported no side effects. Regarding the curves depicting the effect of stimulation vs. sham, it is interesting to see that even the sham group had some benefit, with a decrease in scores. In addition, none of the scores returned to the baseline value in either group [24].

The second randomized trial [25] showed statistical significance in the primary outcome, measured using the VAS. The effect appeared after the fifth stimulation, had a maximum effect after the 10th stimulation, lasted for 15 days, and was absent at the 1-month evaluation. However, the sham group showed some improvement in the VAS and VDS scores. The HAM-D evaluation showed no significant differences between the groups over time in this study population [25].

The third study [26], published in 2020 in the *Journal of Clinical Neuroscience* by a Japanese team, was a randomized pilot trial. Their results are encouraging and demonstrate the potential of rTMS as a treatment for chemotherapy-induced neuropathy, both for pain and dysesthesia. They used different coil orientation angles and found a positive effect in both the postero-anterior (PA) 90% intensity and the lateral-medial (LM) 90% intensity orientation but not in the PA 100% or PA 90% ipsilateral. They showed an amelioration in pain or dysesthesia, mainly in the targeted extremity, and limited modification only on the D-VAS for the non-targeted extremities [26]. Being designed as a pilot trial, it left some unanswered questions. The study was complex, with pain assessment of all four extremities, but it did not provide a concise definition of dysesthesia and how patients define it. They performed a randomized trial with randomization of stimulation sessions rather than of patients. One of the drawbacks is that they did not have a control group, and the meaning for stimulation randomization was not very explicit. It must be noted that the stimulation frequency was lower than that in other studies. In addition, they provided no clear explanation as to why the two other types of coil positioning did not provide any benefit.

The most recent trial was based In China and published in 2022 [27]. Their main endpoint was a decreased pain score, which was achieved with a statistical decrease in NRS in the treatment group from the third day to the third week. Similar to previous studies [24,25], the sham group also showed a decrease in the pain score. Somewhat different from the other two trials, there was no follow-up after the end of stimulation. Secondary endpoints (oral morphine equivalent dose, quality of life, depression, and anxiety) also improved after rTMS. As predicted by Nizard [37], this technique also showed a beneficial role in mood changes, with amelioration in anxiety and depressive symptoms. This is the first study to report unpleasantness, such as scalp numbness or facial muscle twitching in two patients from the rTMS group [27].

3.1.4. Conclusion Regarding rTMS in Cancer Pain

The results are encouraging, with rTMS providing benefits for pain suppression in patients with cancer. This is supported by a recent meta-analysis [21] that included two of the rTMS trials [25,27]. They showed a better effect on pain with rTMS compared to CES and tDCS, but this could be attributed to the fact that tDCS and CES have been represented with only one trial. More data are required to clearly state the role of rTMS in this category of patients. Data on the effectiveness of rTMS on neuropathic pain will hopefully come in the coming years from Colombian and Hong Kong researchers, where clinical trials are open ([NCT05480410] and [NCT04107272]).

3.2. Transcranial Direct Current Stimulation—tDCS

3.2.1. Brief Technique Overview

Transcranial direct current stimulation is another type of non-invasive brain stimulation that uses a low-voltage electric current (maximum of 3 mA). The current is produced by a small device that operates on a battery. It is delivered to the scalp using sponge electrodes. It is safe and easy to use [48].

This technique can be used to modulate neural activity. The current is not powerful enough to produce an action potential but influences the neuronal membrane potential [49]. It has the ability to induce immediate effects with anodal stimulation depolarizing membranes and increasing cortical excitability, whereas cathodal stimulation hyperpolarizes membranes and decreases cortical excitability [49].

New studies have shown that current flows through both outer and inner cortical structures [50]. Motor cortex stimulation has the capacity to modulate the activity of other regions, such as the thalamus, ventrolateral thalamus, insula, anterior cingulate gyrus, and upper brainstem [38,51]. Other mechanisms include endogenous opioid release [38] or activation of the u-opioid system [52].

Studies have proven the efficacy of tDCS in chronic pain [16,53]. The 2018 Cochrane review included 27 studies and 747 patients with chronic pain and found a 0.82 reduction that translates to a 17% reduction in pain in the intervention group. Through a meta-analysis, they reported a positive effect of tDCS on quality of life [14]. The Latin American consensus reviewed 24 tDCS studies and provided the following recommendations: level A for anodal tDCs over M1 in fibromyalgia and level B for neuropathic pain, abdominal pain, and migraine [15]. These recommendations were once again proven in a meta-analysis in 2021 [16]. None of the mentioned guidelines and reviews included studies on chronic pain in patients with cancer.

3.2.2. First Data on tDCS Efficacy in Cancer Pain

There are two published case studies [54,55] using tDCS in cancer patients as a last resort in the treatment of excruciating pain. The first case dates back to 2006 and shows the benefits of tDCS in a patient with pancreatic cancer [54]. A second complex case of bladder cancer with bone metastases had an incredible response to daily stimulation for 20 min with a 1 mA intensity for five consecutive days [55]. Based on their experience, the French team of Nguyen has opened a trial in two hospitals in Nantes, investigating the impact of tDCS on cancer pain in a randomized fashion [56].

3.2.3. Studies on tDCS and Cancer Pain

A database search identified seven studies comprising two pilot studies, one proof-of-concept study, and four randomized clinical trials.

One randomized trial focused primarily on the effect of one tDCS session on cancer-induced nausea and vomiting (CINV), while pain was just one symptom assessed using the Edmonton Symptom Assessment Scale. Their results showed no differences in pain scores between the groups. The lack of benefit was explained by the need for a cumulative effect of brain stimulation on pain impact [57]. This trial is not included in the following discussion.

The first randomized placebo-controlled trial using tDCS for visceral pain was designed in Germany. Finally, it was reported as a pilot study and presented as an abstract in the 2012 World Research Congress of the European Association for Palliative Care [58]. They showed promising results; however, considering the low number of patients, no conclusions were provided.

The second pilot study was conducted by a team from Michigan, USA. Feasibility and safety of tDCS for pain management in patients undergoing chemoradiotherapy for advanced head and neck cancer was researched. A comparison of the five patients in the historical control group showed less weight loss and less dysphagia in the tDCS group. This is the first study to combine tDCS with EEG recording simultaneously [51].

The team continued their work, optimized the protocol, and published in 2022 a proof-of-concept study on two patients with head and neck cancer undergoing radio-chemotherapy [59]. In this study, they used novel devices with remote tDCS, as well as functional near-infrared spectroscopy and EEG. A strict protocol, with multiple visits, clinical measurements, questionnaires, and two neuroimaging techniques, was used to provide the maximum amount of information. With a very well-described method, this study presents a unique type of pain assessment, with both hemodynamic and neurophysiologic input, with data on connections between the bilateral prefrontal and sensory cortices. Imaging revealed a decrease in functional connections between the bilateral prefrontal cortex and sensory cortex, as well as activation of the right prefrontal cortex. With this, they provided further proof that the dorsal lateral prefrontal cortex plays a role in pain perception. Even if just a proof-of-concept study, the study of pain assessment using modern technologies provides a new and optimistic perspective on pain understanding.

Three randomized clinical trials were identified and discussed. Details, as well as the IMMPACT recommendation score, can be found in Table 2. Two of the trials [28,29] have a score of four, while Hanna's article [30] received three points.

The types of pain analyzed in the three randomized trials were diverse, ranging from chronic visceral pain in hepatocellular carcinoma [28] and acute post thoracotomy thoracic pain [29] to neuropathic post mastectomy pain syndrome [30]. The first two trials [28,29] included mostly men, whereas the last trial included only female patients [30]. Chronic pain was defined as pain resistant to medical treatment for at least two months or associated with significant adverse effects, ref. [28], or six months of neuropathic pain in the post mastectomy region, with a DN score of >4 [30]. In the Serbian trial [29], only acute pain was considered, and patients with chronic pain conditions were excluded. The size of the study population was limited, even though the Serbian trial [29] had the largest number of patients (55). Ibrahim [28] and Hanna [30] included 40 and 30 patients, respectively. As an endpoint, the VAS was maintained as the principal measurement of pain relief. Furthermore, the studies reported results based on the VDS, HAM-D, Beck Depression Inventory, morphine dose [29], and measurements of shoulder range of motion using a digital goniometer [30].

The stimulation technique involved placing the anode in the area of the primary motor cortex of the contralateral most painful abdominal area for 30 min, over ten sessions, at 2 mA [28], or the left primary motor cortex for 20 min, over five sessions, at 1.2 mA [29], or was performed bilaterally on M1 for 20 min, over five sessions, at 2 mA [30]. The cathode is usually placed in the contralateral supraorbital region [28,29] or in the ipsilateral supraorbital region [30]. More data are presented in Table 2.

The reported results were encouraging. The Egyptian team of Kehr, in addition to TMS, also took an interest in transcranial direct current stimulation [28]. A very clear and concise results section showed an improvement in pain evaluation as a primary objective but also in the depression score as a secondary outcome for both the active treatment and the sham technique. The effect was seen in both groups starting with the fifth stimulation and lasting to the tenth and then to the one month evaluation, without ever returning to the starting base value. This was valid for both the sham and active groups, with a greater effect in the tDCS group. The difference between the sham and real groups became significant at the fifth evaluation; its maximum was seen on the 10th day of stimulation and remained significant after one month for the VDS and VAS. The effect did not last in the sham group at the last evaluation at one month. For the Hamilton rating scale for depression, a similar effect was observed, but its statistical significance was lower. They reported five mild side effects in terms of skin redness and local burning sensation.

In the Serbian trial [29] performed on patients with lung cancer who underwent thoracotomy, the effect of tDCS combined with morphine was analyzed. A complex pain management protocol for the trial should be complemented because of its rigorousness. Data analyzed from 55 patients who received more than three tDCS stimulations showed that the dose of morphine administered was lower in the active tDCS group. This effect was stronger after the second tDCS session. They proved that tDCS can decrease the total amount of morphine used. As a secondary objective, VAS pain scores were evaluated at specific time points: during rest, in cough, and during movement. The results showed that for the tDCS group, there was a decrease in VAS score with cough. No complications were noted due to the transcranial stimulation procedure. Interestingly, no differences between groups were noted regarding anxiety, mood, depression, or patient-related outcomes, somehow in discordance with studies on chronic pain [29].

The latest [30] randomized trial published in February 2023 came from Egypt and showed a statistical decrease in pain, as well as in the depression score in the group that received stimulation, pre vs. post treatment. Focusing on range of motion, shoulder flexion and extension increased by 4.8% and 5.5%, respectively, in the active stimulation group. Patients were evaluated before the first stimulation and after the last stimulation session, with no further follow-up. This is the only trial that used bilateral cranial stimulation, irrespective of the side of the pain.

3.2.4. Conclusion Regarding tDCS in Cancer Pain

Considering the diversity of pain mechanisms and pathologies, the limited number of patients, and different stimulation parameters, no conclusion can be drawn regarding the efficacy of tDCS in cancer pain. This method is of major interest and is currently under research in this category of patients in a randomized controlled trial, STIMPAL [56], as well as in a Painless PanEuropean Horizon project [60]. A trial of tDCS involving survivors of pediatric bone sarcoma with chronic pain is also underway [NCT05746429]. Future data on better-represented cohorts will provide further information on the role of tDCS in cancer patients.

3.3. Cranial Electrical Stimulation

3.3.1. Brief Technique Overview

Cranial electrical stimulation is another method of neuromodulation. It uses a pulsed current stimulation technique that modifies alpha and beta wave frequencies, increasing the concentration of neurotransmitters, thus having potential neuroplastic and cognitive effects. It does not polarize brain tissue but stimulates it in a rhythmic manner, with potential enhancement of the efficacy of endogenous neurophysiologic activity [32]. This method is recognized as a medical device that is used for the treatment of depression, anxiety, insomnia, and pain. These devices can deliver electrical stimulation through electrodes attached to earlobes. The intensity was <1 mA at 100 Hz. The Cochrane meta-analysis [14] included five studies using CES with 270 patients and showed no statistical effect of CES on pain.

3.3.2. Studies Using CES in Cancer Pain

Through the search, three studies of CES in cancer patients were identified: a prospective, three-group, randomized, double-blinded, longitudinal pilot feasibility study [31], a randomized sham-controlled trial [32], and a non-randomized feasibility study [33]. For further details, refer to Table 3. All three studies had an IMMPACT recommendation score of four. None of the studies discussed below were included in the Cochrane analysis, whereas the 2023 meta-analysis by Chien [21] included Lyon's study published in 2015 [32].

All three studies used the same Alpha-Stim Stress Control System and stimulation parameters. The first study [31] regarding CES dates back to 2010 and investigated the effect of CES on reducing the symptoms of depression, anxiety, fatigue, pain, and sleep disturbances. Their study was a randomized pilot feasibility trial applied to patients with breast cancer receiving chemotherapy. In the interest of concrete results, they used three groups: the active stimulation group, a sham group, and a group that received neither active nor sham. The period of usage was six or eight weeks depending on the timing of the chemotherapy protocols. The protocol was complex, using questionnaires and blood samples to test for inflammatory biomarkers. Their study showed that the method is feasible, as 72% of the eligible patients were enrolled. No adverse events were recorded and none of the participants reported stopping the procedure. The study showed that the devices and the method were safe and acceptable to patients. The results on anxiety, pain, depression, and fatigue were not statistically significant. Authors considered this to be due to the missing data and the disadvantages of the interactive voice response method used for data collection. No conclusion can be drawn from this study regarding the efficacy of CES for cancer pain [31].

The same American team continued their research on CES and published a new article in 2015 [32]. This protocol is somewhat related to the first protocol. They used the same questionnaires but only two groups: sham and active stimulation. Congruent with the first study, they found a certain level of symptoms in breast cancer patients, with fatigue and depression increasing over time. Pain and sleep disturbances fluctuated and anxiety levels decreased over time. Their results were non-significant. It was concluded that CES had no effect on the symptoms of patients with breast cancer during chemotherapy. Their explanation focused on the floor effect, as patients' symptoms were not severe enough to benefit from the intervention [32].

The most recent study on CES [33] was designed as a preliminary study to test the feasibility and efficacy of CES in patients with advanced cancer. The protocol included several questionnaires and saliva samples. The adherence rate was 92%, which revealed good feasibility. Their results showed a statistically significant difference in several symptoms, including pain after the four weeks use of CES. Overall, their results are promising, but the lack of a control group is a major limitation [33].

3.3.3. Conclusion Regarding CES in Cancer Pain

Congruent with the Cochrane meta-analysis [14] that examined non-oncologic patients, the studies discussed could not demonstrate the efficacy of CES in ameliorating pain in patients with cancer. Therefore, further studies are warranted. Currently, no trials involving CES in cancer patients are reported as open on clinicaltrials.gov. The impact of CES in this category of patients remains unknown.

4. Conclusions

Pain is a permanent challenge for oncologists, and new treatment options are constantly being researched. Non-invasive brain stimulation is a relatively new method of neuromodulation that has proven beneficial in relieving chronic pain. With few exceptions, trials regarding pain in patients with cancer were excluded from systematic reviews and guidelines. The role of NIBS in the management of pain in cancer patients remains undefined. There is a paucity of data, with only a handful of studies for each technique, using a limited number of patients and different stimulation parameters. This diversity makes it difficult for medical specialists to assess the potential benefits of NIBS and to integrate them into the therapeutic management of cancer pain. There is an urgent need for more data regarding non-invasive brain neuromodulation techniques in patients with cancer.

Supplementary Materials: The following supporting information can be downloaded at: https://www.mdpi.com/article/10.3390/medicina59111957/s1, Table S1: Major databases search strategies.

Author Contributions: Conceptualization, V.-F.C. and D.-V.M.; methodology, V.-F.C.; resources, V.-F.C., D.C. and D.-V.M.; data curation, V.-F.C.; writing—original draft preparation, V. F.C.; writing—review and editing, V.-F.C., D.C. and D.-V.M.; supervision, D.C. and D.-V.M. All authors have read and agreed to the published version of the manuscript.

Funding: The article processing charge was funded by Transilvania University, Brașov, Romania.

Institutional Review Board Statement: Not applicable.

Informed Consent Statement: Not applicable.

Conflicts of Interest: The authors declare no conflict of interest.

References

1. van den Beuken-van Everdingen, M.H.J.; Hochstenbach, L.M.J.; Joosten, E.A.J.; Tjan-Heijnen, V.C.G.; Janssen, D.J.A. Update on Prevalence of Pain in Patients with Cancer: Systematic Review and Meta-Analysis. *J. Pain Symptom Manag.* **2016**, *51*, 1070–1090.e9. [CrossRef]
2. WHO. *Guidelines for the Pharmacological and Radiotherapeutic Management of Cancer Pain in Adults and Adolescents*; World Health Organization: Geneva, Switzerland, 2018.

3. Smith, T.J.; O'Neil, J. Fundamentals of Cancer Pain Management. In *Supportive Cancer Care*; Springer: Cham, Switzerland, 2016; pp. 111–126. [CrossRef]
4. Meldrum, M. The ladder and the clock: Cancer pain and public policy at the end of the twentieth century. *J. Pain Symptom Manag.* **2005**, *29*, 41–54. [CrossRef] [PubMed]
5. Mamdani, H.; Matosevic, S.; Khalid, A.B.; Durm, G.; Jalal, S.I. Immunotherapy in Lung Cancer: Current Landscape and Future Directions. *Front. Immunol.* **2022**, *13*, 823618. [CrossRef] [PubMed]
6. Greco, M.T.; Roberto, A.; Corli, O.; Deandrea, S.; Bandieri, E.; Cavuto, S.; Apolone, G. Quality of Cancer Pain Management: An Update of a Systematic Review of Undertreatment of Patients with Cancer. *J. Clin. Oncol.* **2014**, *32*, 4149–4154. [CrossRef]
7. Wiffen, P.J.; Wee, B.; Derry, S.; Bell, R.F.; Moore, R.A. Opioids for cancer pain—An overview of Cochrane reviews. *Cochrane Database Syst. Rev.* **2017**, *7*, CD012592. [CrossRef] [PubMed]
8. Corli, O.; Floriani, I.; Roberto, A.; Montanari, M.; Galli, F.; Greco, M.T.; Caraceni, A.; Kaasa, S.; Dragani, T.A.; Azzarello, G.; et al. Are strong opioids equally effective and safe in the treatment of chronic cancer pain? A multicenter randomized phase IV 'real life' trial on the variability of response to opioids. *Ann. Oncol.* **2016**, *27*, 1107–1115. [CrossRef]
9. Bruera, E.; Paice, J.A. Cancer pain management: Safe and effective use of opioids. *Am. Soc. Clin. Oncol. Educ. Book* **2015**, *35*, e593–e599. [CrossRef] [PubMed]
10. Raja, S.N.; Carr, D.B.; Cohen, M.; Finnerup, N.B.; Flor, H.; Gibson, S.; Keefe, F.J.; Mogil, J.S.; Ringkamp, M.; Sluka, K.A.; et al. The revised International Association for the Study of Pain definition of pain: Concepts, challenges, and compromises. *Pain* **2020**, *161*, 1976–1982. [CrossRef]
11. Puretić, M.B.; Demarin, V. Neuroplasticity mechanisms in the pathophysiology of chronic pain. *Acta Clin. Croat.* **2012**, *51*, 425–429. [PubMed]
12. Prinsloo, S.; Gabel, S.; Lyle, R.; Cohen, L. Neuromodulation of cancer pain. *Integr. Cancer Ther.* **2013**, *13*, 30–37. [CrossRef]
13. International Neuromodulation Society [Internet]. Available online: https://www.neuromodulation.com./about-neuromodulation (accessed on 9 July 2023).
14. O'Connell, N.E.; Wand, B.M.; Marston, L.; Spencer, S.; DeSouza, L.H. Non-invasive brain stimulation techniques for chronic pain. *Cochrane Database Syst. Rev.* **2018**, *4*, CD008208. [CrossRef]
15. Baptista, A.F.; Fernandes, A.M.B.; Sá, K.N.; Okano, A.H.; Brunoni, A.R.; Lara-Solares, A.; Iskandar, A.J.; Guerrero, C.; Amescua-García, C.; Kraychete, D.C.; et al. Latin American and Caribbean consensus on noninvasive central nervous system neuromodulation for chronic pain management (LAC2-NIN-CP). *Pain Rep.* **2019**, *4*, e692. [CrossRef]
16. Fregni, F.; El-Hagrassy, M.M.; Pacheco-Barrios, K.; Carvalho, S.; Leite, J.; Simis, M.; Brunelin, J.; Nakamura-Palacios, E.M.; Marangolo, P.; Venkatasubramanian, G.; et al. Evidence-Based Guidelines and Secondary Meta-Analysis for the Use of Transcranial Direct Current Stimulation in Neurological and Psychiatric Disorders. *Int. J. Neuropsychopharmacol.* **2020**, *24*, 256–313. [CrossRef]
17. Lefaucheur, J.-P.; Aleman, A.; Baeken, C.; Benninger, D.H.; Brunelin, J.; Di Lazzaro, V.; Filipović, S.R.; Grefkes, C.; Hasan, A.; Hummel, F.C.; et al. Evidence-based guidelines on the therapeutic use of repetitive transcranial magnetic stimulation (rTMS): An update (2014–2018). *Clin. Neurophysiol.* **2020**, *131*, 474–528. [CrossRef] [PubMed]
18. Wang, M.; Yin, Y.; Yang, H.; Pei, Z.; Molassiotis, A. Evaluating the safety, feasibility, and efficacy of non-invasive neuromodulation techniques in chemotherapy-induced peripheral neuropathy: A systematic review. *Eur. J. Oncol. Nurs.* **2022**, *58*, 102124. [CrossRef]
19. Kahan, B. Cancer pain and current theory for pain control. *Phys. Med. Rehabil. Clin. N. Am.* **2014**, *25*, 439–456. [CrossRef]
20. Chwistek, M. Recent advances in understanding and managing cancer pain. *F1000Research* **2017**, *6*, 945. [CrossRef]
21. Chien, Y.-J.; Chang, C.-Y.; Wu, M.-Y.; Wu, H.-C.; Horng, Y.-S. Noninvasive Brain Stimulation for Cancer Pain Management in Nonbrain Malignancy: A Meta-Analysis. *Eur. J. Cancer Care* **2023**, *2023*, 5612061. [CrossRef]
22. Green, B.N.; Johnson, C.D.; Adams, A. Writing narrative literature reviews for peer-reviewed journals: Secrets of the trade. *J. Chiropr. Med.* **2006**, *5*, 101–117. [CrossRef] [PubMed]
23. Turk, D.C.; Dworkin, R.H.; Burke, L.B.; Gershon, R.; Rothman, M.; Scott, J.; Allen, R.R.; Atkinson, H.J.; Chandler, J.; Cleeland, C.; et al. Developing patient-reported outcome measures for pain clinical trials: IMMPACT recommendations. *Pain* **2006**, *125*, 208–215. [CrossRef]
24. Khedr, E.; Kotb, H.; Mostafa, M.; Mohamad, M.; Amr, S.; Ahmed, M.; Karim, A.; Kamal, S. Repetitive transcranial magnetic stimulation in neuropathic pain secondary to malignancy: A randomized clinical trial. *Eur. J. Pain* **2014**, *19*, 519–527. [CrossRef]
25. Khedr, E.M.; Mostafa, M.G.; Kotb, H.I.; Mohamad, M.F.; Bakry, R.; Kamal, S.M.M. Effect of Repetitive Transcranial Magnetic Stimulation on Malignant Visceral Pain. *Neuroenterology* **2015**, *3*, 1–8. [CrossRef]
26. Goto, Y.; Hosomi, K.; Shimokawa, T.; Shimizu, T.; Yoshino, K.; Kim, S.J.; Mano, T.; Kishima, H.; Saitoh, Y. Pilot study of repetitive transcranial magnetic stimulation in patients with chemotherapy-induced peripheral neuropathy. *J. Clin. Neurosci.* **2020**, *73*, 101–107. [CrossRef] [PubMed]
27. Tang, Y.; Chen, H.; Zhou, Y.; Tan, M.-L.; Xiong, S.-L.; Li, Y.; Ji, X.-H.; Li, Y.-S. Analgesic Effects of Repetitive Transcranial Magnetic Stimulation in Patients with Advanced Non-Small-Cell Lung Cancer: A Randomized, Sham-Controlled, Pilot Study. *Front. Oncol.* **2022**, *12*, 840855. [CrossRef] [PubMed]
28. Ibrahim, N.M.; Abdelhameed, K.M.; Kamal, S.M.M.; Khedr, E.M.H.; Kotb, H.I.M. Effect of Transcranial Direct Current Stimulation of the Motor Cortex on Visceral Pain in Patients with Hepatocellular Carcinoma. *Pain Med.* **2017**, *19*, 550–560. [CrossRef] [PubMed]

29. Stamenkovic, D.M.; Mladenovic, K.; Rancic, N.; Cvijanovic, V.; Maric, N.; Neskovic, V.; Zeba, S.; Karanikolas, M.; Ilic, T.V. Effect of Transcranial Direct Current Stimulation Combined with Patient-Controlled Intravenous Morphine Analgesia on Analgesic Use and Post-Thoracotomy Pain. A Prospective, Randomized, Double-Blind, Sham-Controlled, Proof-of-Concept Clinical Trial. *Front. Pharmacol.* **2020**, *11*, 125. [CrossRef] [PubMed]
30. Hanna, M.H.Z.; RezkAllah, S.S.; Shalaby, A.S.; Hanna, M.Z. Efficacy of transcranial direct current stimulation (tDCS) on pain and shoulder range of motion in post-mastectomy pain syndrome patients: A randomized-control trial. *Bull. Fac. Phys. Ther.* **2023**, *28*, 7. [CrossRef]
31. Lyon, D.E.; Schubert, C.; Taylor, A.G. Pilot study of cranial stimulation for symptom management in breast cancer. *Oncol. Nurs. Forum* **2010**, *37*, 476–483. [CrossRef]
32. Lyon, D.; Kelly, D.; Walter, J.; Bear, H.; Thacker, L.; Elswick, R.K. Randomized sham controlled trial of cranial microcurrent stimulation for symptoms of depression, anxiety, pain, fatigue and sleep disturbances in women receiving chemotherapy for early-stage breast cancer. *SpringerPlus* **2015**, *4*, 369. [CrossRef]
33. Yennurajalingam, S.; Kang, D.-H.; Hwu, W.-J.; Padhye, N.S.; Masino, C.; Dibaj, S.S.; Liu, D.D.; Williams, J.L.; Lu, Z.; Bruera, E. Cranial Electrotherapy Stimulation for the Management of Depression, Anxiety, Sleep Disturbance, and Pain in Patients with Advanced Cancer: A Preliminary Study. *J. Pain Symptom Manag.* **2017**, *55*, 198–206. [CrossRef]
34. Boivie, J.; Meyerson, B.A. A correlative anatomical and clinical study of pain suppression by deep brain stimulation. *Pain* **1982**, *13*, 113–126. [CrossRef] [PubMed]
35. Kakigi, R.; Inui, K.; Tamura, Y. Electrophysiological studies on human pain perception. *Clin. Neurophysiol.* **2005**, *116*, 743–763. [CrossRef] [PubMed]
36. Xiong, H.-Y.; Zheng, J.-J.; Wang, X.-Q. Non-invasive Brain Stimulation for Chronic Pain: State of the Art and Future Directions. *Front. Mol. Neurosci.* **2022**, *15*, 888716. [CrossRef]
37. Nizard, J.; Levesque, A.; Denis, N.; De Chauvigny, E.; Lepeintre, A.; Raoul, S.; Labat, J.-J.; Bulteau, S.; Maillard, B.; Buffenoir, K.; et al. Interest of repetitive transcranial magnetic stimulation of the motor cortex in the management of refractory cancer pain in palliative care: Two case reports. *Palliat. Med.* **2015**, *29*, 564–568. [CrossRef] [PubMed]
38. Garcia-Larrea, L.; Peyron, R. Motor cortex stimulation for neuropathic pain: From phenomenology to mechanisms. *NeuroImage* **2007**, *37*, S71–S79. [CrossRef]
39. Maarrawi, J.; Peyron, R.; Mertens, P.; Costes, N.; Magnin, M.; Sindou, M.; Laurent, B.; Garcia-Larrea, L. Motor cortex stimulation for pain control induces changes in the endogenous opioid system. *Neurology* **2007**, *69*, 827–834. [CrossRef]
40. Nijs, J.; Meeus, M.; Versijpt, J.; Moens, M.; Bos, I.; Knaepen, K.; Meeusen, R. Brain-derived neurotrophic factor as a driving force behind neuroplasticity in neuropathic and central sensitization pain: A new therapeutic target? *Expert Opin. Ther. Targets* **2014**, *19*, 565–576. [CrossRef]
41. Boland, E.G.; Selvarajah, D.; Hunter, M.; Ezaydi, Y.; Tesfaye, S.; Ahmedzai, S.H.; Snowden, J.A.; Wilkinson, I.D. Central pain processing in chronic chemotherapy-induced peripheral neuropathy: A functional magnetic resonance imaging study. *PLoS ONE* **2014**, *9*, e96474. [CrossRef]
42. Lefaucheur, J.-P.; Drouot, X.; Cunin, P.; Bruckert, R.; Lepetit, H.; Créange, A.; Wolkenstein, P.; Maison, P.; Keravel, Y.; Nguyen, J.-P. Motor cortex stimulation for the treatment of refractory peripheral neuropathic pain. *Brain* **2009**, *132*, 1463–1471. [CrossRef]
43. Cha, M.; Um, S.W.; Kwon, M.; Nam, T.S.; Lee, B.H. Repetitive motor cortex stimulation reinforces the pain modulation circuits of peripheral neuropathic pain. *Sci. Rep.* **2017**, *7*, 7986. [CrossRef]
44. Attal, N.; Poindessous-Jazat, F.; De Chauvigny, E.; Quesada, C.; Mhalla, A.; Ayache, S.S.; Fermanian, C.; Nizard, J.; Peyron, R.; Lefaucheur, J.-P.; et al. Repetitive transcranial magnetic stimulation for neuropathic pain: A randomized multicentre sham-controlled trial. *Brain* **2021**, *144*, 3328–3339. [CrossRef] [PubMed]
45. Lefaucheur, J.-P.; André-Obadia, N.; Poulet, E.; Devanne, H.; Haffen, E.; Londero, A.; Cretin, B.; Leroi, A.-M.; Radtchenko, A.; Saba, G.; et al. Recommandations françaises sur l'utilisation de la stimulation magnétique transcrânienne répétitive (rTMS): Règles de sécurité et indications thérapeutiques. *Neurophysiol. Clin.* **2011**, *41*, 221–295. [CrossRef]
46. Lefaucheur, J.-P.; André-Obadia, N.; Antal, A.; Ayache, S.S.; Baeken, C.; Benninger, D.H.; Cantello, R.M.; Cincotta, M.; de Carvalho, M.; De Ridder, D.; et al. Evidence-based guidelines on the therapeutic use of repetitive transcranial magnetic stimulation (rTMS). *Clin. Neurophysiol.* **2014**, *125*, 2150–2206. [CrossRef] [PubMed]
47. Nguyen, N.D.J.P. Value of Repetitive Transcranial Magnetic Stimulation of the Motor Cortex in the Management of Refractory Cancer Pain in Palliative Care: A Case Report. *J. Palliat. Care Med.* **2013**, *3*, 147. [CrossRef]
48. Antal, A.; Alekseichuk, I.; Bikson, M.; Brockmöller, J.; Brunoni, A.R.; Chen, R.; Cohen, L.; Dowthwaite, G.; Ellrich, J.; Flöel, A.; et al. Low intensity transcranial electric stimulation: Safety, ethical, legal regulatory and application guidelines. *Clin. Neurophysiol.* **2017**, *128*, 1774–1809. [CrossRef] [PubMed]
49. Woods, A.J.; Antal, A.; Bikson, M.; Boggio, P.S.; Brunoni, A.R.; Celnik, P.; Cohen, L.G.; Fregni, F.; Herrmann, C.S.; Kappenman, E.S.; et al. A technical guide to tDCS, and related non-invasive brain stimulation tools. *Clin. Neurophysiol.* **2016**, *127*, 1031–1048. [CrossRef]
50. DaSilva, A.F.; Truong, D.Q.; DosSantos, M.F.; Toback, R.L.; Datta, A.; Bikson, M. State-of-art neuroanatomical target analysis of high-definition and conventional tDCS montages used for migraine and pain control. *Front. Neuroanat.* **2015**, *9*, 89. [CrossRef]

51. Hu, X.-S.; Fisher, C.A.; Munz, S.M.; Toback, R.L.; Nascimento, T.D.; Bellile, E.L.; Rozek, L.; Eisbruch, A.; Worden, F.P.; Danciu, T.E.; et al. Feasibility of Non-invasive Brain Modulation for Management of Pain Related to Chemoradiotherapy in Patients with Advanced Head and Neck Cancer. *Front. Hum. Neurosci.* **2016**, *10*, 466. [CrossRef]
52. Dos Santos, M.F.; Love, T.M.; Martikainen, I.K.; Nascimento, T.D.; Fregni, F.; Cummiford, C.; Deboer, M.D.; Zubieta, J.-K.; DaSilva, A.F.M. Immediate effects of tDCS on the μ-opioid system of a chronic pain patient. *Front. Psychiatry* **2012**, *3*, 93. [CrossRef]
53. Lefaucheur, J.-P.; Antal, A.; Ayache, S.S.; Benninger, D.H.; Brunelin, J.; Cogiamanian, F.; Cotelli, M.; De Ridder, D.; Ferrucci, R.; Langguth, B.; et al. Evidence-based guidelines on the therapeutic use of transcranial direct current stimulation (tDCS). *Clin. Neurophysiol.* **2016**, *128*, 56–92. [CrossRef]
54. Silva, G.; Miksad, R.; Freedman, S.D.; Pascual-Leone, A.; Jain, S.; Gomes, D.L.; Amancio, E.J.; Boggio, P.S.; Correa, C.F.; Fregni, F. Treatment of cancer pain with noninvasive brain stimulation. *J. Pain Symptom Manag.* **2007**, *34*, 342–345. [CrossRef] [PubMed]
55. Nguyen, J.-P.; Esnault, J.; Suarez, A.; Dixneuf, V.; Lepeintre, A.; Levesque, A.; Meignier, M.; Lefaucheur, J.-P.; Nizard, J. Value of transcranial direct-current stimulation of the motor cortex for the management of refractory cancer pain in the palliative care setting: A case report. *Clin. Neurophysiol.* **2016**, *127*, 2773–2774. [CrossRef]
56. Nguyen, J.-P.; Gaillard, H.; Suarez, A.; Terzidis-Mallat, É.; Constant-David, D.; Van Langhenhove, A.; Evin, A.; Malineau, C.; Tan, S.V.O.; Mhalla, A.; et al. Bicentre, randomized, parallel-arm, sham-controlled trial of transcranial direct-current stimulation (tDCS) in the treatment of palliative care patients with refractory cancer pain. *BMC Palliat. Care* **2023**, *22*, 15. [CrossRef]
57. Kamal, S.M.; Elhusseini, N.M.; Sedik, M.F.; Mohamad, M.F.; Khedr, E.M.H.; Kotb, H.I.M. Effect of Transcranial Direct Current Brain Stimulation of the Motor Cortex on Chemotherapy-Induced Nausea and Vomiting in Female Patients with Breast Cancer. *Pain Med.* **2021**, *23*, 571–578. [CrossRef] [PubMed]
58. Lowson, E.; Holmes, L.; Addingtonhall, J.; Grande, G.; Payne, S.; Seymour, J.; Hanratty, B. Abstracts of the 7th World Research Congress of the European Association for Palliative Care (EAPC). *Palliat. Med.* **2012**, *26*, 384–674. [CrossRef]
59. Moura, B.d.S.; Hu, X.-S.; DosSantos, M.F.; DaSilva, A.F. Study Protocol of tDCS Based Pain Modulation in Head and Neck Cancer Patients Under Chemoradiation Therapy Condition: An fNIRS-EEG Study. *Front. Mol. Neurosci.* **2022**, *15*, 859988. [CrossRef] [PubMed]
60. Painless Project. Horizon-HLTH-2021-DISEASE-04(2022-2027) Project ID: 101057367. [INTERNET]. Available online: https://palliativeprojects.ru/painless/ (accessed on 18 April 2023).

Disclaimer/Publisher's Note: The statements, opinions and data contained in all publications are solely those of the individual author(s) and contributor(s) and not of MDPI and/or the editor(s). MDPI and/or the editor(s) disclaim responsibility for any injury to people or property resulting from any ideas, methods, instructions or products referred to in the content.

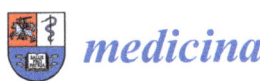

Review

CD34—Structure, Functions and Relationship with Cancer Stem Cells

Petru Radu [1,2], Mihai Zurzu [1,2,*], Vlad Paic [1,2], Mircea Bratucu [1,2], Dragos Garofil [1,2], Anca Tigora [1], Valentin Georgescu [1], Virgiliu Prunoiu [2,3], Costin Pasnicu [1,2], Florian Popa [1,2], Petra Surlin [4], Valeriu Surlin [5] and Victor Strambu [1,2]

1. General Surgery Department, Carol Davila Nephrology Hospital Bucharest, 020021 Bucharest, Romania
2. Tenth Department of Surgery, University of Medicine and Pharmacy "Carol Davila" Bucharest, 050474 Bucharest, Romania
3. Oncological Institute "Prof. Dr. Alexandru Trestioreanu", 022328 Bucharest, Romania
4. Department of Periodontology, University of Medicine and Pharmacy of Craiova, 200349 Craiova, Romania
5. Sixth Department of Surgery, University of Medicine and Pharmacy of Craiova, Craiova Emergency Clinical 7 Hospital, 200642 Craiova, Romania
* Correspondence: zurzu_mihai@yahoo.com

Abstract: The CD34 protein was identified almost four decades ago as a biomarker for hematopoietic stem cell progenitors. CD34 expression of these stem cells has been exploited for therapeutic purposes in various hematological disorders. In the last few decades, studies have revealed the presence of CD34 expression on other types of cells with non-hematopoietic origins, such as interstitial cells, endothelial cells, fibrocytes, and muscle satellite cells. Furthermore, CD34 expression may also be found on a variety of cancer stem cells. Nowadays, the molecular functions of this protein have been involved in a variety of cellular functions, such as enhancing proliferation and blocking cell differentiation, enhanced lymphocyte adhesion, and cell morphogenesis. Although a complete understanding of this transmembrane protein, including its developmental origins, its stem cell connections, and other functions, is yet to be achieved. In this paper, we aimed to carry out a systematic analysis of the structure, functions, and relationship with cancer stem cells of CD34 based on the literature overview.

Keywords: CD34; regenerative stem cell; cancer stem cells

1. Introduction

CD34 represents a transmembrane phosphoglycoprotein present at the cell surface in humans and various animal species and it was first described in hematopoietic stem cells, functioning as an adhesion factor between cells [1,2]. CD34 can likewise mediate the attachment of different stem cells to the extracellular matrix in the bone marrow or straight to the tissue. From a medical perspective, this protein is involved in the process of extracting and enriching hematopoietic stem cells in order to perform bone marrow transplantation [3].

CD34 is primarily known as a biomarker for hematopoietic stem cells (HSCs) and hematopoietic stem precursor cells, but it has also been identified as a marker for several non-hematopoietic cells. For instance, CD34 expression has been observed on endothelial precursors, which are responsible for the formation of blood vessels during development and in response to injury [4]. Additionally, CD34 has been found on fibroblast progenitors, which are involved in the formation and maintenance of connective tissue [5].

According to prior research, CD34 expression has been detected in various types of cells, including hematopoietic stem/progenitor cells, multipotent stromal cells (MSCs), muscle stem cells, interstitial cells, fibrocytes, and endothelial stem cells (Table 1). Nevertheless, the precise role of CD34 in these cells is still a matter of debate and requires further investigation [6,7].

Table 1. CD34 + cells—revised after reference [3].

Cell Type	Differentiation Potential	Morphology	Other Markers
Hematopoietic stem/progenitor cells	- Hematopoietic cells - Hepatocytes - Cardiomyocytes	- Large nucleus - Little cytoplasm - High proliferative capacity	- HLA-DR - CD38 - CD117 - CD45 - CD133
Multipotent stromal cells (MSCs)	- Adipocytes - Chondrocytes - Myocytes - Osteoblats - Angiogenic	- Small cell body - Large round nucleus - Presence of chromatin particles	- Stro-1 - CD73 - CD90 - CD105 - CD146 - CD29 - CD44 - CD271
Muscle stem cells	- Myocytes - Adipocytes - Chondrocytes - Osteoblats	- Presence of myofibril bundles - Large nucleus - Little cytoplasm	- CD56 - Myf5 - Desmin - CD90 - CD106 - Flk-1 - VEGFR - Myod - CD146
Fibrocytes	- Fibroblasts - Adipocytes - Osteogenic, - Osteoblats	- Small spindle shape - Moderate amount of cytoplasm - Small and elongated nucleus	- CD45 - CD80 - CD86 - MHC class I and II
Endothelial cells	- Angiogenesis	- Elongated with filopodia - Lack tight junctions	- CD146, - VE-cadherin - CD133, - CD117, - CD14, - CD31
Interstitial cells	- Unknown	- Triangular or spindle-shaped - Large nucleus - Long cytoplasmic processes	- CD117 - Vimentin - Desmin - Connexin-43 - Pdgfrb

Abbreviation list: ALDH (aldehyde dehydrogenase), CD (cluster of differentiation), CFU-F (colony forming units fibroblast), Flk-1 (fetal liver kinase-1), HF (hair follicle), HLA-DR (human leukocyte antigen-DR), HSC (hematopoietic stem cells), MSC (multipotent mesenchymal stromal cells), Myf5 (myogenic factor 5), MyoD (myogenic differentiation 1), MHC (major histocompatibility complex), PDGFRβ (platelet derived growth factor receptor β), and VEGFR (vascular endothelial growth factor receptor).

There are several different transmembrane proteins that belong to the CD34 family, but among them, the most significant ones are the CD34 hematopoietic antigen, endoglycan, and podocalyxin. These proteins are particularly important because they have been shown to play critical roles in a variety of cellular processes; however, the complete function of CD34 proteins still remains a mystery. According to scientific literature, CD34 proteins are capable of enhancing the proliferation of progenitor cells, which are immature cells that can differentiate into various types of specialized cells, such as blood cells. Furthermore, CD34 proteins have been found to play a role in preventing the differentiation of progenitor cells, which is important for maintaining a pool of immature cells that can continue to develop into different cell types as needed. In addition, CD34 proteins have been shown to improve the migration of cells, which is essential for the movement and distribution of cells throughout the body. Among the CD34 transmembrane proteins, podocalyxin appears to have a particularly significant role in cell development and migration. Research has demonstrated that podocalyxin is involved in regulating cell adhesion and movement, which is crucial for the development and maintenance of various tissues and organs [3,6].

The CD34 molecules are commonly utilized as biomarkers for endothelial, stem, and hematopoietic precursor cells [7,8], as well as podocalyxin, which also shows widespread expression in the previously mentioned cells [9]. Nevertheless, podocalyxin was originally documented as a marker for renal glomerular cells, thus being crucial in the process of renal tissue development [10,11].

Aberrant podocalyxin expression also has immunohistochemical implications in a wide range of malignant tumor pathologies such as breast and prostate cancers [12,13].

Endoglycan is the last member of the CD34 protein family, and it was identified through gene sequencing techniques that showed similarities to the other members of this protein family. Endoglycan is also expressed in a subset of hematopoietic cells, and some studies have suggested that it may be involved in regulating the adhesion and migration of these cells. However, the precise function of endoglycan in hematopoiesis and other physiological processes is not yet fully understood, and further research is needed to elucidate its role [14].

The current challenge in the field of stem cell research and therapy is the potential implications of CD34 markers in cancer pathology. Although these markers have been useful in identifying and isolating stem cells for therapeutic applications, they have also been linked to the development of leukemia and various malignancies [15]. While CD34+ stem cells have shown significant progress in treating blood and immune disorders, recent studies suggest that CD34 markers may also be present on cancer stem cells (CSCs) and promote tumor recurrence and metastasis [15]. Moreover, the presence of CD34 markers on CSCs may interfere with conventional cancer treatments [16]. Therefore, the use of CD34 markers in stem cell research and therapy needs to be carefully managed to improve patient outcomes, and further investigation is necessary to understand their potential limitations and risks.

In this paper, we aimed to carry out a systematic analysis of the structure, functions, and relationship with the cancer stem cells of CD34 based on the literature overview.

2. Structure and Functions of CD34

All three proteins in the CD34 family share similar structural characteristics, including the presence of serine, threonine, and proline residues in their extracellular domains. These domains are heavily glycosylated and sialylated, which gives the proteins an effective size range of 90–170 kDa and defines the CD34 family as a subfamily of sialomucins [10,17,18].

Additionally, for each member of these proteins, the extracellular portion includes: a cysteine globular region, as well as a juxtamembrane region and numerous N-linked glycosylation domains. Further, every protein has a specific and distinctive helix and a cytoplasmic tail that is composed of several phosphorylation domains [6] (Figure 1).

Although CD34 family proteins are generally expected to share highly similar structural domains, the specific differences between them will be outlined in Table 2.

Identifying the binding partners of a novel protein with known functions can provide valuable insights into its biological role. By identifying these partners, researchers can infer the potential pathways and processes in which the novel protein may be involved. This can lead to a better understanding of the protein's function and potential therapeutic applications. In the case of CD34 proteins, the highly conserved cytoplasmic regions suggest the existence of intracellular binding partners. Therefore, in the past, research has been directed towards identifying potential interacting proteins [6].

The first intracellular ligands to be discovered for a CD34 family member were the PDZ-family proteins NHERF and NHERF2, which both interact with podocalyxin, providing a potential link to the actin cytoskeleton [6].

Table 2. Structural characteristics and differences of CD34 family proteins [3,14,19–21].

Structural Characteristics	CD34	Endoglycan	Podocalyxin
Mucin domain length	120 amino acids	350 amino acids	250 amino acids
Cysteine globular domains	Three pairs	Single pair	Two pairs
Cysteine in juxtamembrane region	Absent	Unpaired—involved in its homodimerization	Absent
N-Linked glycosylation sites	Numerous	Numerous	Numerous
Extracellular effective size range (kDa)	90–170	90–170	90–170
Nonglycosylated N-terminal sequences	Absent	Present—high abundance of glutamic acid.	Absent
C-terminal binding pattern	Mildly modified—which has functional implications for intracellular ligand binding	Similar to podocalyxin	Similar to endoglycan

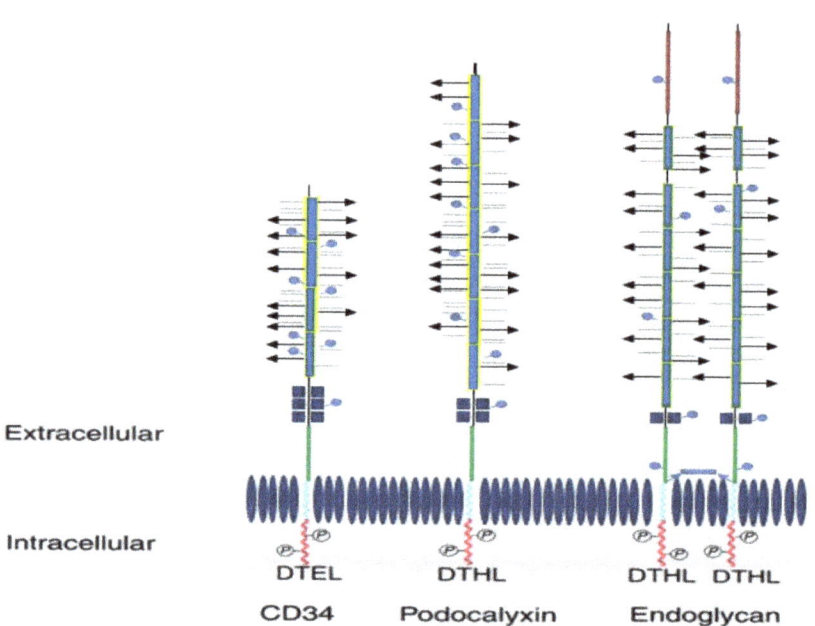

Figure 1. Structure of CD34 family proteins (revised from reference [22]. O-glycosylated (arrows), sialylated (horizontal lines), extracellular mucin domain + sites for N-glycosylation (blue lines with circles), cysteine residues (dark blue square), a juxtamembrane region (green), transmembrane domain (light blue), cytoplasmic tail (red), phosphorylation sites, binding motifs DTEL or DTHL. Endoglycan contains a polyglutamic acid-rich extracellular domain (blue rectangle) and unpaired cysteine residues (dark blue square).

The most well-known ligand is L-selectin. L-selectin is a cell adhesion molecule that is involved in the recruitment of leukocytes to sites of inflammation and infection. CD34 expressed on hematopoietic stem and progenitor cells has been shown to bind to L-selectin expressed on endothelial cells, facilitating the homing of these cells to the bone marrow and other sites of hematopoiesis [3,7].

Furthermore, the adapter protein CRKL has been shown to bind to CD34 in hematopoietic progenitor cells, hinting at a role in signal transduction. These observations suggest that CD34 family members likely have intracellular binding partners that are crucial for their functions [6]. A summarized breakdown of CD 34 protein ligands according to the literature will be provided in Table 3.

Table 3. CD34 family ligands—revised from reference [21].

Ligand	Cell Type	Protein Bound	Interaction
L-selectin	High endothelial venules (HEV)	CD 34 Endoglycan Podocalyxin	Sialyl lewis-x carbohydrate dependent
NRERF-1	Hematopoietic cells	Endoglycan Podocalyxin	C-terminal PDZ interaction
NHERF-2	Podocyte	Podocalyxin	Terminal PDZ interaction
CRKL	Hematopoietic cells	CD 34	Juxtamembrane
ERM	MDCK (Madin-Darby Canine Kidney) cell line	Podocalyxin	Juxtamembrane

The exact functions of CD34 proteins remain a topic of debate, as their roles appear to be complex and multifaceted. Researchers have proposed several potential functions for CD34 proteins, including the ability to promote the proliferation of progenitor cells, inhibit the differentiation of stem cells, and enhance cellular migration and adhesion. CD34 proteins may also play a role in cell morphogenesis. Additionally, studies suggest that CD34 proteins may be involved in immune system regulation, particularly in the adhesion of lymphocytes to blood vessel walls. However, further research is needed to fully understand the many functions of CD34 proteins and how they contribute to various cellular processes [3].

(a) Enhancing proliferation and blocking cell differentiation.

The literature provides several possible explanations for the potential roles of CD34 in promoting cell proliferation and preventing differentiation. One possible reason is its expression in pluripotent hematopoietic progenitor cells, which has been linked to a decrease in adult cell number, suggesting a specific function of CD34 in maintaining the phenotype of progenitor and immature stem cells. However, the precise mechanisms by which CD34 contributes to these processes are still being investigated and are not yet fully understood [23]. Additionally, CD34 has been observed to play a crucial role in regulating hematopoietic precursor stem cell proliferation. Studies using knockout mice have shown that a reduction in CD34 expression results in decreased numbers of these cells in both embryonic and adult tissues, accompanied by defects in their ability to proliferate [24].

Compared to wild-type mice, these particular animals exhibit a substantial reduction in the overall amount of adult precursor cells, along with a small number of embryonic hematopoietic cells and fetal myeloid precursors, although there is certainly no obvious reduction in total adult cell numbers in the hematogenesis system of mature mice [24]. Moreover, past studies have proposed the possibility of the CD34 protein being involved in suppressing cell lineage differentiation, which may have implications for its potential use in cell-based therapies and regenerative medicine [25,26].

(b) Enhance lymphocyte adhesion.

The most well-described function of CD34 proteins is to enhance the adhesion of lymphocytes to specialized endothelial cells in various lymphoid organs. Nowadays, there is a general acceptance that young lymphatic cells are assimilated within secondary lymphoid organs through a multi-step developmental cycle that initially implies their attachment to specialized lymphoid cells in the endothelium (high endothelial venules—HEVs) [27].

When all CD34 proteins are expressed by specialized venules, appropriate glycosylation occurs for interaction with the L-selectin molecule, thus providing ligands for proper cellular interconnection [28,29].

On the other hand, even with extensive vascular display for CD34, podocalyxin, and endoglycan, just these particular venules can properly glycosylate these molecules for the L-selectin ligand, thus rapidly prompting the hypothesis that CD34 proteins possess an overall function in accelerating cellular adhesion [30,31].

(c) Cellular development

It has been proven that podocalyxin is essential for preserving the complex microstructure of renal podocytes [32]. These epithelial cells comprise a cellular body containing numerous extensions (called major processes) as well as several smaller extensions, which arise directly within the main extensions. Podocytes are usually covered with podocalyxin, while Podxl-mice display no evidence of such podocytes at all [32].

The obvious impact of podocalyxin in podocyte embryology and identification of its connection with the actin molecular structure [17] led to further investigations of the involvement of podocalyxin in determining cell form [25].

Podocalyxin is highly expressed on the cell surface, displaying intricate membrane processes. As an example, it has been identified in a subtype of neurons [33]. Like podocytes, neurons have a network-like structure of cytoskeletal components, and cytoskeletal proteins are found in both podocytes and neurons, indicating that comparable processes contribute to the development of extensions in each cell type [34]. Furthermore, megakaryocytes express podocalyxin, which is involved in the formation of their long processes during platelet generation [35].

2.1. CD 34 and Hematopoietic Cells

When used for medical purposes, CD34 levels are monitored in order to ensure quick bone marrow transplantation and may further be applied as a specific label in selective cell sorting in order to enhance an embryonic hematopoietic cell population [36]. Despite the fact that sometimes it is believed that CD34 is only a stem cell indicator, its presence in bone marrow or blood specimens indicates a mixture of both hematopoietic stem and precursor cells [37]. The human hematopoietic cells are subsequently differentiated from CD34+ precursor cells through a decreased level of CD90 and the absence of CD38, human leukocyte antigen, and a range of markers of the adult hematopoietic cells [38].

Human CD34+ hematopoietic cells (HSCs) are also characterized by the ability to differentiate into all hematopoietic lineage cells and possess a high proliferative capacity [38]. Information provided by the literature indicates that CD34+ HSCs and their precursors are able to proliferate into new cell lines, such as cardiomyocytes, respiratory epithelial cells, and hepatocytes [39,40].

2.2. CD 34 Multipotent Mesenchymal Stromal Cells (MSC)

MSCs are located in almost all adult tissues and are a predominant and versatile cell type that is widely researched for therapeutic applications in regenerative medicine [41]. In addition to their well-documented in vitro capacity for mesenchymal differentiation, MSCs have also been shown to possess various other properties. These include their ability to release paracrine factors that promote wound healing, their capacity to create specialized niches within tissues, their ability to modulate immune responses, and their immune privileged status. These properties have made MSCs an attractive therapeutic tool for a wide range of medical applications, including tissue repair, autoimmune disorders, and transplantation [42].

Two past studies have reported CD34 expression in MSCs, both of which focused on fat-derived MSCs [43,44]. While one study focused on the structural characteristics and roles of CD34 protein in association with MSC [44], the other study questioned the hypothesis about CD34 being a specific negative biomarker of multipotent stromal cells [43]. Therefore, Lin et al. reviewed the evidence according to which, CD34 appeared to be an essential marker in the initial MSC investigation, thus pointing to Simmons' investigation, which shows that newly isolated CD34+ bone marrow stem cells build a consistently higher percentage of fibroblastic population comparable to CD34-cells [45].

Additionally, some researchers have proposed that CD34 could potentially serve as a positive biomarker for MSCs with a specific association with vascularization. These cells may be referred to as vascular progenitor cells, suggesting that they have the ability to differentiate into endothelial cells and contribute to blood vessel formation. The potential of CD34+ MSCs as a source for vascular progenitor cells has been explored in various studies, highlighting their potential therapeutic applications for cardiovascular diseases and tissue engineering. However, further research is needed to fully understand the role of CD34 in MSCs and its potential for vascularization [43].

Cells that exhibit CD34 expression constitute at least a fraction of the entire MSC network, while this particular subgroup exhibits particular features. CD34 appears to be linked to a greater efficiency of new cell colony formation and possesses a lasting proliferation capacity [46]. CD34+ MSCs are known to express a range of common stromal cell markers, such as CD90, CD105, and CD73, as well as other markers such as CD271 and Stro-1 that have been identified as MSC-specific markers. Additionally, CD34+ MSCs may also express markers that are associated with other cell types, such as CD45, which is commonly found on hematopoietic cells, and CD133, which is expressed on a variety of progenitor and stem cells. The co-expression of these markers suggests that CD34+ MSCs may represent a heterogeneous population of cells with diverse functional properties [46,47].

CD34+ MSCs have been shown to have a greater pattern of endothelial transdifferentiation [48], which is also observed in embryonic stem cell-derived MSCs, thereby strongly implying that CD34 is a marker of early human MSCs [49].

2.3. CD 34 and Muscle Stem Cells

Muscle satellite cells, also known as muscle stem cells, are small precursor stromal cells that reside in skeletal muscle tissue and have the ability to differentiate into mature muscle cells. CD34 protein is widely used as an indicator for identifying these cells, as it is expressed on the surface of satellite cells, making it a useful marker for identifying and isolating them for further study. The differentiation and proliferation of satellite cells are crucial for muscle growth and regeneration, making them an important focus of research in the field of muscle biology [50].

In vivo, these muscle cells are quiescent until they are stimulated in order to supply myonuclei for muscle fibers during high-intensity physical activity or during muscle injury. The activation of these types of cells, which is believed to be for differentiation, corresponds to a significant upregulation of CD34. Moreover, it is speculated that CD34 may play a fundamental role in regulating muscle progenitor cell differentiation by establishing and sustaining a population of satellite cells [51].

CD34 does not present expression for every satellite muscle cell; however, it is used to identify them along with several other markers, such as CD56 [50]. The first myogenic progenitors studied do not possess the ability to manifest CD34; CD34 expression is first identified as satellite muscle cells develop [52].

Complementary tests further speculate that CD34+ cells may possess the capacity to be more than just muscle progenitors. Separate MSC-like cells that display mesenchymal differentiation were also detected in muscle satellite cells by identifying expression patterns of CD34 [53].

Past studies have also proposed that CD34+ cells found inside the interstitial spaces of muscles may be similar to those from the endothelium based on their expression pattern. Such myoendothelial cells exhibit augmented muscle regeneration capacity when compared to cells that express either muscle stem cells or endothelial patterns [54].

The differences found in the characteristics of satellite muscle cells can be explained by the existence of different subgroups of CD34+ cells with unique differentiation potentials. Markers expressed together with CD34 also affect the differentiation process. As an example, CD34+ cells co-expressing the endothelial marker CD31 exhibit angiogenic differentiation. Nevertheless, CD34+ CD31 cell populations show higher potential for differentiation of adipose and muscle tissue [55].

2.4. CD34 and Endothelial Cells

CD34 is generally considered to be a biomarker for vascular endothelial precursor cells [4]. These bone marrow tissue-derived cells are circulating in the peripheral blood, and their value in proangiogenic therapies has been amply documented [56]. The characteristics of CD34+ endothelial cells are frequently related to those of hematopoietic cells, as these two cell types can be identified and isolated within blood samples by using CD34 as an antigen; therefore, these cells are used in various vascular pathologies [57]. In addition, these cells possess the ability to form new types of cells, such as osteoblasts and cardiomyocytes [58].

Matsumoto suggests from his research the hypothetical presence of an overlap between osteoblasts and endothelial progenitor cells [59]. It is hypothesized that in the bone marrow there are a number of CD34+ precursor cells, which possess the ability to differentiate into endothelial cells as well as osteoblasts. A number of studies have highlighted the use of circulating CD34+ cells for healing broken bones, which frequently have a poor recovery because of insufficient circulation in the area of the fracture [59].

It is believed that there may be a subgroup of mature non-circulating endothelial cells that exhibit CD34 expression and are predominantly situated in the smaller blood vessels, whereas the vast proportion of endothelial cells from larger blood vessels does not exhibit CD34 expression [4]. Unlike the usual biology of endothelial cells, all cells that exhibit CD34 expression have an elongated cell shape without narrow junctions [60].

In the past, research on in vivo cultures has revealed the presence of CD34 protein expression within endothelial cells originating in the umbilical vein; although when grown in vitro, expression is essentially absent and only a small population of cells preserve CD34 expression [4]. These particular cells mentioned previously display unique morphological features as well as numerous filopodia; in addition, CD34 is very well expressed within these filopodia, where angiogenesis is most active, thus highlighting the important functional role of CD34 in progenitor cell activity [60].

2.5. CD 34 and Cancer Stem Cells (CSCs)

Based on information available in the literature, CD34 has been identified in various cancers, such as gastric, breast, thyroid, colorectal, and skin cancer [15]. CD34 has also been utilized as a biomarker to assess angiogenesis in multiple malignancies, such as cervical cancer, gastric cancer, lung cancer, and oral squamous cell carcinoma [15].

In recent years, an increase in CD34 expression, Ang II, and vascular endothelial growth factor has been documented in patients with severe hepatocellular carcinoma [61]. Therefore, as well as for regenerative stem cells, in the case of CD34 expression on cancer cells and CSCs, CD34 was linked with endothelial progenitors and adult cells and angiogenesis. In addition, it is very likely that CD34+ cells found in different mature tissues are endothelial precursor cells, which need future studies to be fully confirmed [15].

In 2006, a group of researchers led by Clarke published a study on the potential involvement of CD34 in tumor development. The study was conducted on mice and involved injecting them with a tumor-promoting substance to induce tumorigenesis. The researchers found that mice lacking the CD34 protein failed to activate angiogenesis, a process that involves the growth of new blood vessels, and therefore developed fewer tumors compared to wild-type mice. CD34 is a protein that is primarily found on the surface of hematopoietic stem cells, which give rise to different types of blood cells. Angiogenesis is a critical process in tumor development, as it provides the growing tumor with a blood supply and nutrients necessary for its survival and growth. Clarke et al.'s findings suggest that CD34 may play a crucial role in angiogenesis and, consequently, tumor development. By comparing CD34 knockout mice with wild-type mice, they were able to demonstrate the importance of CD34 in angiogenesis and tumor growth. Their study provides valuable insights into the molecular mechanisms underlying tumorigenesis and may have implications for the development of new cancer therapies targeting CD34 or related pathways [62].

CSCs are a small subpopulation of cells within a tumor that are believed to be responsible for driving tumor growth and metastasis. These cells possess the ability to regenerate and produce different types of malignant cells that make up the tumor. One of the defining characteristics of CSCs is their expression of certain cell surface biomarkers. These biomarkers are also found in human embryonic cells, adult stem cells, and normal cells. Understanding the biology of CSCs is critical for the development of new cancer treatments that target these cells. By targeting CSCs, it may be possible to eradicate the tumor and prevent its recurrence. However, more research is needed to fully understand the mechanisms underlying CSCs and develop effective therapies that can selectively target them [15,62].

The origin of cancer stem cells is a topic of ongoing debate and speculation in the scientific community. Although the precise source of these cells remains controversial, there are several theories regarding their potential origins, including from precursor cells, stem cells, or even differentiated cells that have undergone reprogramming within the tumor microenvironment. Understanding the origin of CSCs is critical for developing targeted cancer therapies that can effectively eliminate these cells and prevent tumor recurrence [15,63].

Despite significant advances in cancer research, relapse of cancer and/or metastasis remain major challenges in the field. CSCs have been implicated in the development of these phenomena, as they are thought to play a critical role in tumor initiation, growth, and metastasis. Because CSCs are resistant to conventional cancer therapies, they may be responsible for the failure of many treatments to eradicate the disease completely. In recent years, there has been growing interest in the use of CSC-targeted therapies for cancer treatment. By selectively targeting CSCs, it may be possible to eliminate the source of tumor growth and prevent relapse and metastasis. However, there is still much to learn about the biology of CSCs and their role in cancer development, and further research is needed to develop effective treatments that can specifically target these cells while sparing healthy tissue [15].

The expression of various drug resistance receptors in CSC has been linked to chemotherapy resistance. In addition, enhanced DNA repair capabilities in CSC have been linked with the development of radiation resistance in some types of malignancies. Therefore, CSCs were considered promising targets for cancer therapy and medicine discovery. A greater comprehension of cell surface biomarkers expressed on CSCs will allow their isolation and enrichment [15].

The earliest proof of CSCs was demonstrated in acute myeloid leukemia by Lapiod et al. back in 1994 [64]. During the study, Lapiod et al. discovered a specific subpopulation of CSC, characterized by the presence of CD34 and the absence of CD38. To further investigate the role of these cells in the initiation and progression of AML, they were transplanted into mice with severe combined immunodeficiency (SCID). The results of this study confirmed that these CD34+CD38- cells were responsible for initiating leukemia [64].

According to the study conducted by Park et al., hepatic cancer may develop from transformed CD34+ stem cells in the liver, suggesting that stem cells not only play a role in organ and tissue regeneration but may also contribute to the development of cancer. Furthermore, CD34+ cell populations isolated from PLC/PRF/5 liver carcinoma have the ability to generate multiple types of liver cancer in mice. Therefore, this leads to the hypothesis that CD34+ hepatocellular cells may be a subtype of hepatic CSCs [65].

A recent study carried out by Yin P. et al. revealed that a subset of cells found in uterine leiomyoma exhibit characteristics of stem cells. These cells have been classified into three categories based on their expression of CD34: CD34+/CD49b+, CD34+/CD49b-, and CD34-/CD49b-. Among these categories, CD34+/CD49b+ cells were found to be the most prevalent. It is speculated that CD34+ cells, which are known to be endothelial progenitors, may play a role in angiogenesis and contribute to cancer stemness and metastasis in the context of CSCs. The data from the study also suggested that the use of CD34 could be useful in isolating these side population cells for further molecular investigation [66].

The study by Natarajan Aravindan and colleagues aimed to investigate the role of CD34+ cancer stem cells (CSCs) in high-risk neuroblastoma (HR-NB) patients. The researchers found that CD34 expression in NB was associated with MYCN amplification, advanced disease stage, and progressive disease after clinical therapy. CD34+ was also correlated with poor survival in patients with N-MYC-amplified HR-NB. Further analysis of the genetic landscape of CD34+-NB-CSCs identified significant up- and down-modulation of genes compared with NB-CSCs that lack CD34. The study suggests that careful consideration should be exercised for autologous stem-cell rescue with CD34+ selection in NB patients due to the risk of reinfusing NB-CSCs that could lead to post-transplant relapse [67].

2.6. CD34 in Clinical Applications

Despite the potential of embryonic stem cells to differentiate into various cell types during the blastocyst stage, most adult stem cells have limited potential for tissue regeneration. Hematopoietic stem cells are a well-known source of adult stem/progenitor cells. However, CD34+ cells in adult human circulating/peripheral blood have also been found to contain hematopoietic and endothelial progenitor cells, making them an essential source of stem/progenitor cells. Previous research has focused on identifying ways to guide stem cells towards tissue renewal [68]. Past studies have shown that tissue ischemia triggers the mobilization of endothelial precursor cells from the bone marrow into the bloodstream by upregulating cytokines, leading to their migration and incorporation into regions of neovascularization. Based on this breakthrough, multiple studies have demonstrated the therapeutic value of EPCs in various pathologies [68].

The initial investigations into the therapeutic uses of CD34 centered around the transplantation of purified CD34+ hematopoietic progenitor cells for hematopoietic reconstitution. Studies involving irradiated baboons showed that transplantation of these purified CD34 cells resulted in the eventual restoration of normal blood cell numbers [15,69].

Fan-Yen Lee et al. conducted a study to evaluate the effects of circulating CD34+ cells among patients suffering from diffuse coronary artery disease who were not eligible for coronary surgery. The results of this study have significant clinical implications. Intracoronary transfusion of autologous CD34+ cells has been shown to be a safe procedure without any complications. Furthermore, the use of CD34+ cell circulatory therapy has demonstrated efficacy in improving cardiac functions [70].

According to the study by Ahmed El-Badawy et al., stem cell therapy for diabetes mellitus appears to be a reliable and potentially therapeutic alternative. The mobilized marrow CD34+ HSCs exhibited the most encouraging treatment results [71].

Toru Nakamura et al. found that if they transplant CD34+ cells into the hepatic artery in patients with severe liver cirrhosis, the blood flow to the liver will significantly improve. This strongly supports the theory that these cells can differentiate into vascular endothelial cells [15]. In addition to the research mentioned above, another study carried out in mice revealed that transplantation of endothelial stem cells increased hepatic blood flow and reduced portal pressure [72].

According to a study conducted by Quyyumi AA et al. in 2017, which focused on patients with ST-elevation myocardial infarction, the use of CD34+ cells was found to lead to improved myocardial perfusion [73].

3. Discussion

While the CD34 protein has extensive medical uses, its functional roles are not fully clarified. Clinical difficulties encountered with this protein include its variability in expression among different cell types, low expression, and variations in glycosylation models, resulting in challenges in utilizing antibody-based methods to isolate CD34+ cells. Hence, considerable effort has been devoted to better understanding this protein. Despite its reputation as a label for hematopoietic stem cells, its occurrence in other non-hematopoietic cells is still under investigation.

The human CD34 gene is situated in a genomic region that is rich in genes encoding cell adhesion molecules. This intriguing placement has sparked speculation that CD34 may also have a role in cell adhesion, in addition to its well-known function as a marker for hematopoietic stem and progenitor cells. While the molecular mechanisms by which CD34 may regulate cell adhesion are not fully understood, several studies have suggested that it can modulate the activity of integrins, a family of transmembrane adhesion receptors that play crucial roles in cell migration, proliferation, and differentiation. Moreover, recent evidence indicates that CD34 may interact with other adhesion-related proteins, such as selectins, and participate in complex signaling networks that control cell behavior in diverse physiological and pathological contexts.

The nature of CD34 also suggests that this protein participates in a variety of signal transduction pathways, and furthermore, the CD34 protein has been reported to be involved in angiogenesis. Up to now, medical use of CD34 has remained mostly confined to the restoration of the hematopoietic system. The discovery of CD34 expression on a diversity of non-hematopoietic precursor cells will help increase the role of CD34+ cells in the therapy of pathologies beyond blood disorders.

CD34 is commonly used as a marker to identify and isolate CSCs in various types of cancer. CD34-positive CSCs have been identified in leukemia, breast cancer, lung cancer, and other types of tumors. These CD34-positive CSCs have been shown to have enhanced self-renewal ability and increased tumor-initiating capacity compared to CD34-negative cells. However, CD34 expression has been associated with increased tumor aggressiveness and resistance to chemotherapy in some types of cancer. Despite all the information obtained from past studies, the precise mechanisms by which CD34 contributes to cancer development and progression are complex and not yet fully understood.

4. Conclusions

Further research is needed to better understand the functions of CD34 in both normal and malignant cells. This could lead to the development of new targeted therapies that can disrupt the role of CD34 in promoting cancer growth and progression, ultimately improving the prognosis for individuals with cancer.

Author Contributions: Conceptualization, P.R. and M.Z.; methodology, P.R. and V.P. (Vlad Paic); software, M.B.; validation, P.R., F.P. and V.S. (Victor Strambu); formal analysis, D.G. and P.S.; investigation, A.T. and C.P.; resources, V.S. (Valeriu Surlin); data curation, V.P. (Virgiliu Prunoiu) and V.G.; writing—original draft preparation, M.Z. and V.S. (Victor Strambu); writing—review and editing, all authors. All authors have read and agreed to the published version of the manuscript.

Funding: This research received no external funding.

Institutional Review Board Statement: Not applicable.

Informed Consent Statement: Not applicable.

Data Availability Statement: Data sharing is not applicable to this article.

Conflicts of Interest: The authors declare no conflict of interest.

References

1. Tindle, R.W.; Nichols, R.A.; Chan, L.; Campana, D.; Catovsky, D.; Birnie, G.D. A novel monoclonal antibody BI-3C5 recognises myeloblasts and non-B non-T lymphoblasts in acute leukaemias and CGL blast crises, and reacts with immature cells in normal bone marrow. *Leuk. Res.* **1985**, *9*, 1–9. [CrossRef]
2. Civin, C.I.; Strauss, L.C.; Brovall, C.; Fackler, M.J.; Schwartz, J.F.; Shaper, J.H. Antigenic analysis of hematopoiesis. III. A hematopoietic progenitor cell surface antigen defined by a monoclonal antibody raised against KG-1a cells. *J. Immunol.* **1984**, *133*, 157–165. [CrossRef]
3. Sidney, L.E.; Branch, M.J.; Dunphy, S.E.; Dua, H.S.; Hopkinson, A. Concise review: Evidence for CD34 as a common marker for diverse progenitors. *Stem Cells* **2014**, *32*, 1380–1389. [CrossRef] [PubMed]
4. Fina, L.; Molgaard, H.V.; Robertson, D.; Bradley, N.J.; Monaghan, P.; Delia, D.; Sutherland, D.R.; Baker, M.A.; Greaves, M.F. Expression of the CD34 gene in vascular endothelial cells. *Blood* **1990**, *75*, 2417–2426. [CrossRef] [PubMed]
5. Brown, J.; Greaves, M.F.; Molgaard, H.V. The gene encoding the stem cell antigen, CD34, is conserved in mouse and expressed in haemopoietic progenitor cell lines, brain, and embryonic fibroblasts. *Int. Immunol.* **1991**, *3*, 175–184. [CrossRef]
6. Nielsen, J.S.; McNagny, K.M. Novel functions of the CD34 family. *J. Cell Sci.* **2008**, *121*, 3683–3692. [CrossRef]

7. Baumheter, S.; Singer, M.S.; Henzel, W.; Hemmerich, S.; Renz, M.; Rosen, S.D.; Lasky, L.A. Binding of L-selectin to the vascular sialomucin CD34. *Science* **1993**, *262*, 436–438. [CrossRef]
8. Baumhueter, S.; Dybdal, N.; Kyle, C.; Lasky, L.A. Global vascular expression of murine CD34, a sialomucin-like endothelial ligand for L-selectin. *Blood* **1994**, *84*, 2554–2565. [CrossRef]
9. Doyonnas, R.; Nielsen, J.S.; Chelliah, S.; Drew, E.; Hara, T.; Miyajima, A.; McNagny, K.M. Podocalyxin is a CD34-related marker of murine hematopoietic stem cells and embryonic erythroid cells. *Blood* **2005**, *105*, 4170–4178. [CrossRef]
10. Doyonnas, R.; Kershaw, D.B.; Duhme, C.; Merkens, H.; Chelliah, S.; Graf, T.; McNagny, K.M. Anuria, omphalocele, and perinatal lethality in mice lacking the CD34-related protein podocalyxin. *J. Exp. Med.* **2001**, *194*, 13–27. [CrossRef] [PubMed]
11. Kerjaschki, D.; Sharkey, D.J.; Farquhar, M.G. Identification and characterization of podocalyxin—The major sialoprotein of the renal glomerular epithelial cell. *J. Cell Biol.* **1984**, *98*, 1591–1596. [CrossRef] [PubMed]
12. Kelley, T.W.; Huntsman, D.; McNagny, K.M.; Roskelley, C.D.; Hsi, E.D. Podocalyxin: A marker of blasts in acute leukemia. *Am. J. Clin. Pathol.* **2005**, *124*, 134–142. [CrossRef]
13. Casey, G.; Neville, P.J.; Liu, X.; Plummer, S.J.; Cicek, M.S.; Krumroy, L.M.; Curran, A.P.; McGreevy, M.R.; Catalona, W.J.; Klein, E.A.; et al. Podocalyxin variants and risk of prostate cancer and tumor aggressiveness. *Hum. Mol. Genet.* **2006**, *15*, 735–741. [CrossRef]
14. Sassetti, C.; Van Zante, A.; Rosen, S.D. Identification of endoglycan, a member of the CD34/podocalyxin family of sialomucins. *J. Biol. Chem.* **2000**, *275*, 9001–9010. [CrossRef] [PubMed]
15. Kapoor, S.; Shenoy, S.P.; Bose, B. CD34 cells in somatic, regenerative and cancer stem cells: Developmental biology, cell therapy, and omics big data perspective. *J. Cell. Biochem.* **2020**, *121*, 3058–3069. [CrossRef] [PubMed]
16. Dawood, S.; Austin, L.; Cristofanilli, M. Cancer stem cells: Implications for cancer therapy. *Oncology* **2014**, *28*, 1101–1107.
17. Takeda, T. Podocyte cytoskeleton is connected to the integral membrane protein podocalyxin through Na+/H+-exchanger regulatory factor 2 and ezrin. *Clin. Exp. Nephrol.* **2003**, *7*, 260–269. [CrossRef]
18. Hilkens, J.; Ligtenberg, M.J.; Vos, H.L.; Litvinov, S.V. Cell membrane-associated mucins and their adhesion-modulating property. *Trends Biochem. Sci.* **1992**, *17*, 359–363. [CrossRef]
19. Sassetti, C.; Tangemann, K.; Singer, M.S.; Kershaw, D.B.; Rosen, S.D. Identification of podocalyxin-like protein as a high endothelial venule ligand for L-selectin: Parallels to CD34. *J. Exp. Med.* **1998**, *187*, 1965–1975. [CrossRef]
20. He, X.Y.; Antao, V.P.; Basila, D.; Marx, J.C.; Davis, B.R. Isolation and molecular characterization of the human CD34 gene. *Blood* **1992**, *79*, 2296–2302. [CrossRef] [PubMed]
21. Furness, S.G.; McNagny, K. Beyond mere markers: Functions for CD34 family of sialomucins in hematopoiesis. *Immunol. Res.* **2006**, *34*, 13–32. [CrossRef]
22. Nielsen, J.S.; McNagny, K.M. CD34 is a key regulator of hematopoietic stem cell trafficking to bone marrow and mast cell progenitor trafficking in the periphery. *Microcirculation* **2009**, *16*, 487–496. [CrossRef]
23. Krause, D.S.; Fackler, M.J.; Civin, C.I.; May, W.S. CD34: Structure, biology, and clinical utility. *Blood* **1996**, *87*, 1–13. [CrossRef]
24. Cheng, J.; Baumhueter, S.; Cacalano, G.; Carver-Moore, K.; Thibodeaux, H.; Thomas, R.; Broxmeyer, H.E.; Cooper, S.; Hague, N.; Moore, M.; et al. Hematopoietic defects in mice lacking the sialomucin CD34. *Blood* **1996**, *87*, 479–490. [CrossRef]
25. Nielsen, J.S.; McNagny, K.M. Influence of host irradiation on long-term engraftment by CD34-deficient hematopoietic stem cells. *Blood* **2007**, *110*, 1076–1077. [CrossRef] [PubMed]
26. Drew, E.; Merzaban, J.S.; Seo, W.; Ziltener, H.J.; McNagny, K.M. CD34 and CD43 inhibit mast cell adhesion and are required for optimal mast cell reconstitution. *Immunity* **2005**, *22*, 43–57. [CrossRef]
27. Lasky, L.A. Selectins: Interpreters of cell-specific carbohydrate information during inflammation. *Science* **1992**, *258*, 964–969. [CrossRef] [PubMed]
28. Fieger, C.B.; Sassetti, C.M.; Rosen, S.D. Endoglycan, a member of the CD34 family, functions as an L-selectin ligand through modification with tyrosine sulfation and sialyl Lewis x. *J. Biol. Chem.* **2003**, *278*, 27390–27398. [CrossRef] [PubMed]
29. Sarangapani, K.K.; Yago, T.; Klopocki, A.G.; Lawrence, M.B.; Fieger, C.B.; Rosen, S.D.; McEver, R.P.; Zhu, C. Low force decelerates L-selectin dissociation from P-selectin glycoprotein ligand-1 and endoglycan. *J. Biol. Chem.* **2004**, *279*, 2291–2298. [CrossRef]
30. Healy, L.; May, G.; Gale, K.; Grosveld, F.; Greaves, M.; Enver, T. The stem cell antigen CD34 functions as a regulator of hemopoietic cell adhesion. *Proc. Natl. Acad. Sci. USA* **1995**, *92*, 12240–12244. [CrossRef]
31. Larrucea, S.; Butta, N.; Arias-Salgado, E.G.; Alonso-Martin, S.; Ayuso, M.S.; Parrilla, R. Expression of podocalyxin enhances the adherence, migration, and intercellular communication of cells. *Exp. Cell Res.* **2008**, *314*, 2004–2015. [CrossRef] [PubMed]
32. Schnabel, E.; Dekan, G.; Miettinen, A.; Farquhar, M.G. Biogenesis of podocalyxin—The major glomerular sialoglycoprotein—In the newborn rat kidney. *Eur. J. Cell Biol.* **1989**, *48*, 313–326. [PubMed]
33. Vitureira, N.; McNagny, K.; Soriano, E.; Burgaya, F. Pattern of expression of the podocalyxin gene in the mouse brain during development. *Gene Expr. Patterns GEP* **2005**, *5*, 349–354. [CrossRef] [PubMed]
34. Kobayashi, N.; Gao, S.Y.; Chen, J.; Saito, K.; Miyawaki, K.; Li, C.Y.; Pan, L.; Saito, S.; Terashita, T.; Matsuda, S. Process formation of the renal glomerular podocyte: Is there common molecular machinery for processes of podocytes and neurons? *Anat. Sci. Int.* **2004**, *79*, 1–10. [CrossRef] [PubMed]
35. Miettinen, A.; Solin, M.L.; Reivinen, J.; Juvonen, E.; Vaisanen, R.; Holthofer, H. Podocalyxin in rat platelets and megakaryocytes. *Am. J. Pathol.* **1999**, *154*, 813–822. [CrossRef]

36. Berenson, R.J.; Bensinger, W.I.; Hill, R.S.; Andrews, R.G.; Garcia-Lopez, J.; Kalamasz, D.F.; Still, B.J.; Spitzer, G.; Buckner, C.D.; Bernstein, I.D.; et al. Engraftment after infusion of CD34+ marrow cells in patients with breast cancer or neuroblastoma. *Blood* **1991**, *77*, 1717–1722. [CrossRef] [PubMed]
37. Majeti, R.; Park, C.Y.; Weissman, I.L. Identification of a hierarchy of multipotent hematopoietic progenitors in human cord blood. *Cell Stem Cell* **2007**, *1*, 635–645. [CrossRef] [PubMed]
38. Huss, R. Isolation of primary and immortalized CD34-hematopoietic and mesenchymal stem cells from various sources. *Stem Cells* **2000**, *18*, 1–9. [CrossRef]
39. Mao, Q.; Chu, S.; Ghanta, S.; Padbury, J.F.; De Paepe, M.E. Ex vivo expanded human cord blood-derived hematopoietic progenitor cells induce lung growth and alveolarization in injured newborn lungs. *Respir. Res.* **2013**, *14*, 37. [CrossRef]
40. Jang, Y.Y.; Collector, M.I.; Baylin, S.B.; Diehl, A.M.; Sharkis, S.J. Hematopoietic stem cells convert into liver cells within days without fusion. *Nat. Cell Biol.* **2004**, *6*, 532–539. [CrossRef]
41. da Silva Meirelles, L.; Chagastelles, P.C.; Nardi, N.B. Mesenchymal stem cells reside in virtually all post-natal organs and tissues. *J. Cell Sci.* **2006**, *119*, 2204–2213. [CrossRef] [PubMed]
42. Phinney, D.G.; Prockop, D.J. Concise review: Mesenchymal stem/multipotent stromal cells: The state of transdifferentiation and modes of tissue repair—Current views. *Stem Cells* **2007**, *25*, 2896–2902. [CrossRef]
43. Lin, C.S.; Ning, H.; Lin, G.; Lue, T.F. Is CD34 truly a negative marker for mesenchymal stromal cells? *Cytotherapy* **2012**, *14*, 1159–1163. [CrossRef]
44. Scherberich, A.; Di Maggio, N.D.; McNagny, K.M. A familiar stranger: CD34 expression and putative functions in SVF cells of adipose tissue. *World J. Stem Cells* **2013**, *5*, 1–8. [CrossRef] [PubMed]
45. Simmons, P.J.; Torok-Storb, B. CD34 expression by stromal precursors in normal human adult bone marrow. *Blood* **1991**, *78*, 2848–2853. [CrossRef]
46. Quirici, N.; Soligo, D.; Bossolasco, P.; Servida, F.; Lumini, C.; Deliliers, G.L. Isolation of bone marrow mesenchymal stem cells by anti-nerve growth factor receptor antibodies. *Exp. Hematol.* **2002**, *30*, 783–791. [CrossRef] [PubMed]
47. Ferraro, G.A.; De Francesco, F.; Nicoletti, G.; Paino, F.; Desiderio, V.; Tirino, V.; D'Andrea, F. Human adipose CD34+ CD90+ stem cells and collagen scaffold constructs grafted in vivo fabricate loose connective and adipose tissues. *J. Cell. Biochem.* **2013**, *114*, 1039–1049. [CrossRef] [PubMed]
48. De Francesco, F.; Tirino, V.; Desiderio, V.; Ferraro, G.; D'Andrea, F.; Giuliano, M.; Libondi, G.; Pirozzi, G.; De Rosa, A.; Papaccio, G. Human CD34/CD90 ASCs are capable of growing as sphere clusters, producing high levels of VEGF and forming capillaries. *PLoS ONE* **2009**, *4*, e6537. [CrossRef]
49. Kopher, R.A.; Penchev, V.R.; Islam, M.S.; Hill, K.L.; Khosla, S.; Kaufman, D.S. Human embryonic stem cell-derived CD34+ cells function as MSC progenitor cells. *Bone* **2010**, *47*, 718–728. [CrossRef]
50. Sinanan, A.C.; Hunt, N.P.; Lewis, M.P. Human adult craniofacial muscle-derived cells: Neural-cell adhesion-molecule (NCAM.; CD56)-expressing cells appear to contain multipotential stem cells. *Biotechnol. Appl. Biochem.* **2004**, *40*, 25–34. [CrossRef]
51. Beauchamp, J.R.; Heslop, L.; Yu, D.S.; Tajbakhsh, S.; Kelly, R.G.; Wernig, A.; Buckingham, M.E.; Partridge, T.A.; Zammit, P.S. Expression of CD34 and Myf5 defines the majority of quiescent adult skeletal muscle satellite cells. *J. Cell Biol.* **2000**, *151*, 1221–1234. [CrossRef]
52. Cossu, G.; Molinaro, M.; Pacifici, M. Differential response of satellite cells and embryonic myoblasts to a tumor promoter. *Dev. Biol.* **1983**, *98*, 520–524. [CrossRef] [PubMed]
53. Lecourt, S.; Marolleau, J.P.; Fromigue, O.; Vauchez, K.; Andriamanalijaona, R.; Ternaux, B.; Lacassagne, M.N.; Robert, I.; Boumediene, K.; Chereau, F.; et al. Characterization of distinct mesenchymal-like cell populations from human skeletal muscle in situ and in vitro. *Exp. Cell Res.* **2010**, *316*, 2513–2526. [CrossRef] [PubMed]
54. Zheng, B.; Cao, B.; Crisan, M.; Sun, B.; Li, G.; Logar, A.; Yap, S.; Pollett, J.B.; Drowley, L.; Cassino, T.; et al. Prospective identification of myogenic endothelial cells in human skeletal muscle. *Nat. Biotechnol.* **2007**, *25*, 1025–1034. [CrossRef] [PubMed]
55. Dupas, T.; Rouaud, T.; Rouger, K.; Lieubeau, B.; Cario-Toumaniantz, C.; Fontaine-Perus, J.; Gardahaut, M.F.; Auda-Boucher, G. Fetal muscle contains different CD34+ cell subsets that distinctly differentiate into adipogenic, angiogenic and myogenic lineages. *Stem Cell Res.* **2011**, *7*, 230–243. [CrossRef] [PubMed]
56. Brenes, R.A.; Bear, M.; Jadlowiec, C.; Goodwin, M.; Hashim, P.; Protack, C.D.; Ziegler, K.R.; Li, X.; Model, L.S.; Lv, W.; et al. Cell-based interventions for therapeutic angiogenesis: Review of potential cell sources. *Vascular* **2012**, *20*, 360–368. [CrossRef]
57. Mackie, A.R.; Losordo, D.W. CD34-positive stem cells: In the treatment of heart and vascular disease in human beings. *Tex. Heart Inst. J.* **2011**, *38*, 474–485.
58. Tondreau, T.; Meuleman, N.; Delforge, A.; Dejeneffe, M.; Leroy, R.; Massy, M.; Mortier, C.; Bron, D.; Lagneaux, L. Mesenchymal stem cells derived from CD133-positive cells in mobilized peripheral blood and cord blood: Proliferation, Oct4 expression, and plasticity. *Stem Cells* **2005**, *23*, 1105–1112. [CrossRef]
59. Matsumoto, T.; Kuroda, R.; Mifune, Y.; Kawamoto, A.; Shoji, T.; Miwa, M.; Asahara, T.; Kurosaka, M. Circulating endothelial/skeletal progenitor cells for bone regeneration and healing. *Bone* **2008**, *43*, 434–439. [CrossRef]
60. Siemerink, M.J.; Klaassen, I.; Vogels, I.M.; Griffioen, A.W.; Van Noorden, C.J.; Schlingemann, R.O. CD34 marks angiogenic tip cells in human vascular endothelial cell cultures. *Angiogenesis* **2012**, *15*, 151–163. [CrossRef]
61. Ye, G.; Qin, Y.; Lu, X.; Xu, X.; Xu, S.; Wu, C.; Wang, X.; Wang, S.; Pan, D. The association of renin-angiotensin system genes with the progression of hepatocellular carcinoma. *Biochem. Biophys. Res. Commun.* **2015**, *459*, 18–23. [CrossRef]

62. Clarke, M.F.; Dick, J.E.; Dirks, P.B.; Eaves, C.J.; Jamieson, C.H.; Jones, D.L.; Visvader, J.; Weissman, I.L.; Wahl, G.M. Cancer stem cells—Perspectives on current status and future directions: AACR Workshop on cancer stem cells. *Cancer Res.* **2006**, *66*, 9339–9344. [CrossRef] [PubMed]
63. Yang, L.; Shi, P.; Zhao, G.; Xu, J.; Peng, W.; Zhang, J.; Zhang, G.; Wang, X.; Dong, Z.; Chen, F.; et al. Targeting cancer stem cell pathways for cancer therapy. *Signal Transduct. Target. Ther.* **2020**, *5*, 8. [CrossRef] [PubMed]
64. Lapidot, T.; Sirard, C.; Vormoor, J.; Murdoch, B.; Hoang, T.; Caceres-Cortes, J.; Minden, M.; Paterson, B.; Caligiuri, M.A.; Dick, J.E. A cell initiating human acute myeloid leukaemia after transplantation into SCID mice. *Nature* **1994**, *367*, 645–648. [CrossRef] [PubMed]
65. Park, S.C.; Nguyen, N.T.; Eun, J.R.; Zhang, Y.; Jung, Y.J.; Tschudy-Seney, B.; Trotsyuk, A.; Lam, A.; Ramsamooj, R.; Zhang, Y.; et al. Identification of cancer stem cell subpopulations of CD34(+) PLC/PRF/5 that result in three types of human liver carcinomas. *Stem Cells Dev.* **2015**, *24*, 1008–1021. [CrossRef]
66. Yin, P.; Ono, M.; Moravek, M.B.; Coon, J.S.t.; Navarro, A.; Monsivais, D.; Dyson, M.T.; Druschitz, S.A.; Malpani, S.S.; Serna, V.A.; et al. Human uterine leiomyoma stem/progenitor cells expressing CD34 and CD49b initiate tumors in vivo. *J. Clin. Endocrinol. Metab.* **2015**, *100*, E601–E606. [CrossRef]
67. Aravindan, N.; Somasundaram, D.B.; Herman, T.S.; Aravindan, S. Significance of hematopoietic surface antigen CD34 in neuroblastoma prognosis and the genetic landscape of CD34-expressing neuroblastoma CSCs. *Cell Biol. Toxicol.* **2021**, *37*, 461–478. [CrossRef]
68. Kuroda, R.; Matsumoto, T.; Kawakami, Y.; Fukui, T.; Mifune, Y.; Kurosaka, M. Clinical impact of circulating CD34-positive cells on bone regeneration and healing. *Tissue Eng. Part B Rev.* **2014**, *20*, 190–199. [CrossRef]
69. Berenson, R.J.; Andrews, R.G.; Bensinger, W.I.; Kalamasz, D.; Knitter, G.; Buckner, C.D.; Bernstein, I.D. Antigen CD34+ marrow cells engraft lethally irradiated baboons. *J. Clin. Investig.* **1988**, *81*, 951–955. [CrossRef]
70. Lee, F.Y.; Chen, Y.L.; Sung, P.H.; Ma, M.C.; Pei, S.N.; Wu, C.J.; Yang, C.H.; Fu, M.; Ko, S.F.; Leu, S.; et al. Intracoronary Transfusion of Circulation-Derived CD34+ Cells Improves Left Ventricular Function in Patients With End-Stage Diffuse Coronary Artery Disease Unsuitable for Coronary Intervention. *Crit. Care Med.* **2015**, *43*, 2117–2132. [CrossRef]
71. El-Badawy, A.; El-Badri, N. Clinical Efficacy of Stem Cell Therapy for Diabetes Mellitus: A Meta-Analysis. *PLoS ONE* **2016**, *11*, e0151938. [CrossRef] [PubMed]
72. Sakamoto, M.; Nakamura, T.; Torimura, T.; Iwamoto, H.; Masuda, H.; Koga, H.; Abe, M.; Hashimoto, O.; Ueno, T.; Sata, M. Transplantation of endothelial progenitor cells ameliorates vascular dysfunction and portal hypertension in carbon tetrachloride-induced rat liver cirrhotic model. *J. Gastroenterol. Hepatol.* **2013**, *28*, 168–178. [CrossRef] [PubMed]
73. Quyyumi, A.A.; Vasquez, A.; Kereiakes, D.J.; Klapholz, M.; Schaer, G.L.; Abdel-Latif, A.; Frohwein, S.; Henry, T.D.; Schatz, R.A.; Dib, N.; et al. PreSERVE-AMI: A Randomized, Double-Blind, Placebo-Controlled Clinical Trial of Intracoronary Administration of Autologous CD34+ Cells in Patients With Left Ventricular Dysfunction Post STEMI. *Circ. Res.* **2017**, *120*, 324–331. [CrossRef] [PubMed]

Disclaimer/Publisher's Note: The statements, opinions and data contained in all publications are solely those of the individual author(s) and contributor(s) and not of MDPI and/or the editor(s). MDPI and/or the editor(s) disclaim responsibility for any injury to people or property resulting from any ideas, methods, instructions or products referred to in the content.

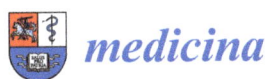 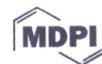

Review

Challenges in the Diagnosis and Individualized Treatment of Cervical Cancer

Melanie Schubert [1,*], Dirk Olaf Bauerschlag [1], Mustafa Zelal Muallem [2], Nicolai Maass [1] and Ibrahim Alkatout [1,*]

1. Department of Obstetrics and Gynecology, University Hospital of Schleswig Holstein, Campus Kiel, 24105 Kiel, Germany
2. Department of Gynecology with Center for Oncological Surgery, Charité–Universitätsmedizin Berlin, Corporate Member of Freie Universität Berlin, Humboldt-Universität zu Berlin, and Berlin Institute of Health, Virchow Campus Clinic, 13353 Berlin, Germany
* Correspondence: melanie.schubert@uksh.de (M.S.); ibrahim.alkatout@uksh.de (I.A.)

Abstract: Cervical cancer is still the fourth most common cancer in women throughout the world; an estimated 604,000 new cases were observed in 2020. Better knowledge of its pathogenesis, gained in recent years, has introduced new preventive and diagnostic approaches. Knowledge of its pathogenesis has made it possible to provide individualized surgical and drug treatment. In industrialized countries, cervical cancer has become a less frequent tumor entity due to the accessibility of the human papilloma virus vaccination, systematic preventive programs/early detection programs, health care infrastructure and the availability of effective therapy options. Nevertheless, globally, neither mortality nor morbidity has been significantly reduced over the past 10 years, and therapy approaches differ widely. The aim of this review is to address recent advances in the prevention, diagnostic investigation and treatment of cervical cancer globally, focusing on advances in Germany, with a view toward providing an updated overview for clinicians. The following aspects are addressed in detail: (a) the prevalence and causes of cervical cancer, (b) diagnostic tools using imaging techniques, cytology and pathology, (c) pathomechanisms and clinical symptoms of cervical cancer and (d) different treatment approaches (pharmacological, surgical and others) and their impact on outcomes.

Keywords: cervical cancer; HPV; nerve-sparing radical hysterectomy; radiochemotherapy; checkpoint inhibitors

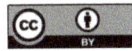

1. Introduction

Ninety percent of cervical cancers occur in low- and middle-income countries (LMIC). It is the fourth most common cancer in women worldwide after breast, colorectal and lung cancer. In 2020, the World Health Organization (WHO) estimated a prevalence of 604,000 new cases and 342,000 deaths worldwide [1]. The median age of women at the initial diagnosis of cervical cancer is currently 55 years and has decreased by 15 years over the past 25 years. In about 25 percent of cases, cervical cancer occurs in women younger than 35 years of age. It is the most common gynecologic malignancy during pregnancy, with an incidence of 0.1–12:10,000 [2].

The introduction of screening examinations by the Papanicolaou smear (Pap smear) since 1971 and the human papillomavirus (HPV) vaccination since 2006 led to a dramatic reduction in the incidence of cervical intraepithelial neoplasms (CIN) and cervical cancer in industrialized countries. Cervical cancer is now the thirteenth most common cancer in women in developed countries such as Germany [3]. However, the past 10 years have witnessed no significant reduction in mortality or morbidity; therapy approaches are still very diverse [2].

2. Pathogenesis and Risk Factors

Eighty percent of cervical cancers are squamous cell carcinomas. However, the incidence of the less common adenocarcinoma of the cervix has been rising over the last decades. Other rare types include adenosquamous, serous papillary and neuroendocrine cervical carcinoma [4].

The carcinogenesis of cervical cancer is considered to be multifactorial. In addition to common cancer risk factors, such as smoking, promiscuity, long-term use of oral contraceptives, low socioeconomic status and immunosuppression caused by infection, such as by the human immunodeficiency virus (HIV) or drug immunosuppressants after organ transplantation, the most relevant factor in the emergence of cervical cancer is HPV [2].

Eighty percent of sexually active women and men are infected by HPV in their lifetimes, but the infection persists in a mere 5–10% and leads to cervical cancer in just 3% [3,5]. A persistent high-risk HPV infection may cause invasive cervical, vulvar, vulvovaginal, penile, anal, oropharyngeal, or head and neck cancer [2]. The developmental phase from HPV infection to cervical cancer is about 20 years [6]. HPV types most commonly responsible for the development of cervical carcinoma include the high-risk HPV types 16, 18, 45, 31, 33, 58, 52, 35, 59, 56, 6, 51, 68, 39, 82, 73, 66 and 70. Cervical cancer arises from the CIN I–III lesions, which are also classified as low-grade squamous intraepithelial lesions (LSIL), high-grade squamous intraepithelial lesions (HSIL) and adenocarcinoma in situ (ACIS) [2]. With an annual regression rate of 15–23% and a regression rate of 55% in 4–6 years, CIN II is less likely to progress to cervical cancer. In contrast, CIN III has an annual progression rate to invasive carcinoma of 0.2–4% [6].

3. Diagnostic Investigation and Prevention

The Pap-only test, the Pap-HPV co-test and the high-risk HPV-only test are the three tests commonly performed for the early detection of cervical cancer. A higher sensitivity, reproducibility and safer prolongation of screening intervals have been proven in several studies for the HPV test compared to conventional cytology or colposcopy [7]. The investigations have demonstrated the safe and sensitive effect of self-sampling for the HPV test, as well as its benefits in LMIC due to its easy and convenient use and its physical and emotional comfort [7,8]. Therefore, HPV self-sampling has been included in the WHO guidelines on self-care interventions for health and well-being published in 2021. The detection of CIN and CIN III by PCR-based self-sampling tests has been demonstrated, but these tests have not been established yet [7].

HPV vaccination is an efficient primary prophylaxis of cervical cancer. In 2007, the recommendations of the Standing Commission on Vaccination (STIKO) imported the precautionary HPV vaccination, which currently advocate vaccination for girls between the ages of 9 and 14 years; since 2018, it has also been recommended for boys of these ages [2]. A prophylactic effect of the HPV vaccination with regard to vaccine-type-specific anogenital diseases has also been shown in women and men aged 14–45 years [9]. The Centers for Disease Control and Prevention (CDC) in the United States recommends a routine HPV vaccination at the age of 11 or 12 years, with the possible start of vaccination at the age of 9 years, a catch-up vaccination to the age of 26 years and a possible vaccination for adults from the age of 27 to 45 years [6].

In terms of tertiary prevention, HPV vaccination was reported to be significantly effective after the surgical treatment of patients with CIN I-III lesions; the risk of developing recurrent CIN was reduced by 58.7% [10]. Despite these data regarding efficacy, the provision of the vaccination on a worldwide basis is still very diverse and worthy of improvement. Less than 30% of LMICs have introduced the HPV vaccination, and only about 20% of women in LMICs have ever been screened for cervical cancer. In contrast, high-income countries have more than an 85% uptake on HPV vaccination, and 60% of women in high-income countries have been vaccinated [11].

Due to the high accessibility and acceptance of vaccines in the population as well as school-based vaccination programs, Portugal, Norway, Iceland, Spain, England and

Sweden have high vaccination rates (95%, 85%, 88%, 80%, 80% and 80%, respectively, in 15-year-old women). The proportion of vaccinated persons in Germany was 44.6% in 2018, and in the United States it was 58.6% in 2020 [2]. The current standard Gardasil 9® vaccine is a nonavalent vaccine for the oncogenic/high-risk HPV types 16, 18, 31, 33, 45, 52 and 58 and for the non-oncogenic/low-risk HPV types 6 and 11 [2,12]. HPV vaccination can prevent up to 70% of HPV-related cervical cancers and up to 90% of genital warts [2].

A new classification was published by the Fédération Internationale de Gynécologie et d'Obstétrique (FIGO) in 2018, which supplements the bimanual palpation examination with magnetic resonance imaging (MRI) of the pelvis/computed tomography (CT) of the chest, abdomen and pelvis, as well as biopsies for clinical staging. MRI provides the best assessment of local tumor spreading in terms of parametrial infiltration (sensitivity 84% [13]), whereas CT is used to rule out distant metastases. Surgical staging permits the best assessment of lymph node involvement through systematic lymphadenectomy (LNE). Histological staging has been performed via the TNM classification from 2010 onward. Because the current treatment recommendations are based on data derived from the application of the old FIGO classification of 2009, the following recommendations in this review are also based on the old FIGO classification. Table 1 and Figure 1 reflect the most recent FIGO classification of 2018 [14].

Table 1. FIGO classification 2018 [14].

Stage			
I			Carcinoma strictly confined to the cervix
	IA		Invasive carcinoma with maximum depth of invasion ≤ 5 mm
		IA1	Stromal invasion ≤ 3 mm in depth
		IA2	Stromal invasion > 3 mm and ≤5 mm in depth
	IB		Deepest invasion > 5 mm; lesion limited to cervix uteri with size measured according to maximum tumor diameter
		IB1	>5 mm depth of stromal invasion and ≤2 cm in greatest dimension
		IB2	>2 cm and ≤4 cm in greatest dimension
		IB3	>4 cm in greatest dimension
II			Invasion beyond the uterus, but no extension into the lower third of the vagina or to the pelvic wall
	IIA		Involvement limited to the upper two thirds of the vagina without parametrial invasion
		IIA1	≤4 cm in greatest dimension
		IIA2	>4 cm in greatest dimension
	IIB		Parametrial invasion but not to the pelvic wall
III			Involvement of the lower third of the vagina and/or extension to the pelvic wall and/or causes hydronephrosis or non-functioning kidney and/or involvement of pelvic and/or para-aortic lymph nodes
	IIIA		Involvement of the lower third of the vagina, with no extension to the pelvic wall
	IIIB		Extension to the pelvic wall and/or hydronephrosis or non-functioning kidney (unless known to be due to another cause)
	IIIC		Involvement of pelvic and/or para-aortic lymph nodes (including micrometastases), irrespective of tumor size and extent
		IIIC1	Pelvic lymph node metastases only
		IIIC2	Para-aortic lymph node metastases
IV			Extension beyond the true pelvis or involvement (biopsy proven) of the mucosa of the bladder or rectum
	IVA		Spread of the growth to adjacent organs
	IVB		Spread to distant organs

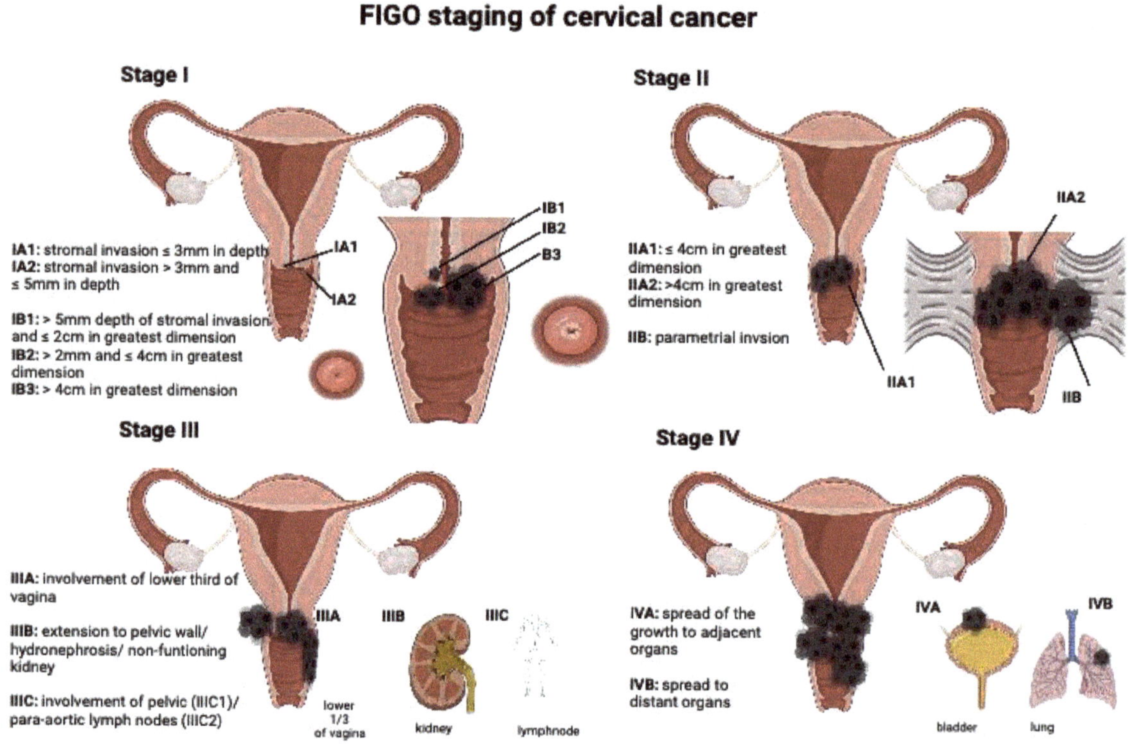

Figure 1. FIGO staging system created with BioRender.com.

4. Surgical Treatment

The therapeutic decision for cervical cancer must be made on an interdisciplinary basis involving gynecologic oncologists, radiation therapists, radiologists, and pathologists. A crucial factor is whether the preservation of fertility is desired and possible. The patient's wishes as well as her general condition, risk factors, menopausal status and life situation must be included in the decision-making process. Surgery and primary radio(chemo)therapy (RCT) are available as curative treatment options. Based on the current recommendations, a multimodal therapy concept should be avoided because of the resulting increase in morbidity. Furthermore, over- or under-therapy should be avoided [2].

The patient's lymph node status is one of the most important prognostic parameters in cervical cancer. The determination of tumor stage, prognosis and the resulting therapy decision is based on the intraoperative assessment of the lymph node status. Preoperative imaging with CT, MRI or PET-CT has been shown to be inferior to the surgical detection of lymph node metastases [15]. A comprehensive algorithm for tumor staging is shown in Figure 2.

One approach to therapy de-escalation in early cervical cancer is the use of a sentinel node biopsy (SNB). The sentinel technique for cervical cancer is recommended in the primary stage pTIa1 L1 and/or pTIA 2 and stage pTIB1 ($\leq$2 cm), and it consists of combined detection with technetium-99 and blue dye or, more commonly used today, with intraoperative visualization with indocyanine green (ICG, Figure 3). Ultrastaging to detect low-volume nodal metastases (isolated tumor cells (ITCs) and micrometastases) is recommended in these cases. SNB is feasible and provides excellent detection rates and sensitivity. SNB reduces morbidity compared to pelvic LNE, especially the incidence of lower limb lymphoedema [16]. The three large phase III studies, the Phenix, SENTICOL III and SENTIX trials, are currently evaluating this technique prospectively and will provide further evidence in connection with this procedure [17–20].

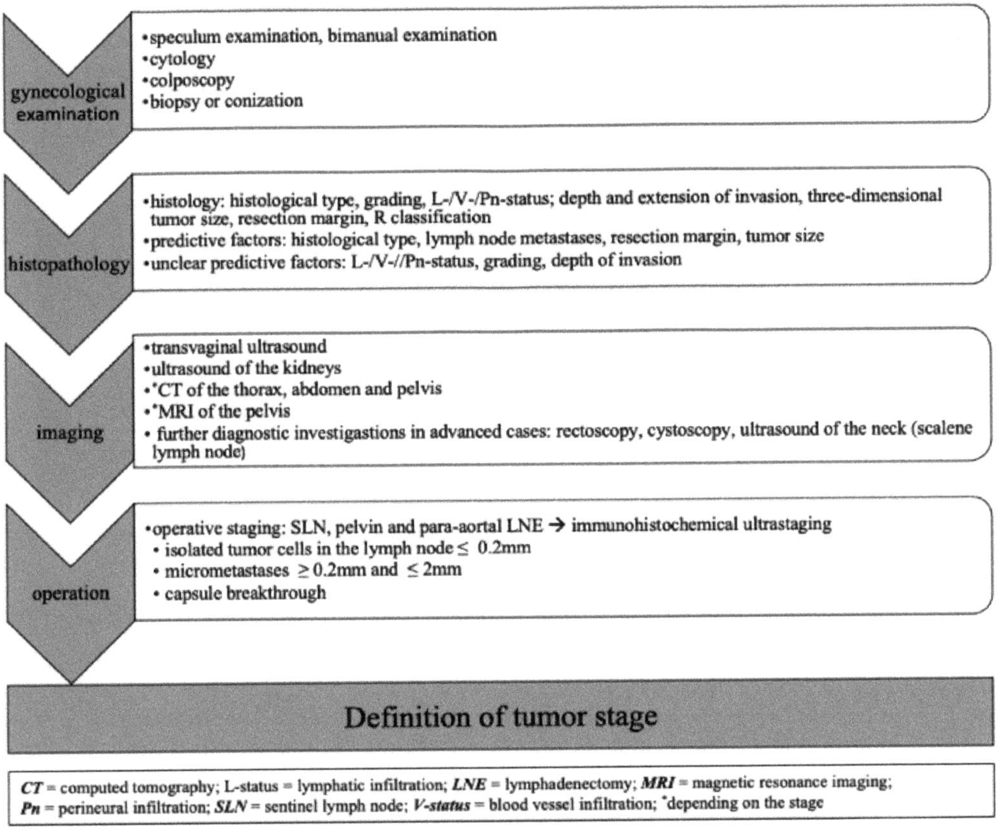

gynecological examination
- speculum examination, bimanual examination
- cytology
- colposcopy
- biopsy or conization

histopathology
- histology: histological type, grading, L-/V-/Pn-status; depth and extension of invasion, three-dimensional tumor size, resection margin, R classification
- predictive factors: histological type, lymph node metastases, resection margin, tumor size
- unclear predictive factors: L-/V-//Pn-status, grading, depth of invasion

imaging
- transvaginal ultrasound
- ultrasound of the kidneys
- *CT of the thorax, abdomen and pelvis
- *MRI of the pelvis
- further diagnostic investigations in advanced cases: rectoscopy, cystoscopy, ultrasound of the neck (scalene lymph node)

operation
- operative staging: SLN, pelvin and para-aortal LNE → immunohistochemical ultrastaging
- isolated tumor cells in the lymph node ≤ 0.2mm
- micrometastases ≥ 0.2mm and ≤ 2mm
- capsule breakthrough

Definition of tumor stage

CT = computed tomography; L-status = lymphatic infiltration; LNE = lymphadenectomy; MRI = magnetic resonance imaging; Pn = perineural infiltration; SLN = sentinel lymph node; V-status = blood vessel infiltration; *depending on the stage

Figure 2. Algorithm of tumor stage definition in cervical cancer, adapted from the German S3 guidelines [2].

In addition to SNB, the sentinel procedure is used as a part of radical systematic LNE to improve the detection of lymph nodes and to avoid the inclusion of lymphatic drainage pathways, which is associated with a higher rate of morbidity. Systematic radical LNE is used to remove all lymph nodes along the vascular pathways of the associated lymphatic drainage area. Fifteen to twenty pelvic lymph nodes and eight to ten para-aortic lymph nodes are considered representative [2].

Data from the Laparoscopic Approach to Cervical Cancer (LACC) trial, a randomized phase III study, especially those obtained in 2018, have called for significant rethinking in the treatment of cervical cancer. The LACC trial showed that patients after laparotomy have a significantly higher rate of disease-free survival (3-year DFS, 97.1% vs. 91.2%; HR 3.74; 95% CI, 1.63 to 8.58) and a significantly better overall survival (3-year OS, 99.0% vs. 93.8%; HR 6.00, 95% CI, 1.77 to 20.30) compared to patients who undergo minimally invasive surgery [21]. The clear superiority of the abdominal approach in terms of OS and DFS was also evident in a recently published final analysis of the LACC trial [22]. The cause is still largely unexplained, which is why cervical cancer should currently be operated on via laparotomy and, only in exceptional cases and after appropriate explanation, via a minimally invasive procedure [14].

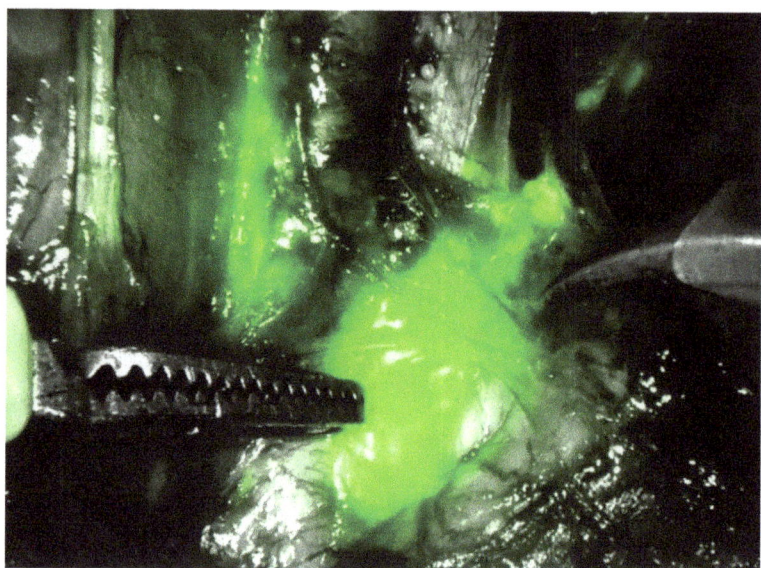

Figure 3. Intraoperative sentinel node visualization with indocyanine green at the Department of Obstetrics and Gynecology, University Hospital of Schleswig Holstein, Campus Kiel, Germany.

Studies aimed at reproving the safety of minimally invasive surgery for cervical cancer have been initiated and are currently in progress. Among the leading points of criticism of the LACC trial are the use of transcervical uterine manipulators, the lack of proper tumor containment at the time of colpectomy leading to peritoneal contamination, non-comparable operators/expertise, a low prevalence of robotic-assisted radical hysterectomy and the lack of proper preoperative imaging and assessment [23–26].

Tumor extirpation by means of previous conization [27,28] or closure using a vaginal cuff showed a comparable DFS and OS in patients treated with a laparoscopy and a laparotomy [24,26]. Ronsini et al. showed, in their meta-analysis, that laparo-assisted vaginal hysterectomies (LARVH) for tumors with a maximum diameter of 2 cm do not appear to affect DFS and OS compared to abdominal radical hysterectomies by using a vaginal cuff to prevent the tumor's spillage and by not using a uterus manipulator. A statement in the subanalysis about tumors > 2 cm could not be made [24].

Comparable OS, DFS and recurrence rates for open and robotic radical hysterectomies were shown in several reports, thus demonstrating the safety of robotic-assisted radical hysterectomies [25,29–33]. Leitao et al. showed, in their recent systematic review and meta-analysis of cancer outcomes, similar OS and DFS rates for robotic-assisted and laparoscopic surgery [1.01 (0.56, 1.80), $p = 0.98$] or open [1.18 (0.99, 1.41), $p = 0.06$] [33]. However, large prospective randomized studies will be needed to cause a change in current guideline recommendations.

The Robot-assisted Approach to Cervical Cancer (RACC) trial, an international, randomized controlled multicenter trial, is currently in progress. Women with early-stage cervical cancer are randomly assigned to robotic-assisted surgery or a laparotomy. The results of this study are eagerly awaited [34]. Likewise, the ongoing Robotic versus Open Radical Hysterectomy for Cervical Cancer (ROCC) trial will provide more detailed insights into this currently critical issue [23].

The different radicality of hysterectomies is classified into the five grades of Piver I–V according to Piver et al., among others, and is listed in Figure 4 [34,35].

4.1. Nerve-Sparing Radical Hysterectomy

The goal of surgical treatment in cervical cancer is not only tumor-free resection but also the preservation of organ functionality and crucial nerves. Modern imaging with MRI provides three-dimensional anatomical information about principal nerves such as the hypogastric nerve (HN), the inferior hypogastric plexus (IHP) and the pelvic splanchnic nerve (PSN). Bladder functionality is achieved through sympathetic nerves for bladder relaxation and parasympathetic innervation for bladder contraction. Therefore, the preservation of the HN, the PSNs, the IHP and the vesical nerve branches must be ensured [36]. A detailed anatomical illustration of these essential nerves is shown in Figure 5.

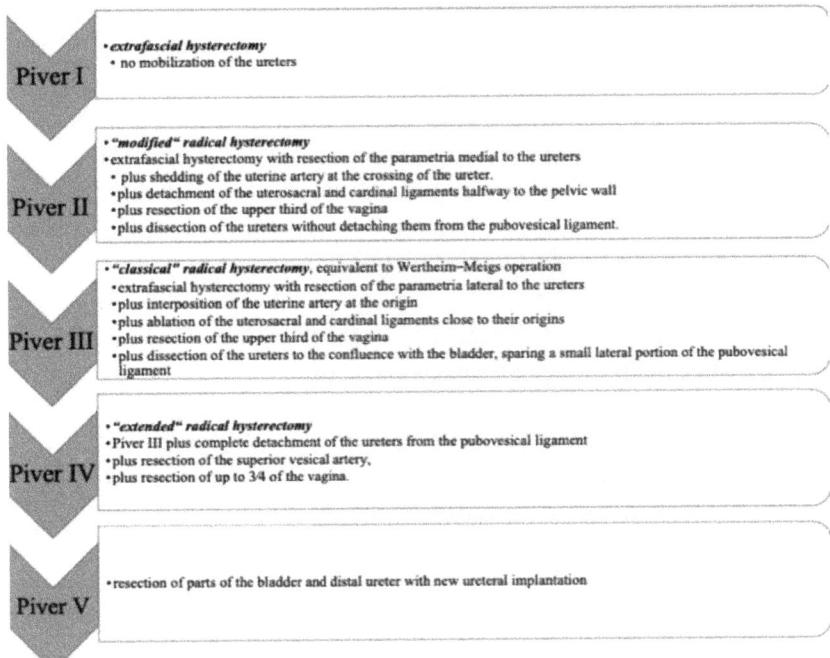

Figure 4. Classification of hysterectomy classified by Piver et al. [35].

A classical radical hysterectomy involves the complete resection of the cardinal ligament along with pelvic splanchnic nerves. In a nerve-sparing radical hysterectomy, the superior HN in conjunction with sympathetic innervation is visualized at the level of the aortic bifurcation, followed by bilateral dissection along the sigmoid colon. The pelvic splanchnic nerve in conjunction with parasympathetic innervation is exposed and spared from the lateral aspect at the same level. Parametrial dissection during a nerve-sparing radical hysterectomy is performed under directed visualization of the contiguous pelvic autonomic nerves. During resection of the dorsal parametrium, the HN in the mesoureter is spared with a previous preparation. The resection of the ventral and lateral parametrium must be performed under the viewing and sparing of the IHP, the bladder branches of the IHP and the PSN [36–39].

It should be mentioned here that nerve-sparing radical hysterectomies are not confined to early-stage cervical cancer. Tumor size plays no role when making the decision about sparing the autonomic nerve system, which must be the standard of care even for tumors > 4 cm in size [38,40].

The classic triad of complications following a radical hysterectomy consists of the lack of bladder sensitivity, a hypo- or non-contractile detrusor and disturbed coordination of detrusor contraction; these should be strictly avoided. Rectal nerve preservation can also prevent slow transit constipation. An underestimated complication of radical hysterectomies is the loss of function of the genital cavernous bodies and the associated vaginal lubrication, which can also be reduced by using the nerve-sparing surgical technique. Nerve-sparing surgery was shown to significantly reduce postoperative morbidity and improve quality of life [38,41–43].

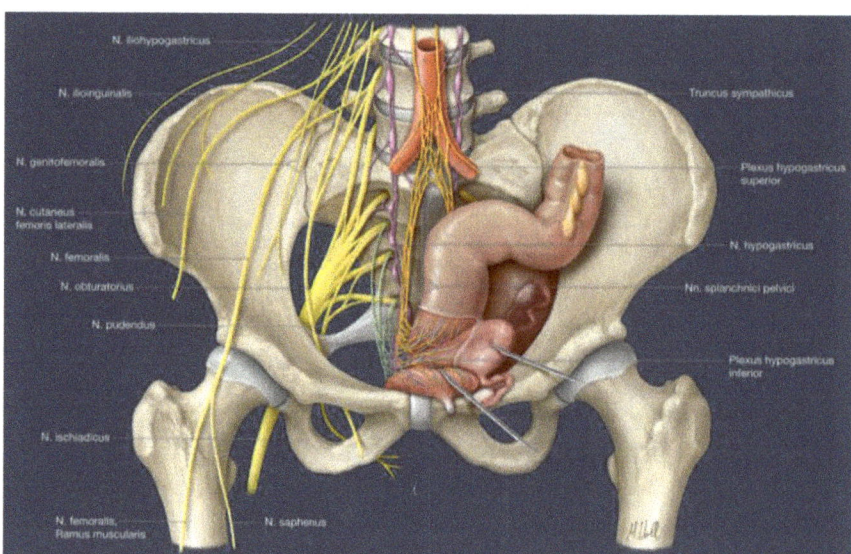

Figure 5. Anatomical illustration of somatic and autonomic pelvic nerves in a female pelvis. Yellow: somatic nerves; orange: sympathetic plexus; purple: sympathetic trunk; green: pelvic splanchnic nerves (PSN), courtesy of Alkatout et al. [44].

4.2. Fertility Preservation

As 40% of patients with cervical cancer are of reproductive age, the preservation of fertility must be taken into account if the patient wishes to preserve her fertility and when such preservation is oncologically justifiable. According to the National Comprehensive Cancer Network (NCCN) guidelines, the European Society of Gynecological Oncology (ESGO)/European Society for Radiotherapy and Oncology (ESTRO)/European Society of Pathology (ESP) guidelines, as well as the German guidelines, fertility-sparing treatment can be offered to patients with stage IA1 to IB1 squamous cell carcinoma and adenocarcinoma of the cervix. Fertility-sparing surgery is not recommended for gastric-type adenocarcinoma, small cell neuroendocrine histology and non-HPV-related adenocarcinomas [2,14,45]. The treatment options for preserving fertility include conization; simple and radical trachelectomy performed abdominally, vaginally or by conventional laparoscopy; or robotic assistance with prophylactic permanent cerclage. Whereas conization or simple trachelectomy is performed with pregnancy rates of 71–75% in stage IA1 and IA2 without risk factors, radical trachelectomy with permanent cerclage should be used as a fertility-preserving procedure in stage IA1 L1 V0, stage IA2 V0 or stage IB1 and IIA1 V0 < 2 cm. From stage IA1 L1 onward, prior histopathological exclusion of lymph node metastases with SNB or LNE is mandatory [2,14,46]. Neoadjuvant chemotherapy can be administered in stage IB1 $\geq$ 2 cm, followed by conization or trachelectomy within studies; this procedure is not recommended as a standard therapy [2].

The selection of patients suitable for fertility preservation should be made on the basis of the pathological extent/stage of the tumor, as well as the patient's comorbidities and her likelihood of becoming pregnant and carrying the pregnancy to term. The patient must be informed in detail about the risks, advantages, and therapy alternatives in a strict sense of shared decision making. Therefore, multidisciplinary consultation with gynecologic oncologists, fertility specialists, pathologists, radiologists and radiation therapists is essential before making therapy decisions. The oncologic safety of these techniques has been proven, but patients must be educated about the fact of a high-risk pregnancy with a higher risk of miscarriage, preterm birth (31–57%) and primary cesarean section after trachelectomy. Similarly, cervical stenosis (5–15%) with associated infertility may occur postoperatively. A hysterectomy need not be performed routinely after completed family planning, but it is recommended in the case of HPV persistence, Pap abnormality, a desire for maximum safety, or limited or abolished accessibility of the cervix [2,46,47].

4.3. Stage-Specific Therapy Guides

The following therapy algorithms for the individual stages of cervical cancer are listed according to the German guidelines [2], the NCCN [46] and the ESGO/ESTRO/ESP guidelines [14].

Patients with stage IA1 without a risk factor should be treated with conization and cervical curettage or a simple hysterectomy in cases of positive margins after conization, completed family planning or a desire for greater safety. In the case of positive margins after conization and the desire to preserve fertility, the patient may be offered re-conization or trachelectomy with prophylactic permanent cerclage. A secondary hysterectomy can be performed in this setting, as mentioned before [2,14,46].

In stage IA1, with the invasion of lymphatic vessels (L1), SNB should be performed in accordance with the same therapy recommendations as those of stage IA1 without L1. SNB is also indicated in stage IA1 with at least two risk factors and in stage IA2 with one risk factor. The involvement of SLN is an indication for systematic LNE followed by RCT, as well as prior ovariopexy with bilateral salpingectomy to preserve intrinsic ovarian function in premenopausal patients. Piver I is performed in cases of disease-free pelvic SLN.

Fertility cannot be preserved in stage IA2 with at least two risk factors. SNB is performed as a part of surgical staging in this setting. In the case of negative SLN, the approach used here is Piver II with bilateral salpingo-oophorectomy if needed [2].

In contrast, the NCCN guidelines for stage IA1 with L1 and stage IA2 recommend a modified radical hysterectomy after previous pelvic LNE or SLN mapping, or in cases of inoperable patients/stage IA2 pelvic external beam radiotherapy (ERBT) with brachytherapy [46]. The ESGO/ESTRO/ESP guidelines recommend adjuvant radiotherapy alone in stage 1A2 with L1, stage 1B1 or stage 2A1 [14].

The international guidelines recommend the use of the Sedlis criteria as a guide for adjuvant treatment decisions in node-negative, margin-negative and parametria-negative cases. The Sedlis criteria include greater than one-third stromal invasion, capillary lymphatic space involvement and a cervical tumor diameter greater than 4 cm [46,48].

In the case of diseased pelvic lymph nodes, surgical staging is again extended to include para-aortic LNE to remove the affected lymph nodes and to determine the radiation field for subsequent RCT [2,14].

Patients with stage IB1 < 2 cm without risk factors should be treated with a radical hysterectomy, Piver II, in the case of negative pelvic SLN [14]. If the patient wishes to preserve her fertility, it would be advisable to perform a radical trachelectomy with prophylactic permanent cerclage. Surgery should only be performed in the absence of an upfront indication for adjuvant radiotherapy [2]. The NCCN or ESGO/ESTRO/ESP guidelines provide no recommendations for a routine secondary hysterectomy [14,46].

Patients with stage IIA1 should be treated with a radical hysterectomy, Piver II, with a tumor-free resection margin of the vaginal cuff. In postmenopausal patients or premenopausal patients with adenocarcinoma, the German guidelines recommend a radical hysterectomy, Piver III, with a tumor-free margin of the vaginal cuff and bilateral salpingo-oophorectomy for stage IB2, IIA2 and IIB with a maximum of two risk factors. RCT is recommended in stage 1B2 and higher with positive margins or residual tumors, including positive lymph nodes on imaging [2,14]. In contrast, the NCCN guidelines give preference to RCT over surgery in stage IB2 and IIA2. The German and ESGO/ESTRO/ESP guidelines advocate RCT rather than surgery in stage IIB and above [2,14]. Whereas the German guidelines recommend surgical lymph node staging via pelvic and para-aortic LNE for stage IB2 and IIA2 tumors with the possible removal of affected lymph nodes, the NCCN guidelines recommend only lymph node staging via radiologic imaging in these stages [2,46].

The recommendation for stage III is surgical staging via systematic LNE with the removal of malignant lymph nodes or radiological assessment of malignancy prior to R(C)T [2]. The ESGO/ESTRO/ESP guidelines advocate for the possibility of para-aortic LNE, at least up to the inferior mesenteric artery with negative para-aortic lymph nodes on imaging and debulking of suspicious pelvic lymph nodes, whereas the NCCN guidelines recommend radiologic staging for stage IB2 and higher [14,46].

In stage IVA, the choices, among others, are R(C)T or primary exenteration in selected cases. In stage IVB, the focus is on symptom-oriented therapy, which consists of radiotherapy or RCT, palliative chemotherapy combined with bevacizumab and with or without pembrolizumab, or best supportive care [2,14,49,50]. Therapy algorithms for the individual tumor stages are shown in Figure 6, adapted according to the German guidelines.

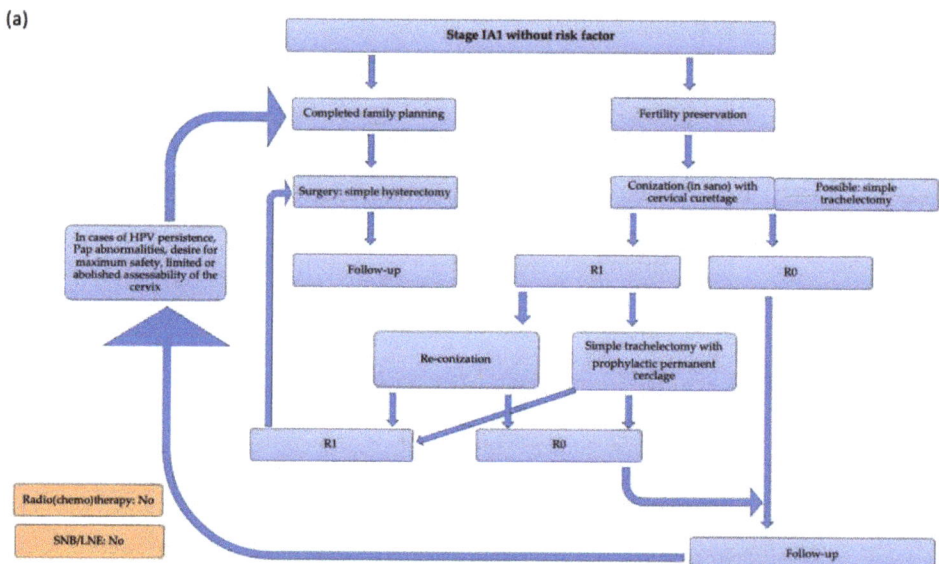

Figure 6. *Cont.*

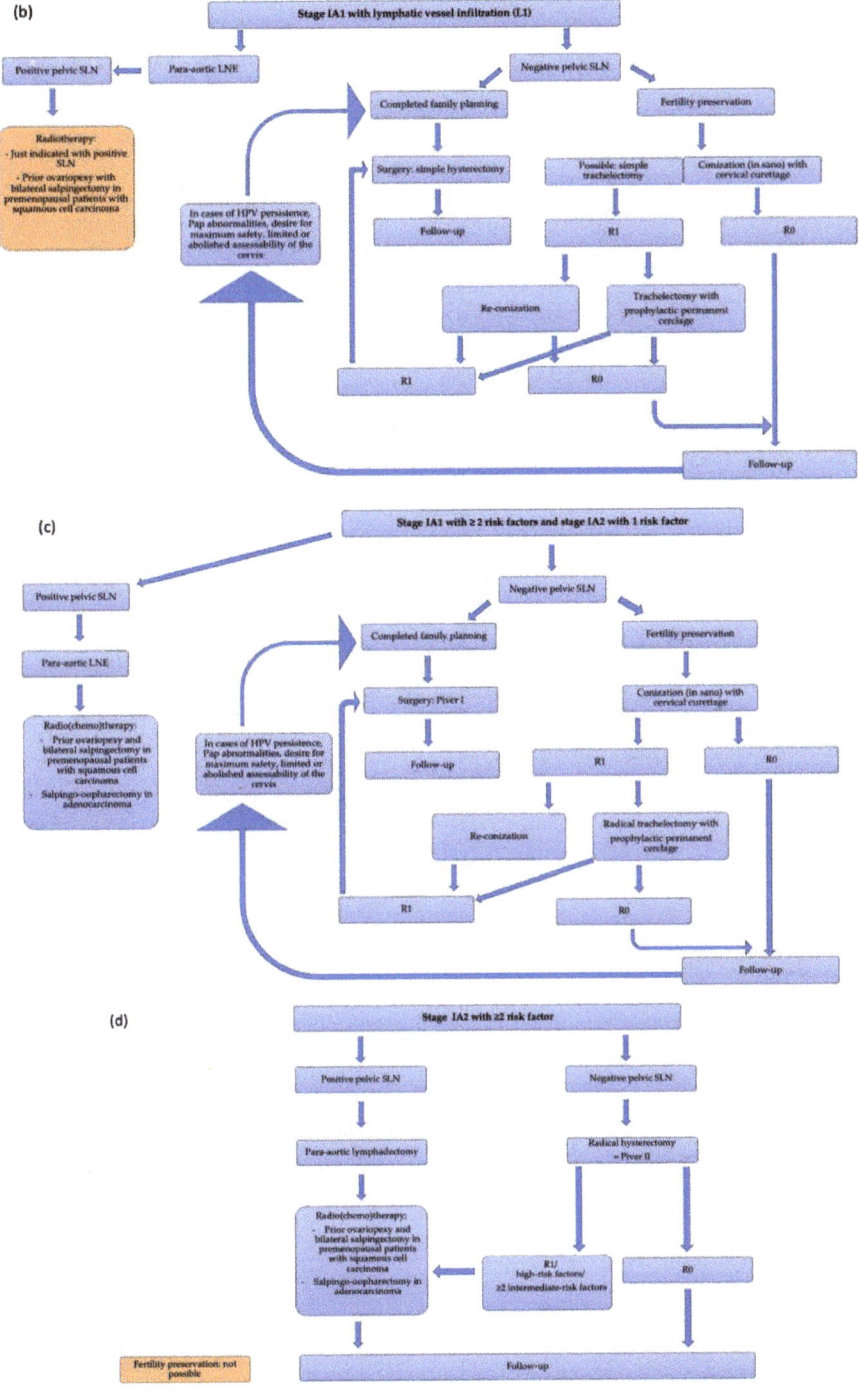

Figure 6. Cont.

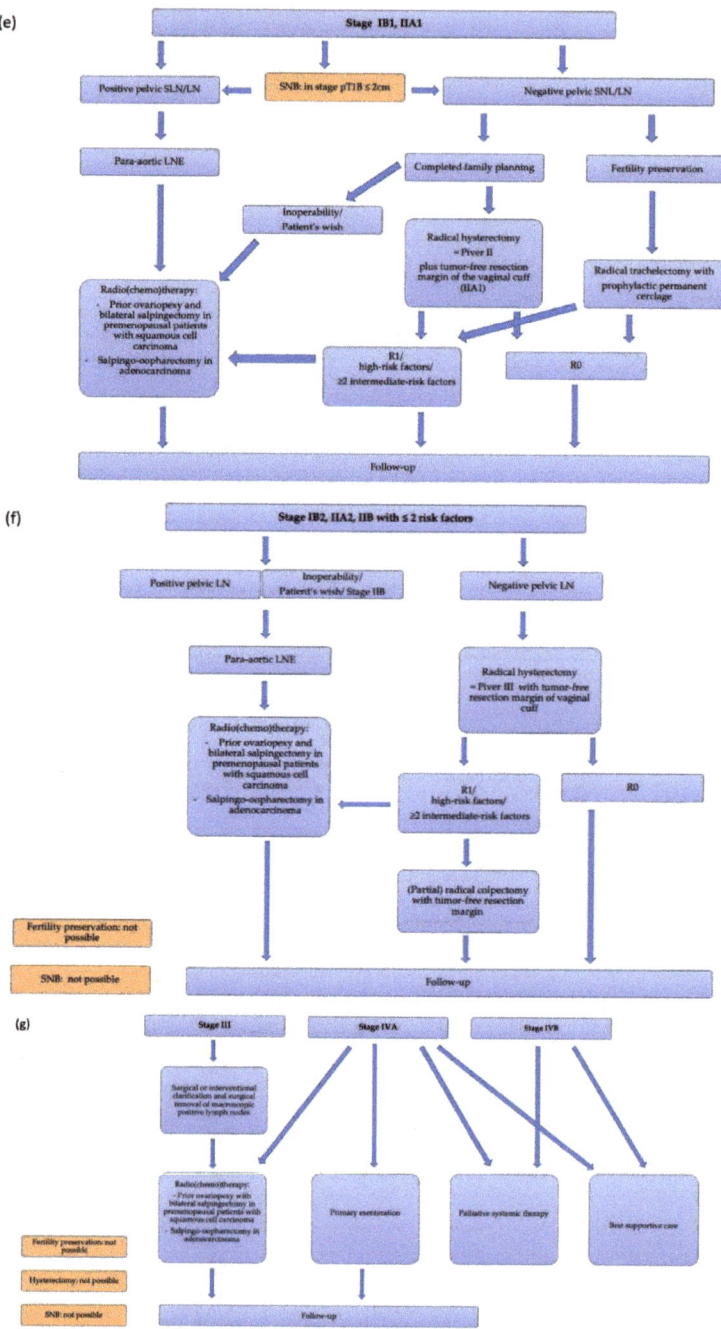

Figure 6. Therapy algorithm for cervical cancer based on the German guidelines: (**a**) Stage IA1 without risk factors; (**b**) Stage IA1 with L1; (**c**) Stage IA1 with ≥2 risk factors and stage IA2 with 1 risk factor; (**d**) Stage IA2 with ≥2 risk factors; (**e**) Stage IB1, IIA1; (**f**) Stage IB2, IIA2, IIB with ≤2 risk factors; (**g**) Stage III, stage IVA, stage IVB [2].

5. Radio(Chemo)Therapy

Intensity-modulated radiotherapy, individualized MRI-guided brachytherapy or image-guided adaptive brachytherapy (IGABIT) should be used in the primary RCT of cervical cancer; this approach provides optimal protection of surrounding tissue by reducing gastrointestinal and urogenital toxicities as well as acute and late therapy-related reactions. The approach also permits the safe use of selective dose escalation or a simultaneous integrated boost [2]. RCT is given with cisplatin 40 mg/m^2 body surface area for 5 weeks as a radiosensitizer and may be administered as a neoadjuvant, primary or adjuvant therapy. In the event of existing contraindications to chemotherapy with cisplatin, such as renal failure, radiation alone is used. Previous LNE may help to define the radiation field, which extends over the pelvic and para-aortic lymphatic drainage area and is referred to as extended-field radiotherapy in the sense of percutaneous radiotherapy when para-aortic lymph nodes are also affected. Brachytherapy must be included if the hysterectomy is not a part of the primary operative therapy/staging procedure. Percutaneous radiation of the primary tumor and lymph nodes is primarily performed with combined cisplatin-containing chemotherapy, followed by brachytherapy of the primary tumor [2,14,46]. Adjuvant RCT should be given to patients with histologically confirmed postoperative high-risk factors, such as lymph node metastases and parametrial infiltration, as well as positive resection margins. Adjuvant radiotherapy alone is the adjuvant therapy of choice for intermediate-risk factors or positive Sedlis criteria, such as lymphovascular space invasion, invasion of more than a third of cervical stromal and tumor size > 4 cm [51]. Clearly, the high morbidity of adjuvant RCT after surgery should be considered and discussed with the patient [46].

6. Medical Therapy

In addition to surgical and radiologic (lymph node) staging, the current standard therapy for locally advanced cervical cancer is primary simultaneous RCT with cisplatin [2,14,46]. Patients with recurrent, persistent or metastatic cervical cancer should be treated with a combination of cisplatin/topotecan or cisplatin/paclitaxel and bevacizumab. This combination has shown benefits in terms of survival (8.2 months vs. 6 months; HR 0.68 [95% CI 0.56–0.84]; $p = 0.0002$), DFS (13.3 months vs. 16.8 months; HR 0.77 [95% CI 0.062–0.95]; $p = 0.007$) and response rates (49% vs. 36%; $p = 0.003$) in a GOG 240 study [45,50]. A randomized phase III JCOG0505 trial showed equal efficacy; carboplatin can be used instead of cisplatin to prevent nephrotoxicity and neutropenia [52]. More recent data from the phase II CECILIA trial showed that the combination of carboplatin with paclitaxel and bevacizumab achieves comparable efficacy and has a favorable side effect profile [53]. Nab-paclitaxel, vinorelbine, ifosfamide, topotecan, pemetrexed or irinotecan can be used in second-line therapy [2].

Analogous to the treatment of endometrial cancer, new data have been obtained for cervical cancer in regard to immune checkpoint inhibitors. The largely HPV-dependent carcinogenesis of cervical cancer explains the high immunogenicity of these tumors. Thus, immunotherapy could be successful in this setting. The programmed cell death ligand PD-1/PD-L1 system is particularly important for the course of the disease and is involved in carcinogenesis. A KEYNOTE 158 trial revealed a response rate of 15% and promising OS rates (median, 9.4 months for the entire study population and 11.0 months for the PD-L1-positive population) in patients with advanced cervical cancer and PD-L1 positivity of tumor tissue. This is roughly comparable to established therapies. What is outstanding, however, is the favorable response rate within 2.1 months and the pronounced duration of the response [54].

A randomized, placebo-controlled, double-blind phase 3 (KEYNOTE 826) trial yielded notable results. Adding pembrolizumab (200 mg every 3 weeks), a humanized monoclonal PD-1 antibody, to cisplatin or carboplatin/paclitaxel with or without additional bevacizumab, a recombinant monoclonal antibody to human vascular endothelial-derived growth factor (VEGF), in patients with advanced cervical cancer and a positive PD-L1 status (combined positive score (CPS) ≥ 1) demonstrated a significant improvement in median OS (not reached vs. 16.3 months; HR 0.64; $p = 0.0001$) and median DFS (10.4 vs. 8.2 months;

HR 0.62; $p < 0.0001$). Compared to the placebo group, the treatment with pembrolizumab yielded an objective response rate of 68% vs. 50%, as well as a median response duration of 18.0 vs. 10.4 months [49,55]. Based on these data, the Food and Drug Administration (FDA) approved pembrolizumab 2021 as first-line therapy in combination with chemotherapy, with or without bevacizumab, for the treatment of patients with persistent, recurrent or metastatic cervical cancer whose tumors express PD-L1 (CPS $\geq$ 1). Pembrolizumab has also been approved as a sole therapy in patients with recurrent or metastatic cervical cancer who are progressive on chemotherapy.

Currently, the effect of pembrolizumab in addition to concurrent RCT in primary advanced cervical cancer is being investigated in an ENGOT-cx11/KEYNOTE-A18 trial. Completion of the trial is anticipated in December 2024 [56].

Nivolumab (anti-PD-1) and ipilimumab (cytotoxic T-lymphocyte antigen 4 antibody; anti-CTLA4) are other forward-looking compounds. Monotherapy with nivolumab and in combination with ipilimumab are being tested in the ongoing CheckMate 358, a multicenter, multicohort phase I/II trial. The treatment response ranged between 26.3% (nivolumab treatment, 95% CI, 9.1 to 51.2) and 38.4% (nivolumab and ipilimumab) in non-pretreated patients. Even patients with prior lines of treatment achieved a response rate of 34.9%. These studies showed that, in patients who responded, the response was of a rather long duration compared to that of conventional therapy. The median OS was 21.6 months (95% CI 8.3–46.9), 15.2 months (95% CI 9.0–36.2) and 20.9 months (95% CI 14.4–32.8), and the median PFS was 5.1 months (95% CI 1.9–9.1), 3.8 months (95% CI 2.1–10.3) and 5.8 months (95% CI 3.8–9.3) in patients treated with nivolumab monotherapy, a combination of nivolumab 3 mg/kg and ipilimumab 1 mg/kg every 2 weeks, and a combination of nivolumab 1 mg/kg and ipilimumab 3 mg/kg every 6 weeks, respectively [57].

Another promising antibody tested and proven in an EMPOWER-Cervical 1/GOG-3016/ENGOT-cx9 study, an open-label, multicenter, phase 3 trial, is cemiplimab (anti-PD-1), which most recently achieved a 3.5 month improvement in OS with an acceptable side effect profile as a monotherapy, regardless of PD-L1 status, in advanced cervical cancer [58]. Cemiplimab was recently approved as a monotherapy by the European Medicines Agency in patients with recurrent or metastatic cervical cancer whose disease progressed on or after platinum-based chemotherapy.

Tisotumab vedotin, another new substance, is a tissue factor-directed antibody–drug conjugate (ADC) and showed good efficacy in a multicenter, phase II innovaTV 204/GOG-3023/ENGOT-cx6 trial; further testing in phase III studies will be needed [59]. The therapy mechanism of tisotumab vedotin is based on its complex formation with tissue factors and the subsequent intracellular release of monomethyl auristatin E, a microtubule-disrupting agent, which leads to cell cycle arrest and apoptotic cell death.

In addition to the mentioned immunotherapies for cervical cancer, further promising immunotherapy strategies such as the engineered T cell receptor (TCR)-like antibody therapy and engineered chimeric antigen receptor (CAR) T cell therapy have yielded promising outcomes in terms of cytotoxicity and cervical tumor regression. Resistance to T-cell-mediated recognition, toxicity, patient specificity (genetically engineered T cells, no standard treatment) and high costs are current hurdles that still need to be overcome [60,61].

Neoadjuvant Chemotherapy

Currently, neoadjuvant chemotherapy (NACT) is not a standard of care in cervical cancer but may result in operable findings in selected patient. Although no improvements have been shown yet in PFS and OS, the following advantages have been noted: potential preservation of fertility, a significantly lower incidence of lymph node metastases and parametrial invasion and a lesser need for adjuvant RCT [62–64]. Therefore, platinum-based NACT followed by a radical hysterectomy represents a therapy option, especially for selected patients with stage Ib2-IIb. However, the side effects of chemotherapy must be weighed against its benefits. Trifanescu et al., in a retrospective study of 108 patients treated with neoadjuvant radiotherapy $\pm$ chemotherapy followed by robotic-assisted radical hysterectomy, reported a pathological complete response rate of 66% and a DFS of 100% at 36 months in early-stage patients with stage IB-IIA, and 80% in advanced-stage stage IIB-IVA [32]. Nevertheless, compared to cisplatin-based RCT, this treatment option is inferior in OS and PFS. The number of patients who remain inoperable and require definitive chemoradiation is about 25–30%. The value of NACT compared to cisplatin-based RCT remains a subject of ongoing investigation [65–68].

7. Conclusions

Important data have been obtained recently about the prevention, diagnosis and treatment of cervical cancer. The three pillars of therapy are surgery, RCT and medical therapy. The effectiveness of the HPV vaccination has been established. However, we face barriers in the achievement of high vaccination rates, especially in LMICs.

Screening programs for cervical dysplasia and cervical cancer have become widely established. Rhythmic screening for HPV and the PAP smear, if necessary, with a colposcopy for further clarification, have already been successful in terms of minimizing cervical dysplasia. However, the effective implementation of these programs in LMICs—countries with the highest incidence of cervical cancer—remains unresolved. The results of the LACC trial, which yielded proof of a higher rate of recurrence, a lower rate of DFS and a lower OS among patients undergoing minimally invasive surgery, have led clinicians to reconsider their view about the surgical approach.

Immune checkpoint inhibitors in particular could serve as a relatively well-tolerated therapy option, with a very prolonged response in patients with advanced cervical cancer whose disease prognosis is predictably poor.

The goal is not only to generate global accessibility for the effective prevention of cervical cancer, but also to include patients in randomized, prospective trials and to standardize evidence-based recommendations for all patients in order to improve disease-free survival, overall survival and quality of life.

Author Contributions: Conceptualization, M.S. and I.A.; Project administration, I.A.; Supervision, I.A. and D.O.B.; Visualization, I.A., M.Z.M., N.M. and D.O.B.; Writing—original draft preparation, M.S.; Writing—review and editing, I.A. and D.O.B. All authors have read and agreed to the published version of the manuscript.

Funding: This research received no external funding.

Institutional Review Board Statement: All procedures involving human participants were performed in accordance with the ethical standards of the institutional and/or national research committee, as well as the 1964 Helsinki Declaration and its later amendments or comparable ethical standards.

Informed Consent Statement: Informed consent was obtained from all subjects involved in the study.

Data Availability Statement: The datasets analyzed for the current study are available from the corresponding author upon reasonable request.

Acknowledgments: We acknowledge financial support by Land Schleswig-Holstein within the funding program Open Access Publication Fond (DFG-OA-Fonds).

Conflicts of Interest: The authors declare that there are no conflict of interest.

Abbreviations

ACIS	adenocarcinoma in situ
ADC	antibody–drug conjugate
Anti-CTLA4	cytotoxic T-lymphocyte antigen 4 antibody
CIN	cervical intraepithelial neoplasm
CDC	Centers for Disease Control and Prevention
CPS	combined positive score

CT	computed tomography
DFS	disease-free survival
ERBT	pelvic external beam radiotherapy
ESGO	European Society of Gynaecological Oncology
ESRO	European Society for Radiotherapy and Oncology
ESP	European Society of Pathology
FDA	Food and Drug Administration
FIGO	Fédération Internationale de Gynécologie et d'Obstétrique
HIV	human immune deficiency virus
HPV	human papilloma virus
HN	hypogastric nerve
HSIL	high-grade squamous intraepithelial lesion
ICG	indocyanine green
IGABIT	image-guided adaptive brachytherapy
IHO	inferior hypogastric plexus
ITC	isolated tumor cells
LACC	Laparoscopic Approach to Cervical Cancer
LARVH	laparo-assisted vaginal hysterectomy
LMIC	low- and middle-income countries
LNE	lymphadenectomy
LSIL	low-grade squamous intraepithelial lesion
MRI	magnetic resonance imaging
NACT	neoadjuvant chemotherapy
NCCN	National Comprehensive Cancer Network
PAP	Papanicolaou
PD/PD-L1	programmed cell death/programmed cell death ligand 1
PSN	pelvic splanchnic nerve
RACC	Robot-assisted Approach to Cervical Cancer
RCT	radiochemotherapy
ROCC	Robotic versus Open Radical Hysterectomy for Cervical Cancer
SLN	sentinel lymph node
SNB	sentinel node biopsy
STIKO	Standing Commission on Vaccination
TCR	T cell receptor
VEGF	vascular endothelial-derived growth factor
WHO	World Health Organization

References

1. Sung, H.; Ferlay, J.; Siegel, R.L.; Laversanne, M.; Soerjomataram, I.; Jemal, A.; Bray, F. Global Cancer Statistics 2020: GLOBOCAN Estimates of Incidence and Mortality Worldwide for 36 Cancers in 185 Countries. *CA Cancer J. Clin.* **2021**, *71*, 209–249. [CrossRef] [PubMed]
2. Leitlinienprogramm Onkologie (Deutsche Krebsgesellschaft, Deutsche Krebshilfe, AWMF): S3-Leitlinie Diagnostik, Therapie und Nachsorge der Patientin mit Zervixkarzinom, Langversion, 2.2. 2022; AWMF-Registernummer: 032/033OL. Available online: https://www.leitlinienprogramm-onkologie.de/leitlinien/zervixkarzinom/ (accessed on 17 August 2022).
3. Chrysostomou, A.C.; Stylianou, D.C.; Constantinidou, A.; Kostrikis, L.G. Cervical Cancer Screening Programs in Europe: The Transition Towards HPV Vaccination and Population-Based HPV Testing. *Viruses* **2018**, *10*, 729. [CrossRef] [PubMed]
4. Raspollini, M.R.; Lax, S.F.; McCluggage, W.G. The central role of the pathologist in the management of patients with cervical cancer: ESGO/ESTRO/ESP guidelines. *Virchows Arch.* **2018**, *473*, 45–54. [CrossRef] [PubMed]
5. Schiffman, M.; Wentzensen, N.; Wacholder, S.; Kinney, W.; Gage, J.C.; Castle, P.E. Human papillomavirus testing in the prevention of cervical cancer. *J. Natl. Cancer Inst.* **2011**, *103*, 368–383. [CrossRef] [PubMed]
6. Kopp, S.A.; Turk, D.E. Human Papillomavirus Vaccinations: Provider Education to Enhance Vaccine Uptake. *Clin. Pediatr.* **2023**, onlinefirst. [CrossRef] [PubMed]
7. Serrano, B.; Ibáñez, R.; Robles, C.; Peremiquel-Trillas, P.; de Sanjosé, S.; Bruni, L. Worldwide use of HPV self-sampling for cervical cancer screening. *Prev. Med.* **2022**, *154*, 106900. [CrossRef]
8. Gizaw, M.; Teka, B.; Ruddies, F.; Abebe, T.; Kaufmann, A.M.; Worku, A.; Wienke, A.; Jemal, A.; Addissie, A.; Kantelhardt, E.J. Uptake of Cervical Cancer Screening in Ethiopia by Self-Sampling HPV DNA Compared to Visual Inspection with Acetic Acid: A Cluster Randomized Trial. *Cancer Prev. Res.* **2019**, *12*, 609–616. [CrossRef]

9. Wang, R.; Pan, W.; Jin, L.; Huang, W.; Li, Y.; Wu, D.; Gao, C.; Ma, D.; Liao, S. Human papillomavirus vaccine against cervical cancer: Opportunity and challenge. *Cancer Lett.* **2020**, *471*, 88–102. [CrossRef]
10. Karimi-Zarchi, M.; Allahqoli, L.; Nehmati, A.; Kashi, A.M.; Taghipour-Zahir, S.; Alkatout, I. Can the prophylactic quadrivalent HPV vaccine be used as a therapeutic agent in women with CIN? A randomized trial. *BMC Public Health* **2020**, *20*, 274. [CrossRef]
11. Brisson, M.; Kim, J.J.; Canfell, K.; Drolet, M.; Gingras, G.; Burger, E.A.; Martin, D.; Simms, K.T.; Bénard, É.; Boily, M.C.; et al. Impact of HPV vaccination and cervical screening on cervical cancer elimination: A comparative modelling analysis in 78 low-income and lower-middle-income countries. *Lancet* **2020**, *395*, 575–590. [CrossRef]
12. Hillemanns, P.; Kampers, J.; Hachenberg, J.; Jentschke, M. Vaccination against human papillomavirus. *Internist* **2021**, *62*, 816–826. [CrossRef]
13. Thomeer, M.G.; Gerestein, C.; Spronk, S.; van Doorn, H.C.; van der Ham, E.; Hunink, M.G. Clinical examination versus magnetic resonance imaging in the pretreatment staging of cervical carcinoma: Systematic review and meta-analysis. *Eur. Radiol.* **2013**, *23*, 2005–2018. [CrossRef]
14. Cibula, D.; Pötter, R.; Planchamp, F.; Avall-Lundqvist, E.; Fischerova, D.; Haie Meder, C.; Köhler, C.; Landoni, F.; Lax, S.; Lindegaard, J.C.; et al. The European Society of Gynaecological Oncology/European Society for Radiotherapy and Oncology/European Society of Pathology Guidelines for the Management of Patients with Cervical Cancer. *Int. J. Gynecol. Cancer* **2018**, *28*, 641–655. [CrossRef] [PubMed]
15. Selman, T.J.; Mann, C.; Zamora, J.; Appleyard, T.L.; Khan, K. Diagnostic accuracy of tests for lymph node status in primary cervical cancer: A systematic review and meta-analysis. *CMAJ* **2008**, *178*, 855–862. [CrossRef] [PubMed]
16. Balaya, V.; Guani, B.; Morice, P.; Querleu, D.; Fourchotte, V.; Leblanc, E.; Daraï, E.; Baron, M.; Marret, H.; Levêque, J.; et al. Long-term oncological safety of sentinel lymph node biopsy in early-stage cervical cancer: A post-hoc analysis of SENTICOL I and SENTICOL II cohorts. *Gynecol. Oncol.* **2022**, *164*, 53–61. [CrossRef] [PubMed]
17. Lecuru, F.R.; McCormack, M.; Hillemanns, P.; Anota, A.; Leitao, M.; Mathevet, P.; Zweemer, R.; Fujiwara, K.; Zanagnolo, V.; Zahl Eriksson, A.G.; et al. SENTICOL III: An international validation study of sentinel node biopsy in early cervical cancer. A GINECO, ENGOT, GCIG and multicenter study. *Int. J. Gynecol. Cancer* **2019**, *29*, 829–834. [CrossRef]
18. Cibula, D.; Dusek, J.; Jarkovsky, J.; Dundr, P.; Querleu, D.; van der Zee, A.; Kucukmetin, A.; Kocian, R. A prospective multicenter trial on sentinel lymph node biopsy in patients with early-stage cervical cancer (SENTIX). *Int. J. Gynecol. Cancer* **2019**, *29*, 212–215. [CrossRef]
19. Cibula, D.; Kocian, R.; Plaikner, A.; Jarkovsky, J.; Klat, J.; Zapardiel, I.; Pilka, R.; Torne, A.; Sehnal, B.; Ostojich, M.; et al. Sentinel lymph node mapping and intraoperative assessment in a prospective, international, multicentre, observational trial of patients with cervical cancer: The SENTIX trial. *Eur. J. Cancer* **2020**, *137*, 69–80. [CrossRef]
20. Tu, H.; Huang, H.; Xian, B.; Li, J.; Wang, P.; Zhao, W.; Chen, X.; Xie, X.; Wang, C.; Kong, B.; et al. Sentinel lymph node biopsy versus pelvic lymphadenectomy in early-stage cervical cancer: A multi-center randomized trial (PHENIX/CSEM 010). *Int. J. Gynecol. Cancer* **2020**, *30*, 1829–1833. [CrossRef]
21. Ramirez, P.T.; Frumovitz, M.; Pareja, R.; López, A.; Vieira, M.d.A.; Ribeiro, R. Phase III randomized trial of laparoscopic or robotic versus abdominal radical hysterectomy in patients with early-stage cervical cancer: LACC Trial. *Gynecol. Oncol.* **2018**, *149*, 245. [CrossRef]
22. Melamed, A.; Ramirez, P.T. Changing treatment landscape for early cervical cancer: Outcomes reported with minimally invasive surgery compared with an open approach. *Curr. Opin. Obstet. Gynecol* **2020**, *32*, 22–27. [CrossRef] [PubMed]
23. Bixel, K.L.; Leitao, M.M.; Chase, D.M.; Quick, A.; Lim, P.C.; Eskander, R.N.; Gotlieb, W.H.; LoCoco, S.; Martino, M.A.; McCormick, C.; et al. ROCC/GOG-3043: A randomized non-inferiority trial of robotic versus open radical hysterectomy for early-stage cervical cancer. *J. Clin. Oncol.* **2022**, *40*, TPS5605. [CrossRef]
24. Ronsini, C.; Köhler, C.; de Franciscis, P.; La Verde, M.; Mosca, L.; Solazzo, M.C.; Colacurci, N. Laparo-assisted vaginal radical hysterectomy as a safe option for minimal invasive surgery in early stage cervical cancer: A systematic review and meta-analysis. *Gynecol. Oncol.* **2022**, *166*, 188–195. [CrossRef] [PubMed]
25. Alfonzo, E.; Wallin, E.; Ekdahl, L.; Staf, C.; Rådestad, A.F.; Reynisson, P.; Stålberg, K.; Falconer, H.; Persson, J.; Dahm-Kähler, P. No survival difference between robotic and open radical hysterectomy for women with early-stage cervical cancer: Results from a nationwide population-based cohort study. *Eur. J. Cancer* **2019**, *116*, 169–177. [CrossRef] [PubMed]
26. Fusegi, A.; Kanao, H.; Ishizuka, N.; Nomura, H.; Tanaka, Y.; Omi, M.; Aoki, Y.; Kurita, T.; Yunokawa, M.; Omatsu, K.; et al. Oncologic Outcomes of Laparoscopic Radical Hysterectomy Using the No-Look No-Touch Technique for Early Stage Cervical Cancer: A Propensity Score-Adjusted Analysis. *Cancers* **2021**, *13*, 6097. [CrossRef]
27. Casarin, J.; Bogani, G.; Papadia, A.; Ditto, A.; Pinelli, C.; Garzon, S.; Donadello, N.; Laganà, A.S.; Cromi, A.; Mueller, M.; et al. Preoperative Conization and Risk of Recurrence in Patients Undergoing Laparoscopic Radical Hysterectomy for Early Stage Cervical Cancer: A Multicenter Study. *J. Minim. Invasive Gynecol.* **2021**, *28*, 117–123. [CrossRef]
28. Chacon, E.; Manzour, N.; Zanagnolo, V.; Querleu, D.; Núñez-Córdoba, J.M.; Martin-Calvo, N.; Căpîlna, M.E.; Fagotti, A.; Kucukmetin, A.; Mom, C.; et al. SUCCOR cone study: Conization before radical hysterectomy. *Int. J. Gynecol. Cancer* **2022**, *32*, 117–124. [CrossRef]
29. Li, J.; Gong, X.; Li, P.; Xiao, L.; Chang, X.; Ouyang, X.; Tang, J. Application of Da Vinci robotic surgery system in cervical cancer: A single institution experience of 557 cases. *Asian J. Surg.* **2022**, *45*, 707–711. [CrossRef]

30. Sekhon, R.; Naithani, A.; Makkar, P.; Pratima, R.; Sharma, P.; Rawal, S.; Goyal, Y.; Mitra, S.; Sharma, A.; Mehta, A. Robotic radical hysterectomy versus open radical hysterectomy for cervical cancer: A single-centre experience from India. *J. Robot. Surg.* **2022**, *16*, 935–941. [CrossRef]
31. Uwins, C.; Patel, H.; Prakash Bhandoria, G.; Butler-Manuel, S.; Tailor, A.; Ellis, P.; Chatterjee, J. Laparoscopic and Robotic Surgery for Endometrial and Cervical Cancer. *Clin. Oncol.* **2021**, *33*, e372–e382. [CrossRef]
32. Trifanescu, O.G.; Gales, L.N.; Serbanescu, G.L.; Zgura, A.F.; Iliescu, L.; Mehedintu, C.; Anghel, R.M. Long-term oncological outcome in patients with cervical cancer after 3 trimodality treatment (radiotherapy, platinum-based chemotherapy, and robotic surgery). *Medicine* **2021**, *100*, e25271. [CrossRef]
33. Leitao, M.M.J.; Kreaden, U.S.; Laudone, V.; Park, B.J.; Pappou, E.P.; Davis, J.W.; Rice, D.C.; Chang, G.J.; Rossi, E.C.; Hebert, A.E.; et al. The RECOURSE Study: Long-term Oncologic Outcomes Associated With Robotically Assisted Minimally Invasive Procedures for Endometrial, Cervical, Colorectal, Lung, or Prostate Cancer: A Systematic Review and Meta-analysis. *Ann. Surg.* **2023**, *277*, 387–396. [CrossRef] [PubMed]
34. Falconer, H.; Palsdottir, K.; Stalberg, K.; Dahm-Kähler, P.; Ottander, U.; Lundin, E.S.; Wijk, L.; Kimmig, R.; Jensen, P.T.; Zahl Eriksson, A.G.; et al. Robot-assisted approach to cervical cancer (RACC): An international multi-center, open-label randomized controlled trial. *Int. J. Gynecol. Cancer* **2019**, *29*, 1072–1076. [CrossRef] [PubMed]
35. Piver, M.S.; Rutledge, F.; Smith, J.P. Five classes of extended hysterectomy for women with cervical cancer. *Obstet. Gynecol.* **1974**, *44*, 265–272. [CrossRef]
36. Sakuragi, N.; Murakami, G.; Konno, Y.; Kaneuchi, M.; Watari, H. Nerve-sparing radical hysterectomy in the precision surgery for cervical cancer. *J. Gynecol. Oncol.* **2020**, *31*, e49. [CrossRef]
37. Kietpeerakool, C.; Aue-Aungkul, A.; Galaal, K.; Ngamjarus, C.; Lumbiganon, P. Nerve-sparing radical hysterectomy compared to standard radical hysterectomy for women with early stage cervical cancer (stage Ia2 to IIa). *Cochrane Database Syst. Rev.* **2019**, *2*, Cd012828. [CrossRef]
38. Muallem, M.Z.; Armbrust, R.; Neymeyer, J.; Miranda, A.; Muallem, J. Nerve Sparing Radical Hysterectomy: Short-Term Oncologic, Surgical, and Functional Outcomes. *Cancers* **2020**, *12*, 483. [CrossRef]
39. Muallem, M.Z.; Jöns, T.; Seidel, N.; Sehouli, J.; Diab, Y.; Querleu, D. A Concise Paradigm on Radical Hysterectomy: The Comprehensive Anatomy of Parametrium, Paracolpium and the Pelvic Autonomic Nerve System and Its Surgical Implication. *Cancers* **2020**, *12*, 1839. [CrossRef]
40. Muallem, M.Z. A New Anatomic and Staging-Oriented Classification of Radical Hysterectomy. *Cancers* **2021**, *13*, 3326. [CrossRef]
41. Cibula, D.; Velechovska, P.; Sláma, J.; Fischerova, D.; Pinkavova, I.; Pavlista, D.; Dundr, P.; Hill, M.; Freitag, P.; Zikan, M. Late morbidity following nerve-sparing radical hysterectomy. *Gynecol. Oncol.* **2010**, *116*, 506–511. [CrossRef]
42. Plotti, F.; Ficarola, F.; Messina, G.; Terranova, C.; Montera, R.; Guzzo, F.; de Cicco Nardone, C.; Rossini, G.; Schirò, T.; Gatti, A.; et al. Tailoring parametrectomy for early cervical cancer (Stage IA-IIA FIGO): A review on surgical, oncologic outcome and sexual function. *Minerva Ginecol.* **2021**, *73*, 149–159. [CrossRef]
43. Yamamoto, A.; Kamoi, S.; Ikeda, M.; Yamada, T.; Yoneyama, K.; Takeshita, T. Effectiveness and Long-term Outcomes of Nerve-Sparing Radical Hysterectomy for Cervical Cancer. *J. Nippon. Med. Sch.* **2021**, *88*, 386–397. [CrossRef] [PubMed]
44. Alkatout, I.; Wedel, T.; Pape, J.; Possover, M.; Dhanawat, J. Review: Pelvic nerves - from anatomy and physiology to clinical applications. *Transl. Neurosci.* **2021**, *12*, 362–378. [CrossRef] [PubMed]
45. Abu-Rustum, N.R.; Yashar, C.M.; Bean, S.; Bradley, K.; Campos, S.M.; Chon, H.S.; Chu, C.; Cohn, D.; Crispens, M.A.; Damast, S.; et al. NCCN Guidelines Insights: Cervical Cancer, Version 1.2020: Featured Updates to the NCCN Guidelines. *J. Natl. Compr. Cancer Netw.* **2020**, *18*, 660–666. [CrossRef] [PubMed]
46. Koh, W.J.; Abu-Rustum, N.R.; Bean, S.; Bradley, K.; Campos, S.M.; Cho, K.R.; Chon, H.S.; Chu, C.; Clark, R.; Cohn, D.; et al. Cervical Cancer, Version 3.2019, NCCN Clinical Practice Guidelines in Oncology. *J. Natl. Compr. Cancer Netw.* **2019**, *17*, 64–84. [CrossRef] [PubMed]
47. Nezhat, F.; Erfani, H.; Nezhat, C. A systematic review of the reproductive and oncologic outcomes of fertility-sparing surgery for early-stage cervical cancer. *J. Turk.-Ger. Gynecol. Assoc.* **2022**, *23*, 287–313. [CrossRef]
48. Chu, R.; Zhang, Y.; Qiao, X.; Xie, L.; Chen, W.; Zhao, Y.; Xu, Y.; Yuan, Z.; Liu, X.; Yin, A.; et al. Risk Stratification of Early-Stage Cervical Cancer with Intermediate-Risk Factors: Model Development and Validation Based on Machine Learning Algorithm. *Oncologist* **2021**, *26*, e2217–e2226. [CrossRef]
49. Shapira-Frommer, R.; Alexandre, J.; Monk, B.; Fehm, T.N.; Colombo, N.; Caceres, M.V.; Hasegawa, K.; Dubot, C.; Li, J.J.; Stein, K.; et al. KEYNOTE-826: A phase 3, randomized, double-blind, placebo-controlled study of pembrolizumab plus chemotherapy for first-line treatment of persistent, recurrent, or metastatic cervical cancer. *J. Clin. Oncol.* **2019**, *37*, TPS5595. [CrossRef]
50. Tewari, K.S.; Sill, M.W.; Penson, R.T.; Huang, H.; Ramondetta, L.M.; Landrum, L.M.; Oaknin, A.; Reid, T.J.; Leitao, M.M.; Michael, H.E.; et al. Bevacizumab for advanced cervical cancer: Final overall survival and adverse event analysis of a randomised, controlled, open-label, phase 3 trial (Gynecologic Oncology Group 240). *Lancet* **2017**, *390*, 1654–1663. [CrossRef]
51. Sedlis, A.; Bundy, B.N.; Rotman, M.Z.; Lentz, S.S.; Muderspach, L.I.; Zaino, R.J. A randomized trial of pelvic radiation therapy versus no further therapy in selected patients with stage IB carcinoma of the cervix after radical hysterectomy and pelvic lymphadenectomy: A Gynecologic Oncology Group Study. *Gynecol. Oncol.* **1999**, *73*, 177–183. [CrossRef]

52. Kitagawa, R.; Katsumata, N.; Shibata, T.; Kamura, T.; Kasamatsu, T.; Nakanishi, T.; Nishimura, S.; Ushijima, K.; Takano, M.; Satoh, T.; et al. Paclitaxel Plus Carboplatin Versus Paclitaxel Plus Cisplatin in Metastatic or Recurrent Cervical Cancer: The Open-Label Randomized Phase III Trial JCOG0505. *J. Clin. Oncol.* **2015**, *33*, 2129–2135. [CrossRef] [PubMed]
53. Redondo, A.; Colombo, N.; McCormack, M.; Dreosti, L.; Nogueira-Rodrigues, A.; Scambia, G.; Lorusso, D.; Joly, F.; Schenker, M.; Ruff, P.; et al. Primary results from CECILIA, a global single-arm phase II study evaluating bevacizumab, carboplatin and paclitaxel for advanced cervical cancer. *Gynecol. Oncol.* **2020**, *159*, 142–149. [CrossRef]
54. Chung, H.C.; Ros, W.; Delord, J.P.; Perets, R.; Italiano, A.; Shapira-Frommer, R.; Manzuk, L.; Piha-Paul, S.A.; Xu, L.; Zeigenfuss, S.; et al. Efficacy and Safety of Pembrolizumab in Previously Treated Advanced Cervical Cancer: Results From the Phase II KEYNOTE-158 Study. *J. Clin. Oncol.* **2019**, *37*, 1470–1478. [CrossRef]
55. Colombo, N.; Dubot, C.; Lorusso, D.; Caceres, M.V.; Hasegawa, K.; Shapira-Frommer, R.; Tewari, K.S.; Salman, P.; Hoyos Usta, E.; Yañez, E.; et al. Pembrolizumab for Persistent, Recurrent, or Metastatic Cervical Cancer. *N. Engl. J. Med.* **2021**, *385*, 1856–1867. [CrossRef] [PubMed]
56. Lorusso, D.; Colombo, N.; Coleman, R.L.; Randall, L.M.; Duska, L.R.; Xiang, Y.; Hasegawa, K.; Rodrigues, A.N.; Cibula, D.; Mirza, M.R.; et al. ENGOT-cx11/KEYNOTE-A18: A phase III, randomized, double-blind study of pembrolizumab with chemoradiotherapy in patients with high-risk locally advanced cervical cancer. *J. Clin. Oncol.* **2020**, *38*, TPS6096. [CrossRef]
57. Naumann, R.W.; Hollebecque, A.; Meyer, T.; Devlin, M.-J.; Oaknin, A.; Kerger, J.; López-Picazo, J.M.; Machiels, J.-P.; Delord, J.-P.; Evans, T.R.J.; et al. Safety and Efficacy of Nivolumab Monotherapy in Recurrent or Metastatic Cervical, Vaginal, or Vulvar Carcinoma: Results From the Phase I/II CheckMate 358 Trial. *J. Clin. Oncol.* **2019**, *37*, 2825–2834. [CrossRef]
58. Tewari, K.S.; Monk, B.J.; Vergote, I.; Miller, A.; de Melo, A.C.; Kim, H.-S.; Kim, Y.M.; Lisyanskaya, A.; Samouëlian, V.; Lorusso, D.; et al. Survival with Cemiplimab in Recurrent Cervical Cancer. *N. Engl. J. Med.* **2022**, *386*, 544–555. [CrossRef] [PubMed]
59. Coleman, R.L.; Lorusso, D.; Gennigens, C.; González-Martín, A.; Randall, L.; Cibula, D.; Lund, B.; Woelber, L.; Pignata, S.; Forget, F.; et al. Efficacy and safety of tisotumab vedotin in previously treated recurrent or metastatic cervical cancer (innovaTV 204/GOG-3023/ENGOT-cx6): A multicentre, open-label, single-arm, phase 2 study. *Lancet Oncol.* **2021**, *22*, 609–619. [CrossRef]
60. Dass, S.A.; Selva Rajan, R.; Tye, G.J.; Balakrishnan, V. The potential applications of T cell receptor (TCR)-like antibody in cervical cancer immunotherapy. *Hum. Vaccines Immunother.* **2021**, *17*, 2981–2994. [CrossRef]
61. Doran, S.L.; Stevanović, S.; Adhikary, S.; Gartner, J.J.; Jia, L.; Kwong, M.L.M.; Faquin, W.C.; Hewitt, S.M.; Sherry, R.M.; Yang, J.C.; et al. T-Cell Receptor Gene Therapy for Human Papillomavirus-Associated Epithelial Cancers: A First-in-Human, Phase I/II Study. *J. Clin. Oncol.* **2019**, *37*, 2759–2768. [CrossRef]
62. Rydzewska, L.; Tierney, J.; Vale, C.L.; Symonds, P.R. Neoadjuvant chemotherapy plus surgery versus surgery for cervical cancer. *Cochrane Database Syst. Rev.* **2012**, *12*, Cd007406. [CrossRef] [PubMed]
63. Peng, Y.H.; Wang, X.X.; Zhu, J.S.; Gao, L. Neo-adjuvant chemotherapy plus surgery versus surgery alone for cervical cancer: Meta-analysis of randomized controlled trials. *J. Obstet. Gynaecol. Res.* **2016**, *42*, 128–135. [CrossRef] [PubMed]
64. Kim, H.S.; Sardi, J.E.; Katsumata, N.; Ryu, H.S.; Nam, J.H.; Chung, H.H.; Park, N.H.; Song, Y.S.; Behtash, N.; Kamura, T.; et al. Efficacy of neoadjuvant chemotherapy in patients with FIGO stage IB1 to IIA cervical cancer: An international collaborative meta-analysis. *Eur. J. Surg. Oncol.* **2013**, *39*, 115–124. [CrossRef] [PubMed]
65. Cosio, A.G.S. Neoadjuvant Chemotherapy in Locally Advanced Cervical Cancer: Review of the Literature and Perspectives of Clinical Research. *Anticancer. Res.* **2020**, *40*, 4819–4828. [CrossRef]
66. Gupta, S.; Maheshwari, A.; Parab, P.; Mahantshetty, U.; Hawaldar, R.; Sastri Chopra, S.; Kerkar, R.; Engineer, R.; Tongaonkar, H.; Ghosh, J.; et al. Neoadjuvant Chemotherapy Followed by Radical Surgery Versus Concomitant Chemotherapy and Radiotherapy in Patients With Stage IB2, IIA, or IIB Squamous Cervical Cancer: A Randomized Controlled Trial. *J. Clin. Oncol.* **2018**, *36*, 1548–1555. [CrossRef]
67. Miriyala, R.; Mahantshetty, U.; Maheshwari, A.; Gupta, S. Neoadjuvant chemotherapy followed by surgery in cervical cancer: Past, present and future. *Int. J. Gynecol. Cancer* **2022**, *32*, 260–265. [CrossRef]
68. Kenter, G.; Greggi, S.; Vergote, I.; Katsaros, D.; Kobierski, J.; Massuger, L.; van Doorn, H.C.; Landoni, F.; Van Der Velden, J.; Reed, N.S.; et al. Results from neoadjuvant chemotherapy followed by surgery compared to chemoradiation for stage Ib2-IIb cervical cancer, EORTC 55994. *J. Clin. Oncol.* **2019**, *37*, 5503. [CrossRef]

Disclaimer/Publisher's Note: The statements, opinions and data contained in all publications are solely those of the individual author(s) and contributor(s) and not of MDPI and/or the editor(s). MDPI and/or the editor(s) disclaim responsibility for any injury to people or property resulting from any ideas, methods, instructions or products referred to in the content.

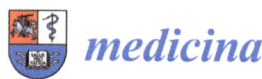 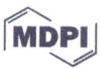

Review

Colorectal Cancer—The "Parent" of Low Bowel Obstruction

Valentin Titus Grigorean [1,2,†], Anwar Erchid [2,*], Ionuț Simion Coman [1,2,†] and Mircea Lițescu [1,3]

1. General Surgery Department, "Carol Davila" University of Medicine and Pharmacy, 37 Dionisie Lupu Street, 020021 Bucharest, Romania; grigorean.valentin@yahoo.com (V.T.G.); ionut.coman@umfcd.ro (I.S.C.); mircealitescu@gmail.com (M.L.)
2. General Surgery Department, "Bagdasar-Arseni" Clinical Emergency Hospital, 12 Berceni Road, 041915 Bucharest, Romania
3. General Surgery Department, "Sf. Ioan" Clinical Emergency Hospital, 13 Vitan-Bârzești Road, 042122 Bucharest, Romania
* Correspondence: erchid.anwar@yahoo.com
† The authors Valentin Titus Grigorean and Ionuț Simion Coman contributed equally to this work.

Abstract: *Introduction*: Despite the improvement of early diagnosis methods for multiple pathological entities belonging to the digestive tract, bowel obstruction determined by multiple etiologies represents an important percentage of surgical emergencies. *General data*: Although sometimes obstructive episodes are possible in the early stages of colorectal cancer, the most commonly installed intestinal obstruction has the significance of an advanced evolutionary stage of neoplastic disease. *Development of Obstructive Mechanism*: The spontaneous evolution of colorectal cancer is always burdened by complications. The most common complication is low bowel obstruction, found in approximately 20% of the cases of colorectal cancer, and it can occur either relatively abruptly, or is preceded by initially discrete premonitory symptoms, non-specific (until advanced evolutionary stages) and generally neglected or incorrectly interpreted. Success in the complex treatment of a low neoplastic obstruction is conditioned by a complete diagnosis, adequate pre-operative preparation, a surgical act adapted to the case (in one, two or three successive stages), and dynamic postoperative care. The moment of surgery should be chosen with great care and is the result of the experience of the anesthetic-surgical team. The operative act must be adapted to the case and has as its main objective the resolution of intestinal obstruction and only in a secondary way the resolution of the generating disease. *Conclusions*: The therapeutic measures adopted (medical-surgical) must have a dynamic character in accordance with the particular situation of the patient. Except for certain or probably benign etiologies, the possibility of colorectal neoplasia should always be considered, in low obstructions, regardless of the patient's age.

Keywords: cancer; colorectal; obstruction

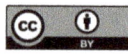

1. Introduction

Despite the improvement of early diagnosis methods for multiple pathological entities belonging to the digestive tract, bowel obstruction determined by multiple etiologies represents an important percentage of surgical emergencies, accounting for approximately 20–30% of the cases diagnosed with acute abdomen [1]. Efforts made to identify and treat inflammatory diseases of the small intestine and colon, diagnosis of colic and rectal neoplasms in early stages, or the surgical resolution of parietal defects in uncomplicated stage have brought improvements regarding the precipitation of an obstructive episode of various etiologies [2].

This research focuses on the determinism, the physiological mechanisms, and the treatment particularities of obstructive colorectal cancer, an entity representing 60–80% of low bowel obstructions [3,4].

2. General Data

Intestinal obstruction is commonly found in surgical services, as a stand-alone entity (with impressive etiological, pathogenic, and topographic diversity), or as an epiphenomenon of other medical or surgical conditions (basal pneumonia, acute appendicitis, acute pancreatitis, etc.). Although the clinic is generally sufficient for positive and topographic diagnosis, the etiological and pathogenic details cannot be clearly outlined, losing their specificity due to an intricate clinic with a spectacular dynamic of the suggestive elements for certain generating causes. With the exception of obstructions with ischemic mechanism from the beginning (complicated parietal defects, intestinal intussusceptions and volvulus, internal hernias, etc.), those of the simple obstructive type present a clinical, dynamic mosaic, which frequently fails the attempts of systematization, creating taxonomic controversies, but justifies hydro-electrolytic, acid-base and nutritional rebalancing measures and finally the surgical procedure [5].

The contribution of paraclinical and laboratory investigations is extremely useful, but even in these conditions a lot of cases remain etiologically obscure [3,6]. Clinical aspects are even more nuanced when the obstructive accident occurs after surgery. The interplay of anatomical and functional causative elements, as well as clinical atypia, explains the diagnostic difficulties and medical-surgical treatment that is difficult to standardize [7].

A serious clinical entity by itself, intestinal obstruction can also be complicated (abscessed tumors, bleeding, diastatic perforations, etc.) which produces an exponential worsening generating mortality rates comparable to severe digestive bleeding, severe pancreatitis, or major sepsis [8].

Distal bowel obstructions (colorectal) have a simple obstruction (except volvulus) as their established mechanism. Symptoms are more indefinite, and the worsening of the general condition occurs more slowly. These so-called "advantages" are nullified by factors, such as age, etiology (often malignant), and multiple complications (most commonly septic). The decompressing factor that the small intestine can have in distal obstructions can be canceled by a pressure-competent ileocecal valve, transforming the colon into a closed, under-pressure loop (double obturated) [9]. Massive and polymorphic bacterial translocation, colic perforations (adjacent to the tumor or diastatic), or diffuse parietocolic necrosis are factors that can lead to rapid, sometimes irreversible worsening. The massive release of endotoxins and digestive enzymes in conditions of compromised mucous-epithelial barrier and microbial populations with exacerbated pathogenicity, explains the initiation of harmful systemic effects, even in the absence of intestinal perforation. The existence and severity of this pathogenic link are confirmed by toxico-septic phenomena being maintained even after the surgical removal of the lesion that generated bowel obstruction [10,11].

Ischemic-type rheologic changes have multiple pathogenies. The cumulative effect of colic parietal vessel elongation (as a result of progressive intestinal distension), the ischemia produced by direct tissue pressure (brides or lateral obstructions), extensive hemorrhagic intraparietal changes (as a result of the rupture of the vessels in the colic wall), or hypovolemic parietal hypoxia contribute to the premature alteration of the mucous-epithelial barrier, and then to colic perforation [3].

Massive fluid-electrolyte intersectoral redistributions, with the formation of the IIIrd surgical space, associated with hydro-electrolyte losses through vomiting, contribute to the establishment of the dysvolemic status (up to critical hypovolemia), which in association with the installed toxic-septic status, represent a powerful pathogenic association [12].

The first pathogen that occurs is the impairment of lumen freedom, with upstream storage of gas and stercoral content. Secondarily, enteral motility disorders are installed as a result of cholic distension and episodic appearance of hyperperistaltism for evacuation purposes ("fighting colic"). The tertiary element that occurs is the modification of intestinal wall viability with the addition of infectious factor (tumor abscess) or juxtatumoral or diastatic colic perforations. Low digestive malignancy, along with progressive lumen obstruction, can precipitate the obstructive episode through other mechanisms: invagination of pediculate tumors, extrinsic parietal invasions, obstructive carcinomatosis, the association of ischemic colic sufferings, etc. From this perspective, mechanical intestinal occlusion presents an initiator of pathogenic mechanisms (the obstacle in the colic lumen) and a systemic resonator (the set of general changes) that worsens itself by dysvolemia and sepsis [13].

Although sometimes obstructive episodes are possible in the early stages of colorectal cancer, the most commonly installed intestinal obstruction has the significance of an advanced evolutionary stage of neoplastic disease. Malignant colorectal obstructions generally evolve with an afebrile state. "Warm" obstructions suggest the appearance of septic, ischemic or co-existence of multiple metastases with hyperpyrexia, accentuated in the context of intersectoral dehydration [14].

A therapeutic attitude in confirmed or intuited non-ischemic cases begins with measures aimed at hydro-electrolyte, acid-base, metabolic rebalancing, and measures to release the intestinal territory proximal to the stenosis through sustained digestive aspiration (less effective in distal obstacles) and retrograde rectocolic lavage. The rhythm and duration of these measures remain an equation with multiple unknowns and traps, but aim at reconfiguring the general state, correcting the installed imbalances (most often partial), impregnating with antibiotic and possibly anticoagulant, cardiac tonic, etc. [13].

Depending on the specific situation, these measures can be adopted regulated or ultra-quickly. In the case of a favorable response, this period can be extended, hoping for complete release, which would allow a safer and more comfortable surgical act, in elective conditions. Failure to respond requires emergency surgery. The surgical attitude cannot be standardized considering the multitude of factors involved, but it ranges from large-scale surgical interventions aimed at solving the generating injury (tumor) as well as the complication (obstruction), to minimal surgical gestures that can contribute to the resolution of the obstruction (cecostomy) [15,16].

Although there is no unity of opinion regarding surgical strategies depending on topography, for the right colon, the right hemicolectomy followed by ileo-transverse anastomosis maintains a leading position, while for tumors located under the splenic flexure of the colon, the interventions in two or three times with different types of stomas upstream are valid, practiced for reasons of safety or necessity.

Quality pre-operative preparation, a well-conducted and adapted surgical act and meticulous postoperative care can bring good results with the resolution of the underlying disease (neoplasm) and its complication (obstruction). However, this morbid association represents a severe pathological circumstance, in front of which optimism must remain moderate and circumspect [17,18].

3. Determinism of Colorectal Cancer

Although there are embryological, anatomical, histological, and functional differences between colic and rectal locations respectively, we note the existence of some common elements between the neoplasms of these segments.

3.1. Embryological Factor

The middle portion of the primitive intestine (mesenteron) generates the upper structures of the digestive tract (duodenum, jejunum, ileum), but also cecum, appendix vermiform, ascending colon, and right half of the transverse colon. The metenteron (embryonic posterior intestine) will develop the distal half of the transverse colon, descendant, sigmoid, rectum and upper portion of the anal canal. Studies on the different embryological origins of malignant colorectal segments suggest possible connections between embryology and carcinogenesis, this area of research being of high interest and requiring further studies [19].

3.2. Genetic Factor

The involvement of genetic factors with autosomal dominant transmission was confirmed with the identification of hereditary nonpolyposis neoplasm (Lynch Syndrome I and II) and adenomatous familial polyposis [20,21].

In addition, it is important to mention the adenoma-carcinoma sequence, which is defined by a set of recurrent driver mutations in a series of genes (KRAS, APC, SMAD4, TP53) that accumulate in the process of adenoma formation and progression to sporadic colorectal cancer [22].

3.3. Histological Factor

The entire colon and rectum above the pectinated line is lined with one layered columnar epithelium. Below this level, up to the Hilton's white line, the rectal epithelium is a non-keratinized, pluristratified pavement. In the area of interference between the two territories, histologists describe a state of "cellular unrest", which predisposes to phenomena of metaplasia and even malignant degeneration. Gland structures with different morphology and function can contribute to oncogenesis [23].

3.4. Environmental Factors

The geographical distribution of colorectal cancer is uneven between different countries or continents. The migration of some population groups to regions with high incidence increases the frequency of this pathology, suggesting the influence of some environmental factors [24].

3.5. Age and Gender

The distribution of colorectal cancer between the two genders is relatively equal, with the prevalence on the right colon in women and on the left colon in men. The maximum incidence is recorded at 60–70 years of age, although it is more and more common at a young age [25]. In the case of obstructive colorectal cancer, the proportions are also similar, with various studies showing heterogeneous results, some of them highlighting a slightly higher frequency in men and others in women [26–29].

3.6. Precancerous Colorectal Disorders

Inflammatory bowel diseases (Crohn's disease, ulcerative colitis) and diffuse colic polyposis, register a significant percentage of malignant degeneration in the absence of treatment or in conditions of insufficient or incorrectly conducted treatment [24,30]. The risk of colorectal cancer may vary between 0.06% and 0.2% reported annual incidence, between 2.5% and 8% reported cumulative incidence of 20 years, and between 7.5% and 18% reported cumulative incidence of 30 years of inflammatory bowel disease [31–33].

3.7. Diet

The low intake of vegetables and cellulose fibers and the excess of animal fats, carbohydrates, and alcohol predisposes to the development of colorectal neoplasia [34].

3.8. Hepatobiliary Disorders and Cholecystectomy

The excessive presence of secondary bile acids (deoxycholic and lithocholic) in the digestive tract promotes carcinogenesis. The effect seems mediated by the excessive fixation of dietary calcium, which causes punctual peeling of the cholic mucosa, favoring the appearance of metaplastic changes. Large bile discharges into the digestive tract post-cholecystectomy raised the suspicion that this surgery predisposes to colorectal cancer [35,36].

3.9. Various Factors

Obesity, sedentary lifestyle, smoking, diabetes, abdominal radiotherapy, racial factor, etc., are other factors that can leave their mark on colorectal carcinogenesis [37–41].

3.10. Drug-Related Factors

Vitamins A, C, E, beta carotene, aspirin, and non-steroidal anti-inflammatory drugs seem to have a protective role, noting a higher incidence of colorectal neoplasm in those with vitamin deficiencies [42,43].

4. Development of the Obstructive Mechanism

The spontaneous evolution of colorectal cancer is always burdened by complications. Their variety is very large. Among the local complications, the most common are: loco-regional invasion with possible inter-visceral or external fistulas, tumor infection with adjacent sclerolipomatous reaction or abscesses, peritonitis by evacuation of tumor abscesses or intestinal perforations, intestinal obstructions, lower digestive bleeding, etc. General complications are represented by anemia, paraneoplastic venous thrombosis, multiple metastases, hepatic abscesses with systemic sepsis, etc. [44,45].

The most common complication is low bowel obstruction, found in approximately 20% of the cases of colorectal cancer and can occur either relatively abruptly, or is preceded by initially discrete premonitory symptoms, non-specific (until advanced evolutionary stages), and generally neglected or incorrectly interpreted [18,46].

The common obstructive mechanism is simple obstruction and is specific to situations with preceding manifestations (transit disorders, anemia, weight loss, etc.). For forms with sudden onset may occur intussusceptions (rare at the colic level and non-existent at the rectal level), volvuluses of supratumoral mobile segments and the association of peritoneal carcinomatosis or enteral ischemic phenomena. Colic volvulus is favored by the increased weight of endoluminal content and hypermobility, with fixed points of the extremities as close as possible. In intestinal volvuluses, necrosis is not directly correlated with the number of rotations of the loop, but with the degree of "constriction of the affected mesenteries" [29,47].

Low bowel obstruction due to neoplastic cause (colon and rectal cancer) presents anatomical and functional characteristics important in stage, pathogenic, topographic, and etiological diagnosis, orienting therapeutic consequences.

4.1. Anatomical Factors

4.1.1. The Diameter of the Colorectal Segments

The simple obstructive mechanism is installed later in colic segments with large caliber. Subsequently, the ileocecal valve follows the segment with the largest diameter (the cecum and the ascending colon), which explains the lower frequency of right colon occlusions if the Bauhin valve is not interested. The diameter of the colic lumen decreases discreetly to the distal segments (except the rectal ampulla). Peritumoral sclerolipomatosis and anemia are more common in the right colon, contributing to the shaping of the characteristics specific to this level of tumor location [48,49].

4.1.2. The Thickness of the Colic Wall

The thickness of the colic wall has less importance regarding the frequency of colorectal neoplasms on certain topographies but has profound relevance in relation to retrograde diastatic perforations (Laplace's law) (Figure 1). The large colic caliber associated with the reduced thickness of the wall allows the development of lateral rupture pressure that makes the cecum and ascending colon wall vulnerable (the rupture pressure at this level is approximately 80–100 cm H_2O, compared to the one in the small intestine where it is approximately 200–300 cm H_2O) [50–53].

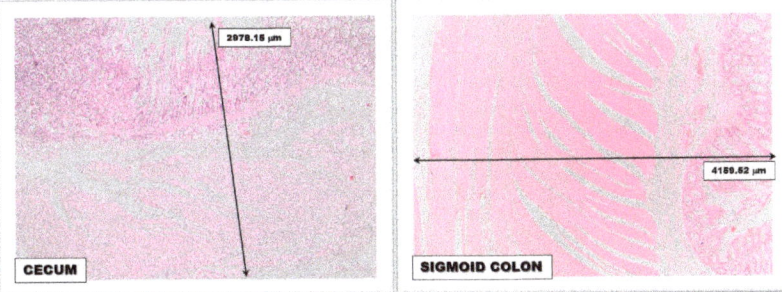

Figure 1. Microscopic image revealing the difference between the thickness of the normal cecal wall and the normal sigmoid colon wall; magnifying glass, 4× (obtained from the Histopathology Department, "Bagdasar-Arseni" Clinical Emergency Hospital from Bucharest).

4.1.3. Colorectal Vascularization

Although it enjoys two important arterial sources (upper mesenteric artery for the right colon and lower mesenteric artery for the left colon) and marginal arches Drummond and Riolan-Haller and inconstant central intermesenteric anastomosis Huard, the colon does not benefit through long and short vasa recta arteries of a generous arterial flow comparable to the upper segments of the tract digestive system (stomach and small intestine). Mesenteric arteries are the preferred territories for the phenomenon of atheromatosis contributing to the progressive decrease of blood flow in irrigated territories. Elongation of vasa recta in the distended colic wall favors ischemia and parietal microthromboses, precipitating colic perforation. The closing of the venous network (a consequence of parietal pressure) is an additional factor in the irreversibility of parietal lesions [54,55].

4.1.4. Anatomical and Functional Sphincters

The colorectal area stretches between the ileocecal valve and the anal sphincter. The latter is of limited importance in low intestinal obstruction, being most commonly located under the obstacle. The ileocecal valve is deeply involved in the pressure play and dynamics of the cholic stasis content in low intestinal obstruction. A "permissive" valve can favor the reflux of stercoral content towards the ileal and then jejunal territory, tempering for the moment the axial and lateral pressures from the obstructed colon. Its increased pressure competence can close the possibility of retrograde reflux, with the exponential increase of intracolic pressures.

The functional sphincters of the colon (Cannon-Boehm, Payr, Moutier, and Obiern) are limited areas with better represented circular musculature and may have a limited role in colon dynamics in the early stages of the obstruction evolution. It can be concluded that Laplace's physical law may be influenced by cholic morphofunctional characteristics [56,57].

4.1.5. The Mobility of Colic Segments

The mobility of colic segments can influence the dynamics of the obstructive process. If the fixed segments are the site of tumor development, they will suffer a simple process of obstruction, while for mobile segments other obstructive mechanisms may overlap (intussusceptions, volvuluses, etc.) [58].

4.1.6. Tumor Morphopathology

Obstruction of the colic lumen is more common in ulcer-vegetative (Figure 2), exophytic, and polypoid forms. Diffuse infiltrative forms can also be incriminated, especially in situations where the axial extension of the tumor is very large [59].

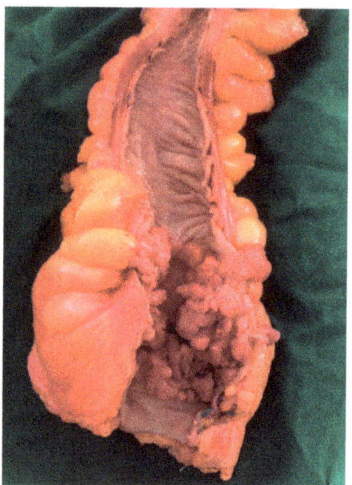

Figure 2. Postoperative specimen of a tumor located in the colorectal junction (collection of General Surgery Department—"Bagdasar-Arseni" Clinical Emergency Hospital from Bucharest).

4.2. Functional Factors

4.2.1. Colic Peristalsis

Colic innervation is vegetative, receptor and effector. The Meissner submucous plexus and axons of neurons in the posterior root node of the spinal nerves T11-L1 are responsible for visceral sensitivity. The secretive and motor activities are modulated by the Auerbach myenteric plexus, unequally represented for the right colon (related to the upper mesenteric plexus) and the left colon (dependent on the lower mesenteric plexus). The poor representation of the myenteric plexus is associated with a diminished peristaltic accompanied by a background distension of the left colon (megadolichocolon), decompensated early in the obstacles of colorectal junction or below this level. Colic hyperdistension makes the action of pharmacological active factors (acetylcholine, neostigmine) ineffective on tonus and peristalsis [60,61].

4.2.2. Other Functional Factors

Other functional factors involved in the pathogenic mechanisms of low intestinal obstruction depend on the individual characteristics of each patient, or derive from anatomical considerations: cholic resorptive function, dramatically extracted dysmicrobisms [62,63], nutrition prior to the installation of the obstruction, degree of damage to the mucus-epithelium barrier [64], associated diseases that amplify the effects of dysvolemia and sepsis, various reflex factors, etc. [65,66].

Success in the complex treatment of a low neoplastic obstruction is conditioned by a complete diagnosis, adequate pre-operative preparation, a surgical act adapted to the case (in one, two or three successive stages) and dynamic postoperative care. Diagnostic errors consist both in overestimating the case (sometimes practicing exploratory laparotomy in medical conditions that evolve with intestinal paresis), but especially in the negative (assessment of the case as a non-surgical emergency, failure to identify cases with initial ischemic mechanism, not performing intraoperatively the diagnosis of all obstructive mechanisms involved and incomplete, inadequate or with potential for relapse surgical solutions). Etiological clarification is only possible sometimes, but this aspect is not a major drawback given the indication of surgical exploration, which will clarify this aspect as well.

Preoperative management of patients diagnosed with bowel obstruction involves, even from the emergency room, the placement of a peripheral venous catheter and starting the infusion of crystalloid solutions such as saline or Ringer solution. Acid-base and electrolyte rebalancing is a priority, often requiring repeated assessments of serum ions and pH. Considering the potential for dehydration and the rapid evolution of the disease, a urinary catheter is necessary for monitoring diuresis. In patients with severe cardiac, renal, or pulmonary failure, monitoring of fluid and electrolyte rebalancing using central Swan-Ganz catheters may be helpful. Preoperative hematological imbalances such as severe anemic syndromes can be adjusted by blood transfusions and severe thrombocytopenia by administering platelet masses. In the case of coagulopathy (liver cirrhosis, hematological disorders) or in case of changes in coagulation parameters due to treatments for various cardiologic disorders, prompt administration of plasma or vitamin K is necessary. Antibiotherapy, thromboembolic prophylaxis, and treatment of associated diseases are equally important [52,67–70].

The moment of surgery should be chosen with great care and is the result of the experience of the anesthetic-surgical team. The operative act must be adapted to the case and has as its main objective the resolution of intestinal obstruction and only in a secondary way the resolution of the generating disease. The resection of the involved colorectal segment is performed (right or left colectomy, segmental colectomy, rectocolectomy), respecting oncological principles. Afterward, anastomosis is taken into account when the proximal segment shows no structural changes. Otherwise, to avoid a digestive fistula, it is recommended to close the distal segment and perform an ostomy at the level of the proximal one [71].

Often, the surgical procedure does not involve the removal of the obstructive process, but only the restoration of the digestive transit. This involves cases in which is intended to shorten the duration of the surgical intervention due to the patient's comorbidities and the general condition at the time or procedures performed for palliative purposes, for advanced neoplasia. In the case of external digestive derivations without removal of the obstructive process, it is recommended to perform a continuous ostomy, in order to avoid a "closed loop" [72].

"The patient with intestinal obstruction is in the situation of a rescued from drowning. This is not the case for a swimming lesson"—Wangensteen.

The postoperative stage can crown the effort made to save the patient or compromise the previous efforts and should be managed by a multidisciplinary team. Analgesic, antibiotic, prokinetic, and anticoagulation therapy in the case of prolonged immobilization should be taken into account. Diuresis and intestinal transit will be monitored, and oral nutrition will be gradually resumed. Local complications (wound abscess, necrosis, evisceration, ostomy dehiscence or parastomal abscess) or general complications, such as cardiorespiratory, renal, or hepatic failures, should be closely monitored and treated promptly [73].

5. Conclusions

- The main cause of low bowel obstruction is colorectal cancer.
- Preceded by early or sudden signs, low neoplastic obstruction generally has the meaning of a neoplasm in an advanced evolutionary stage.
- The therapeutic measures adopted (medical-surgical) must have a dynamic character in accordance with the particular situation of the patient.
- Except for certain or probably benign etiologies, the possibility of colorectal neoplasia should always be considered, in low obstructions, regardless of the patient's age.
- A "truce" in the fight against the obstruction can be deceptive.

Author Contributions: Conceptualization, V.T.G. and I.S.C.; methodology, M.L.; software, A.E.; validation, V.T.G., I.S.C. and M.L.; formal analysis, A.E.; investigation, I.S.C.; resources, A.E.; data curation, M.L.; writing—original draft preparation, V.T.G. and I.S.C.; writing—review and editing, A.E. and M.L.; visualization, A.E.; supervision, V.T.G.; project administration, I.S.C. All authors have read and agreed to the published version of the manuscript.

Funding: This research received no funding.

Institutional Review Board Statement: The study was conducted in accordance with the Declaration of Helsinki, and approved by the Ethics Committee of "Bagdasar-Arseni" Clinical Emergency Hospital from Bucharest.

Informed Consent Statement: Informed consent was obtained from all subjects involved in the study.

Data Availability Statement: Data is unavailable due to privacy or ethical restrictions.

Conflicts of Interest: The authors declare no conflict of interest.

References

1. Bancu, S. Bowel obstructions. In *Surgical Textbook*; Popescu, I., Ed.; Romanian Academy Publishing: Bucharest, Romania, 2008; p. 1094.
2. Koşar, M.N.; Görgülü, Ö. Incidence and mortality results of intestinal obstruction in geriatric and adult patients: 10 years retrospective analysis. *Turk. J. Surg.* **2021**, *37*, 363–370. [CrossRef] [PubMed]
3. Jaffe, T.; Thompson, W.M. Large-Bowel Obstruction in the Adult: Classic Radiographic and CT Findings, Etiology, and Mimics. *Radiology* **2015**, *275*, 651–663. [CrossRef] [PubMed]
4. Biondo, S.; Parés, D.; Frago, R.; Martí-Ragué, J.; Kreisler, E.; De Oca, J.; Jaurrieta, E. Large Bowel Obstruction: Predictive Factors for Postoperative Mortality. *Dis. Colon Rectum* **2004**, *47*, 1889–1897. [CrossRef]
5. Neri, V.; Neri, V. Management of Intestinal Obstruction. In *Actual Problems of Emergency Abdominal Surgery*; IntechOpen: London, UK, 2016.
6. Paulson, E.K.; Thompson, W.M. Review of Small-Bowel Obstruction: The Diagnosis and When to Worry. *Radiology* **2015**, *275*, 332–342. [CrossRef] [PubMed]
7. Smith, D.A.; Kashyap, S.; Nehring, S.M. Bowel Obstruction. Available online: https://www.ncbi.nlm.nih.gov/books/NBK441975/ (accessed on 6 March 2023).
8. Alese, O.B.; Kim, S.; Chen, Z.; Owonikoko, T.K.; El-Rayes, B.F. Mortality from malignant bowel obstruction in hospitalized U.S. cancer patients. *J. Clin. Oncol.* **2014**, *32*, 9626. [CrossRef]
9. Johnson, W.R.; Hawkins, A.T. Large Bowel Obstruction. *Clin. Colon Rectal Surg.* **2022**, *34*, 233–241. [CrossRef]
10. Sagar, P.M.; MacFie, J.; Sedman, P.; May, J.; Mancey-Jones, B.; Johnstone, D. Intestinal obstruction promotes gut translocation of bacteria. *Dis. Colon Rectum* **1995**, *38*, 640–644. [CrossRef]
11. MacFie, J. Current status of bacterial translocation as a cause of surgical sepsis. *Br. Med. Bull.* **2005**, *71*, 1–11. [CrossRef]
12. Kanat, B.H.; Eröz, E.; Saçli, A.; Kutluer, N.; Gençtürk, M.; Sözen, S. Surgical Recovery of Intestinal Obstructions: Pre- and Postoperative Care and How Could it Be Prevented? In *Surgical Recovery*; IntechOpen: London, UK, 2020. [CrossRef]
13. Tuca, A.; Guell, E.; Martinez-Losada, E.; Codorniu, N. Malignant bowel obstruction in advanced cancer patients: Epidemiology, management, and factors influencing spontaneous resolution. *Cancer Manag. Res.* **2012**, *4*, 159–169. [CrossRef]
14. Podnos, Y.D.; Jimenez, J.C.; Wilson, S.E. Intra-abdominal Sepsis in Elderly Persons. *Clin. Infect. Dis.* **2002**, *35*, 62–68. [CrossRef]
15. Perrier, G.; Peillon, C.; Liberge, N.; Steinmetz, L.; Boyet, L.; Testart, J. Cecostomy is a useful surgical procedure: Study of 113 colonic obstructions caused by cancer. *Dis. Colon Rectum* **2000**, *43*, 50–54. [CrossRef] [PubMed]
16. Sommeling, C.A.; Haeck, L. Caecostomy in the management of acute left colonic obstruction. *Acta Chir. Belg.* **1997**, *97*, 217–219. [PubMed]
17. Sawai, R.S. Management of Colonic Obstruction: A Review. *Clin. Colon Rectal Surg.* **2012**, *25*, 200–203. [CrossRef] [PubMed]
18. Webster, P.J.; Aldoori, J.; Burke, D.A. Optimal management of malignant left-sided large bowel obstruction: Do international guidelines agree? *World J. Emerg. Surg.* **2019**, *14*, 1–8. [CrossRef]
19. Kostouros, A.; Koliarakis, I.; Natsis, K.; Spandidos, D.A.; Tsatsakis, A.; Tsiaoussis, J. Large intestine embryogenesis: Molecular pathways and related disorders (Review). *Int. J. Mol. Med.* **2020**, *46*, 27–57. [CrossRef]
20. Ahadova, A.; Seppälä, T.T.; Engel, C.; Gallon, R.; Burn, J.; Holinski-Feder, E.; Steinke-Lange, V.; Möslein, G.; Nielsen, M.; Ten Broeke, S.W.; et al. The "unnatural" history of colorectal cancer in Lynch syndrome: Lessons from colonoscopy surveillance. *Int. J. Cancer* **2021**, *148*, 800–811. [CrossRef]
21. Stec, R.; Pławski, A.; Synowiec, A.; Mączewski, M.; Szczylik, C. Colorectal cancer in the course of familial adenomatous polyposis syndrome ("de novo" pathogenic mutation of APC gene): Case report, review of the literature and genetic commentary. *Arch. Med. Sci.* **2010**, *6*, 283. [CrossRef]
22. Smit, W.L.; Spaan, C.N.; de Boer, R.J.; Ramesh, P.; Garcia, T.M.; Meijer, B.J.; Vermeulen, J.L.M.; Lezzerini, M.; MacInnes, A.W.; Koster, J.; et al. Driver mutations of the adenoma-carcinoma sequence govern the intestinal epithelial global translational capacity. *Proc. Natl. Acad. Sci. USA* **2020**, *117*, 25560–25570. [CrossRef]
23. Fleming, M.; Ravula, S.; Tatishchev, S.F.; Wang, H.L. Colorectal carcinoma: Pathologic aspects. *J. Gastrointest. Oncol.* **2012**, *3*, 153–173. [CrossRef]
24. Arturo Pacheco-Pérez, L.; Judith Ruíz-González, K.; César de-la-Torre-Gómez, A.; Carlos Guevara-Valtier, M.; Azucena Rodríguez-Puente, L.; Mercedes Gutiérrez-Valverde, J. Environmental factors and awareness of colorectal cancer in people at familial risk*. *Rev. Lat. Am. Enferm.* **2019**, *27*, e3195.

25. Kim, S.E.; Paik, H.Y.; Yoon, H.; Lee, J.E.; Kim, N.; Sung, M.K. Sex- and gender-specific disparities in colorectal cancer risk. *World J. Gastroenterol.* **2015**, *21*, 5167. [CrossRef] [PubMed]
26. Luis Márquez Coronel, J.; Enmil, J.; Carvajal, S.; Castro, T.T. Prevalence of intestinal obstruction in patients with colon cancer: A single-center cross-sectional study. Prevalence of intestinal obstruction in patients with colon cancer: A single-center observational study. *Rev. Oncol. Ecu.* **2022**, *32*, 300–309.
27. Alese, O.B.; Kim, S.; Chen, Z.; Owonikoko, T.K.; El-Rayes, B.F. Management patterns and predictors of mortality among US patients with cancer hospitalized for malignant bowel obstruction. *Cancer* **2015**, *121*, 1772–1778. [CrossRef]
28. Winner, M.; Mooney, S.J.; Hershman, D.L.; Feingold, D.L.; Allendorf, J.D.; Wright, J.D.; Neugut, A.I. Management and outcomes of bowel obstruction in patients with stage IV colon cancer: A population-based cohort study. *Dis. Colon Rectum* **2013**, *56*, 834–843. [CrossRef] [PubMed]
29. Machicado Zuñiga, E.; Giraldo Casas, R.C.; Fernández, K.F.E.; Geng Cahuayme, A.A.A.; García Dumler, D.; Fernández Concha Llona, I.; Fisher Alvarez, M.; Cano Córdova, A.S. Localización y clínica asociada al cáncer de colon: Hospital Nacional Arzobispo Loayza: 2009–2013. *Horiz. Méd.* **2015**, *15*, 49–55. [CrossRef]
30. Stidham, R.W.; Higgins, P.D.R. Colorectal Cancer in Inflammatory Bowel Disease. *Clin. Colon Rectal Surg.* **2018**, *31*, 168–178.
31. Winther, K.V.; Jess, T.; Langholz, E.; Munkholm, P.; Binder, V. Long-term risk of cancer in ulcerative colitis: A population-based cohort study from Copenhagen County. *Clin. Gastroenterol. Hepatol.* **2004**, *2*, 1088–1095. [CrossRef]
32. Eaden, J.A.; Abrams, K.R.; Mayberry, J.F. The risk of colorectal cancer in ulcerative colitis: A meta-analysis. *Gut* **2001**, *48*, 526–535. [CrossRef]
33. Lakatos, P.L.; Lakatos, L. Risk for colorectal cancer in ulcerative colitis: Changes, causes and management strategies. *World J. Gastroenterol.* **2008**, *14*, 3937. [CrossRef]
34. Thanikachalam, K.; Khan, G. Colorectal Cancer and Nutrition. *Nutrients* **2019**, *11*, 164. [CrossRef]
35. Nguyen, T.T.; Ung, T.T.; Kim, N.H.; Jung, Y.D. Role of bile acids in colon carcinogenesis. *World J. Clin. Cases* **2018**, *6*, 577–588. [CrossRef]
36. Režen, T.; Rozman, D.; Kovács, T.; Kovács, P.; Sipos, A.; Bai, P.; Mikó, E. The role of bile acids in carcinogenesis. *Cell. Mol. Life Sci.* **2022**, *79*, 243. [CrossRef]
37. Bardou, M.; Barkun, A.N.; Martel, M. Obesity and colorectal cancer. *Gut* **2013**, *62*, 933–947. [CrossRef] [PubMed]
38. Cong, Y.J.; Gan, Y.; Sun, H.L.; Deng, J.; Cao, S.Y.; Xu, X.; Lu, Z.X. Association of sedentary behaviour with colon and rectal cancer: A meta-analysis of observational studies. *Br. J. Cancer* **2014**, *110*, 817–826. [CrossRef] [PubMed]
39. Gram, I.T.; Park, S.-Y.; Wilkens, L.R.; Haiman, C.A.; Le Marchand, L. Smoking-Related Risks of Colorectal Cancer by Anatomical Subsite and Sex. *Am. J. Epidemiol.* **2020**, *189*, 543–553. [CrossRef]
40. Yao, C.; Nash, G.F.; Hickish, T. Management of colorectal cancer and diabetes. *J. R. Soc. Med.* **2014**, *107*, 103–109. [CrossRef]
41. Lewandowska, A.; Rudzki, G.; Lewandowski, T.; Stryjkowska-Góra, A.; Rudzki, S. Risk Factors for the Diagnosis of Colorectal Cancer. *Cancer Control* **2022**, *29*, 1–15. [CrossRef]
42. Song, M.; Garrett, W.S.; Chan, A.T. Nutrients, Foods, and Colorectal Cancer Prevention. *Gastroenterology* **2015**, *148*, 1244. [CrossRef] [PubMed]
43. Maniewska, J.; Jeżewska, D. Non-Steroidal Anti-Inflammatory Drugs in Colorectal Cancer Chemoprevention. *Cancers* **2021**, *13*, 594. [CrossRef]
44. Yang, X.-F.; Pan, K. Diagnosis and management of acute complications in patients with colon cancer: Bleeding, obstruction, and perforation. *Chin. J. Cancer Res.* **2014**, *26*, 331–340. [CrossRef]
45. Kirchhoff, P.; Clavien, P.-A.; Hahnloser, D. Complications in colorectal surgery: Risk factors and preventive strategies. *Patient Saf. Surg.* **2010**, *4*, 5. [CrossRef]
46. Roeland, E.; Gunten, C.F. Current concepts in malignant bowel obstruction management. *Curr. Oncol. Rep.* **2009**, *11*, 298–303. [CrossRef] [PubMed]
47. Winner, M.; Mooney, S.J.; Hershman, D.L.; Feingold, D.L.; Allendorf, J.D.; Wright, J.D.; Neugut, A.I. Incidence and Predictors of Bowel Obstruction in Elderly Patients with Stage IV Colon Cancer: A Population-Based Cohort Study. *JAMA Surg.* **2013**, *148*, 715–722. [CrossRef]
48. Demb, J.; Earles, A.; Martínez, M.E.; Bustamante, R.; Bryant, A.K.; Murphy, J.D.; Liu, L.; Gupta, S. Risk factors for colorectal cancer significantly vary by anatomic site. *BMJ Open Gastroenterol.* **2019**, *6*, e000313. [CrossRef] [PubMed]
49. Gainant, A. Emergency management of acute colonic cancer obstruction. *J. Visc. Surg.* **2012**, *149*, e3–e10. [CrossRef]
50. Rubin, J.; Principe, D.R.; Movitz, B.; Ng, M.; Kochar, K. Cecum perforation secondary to plunger-induced barotrauma. *J. Surg. Case Rep.* **2019**, *2019*, rjz077. [CrossRef]
51. Pouli, S.; Kozana, A.; Papakitsou, I.; Daskalogiannaki, M.; Raissaki, M. Gastrointestinal perforation: Clinical and MDCT clues for identification of aetiology. *Insights Into Imaging* **2020**, *11*, 1–19. [CrossRef] [PubMed]
52. Shao, J.; Sun, L.; Fu, Q. Small Bowel Perforation Due to Blunt Trauma of Left Leg with an Incarcerated Inguinal Hernia: A Case Report. *Front. Surg.* **2021**, *8*, 710417. [CrossRef]
53. Baer, C.; Menon, R.; Bastawrous, S.; Bastawrous, A. Emergency Presentations of Colorectal Cancer. *Surg. Clin. N. Am.* **2017**, *97*, 529–545. [CrossRef] [PubMed]

54. Wang, S.C.; Schulman-Marcus, J.; Fantauzzi, J.; Bevington, T.; Sayegh, A.; Lee, E.; Ata, A.; Kambam, M.; Sidhu, M.; Lyubarova, R. Colon cancer laterality is associated with atherosclerosis and coronary artery disease. *J. Gastrointest. Oncol.* **2019**, *10*, 30–36. [CrossRef]
55. Yamaji, Y.; Yasunaga, H.; Hirata, Y.; Yamada, A.; Yoshida, S.; Horiguchi, H.; Fushimi, K.; Koike, K. Association Between Colorectal Cancer and Atherosclerotic Diseases: A Study Using a National Inpatient Database in Japan. *Dig. Dis. Sci.* **2016**, *61*, 1677–1685. [CrossRef]
56. Gagliardi, J.A.; Radvany, M.G.; Kilkenny, T.E.; Russo, R.D. Colonic sphincters revisited: Simulators of organic disease. *Hawaii Med. J.* **1994**, *53*, 278–282. [PubMed]
57. McKnight, S.T.; Myers, A.; Canon, C.L.; Hawn, M. A functional colonic obstruction: Cannon's point. *Radiol. Case Rep.* **2011**, *6*, 557. [CrossRef]
58. McCullough, J.; Engledow, A. Treatment Options in Obstructed Left-sided Colonic Cancer. *Clin. Oncol.* **2010**, *22*, 764–770. [CrossRef]
59. Marzouk, O.; Schofield, J. Review of Histopathological and Molecular Prognostic Features in Colorectal Cancer. *Cancers* **2011**, *3*, 2767–2810. [CrossRef]
60. Duan, H.; Cai, X.; Luan, Y.; Yang, S.; Yang, J.; Dong, H.; Zeng, H.; Shao, L. Regulation of the Autonomic Nervous System on Intestine. *Front. Physiol.* **2021**, *12*, 700129. [CrossRef]
61. Lin, Y.-M.; Fu, Y.; Winston, J.; Radhakrishnan, R.; Sarna, S.K.; Huang, L.-Y.M.; Shi, X.-Z. Pathogenesis of abdominal pain in bowel obstruction: Role of mechanical stress-induced upregulation of nerve growth factor in gut smooth muscle cells. *Pain* **2017**, *158*, 583–592. [CrossRef]
62. Artemev, A.; Naik, S.; Pougno, A.; Honnavar, P.; Shanbhag, N.M. The Association of Microbiome Dysbiosis with Colorectal Cancer. *Cureus* **2022**, *14*, e22156. [CrossRef] [PubMed]
63. Gao, Z.; Guo, B.; Gao, R.; Zhu, Q.; Qin, H. Microbiota disbiosis is associated with colorectal cancer. *Front. Microbiol.* **2015**, *6*, 20. [CrossRef] [PubMed]
64. Chia-Hui Yu, L. Microbiota dysbiosis and barrier dysfunction in inflammatory bowel disease and colorectal cancers: Exploring a common ground hypothesis. *J. Biomed. Sci.* **2018**, *25*, 79.
65. Hegde, S.; Lin, Y.-M.; Golovko, G.; Khanipov, K.; Cong, Y.; Savidge, T.; Fofanov, Y.; Shi, X.-Z. Microbiota dysbiosis and its pathophysiological significance in bowel obstruction. *Sci. Rep.* **2018**, *8*, 1–12. [CrossRef] [PubMed]
66. Stefano Corazziari, E. Intestinal mucus barrier in normal and inflamed colon. *J. Pediatr. Gastroenterol. Nutr.* **2009**, *48*, S54–S55. [CrossRef] [PubMed]
67. Pisano, M.; Zorcolo, L.; Merli, C.; Cimbanassi, S.; Poiasina, E.; Ceresoli, M.; Agresta, F.; Allievi, N.; Bellanova, G.; Coccolini, F.; et al. 2017 WSES guidelines on colon and rectal cancer emergencies: Obstruction and perforation. *World J. Emerg. Surg.* **2018**, *13*, 1–27. [CrossRef]
68. Yoo, R.-N.; Cho, H.-M.; Kye, B.-H. Management of obstructive colon cancer: Current status, obstacles, and future directions. *World J. Gastrointest. Oncol.* **2021**, *13*, 1850–1862. [CrossRef] [PubMed]
69. Adler, D.G. Management of malignant colonic obstruction. *Curr. Treat. Options Gastroenterol.* **2005**, *8*, 231–237. [CrossRef]
70. Soybel, D.; Santos, A. Ileus and bowel obstruction. In *Greenfield's Surgery. Scientific Principles and Practice*, 6th ed.; Mulholland, M., Lillemoe, K., Doherty, G., Upchurch, G., Jr., Alam, H., Pawlik, T., Eds.; Wolters Kluwer: Philadelphia, PA, USA, 2017; pp. 782–808.
71. Stoyanov, H.; Julianov, A.; Valtchev, D.; Matev, A. Results of the treatment of colorectal cancer complicated by obstruction. *Wien. Klin. Wochenschr.* **1998**, *110*, 262–265.
72. Fabrizio, A.; Wick, E. The Management of Large Bowel Obstruction. In *Current Surgical Therapy*, 12th ed.; Cameron, J., Cameron, A., Eds.; Elsevier: Philadelphia, PA, USA, 2016; pp. 180–182.
73. Angelescu, N. *Bowel Obstructions*; Surgical Textbook; Editura Medicala: Bucharest, Romania, 2003; pp. 2168–2184.

Disclaimer/Publisher's Note: The statements, opinions and data contained in all publications are solely those of the individual author(s) and contributor(s) and not of MDPI and/or the editor(s). MDPI and/or the editor(s) disclaim responsibility for any injury to people or property resulting from any ideas, methods, instructions or products referred to in the content.

Review

Mass Spectrometry Contribution to Pediatric Cancers Research

Marco Agostini, Pietro Traldi * and Mahmoud Hamdan

Istituto di Ricerca Pediatrica Città della Speranza, Corso Stati Uniti 4, 35100 Padova, Italy
* Correspondence: p.traldi@irpcds.org

Abstract: For over four decades, mass spectrometry-based methods have provided a wealth of information relevant to various challenges in the field of cancers research. These challenges included identification and validation of novel biomarkers for various diseases, in particular for various forms of cancer. These biomarkers serve various objectives including monitoring patient response to the various forms of therapy, differentiating subgroups of the same type of cancer, and providing proteomic data to complement datasets generated by genomic, epigenetic, and transcriptomic methods. The same proteomic data can be used to provide prognostic information and could guide scientists and medics to new and innovative targeted therapies The past decade has seen a rapid emergence of epigenetics as a major contributor to carcinogenesis. This development has given a fresh momentum to MS-based proteomics, which demonstrated to be an unrivalled tool for the analyses of protein post-translational modifications associated with chromatin modifications. In particular, high-resolution mass spectrometry has been recently used for systematic quantification of chromatin modifications. Data generated by this approach are central in the search for new therapies for various forms of cancer and will help in attempts to decipher antitumor drug resistance. To appreciate the contribution of mass spectrometry-based proteomics to biomarkers discovery and to our understanding of mechanisms behind the initiation and progression of various forms of cancer, a number of recent investigations are discussed. These investigations also include results provided by two-dimensional gel electrophoresis combined with mass spectrometry.

Keywords: pediatric cancer; two-dimensional gel electrophoresis; MS-based proteomics; metabolomics; pharmacokinetics of anticancer drugs; epigenetics; chromatin modifications

1. Introduction

Despite impressive advances in the genomic, epigenetic, and proteomic fields, various forms of cancer continue to exact unacceptable price in terms of deaths and the quality of life throughout the world. On the other hand, the last three decades have witnessed intense research activities both at the clinical and at the academic levels to identify reliable biomarkers, more targeted and less toxic therapies, and diagnostic strategies which can help in the early diagnosis and better prognosis of these devastating diseases. One major line of investigation concentrated on the identification of proteins which under disease conditions may experience significant change in their levels of expression. These studies involved both adult and pediatric patients delivering much needed information, which may lead to new drug targets. It is worth pointing out that these proteomic studies assume more relevance in the case of pediatric patients, because pediatric cancers tend to have less genomic alterations compared to adults, while proteomic changes are comparable to those observed in adult cancers. These proteomic analyses can be performed either on tissue samples [1,2] or on biofluids [3,4]; the latter approach is commonly referred to as liquid biopsy. A wide range of liquid samples used in this approach can be obtained in a non-invasive manner, which renders it highly attractive in clinical investigations, particularly in pediatric analyses. The most commonly analyzed biofluids are blood (plasma, serum) and urine, but other biofluids have been examined by MS-based proteomics including expressed prostatic secretions [5], saliva [6], tears [7], and cerebrospinal fluid (CSF) [8].

In a recent review by McEachron and Helman [9], the authors underlined the emerging role of liquid biopsy as a versatile source for various biomarkers, which are necessary for monitoring and management of disease both in adults and in pediatric patients. According to the authors, the increasing use of this approach removed the obstacle of performing serial biopsies in pediatric patients. Such serial analyses allow monitoring and management of solid and CNS tumors by using minimally invasive tests. These analyses can detect both cellular and molecular biomarkers of a given disease, including cell-free DNA, circulating tumor cells, micro RNAs, proteins, and metabolites.

Currently, the identification of the observed proteins may be established by monitoring DNA and mRNA sequences. However, such approach carries two relevant limitations. First, it cannot provide accurate information on the levels of expression of the proteins in question [10,11], and second, it does not furnish information on their stability or on any possible post-translational modifications [12,13]. Such limitations underlined the need for an alternative, yet complementary approach to protein assessment based on transcripts. MS-based proteomic techniques provide such second approach in which various proteomic strategies can be used to assess protein expression, assign function(s), and identify possible post-translational modifications, which a given protein may experience. These strategies employ a wide range of MS-based methodologies and a variety of separation and sample preparation protocols. It is relevant to point out that such strategies are not exclusively designed to identify proteins as biomarkers. Other biological molecules present in blood, cerebrospinal fluid, and tissues can have an equally important role as possible biomarkers of various forms of cancer. In the last thirty years, a battery of separation methods coupled to high-resolution mass spectrometry detection have been used to explore the molecular mechanisms responsible for the initiation and progression of various forms of cancer. The capability of some of these separation methods has been enhanced through the additional use of purification, fractionation, metabolic labelling, and dominant proteins depletion to favor the detection of low-copy proteins.

The recent review by McEachron and Helman [9] described the present status of key aspects of pediatric cancer research, focusing on genetic and epigenetic drivers of disease, cellular origins of various pediatric cancers, and cellular immunotherapies. The conclusions by these authors are highly informative and deserve to be underlined in the present work: First, at the genetic level, the authors argued that many genetic changes identified in pediatric cancers are distinct from adult cancers and will require unique interventions. Second, it is becoming clear that pediatric tumors appear to have a high degree of epigenetic changes that lead to a widespread alteration in gene expression secondary to these changes, understanding such alterations may lead to the discovery and development of novel therapies. Third, germline genetic variations associated with predisposition to cancer appear to occur at a higher frequency in pediatric patients compared to adult cancer patients.

Over the last two decades, a strong body of evidence has emerged confirming that the initiation and progression of cancer is controlled by both genetic and epigenetic events. Unlike genetic alterations, which are almost impossible to reverse, epigenetic aberrations are potentially reversible, allowing the diseased cell population to return to its normal state. The X-ray crystal structure of chromatin [14] revealed a structure made of repeating units of nucleosomes, which consist of ~146 base pairs of DNA wrapped around an octamer of 4 core histone proteins (H3, H4, H2A, and H2B) (Figure 1).

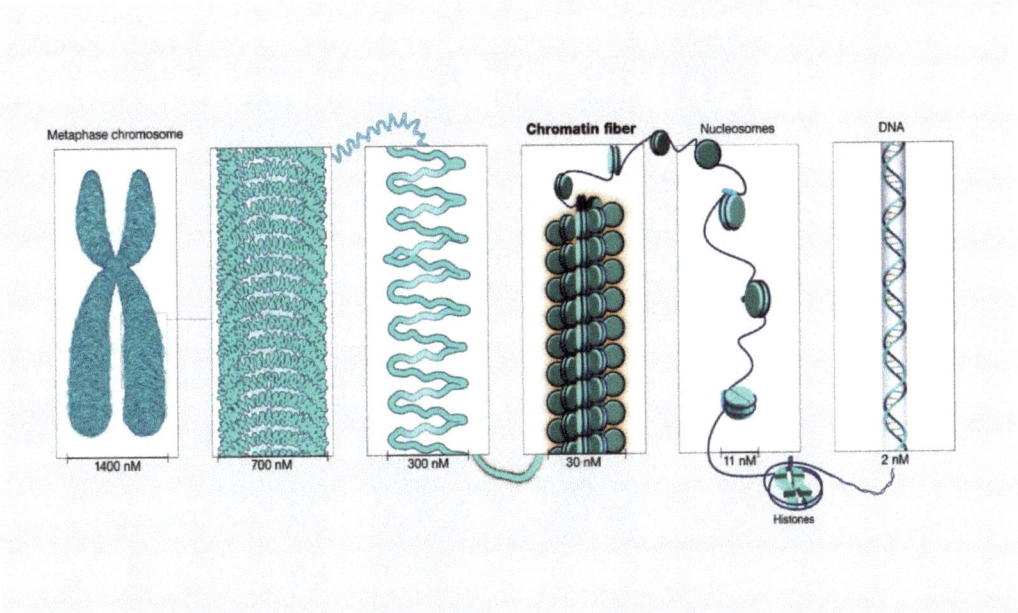

Figure 1. The structure of chromatin within a chromosome. Chromatin refers to a mixture of DNA and proteins that form the chromosomes found in the cells of humans and other higher organisms. Many of the proteins, namely histones, package the massive amount of DNA in a genome into a highly compact form that can fit in the cell nucleus. Courtesy: National Human Genome Research Institute.

Genetic and epigenetic investigations that followed provided sufficient information to suggest that chromatin structure can be modified in a number of ways. The recent literature cites at least eight distinct types of modifications found on histones, where a major part of available information regards small covalent modifications: methylation, acetylation, and phosphorylation [15]. MS-based strategies are the methods of choice for the analyses and quantification of protein post-translational modifications (PTMs), including those associated with histones. Currently, "shot gun" MS-based strategy is the preferred choice for the analyses and identification of histones PTMs. This strategy encompasses three different methods: In bottom-up method, histones are enzymatically digested, and the resulting peptides mixture is subjected to reversed-phase liquid chromatography (LC) separation prior to MS and MS/MS analyses. The LC step is highly critical, in which various gradients have to be used to separate a high percentage of isobaric peptides present in the investigated digests [16]. The main limitation of this method is due to the presence of a high number of basic residues within the histone sequence. This limitation is often resolved by using Arg-C protease instead of trypsin [17]. Top-down or middle-down are two MS-based methods, which can be used for the analyses of intact histones or large protein fragments, respectively [18]. In top-down, intact histones are chromatographically separated and directly analyzed, while in middle-down, long histone peptides (>5 kDa) are obtained through enzymatic digestion with proteases that cleave at less frequently occurring residues, such as Glu-C and Asp-N, and are usually separated using weak-cation exchange combined with hydrophilic interaction liquid chromatography [19]. One of the major challenges for both methods is the ability to distinguish isobaric peptides, a problem that becomes more relevant for the larger molecules analyzed in middle- and top-down methods. Using these methods, isobaric species are often co-isolated and fragmented at the MS/MS level, and as a consequence, they cannot be discriminated. Another issue related to top- and middle-down methods is that long peptides have much wider charge state distributions than bottom-up peptides, which reduces the overall signal intensity of each charged state. This sensitivity issue may be partially mitigated for middle-down method by prefractionation of the digested mixture. In this article, an attempt is made to underline the contribution of MS-based strategies to cancers research. The authors cite and discuss both early as well as recent studies in which the use of mass spectrometry contributed to the discovery of potential cancer biomarkers, understanding of the progression, and the biology of various tumors. A particular emphasis is given to the role of MS-based studies of chromatin modifications, which are central to the understanding of various mechanisms responsible for different epigenetic alterations.

2. MS-Based Proteomic Analyses

2.1. Two-Dimensional Gel Electrophoresis Combined with Mass Spectrometry

Currently, there are two main strategies for the analyses and identification of proteins (proteoforms) present in complex biological samples: liquid chromatography coupled to mass spectrometry (LC-MS, MS-MS) and two-dimensional polyacrylamide gel electrophoresis in combination with mass spectrometry (2D-PAGE-MS). The first approach is commonly called shotgun proteomics, which encompasses the methods of top-down, middle-down, and bottom-up [20]. Before discussing some data generated by the two strategies, the following observations are of interest: (i) It is not always appreciated that the two strategies are complementary (see Figure 2).

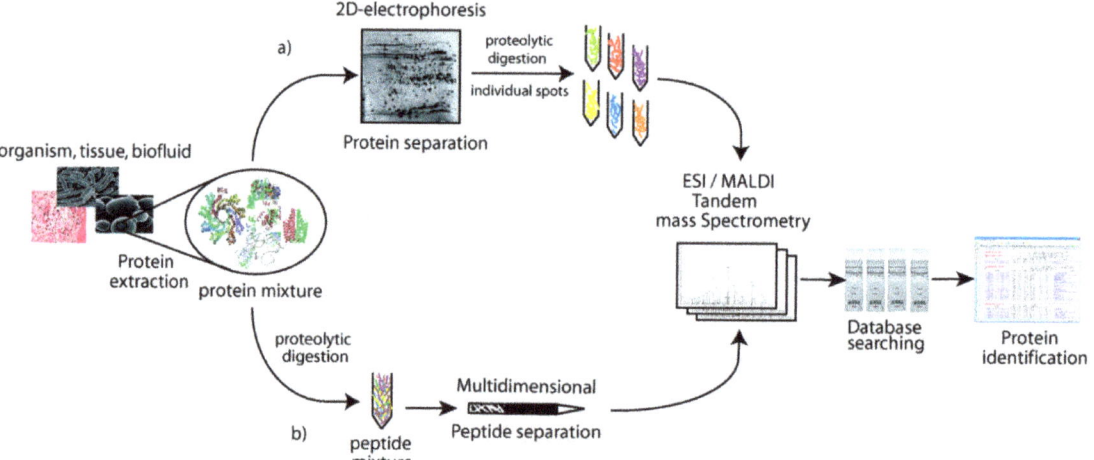

Figure 2. The main steps in bottom-up analyses of a protein mixture, Two routes of analysis: the upper shows digestion of individual proteins separated by 2D-PAGE, while the lower route shows the digestion and analysis of protein mixture. (Reprinted with permission from Fournier ML, Gilmore JM, Martin-Brown SA, Washburn MP. Multidimensional separations-based shotgun proteomics. *Chem. Rev.* **2007**, *107*, 3654–3686. Copyright {2007} American Chemical Society).

The intact proteins separated by 2D-PAGE are often digested into peptides to be separated and identified by LC/MS, MS-MS. (ii) Two-dimensional gel electrophoresis was instrumental in the birth of modern proteomics over 40 years ago, an observation which explains why some research scientists consider such approach as outdated technique for current proteomic analyses. The authors will not enter into the technical details, advantages, and drawbacks of both strategies. Instead, a well-written review on what two-dimensional gel electrophoresis can offer in present-day proteomics is worth reading [21].

Polyacrylamide gel electrophoresis (2D-PAGE) [22] remains one of the main players in the investigation of complex proteomic systems. A modified version of this technique is known as two-dimensional differential in gel electrophoresis (2D-DIGE) [23], where the proteins are pre-labelled with up to three fluorescent dyes. This labelling procedure allows different protein samples to be run on the same gel with the direct consequence of a better reproducibility and easier quantification when compared with 2D-PAGE. This technique combined with MALDI-MS was used by Braoudaki et al. [24] to investigate the proteomic profiles of pediatric patients of acute lymphoblastic leukemia (ALL). The scope of the study was the search for candidate biomarkers in low- and high-risk patients, which could be used for diagnosis, prognosis, and patient-targeted therapy. The authors used Western blot analyses to confirm the differential expression of a number of the detected proteins. Bone marrow and peripheral blood plasma and cell lysates samples were obtained from pediatric patients with low- and high-risk ALL. To favor the detection of low-abundant proteins, depletion of dominant proteins was performed. This study identified a number of proteins, which the authors described as potential biomarkers for the stratification of ALL. There are two interesting elements in this study, which should be underlined: First, proteins depletion in complex biological samples helps in the detection of low-copy proteins. Second, differentially expressed proteins, identified in the same study, were used for pathway analysis. For this purpose, the Swiss-Prot accession numbers were inserted into the search tool for the retrieval of interacting genes/proteins. Second, differentially expressed proteins detected in 2D-PAGE and in MALDI-MS analyses were further confirmed by Western blot analyses.

Cancer cell resistance to chemotherapy is still considered a major factor in the failure of treatment of different forms of pediatric cancer, in particular high-risk forms of the disease. A number of works have shown that such failure can have various forms. For example, some forms of cancer can be intrinsically resistant and unlikely to respond to such treatment, whereas other forms show initial response to such treatment but then regrow to become resistant. The question of chemoresistance remains central for the success or failure of a given treatment and more concentrated efforts are needed to understand the main factors/molecules which may trigger such resistance.

In one of the early studies by Sinha et al. [25], 2D-PAGE in combination with MALDI-TOF-MS was used to investigate chemoresistance development in melanoma cell lines. The authors used a panel of human melanoma cell variants exhibiting low and high level of resistance to four commonly used anticancer drugs in melanoma treatment. The authors reported that a number of proteins have experienced differential expression. For example, in most cell variants, upregulation of heat shock protein isoforms HSP60 and HSP70 was observed. The same study reported an increased expression of the small stress protein HSP27. It is interesting to note that in an earlier study by Sarto et al. [26], it was reported that upon cell stimulation in leukemia, HSP27 was frequently the target of phosphorylation. The same protein has been frequently associated with the inhibition of apoptosis induced by different chemotherapeutics.

It is well established that cisplatin-based chemotherapy is one of the main treatments for various forms of tumors in advanced stage. Although the rate of initial response to the treatment is usually high, relapse with cisplatin-resistant cells occurs in the majority of patients. It is now well recognized that chemoresistance is a major problem in cancer treatment; therefore, proteomic analyses, which can shed some light on the role of different proteins involved in such resistance, are much needed. A number of studies have demonstrated that cisplatin-based agents are known to target DNA, with which can form both inter-strand and intra-strand crosslinks [27]. Further studies have also found that mitochondria were associated with the cisplatin resistance. Mitochondrial DNA and membrane proteins were reported as preferential targets of cisplatin. It was also shown by several groups that mitochondria impairment appeared to play an important role in the platinum resistance of ovarian cancer cells. Using 2D-DIGE combined with MALDI-TOF-MS, Dai et al. [28] investigated the mitochondrial proteins difference between platinum-sensitive human ovarian cancer cell with that of four platinum-resistant variants. The authors reported a number of proteins observed in the resistant cells, which have experienced up or downregulation. The same study reported that some proteins in the resistant cells were upregulated more than three folds compared to their counterparts in platinum-sensitive cells. It is also fair to say that regardless of its entity, cancer is a highly complex disease composed of cancer cells, stromal cells, and the extracellular matrix. It is now commonly accepted that the genetic and epigenetic alterations could be responsible for the initial growth and progression in various types of cancer. However, it is not clear yet whether the microenvironment (stromal cells, extracellular matrix) plays a role in the resistance to cell apoptosis. If that is the case, then it would not be unreasonable to assume that the microenvironment of a given cancer can influence its progression, its drug resistance, and metastasis. A recent review by Dzobo [29] has given an account on how deciphering the role(s) of the tumor microenvironment could lead to more effective cancer therapies. The author argued that therapies targeting exclusively cancer cells are usually insufficient when the stromal component of the microenvironment causes therapy resistance. In other words, the therapy is likely to be more successful if the anticancer drug can be designed to target both cancer as well as stromal cells.

2D-PAGE, DIGE in combination with mass spectrometry have furnished extensive experimental data on the role of proteomics in the understanding of various diseases, in particular various forms of cancer. Having said that, this powerful analytical tool like many others has its limitations, which are mainly due to extensive heterogeneity and a wide dynamic range of proteins present in a given proteomic system. Other limitations are associated with sample load in 2D gel analyses and the width of the pH range in which the separation takes place. In a well-designed study, Gygi et al. [30] evaluated the capability of 2D-PAGE in detecting low abundance proteins in yeast proteome. The authors used this technique to separate and visualize proteins followed by mass spectrometry for their identification. The main conclusion of this study was that despite the high sample load and extended electrophoretic separation, proteins from genes with codon bias values of <0.1 (low abundance proteins) were not found; this is despite existing data indicating that at least half of all yeast genes fall into that range. Low abundance proteins were however detected when higher sample loads were used. This included beginning with 50 mg of total yeast protein as well as using a strategy that included SDS/PAGE, in-gel digestion, strong cation exchange chromatography separation, and on-line microcapillary LC-MS/MS techniques.

The results of this study are in line with other investigations, which highlighted the complexity of proteins heterogeneity in terms of the range of their isoelectric points, molecular masses, and abundances, which can challenge the most powerful and high-resolution techniques including 2D-PAGE. It is sufficient to recall that in a standard human cell, the most abundant protein is often actin, which is present at roughly 10^8 molecules per cell compared with some cellular receptors or transcription factors, which are probably present at 10^2–10^3 molecules per cell [31]. The situation can be more challenging in sera, where albumin is at 40 mg/mL, while cytokines are present at pg/mL levels. It has been known for a number of years that to detect low-copy proteins in a proteome using 2D-PAGE, enrichment or prefractionation strategies are needed. What these and other similar studies tell us is that the combination of 2DE-MS can separate and identify hundreds of proteins in a single analysis; however, to reach low copy proteins within the same analysis, other strategies have to be adapted, including fractionation and enrichment on the 2DE side, while the MS component has to adapt all recent developments not only on the MS side but also on the chromatography of the digested proteins separated by the 2DE.

Drug resistance remains one of the big challenges in oncology, particularly for cytotoxic chemotherapy. In the last few years, the use of 2D-DIGE to investigate drug resistance has diminished in favor of LC/MS, MS-MS and mass spectrometry imaging (MSI) using MALDI ionization. MSI is a label-free method that is used to map the distribution of a wide range of molecules in different biological samples. One of the key features of MALDI-MSI that makes its use appealing is the ability to detect and study the distribution of multiple compounds simultaneously without the need for labelling. It is of interest to note that the powerful and widely used LC/MS-MS lacks information on spatial distribution, which is highly important in the analyses of heterogeneous biological samples. Compared with traditional clinical imaging methods requiring the use of indirect labels such as radiolabels or probes, MSI not only has high spatial resolution in low micrometer scale but also can simultaneously detect the spatial distribution of a drug and its resulting metabolites; both features are relevant in studies related to drug mechanisms of action and related drug resistance [32]. Traditional imaging methods, including whole body autoradiography (WBA), positron emission tomography (PET), and fluorescence microscopy (FM), have all been used to study drug distribution in pre-clinical models and occasionally in patients. These methods have the advantage of being less invasive than biopsy-based assays, but both WBA and PET have low spatial resolution and require radiolabeled drugs. FM allows the study of drug distribution at a cellular level but is limited to drugs that have intrinsic fluorescence; otherwise, fluorescent labels have to be introduced. Such labelling procedure has its drawbacks, where the resulting images fail to distinguish between the parent drug and its metabolites. Like any other analytical technique, MSI has a number of critical steps, which have to be rigorously implemented before this relatively young technique can deliver on its potential. The choice of the matrix and its application to the sample are critical steps for the success of analyses. Interference of the matrix ions with those of the sample, particularly at low m/z values, is a well-known defect of MALDI. This defect is normally addressed by high-resolution MS to investigate the suspected ions; in the absence of such option, the use of different matrices may provide a partial solution. MSI generate impressive amounts of data, which have to be carefully analyzed and interpreted, a step requiring experience together with powerful informatic tools, including suitable algorithms.

There is an ever-growing body of evidence suggesting that epigenetic mechanisms play an important role in bringing about drug resistance in cancer cells. Furthermore, a number of recent studies have shown some correlation between antitumor drug resistance and some epigenetic alterations [33,34]. Pediatric acute lymphoblastic leukemia (ALL) is a representative example on how these recent data are going to impact our understanding of antitumor drug resistance. Survival rates for children diagnosed with ALL have improved substantially, but patients who relapse continue to face an unacceptable prognosis. Genomic research allowed for considerable advances in risk stratification of ALL and have contributed to the development of novel therapeutic strategies. These strategies have been enhanced and extended by the new discoveries in epigenetic research. Such discoveries indicate an important role for the epigenome as a mediator of disease relapse and chemoresistance. Furthermore, genome-wide approaches to interrogate the epigenetic landscape have revealed relapse-specific patterns of epigenetic aberrations that tightly correlate with gene expression. Evidently, further studies are needed to better understand the correlation between these epigenetic alterations and leukemogenesis and how these abnormalities contribute to differences in chemotherapy sensitivity. Many preclinical and early phase studies have concentrated on the reversal of the epigenetic alterations. Some of these studies have demonstrated the validity of such approach; however, the application of this approach at the clinical level only had a partial success, mainly because of undesired side effects [35]. Considering the fast progress in the area of novel epigenetic modulators, there is a high potential for near future discovery of more efficient agents necessary to apply this epigenetic therapeutic approach in ALL.

Gel electrophoresis in combination with mass spectrometry have furnished extensive experimental data on the role of proteomics in the understanding of various diseases, in particular various forms of cancer. Having said that, this powerful analytical tool like many others has its limitations, which are mainly due to extensive heterogeneity and a wide dynamic range of proteins present in a given proteomic system. Other limitations are associated with sample load and the width of the pH range in which the separation takes place. In a well-designed study, Gygi et al. [30] evaluated the capability of 2D-PAGE in detecting low abundance proteins in yeast proteome. The authors used this technique to separate and visualize proteins followed by mass spectrometry for their identification. The main conclusion of this study was that despite the high sample load and extended electrophoretic separation, proteins from genes with codon bias values of <0.1 (low abundance proteins) were not found; this is despite existing data indicating that at least half of all yeast genes fall into that range. Low abundance proteins were however detected when higher sample loads were used. This included beginning with 50 mg of total yeast protein as well as using a strategy that included SDS/PAGE, in-gel digestion, strong cation exchange chromatography separation, and on-line microcapillary LC-MS/MS techniques.

The results of this study are in line with other investigations, which highlighted the complexity of proteins heterogeneity in terms of the range of their isoelectric points, molecular masses, and abundances, which can challenge the most powerful and high-resolution techniques. It is sufficient to recall that in a standard human cell, the most abundant protein is often actin, which is present at roughly 10^8 molecules per cell compared with some cellular receptors or transcription factors, which are probably present at 10^2–10^3 molecules per cell [31]. The situation can be more challenging in sera, where albumin is at 40 mg/mL, while cytokines are present at pg/mL levels. It has been known for a number of years that to detect low-copy proteins in a proteome using 2D-PAGE, enrichment or prefractionation strategies are needed. What these and other similar studies tell us is that the combination of 2D-PAGE-MS can separate and identify hundreds of proteins in a single analysis; however, to reach low copy proteins within the same analysis, other strategies have to be adapted, including fractionation and enrichment.

2.2. Mass Spectrometry Analyses of Biofluids

The invasive nature of surgical biopsies prevents their sequential application to monitor disease, particularly for pediatric patients. Currently, there is enough evidence to suggest that these single biopsies fail to reflect cancer progression, intratumor heterogeneity, and drug sensitivities, which tend to change over time. While tissue samples have the potential to provide novel biological insights, many clinical proteomic studies have chosen clinical samples that are obtainable in a non-invasive or minimally invasive manner, as in the case of liquid biopsies. In recent years, liquid biopsy has assumed an important role in disease monitoring both in adult and in pediatric patients. Furthermore, it is becoming more evident that such monitoring is central in the management of various forms of cancer, particularly in the pediatric population. The recent and unmistakable increase in the use of this powerful analytical tool is due to its minimally invasive tests that can be performed on easily accessible body fluids. Prior to the development of this tool, the repetition of surgical biopsies in pediatric patients was discouraged unless considered medically necessary. Such limitation hindered the search for reliable biomarkers associated with the development of certain diseases. Such lack of reliable biomarkers was more evident in studies related to CNS and solid tumors in children. The recent literature suggests that the use of liquid biopsies could greatly reduce sampling limitations and thus allowing time-dependent assessment of disease evolvement. Encouraging data generated by liquid biopsy sampling has been reported recently, where the detection and quantification of cfDNA have been revealed in various solid and CNS tumors of childhood [36].

Chromatography coupled to high-resolution mass spectrometry is one of the principal tools for the analyses of samples derived from biofluids. Because of the very complex nature of many biological samples, efficient sample preparation protocols to remove unwanted components and to selectively extract the compounds of interest are an essential part of almost every bioanalytical workflow. The proteomes of biofluids, including serum, saliva, cerebrospinal fluid, and urine, are rich with proteins and other biomolecules varying depending on the physiological and/or pathophysiological of the subject. Advances in mass spectrometric technologies have facilitated the in-depth characterization of biofluid proteomes which are now considered hosts of a wide array of clinically relevant biomarkers for a number of diseases [37]. Currently, there are two main strategies in the proteomic analyses of biofluids [38]. The strategy for biomarkers discovery requires multidimensional fractionation in combination with high-resolution mass spectrometry methods, including tandem mass spectrometry (MS/MS). While this approach provides a large amount of data and can identify hundreds of proteins, it remains time consuming and limited in the number of comparisons that can be made. On the other hand, the high throughput nature of the diagnostic development approach (see Figure 3) has made it highly popular.

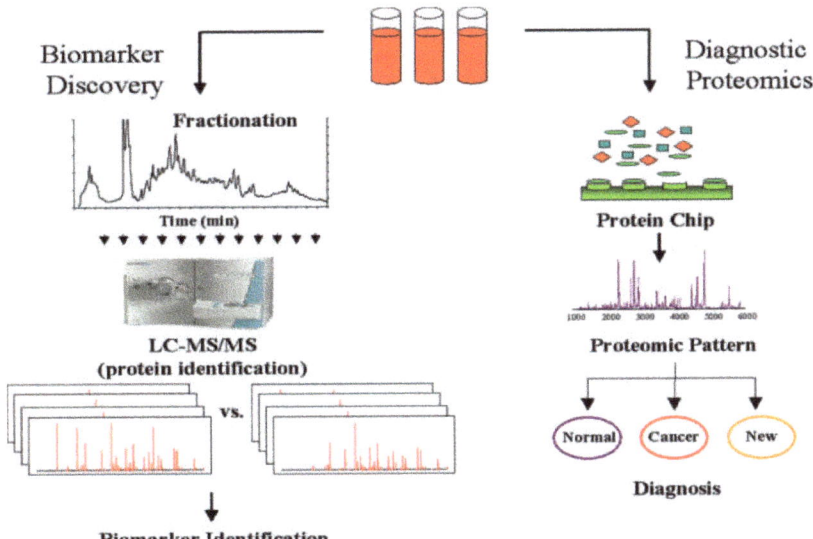

Figure 3. MS-based methods for biomarker discovery (left side) and pattern-based diagnostic proteomics (right side). (Reprinted/adapted with permission from Ref [38]. Copyright year 2005).

In this method, biofluids from hundreds of patients and controls are analyzed by LC/MS, MS/MS. Information on the detected proteins can be rapidly obtained, while the use of sophisticated algorithms facilitates the recognition of various peaks within a multitude of spectra that allow the source of the biofluids (i.e., disease-afflicted or healthy individual) to be established. Although this approach has shown remarkable ability to correctly diagnose patients in blind validation studies, it lacks the capability to directly identify specific proteins associated with the peaks that indicate the source of the biofluids. In cases where the diagnostic protein peaks have been identified, their relationship to the disease condition is not clear because the proteins within the peak are not identified.

It can be said that one of the main objectives of various MS-based proteomic analyses of biofluids is to detect and possibly identify molecular entities associated with a given disease condition. These (entities can be protein(s), metabolite(s), lipids, cfDNA, or other biomolecules present in the investigated sample. Some of these molecules are further investigated to establish their potential as valid biomarkers for a given disease. This phase of discovery is commonly followed by a phase of validation and clinical testing of these potential biomarkers. It has to be emphasized that a successful conclusion of both phases requires highly strict standard operating procedures. The application of such procedures becomes fundamental in metabolic analyses, where a wide spectrum of methods is used in different metabolomics laboratories. In view of this, the Metabolomics Society has set up the "metabolomics Standards Initiative Committee that has established rules to standardize metabolomics systems [39]. Quality control and standard operating procedures should be carefully followed to reduce pre-analyses errors.

Research efforts over the last two decades have provided strong evidence to suggest that various forms of cancer can be attributed to metabolic alterations in various cellular systems. These emerging data have been supported by recent research efforts in which new technologies including high-resolution mass spectrometry have been employed. A representative example of such efforts has been recently reported by Petrik et al. [40]. In their study, the authors used high-resolution negative-ion electrospray mass spectrometry to analyze blood spots taken from newborns. Untargeted metabolomic analyses were performed on 48 archived blood spots from newborns who later developed AML as well as samples taken from 46 healthy controls. Before considering the main conclusions of this study, the following considerations should be underlined: First, ongoing research activities that consider cancer as a disease of highly altered cellular metabolism have accelerated interest in snapshot metabolomics in various human tissues. Second, the chemistry of the endogenous metabolites is fairly complex, which ranges from charged inorganic molecules to hydrophobic lipids to hydrophilic carbohydrates. Because of such complexity, no single analytical method can capture the full range of endogenous metabolites. This chemical complexity required the combination of two powerful analytical tools: high-resolution mass spectrometry and liquid chromatography. The chromatography component allows the separation of various chemical entities, which happen to have different chemical properties (different hydrophobicity/hydrophilicity), while high-resolution mass spectrometry provides accurate molecular weight assignments of the separated metabolites. The authors concluded that metabolic profiles of newborns' dried blood spots could discriminate between newborns that later developed acute myeloid leukemia (AML) from those that did not, and that these profiles were sex specific. Furthermore, predictive metabolites in females suggested that several biological pathways may be involved in AML initiation. One pathway contained four ceramide metabolites positively associated with AML risk, while another pathway in females may be linked with protective effects of breastfeeding. Metabolite predictors in males were more heterogeneous and showed no relationship with the available covariate risk factors, suggesting that etiology in males may be more multifactorial than females. The authors also acknowledged that the sample size was limited in accordance with the rarity of pediatric AML. Furthermore, annotations of the metabolite predictors were limited by the absence of tandem mass spectrometry data for confirmation.

In a more recent study [41], LC/MS was used to investigate metabolites in urine samples taken from medulloblastoma (MB) patients. Samples were taken from over 100 (MB) patients and from a similar number of healthy controls. These analyses concluded that among all differentially identified metabolites, four metabolites (tetrahydrocortisone, cortolone, urothion, and 20-oxo-leukotriene E4) were specific to MB. Furthermore, the analysis of these four metabolites in pre- and postoperative MB urine samples showed that their levels returned to a healthy state after the operation (especially after one month), showing the potential specificity of these metabolites for MB.

3. Investigation of Pediatric Leukemia by Mass Spectrometry-Based Methods

3.1. Acute Myeloid Leukemia

Acute lymphocytic (lymphoblastic) leukemia (ALL) is the more diffused form of leukemia, where three out of four childhood cases are attributed to this form, in which the predominant phenotype is B-cell precursor ALL. It affects children in the age from 2 to 5 years, while the less common T-cell phenotype tends to increase with age (United States SEER program 1975–1995 Vol. vi). B-cell precursor ALL tends to have numerical and structural chromosomal abnormalities such as high hyper diploidy (defined by the presence of 51–67 chromosomes, referred to as 51+). Acute myeloid leukemia (AML) is rare in children and occurs uniformly across all ages. This form of leukemia is often characterized by recurrent chromosomal abnormalities such as MLL fusions located at chromosome 11q23 [42]. It is useful to emphasize that world-wide clinical investigations have demonstrated that ALL is an intrinsically lethal form of cancer. Having said that, it is encouraging to note that current cure rates for ALL using combination chemotherapy are around 90%, making such achievement one of the success stories of oncology.

Almost 50 years ago, French-American-British (FAB) Co-operative Group published proposals for the classification of the acute leukemias [43]. These proposals based on conventional morphological and cytochemical methods were suggested following the study of peripheral blood and bone marrow films from some 200 cases of acute leukemia by a group of French, American, and British hematologists. These proposals were later enriched by classifications provided by the World Health Organization (WHO), which combined the analyses of morphology, immunophenotyping, cytogenetics, and molecular genetics of acute leukemia cells [44].

3.2. Leukemia Subgroups

Based on the type and degree of maturity of the leukemic cell population (blast), which are defined by French-American-British (FAB) classification, AML is further divided into eight subgroups (M0 to M7), including subgroups from granulocytic- or myeloid-derived progenitors (M0 to M3), subgroups from monocytic myeloid-derived progenitors (M4 and M5), and the relatively rare leukemias deriving from megakaryocytic and erythroid progenitors (M6 and M7). The (FAB) classifications provide important guidelines for the diagnosis, treatment, and prognostic prediction of acute leukemia; however, the same classifications fail to provide accurate differentiation between all indicated subtypes, and do not correlate well with the clinical outcomes. The identification of reliable protein biomarkers for acute myeloid leukemia (AML) that could help in diagnosis and prognosis, treatment, and the selection for bone marrow transplant requires substantial comparative proteomic studies and a high number of samples suitable for use in present-day technologies. These efforts have been given new momentum by the more frequent use of high-resolution mass spectrometry combined with newly developed enrichment and labelling schemes to favor the detection and quantification of post-translational modifications. There is no shortage of proteomic studies in the search for protein biomarkers for the diagnosis and classification of AML. That being said, the current literature shows that a major part of these studies has used low-resolution mass spectrometry, low number of investigated samples without follow-up investigations, involving a major number of samples to validate the findings of the initial analyses. However, more recent reports on this argument show that proteomic and phosphoproteomic investigations are taking advantage of more access to large cohorts of AML patients to sample from. It should be pointed out that such proteomic efforts are not limited to biomarkers discovery; a variety of MS-based methods and technologies now play valuable and expanding roles in the diagnosis and monitoring of acute leukemia, as well as in identification of therapeutic targets and biomarkers, drug discovery, and other important areas of leukemia research [45].

MS-based approaches to identify and quantify proteins in complex biological samples require a multistep workflow that includes sample preparation, liquid chromatography tandem mass spectrometry (LC-MS/MS), data analysis, and results interpretation. In sample preparation stage, cells are lysed, sulphur bridges reduction, cystine alkylation, protein digestion, and desalting to remove chemicals and residual intact proteins before introducing the sample for LC/MS-MS analysis (see Figure 4).

To perform protein quantification, it is necessary to perform some form of labelling. Stable isotope labeling by amino acids (SILAC) is a metabolic labeling technique that introduces light and heavy versions of amino acids (the most commonly used are arginine and lysine) to whole cells through the growth medium containing the desired amino acid form [46]. Other less used labelling methods include isobaric tags for relative and absolute quantification (iTRAQ) and tandem mass tag (TMT). These two techniques are often used for quantitative biomarker discovery studies where SILAC is not applicable [47].

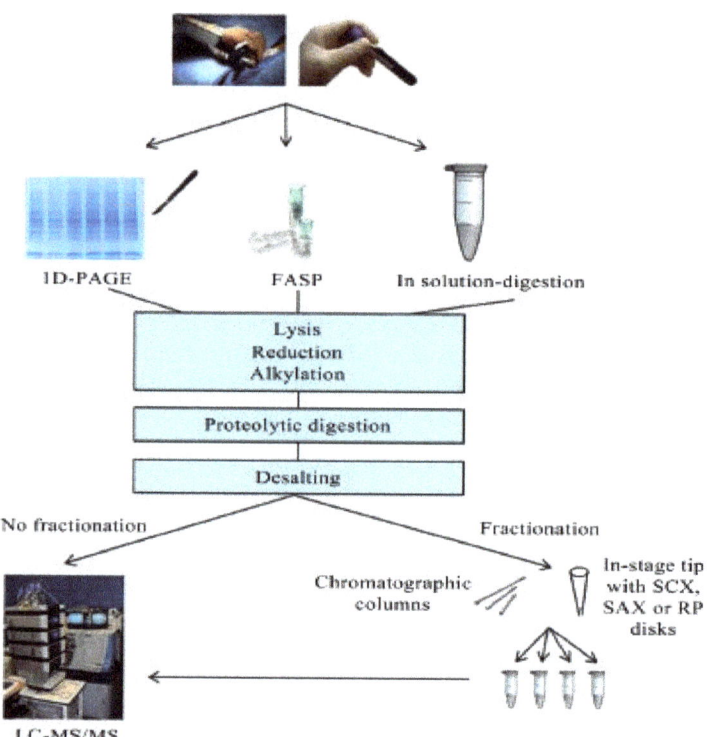

Figure 4. Proteomic workflow comprising three approaches for sample preparation, including filter-assisted sample preparation (FASP). (From Aasebø, E.; Forthun, R.B.; Berven, F.; Selheim, F.; Hernandez-Valladares, M. Global Cell Proteome Profiling, Phospho-signaling and Quantitative Proteomics for Identification of New Biomarkers in Acute Myeloid Leukemia Patients. *Curr. Pharm. Biotechnol.* **2016**, *17*, 52–70).

It is now fairly accepted that AML patients do not exhibit clinical indications, which could help clinicians to predict risk. MS-based proteomics can contribute to the discovery of new prognostic and risk stratifying biomarkers to complement existing morphological, cytogenetic, and molecular risk factors. Several groups have used MS-based proteomics to optimize the cytogenetic classification of AML. An investigation by Nicolas et al. [48] reported the use of protein profiles to subdivide the intermediate and unfavorable cytogenetic groups into subgroups with significantly different survival rates. The same study reported that the most discriminating protein between survival and death was S10A8, which was verified as a biomarker for poor prognosis in a different patient cohort, and found to predict death (during the follow-up period of 57 months) with 85% sensitivity and 72% specificity. Based on these results, the authors suggested that the increased expression of this protein may be used as a high-risk prognostic AML biomarker. In another study, profiling of serum peptides has been performed on samples from 72 AML patients, 72 healthy controls, 37 AML patients with complete remission, and 30 refractory and relapse AML patients [49]. The samples were analyzed with MALDI-TOF and LC-ESI-MS/MS spectrometry to identify candidate biomarkers, followed by immunoblotting for validation studies. Three proteins, ubiquitin-like modifier activating enzyme 1 (UBA1), isoform 1 of fibrinogen alpha chain precursor (FIBA), and platelet factor 4 (PLF4), correlated with AML clinical outcome and could possibly be used for predicting AML relapse, monitoring minimal residual disease, and predicting prognosis in clinical practice. The increase in the availability of AML samples directly from patients or from biobanks, suitable for proteomic analyses, promises new validated protein biomarkers. Furthermore, the increasing use of peptide and modified peptide signatures based on MS data may result in clinical strategies to differentiate AML subgroups and to predict prognosis or treatment response [50].

4. Mass Spectrometry in the Study of Solid Tumors in Children

Solid tumors account for about 60% of all pediatric malignant neoplasms. The spectrum of tumor types that occur in children is much different from that observed in adults. Pediatric neoplasms include tumors of the central nervous system (35%), soft sarcoma, including rhabdomyosarcoma (7%), Wilms tumor (6%), bone tumors, including osteosarcoma and Ewing sarcoma (8%), retinoblastoma (5%), and miscellaneous tumors, including hepatoblastoma, germ cell tumors, and melanoma (17%) [51]. Substantial progress has been made in the diagnosis and management of these tumors since the original demonstration of the chemosensitivity of Wilms tumor to actinomycin D in 1966. Cure rates for most childhood solid tumors have increased by as much as 50% since the mid-1970s. Such increase is attributed largely to improved understanding of prognostically important biological and clinical features, enhanced precision of clinical staging systems, consistent use of supportive care, and development of more effective treatment, often incorporating a combination of chemotherapy, surgery, and radiation.

4.1. Medulloblastoma

Medulloblastoma (MB) is the most common malignant pediatric brain tumor known to be characterized by high incidence of metastasis of the central nervous system, a characteristic which calls for highly aggressive cure, including prophylactic radiation administered to the entire brain and spine. Unfortunately, such highly aggressive regime leaves the majority of long-term survivors with permanent and debilitating neurocognitive impairments, while the remaining patients relapse with terminal metastatic disease. This dramatic scenario underlines the need for a more targeted and possibly more effective therapies. It goes without saying that to achieve such tantalizing objective, a further understanding of the various mechanisms regulating this disease, particularly the process of metastasis, is necessary. Mass spectrometry-based methods can give a valuable contribution to realize such goal. A recent work by Paine et al. [52] is a representative example in this direction. The authors used MALDI-mass spectrometry imaging to examine whole brains from SmoA1 mice. The authors reported that the disease progression in these species faithfully recapitulates the pattern of tumor progression in humans. Briefly, six mice brains were collected under identical conditions: three brains containing non-metastasizing primary tumor and three brains containing a metastasizing primary tumor. These brains were segmented into three main regions and examined by MALDI-TOF operating in negative ion mode. The mean mass spectra for the three segmented regions from both non-metastasizing and metastasizing MB mouse brains are shown in Figure 5.

The authors identified ten lipids that were differentially expressed within non-metastasizing and metastasizing MB primary tumors. The low abundance and the heterogeneity of these lipids required the imaging of the full 3D volume of the brain and the segmentation of the tumor regions. These lipids were identified as having significant differences in TIC normalized relative abundances between the two groups. Chemical structures of these lipids were obtained using accurate mass measurements and MS/MS experiments.

Among the lipids observed to increase in metastasizing primary tumors are the phosphatidylinositol and two phosphoinositides. These three lipids are all structurally related, containing the same fatty acyl chain composition and core head group, and differing only by the degree of phosphorylation on the inositol moiety. PIPs are generated by phosphoinositide kinases (PIKs) to convey signals from the cell surface to the cytoplasm and are downstream effectors on multiple pathways involved in the survival and growth of normal cells. Dysregulation of the PI3K signaling pathway, most commonly caused by alteration of the PTEN gene, has been widely associated with oncogenesis in humans due to unbridled cell growth and proliferation. All three lipids—participants in the same signaling pathway—were observed to be elevated in metastasizing tumors compared to their non-metastasizing counterparts, therefore providing strong evidence that this pathway is upregulated in medulloblastoma metastasizing tissue. According to the authors, the ten lipids identified represent prime candidates for validation in human MB tissues and for further investigation with respect to the potential functional mechanism of these lipids in the promotion of metastasis in human and murine SHH MB.

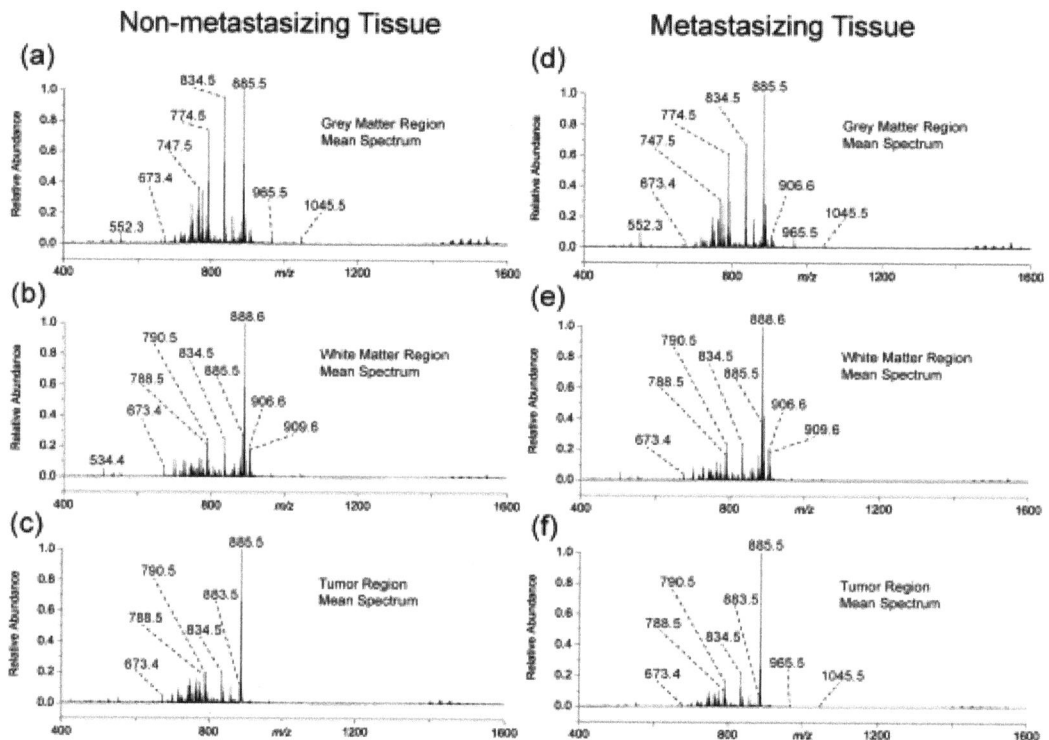

Figure 5. The calculated mean spectra for tumor regions mouse brain containing a non-metastasizing medulloblastoma primary tumor (**a–c**) and tumor regions in a mouse brain containing a metastasizing medulloblastoma primary tumors (**d–f**). (From Paine et al., *Sci. Rep.* 2019).

Considering the results reported above, the following observations can be made: (i) Mass spectrometry imaging on its own (without prior separation/fractionation or labelling) can detect specific molecular changes in complex biological samples. (ii) The difference in lipid profiles between metastasizing and none reported in this study is an important contribution to current attempts to understand the mechanism(s) regulating the metastasize and the tumor progression in MB. (iii) Phosphatidylinositol-3 kinases (PI3Ks) constitutes a lipid kinase family characterized by their ability to phosphorylate inositol ring 3'-OH group in inositol phospholipids to generate the second messenger phosphatidylinositol-3,4,5-triphosphate (PIP3) at the inner side of the membrane. It is relevant to point out that PI3K and AKT has gained a relatively recent recognition as an important regulator of mammalian cell proliferation and survival. The dysregulation of several components of this pathway in a wide spectrum of human cancers is one of the reasons why PI3K-AKT has gained a prominent status in cancer research.

Another recent study demonstrating the use of MS imaging to investigate brain tumors has been reported by Clark et al. [53]. The aim of the study was to identify lipid profiles capable of differentiating medulloblastoma (MB), which originates in the posterior fossa of the brain, from pineoblastoma (PB), which originates within the pineal gland. Medulloblastoma and pineoblastoma exhibit overlapping clinical features and have similar histopathological characteristics. Histopathological similarities confound rapid diagnoses of these two tumor types. The authors used high-resolution Fourier transform ion cyclotron resonance (FT-ICR) equipped with MALDI to examine archived frozen human tumor specimens (eight medulloblastoma and three pineoblastoma tissue samples). The acquired datasets were examined with multivariate statistical analyses to generate classifiers capable of distinguishing the two tumor types. Furthermore, the discriminative molecules were queried against the lipid maps database and identified. The authors concluded that imaging MS identified a number of lipids which could distinguish the two forms of brain cancer. Glycerophosphoglycerols were identified as the classifiers of MB, while sphingolipids were identified as the top classifiers of PB. This study revealed a number of elements which merit further considerations. First, the two investigated forms of cancer are known to exhibit overlapping clinical features and have similar histopathological characteristics, which renders the reported conclusions highly valuable. Second, these conclusions are based on a fairly limited number of samples and therefore, and as suggested by the authors, verification and possible validation of the reported classifiers require further investigations, where much higher number of samples should be used. Third, one of the interesting elements in the same study is that the MS images were serially acquired using alternating positive and negative ion modes. This approach enhances the chances of capturing molecules, which ionizes more efficiently in positive ion mode but not in negative ion mode and vice versa. The authors have used high-resolution MS imaging, which is highly suitable for spatially resolved molecules within a given sample allowing for label free molecular images. This characteristic allows these images to be compared with more traditional histopathology and immunohistochemistry assessment for initial validation.

In a study by Woolman et al. [54], Picosecond infrared laser desorption mass spectrometry (PIRL-MS) was used to generate molecular signatures, which could be used for MB subgroups classification. The authors used in excess of a hundred tissue samples supplied by a local biobank. Each sample was subjected to 10 to 15 s PIRL-MS data collection and principal component analysis with linear discriminant analysis (PCA-LDA). The MB subgroups model was established from 72 independent samples; the remaining 41 samples were classified as unknown tumors and further subjected to multiple 10 s PIRL-MS sampling and real-time PCA-LDA analyses using the above model. The resultant 124 PIRL-MS spectra from each sampling event, after the application of a 95% PCA-LDA prediction probability threshold, yielded a 98.9% correct classification rate. Post-ablation histopathologic analyses suggested that heterogeneity or sample damage prior to PIRL-MS sampling at the site of laser ablation was responsible for the failure of the classification.

4.2. Neuroblastoma

Neuroblastoma is the most common extracranial solid tumor in childhood and the most frequently diagnosed neoplasm during infancy. The disease is known for its broad spectrum of clinical behavior and efforts to tailor treatment according to the predicted clinical aggressiveness of the tumor have been ongoing for decades. Neuroblastoma patients are classified according to disease stage and molecular alterations into three groups: low, intermediate, and high risk. Although the first two groups show five-year survival rates greater than 90%, the survival of high-risk patients remains poor at approximately 40%. Despite aggressive treatment consisting of surgery and a combination of high-dose chemotherapy, radiotherapy, and immunotherapy, the survival rate of high-risk neuroblastoma remains notably low [55,56], which renders high-risk NB a good candidate for epigenetic therapies to overcome drug resistance. In fact, epigenetic therapies are an emerging option for overcoming NB drug resistance. This approach proposes targeting of epigenetic regulators, which are proteins involved in the creation, detection, and interpretation of epigenetic signals. Currently, most epigenetic drugs act at three main levels: (i) DNA methylation, which can be modulated by targeting of DNA methyltransferases (DNMT); (ii) histone modifications, such as acetylation and methylation, which can be targeted by inhibiting the enzymes responsible for these chemical changes; and (iii) blockage of the interpretation of these modifications by targeting epigenetic readers, among which proteins containing bromodomains are the most thoroughly characterized.

It is important to point out that there is an unidentified subset of low-risk and intermediate-risk children who would benefit from treatment reduction while maintaining high survival rates. However, current classification fails to distinguish those high-risk NB that will not respond to initial therapy or will relapse after treatment. Thus, a refinement in risk group classification at the time of diagnosis is crucial to guide therapy and identify those patients who will not respond to standard treatments. Increasingly accurate risk classification and refinements in treatment stratification strategies have been achieved with the more recent discovery of robust genomic and molecular biomarkers. The last few years have witnessed increasing use of MS-based strategies in the search for such markers. Two examples, which use such strategies, are considered here. In a study by Quintàs et al. [57], plasma samples collected from 110 NB patients were analyzed by ultra-performance liquid chromatography-time of flight mass spectrometry (UPLC-TOF-MS); the potential of plasma metabolomic profiling to improve current NB risk-group stratification and predict response to therapy was evaluated. Plasma samples were analyzed in positive electrospray ionization mode. A sample aliquot was also analyzed using the auto MS/MS method. The analyses were able to identify different plasma metabolic profiles in high- and low-risk NB patients at diagnosis. According to the authors, the metabolic model correctly classified 16 high-risk and 15 low-risk samples in an external validation set providing 84.2% sensitivity and 93.7% specificity. Metabolomic profiling could also discriminate high-risk patients with active disease from those in remission. Notably, a plasma metabolomic signature at diagnosis identified a subset of high-risk NB patients who progressed during treatment. The main conclusion of this study was the ability of the metabolic profiling to potentially predict those patients with high-risk neuroblastoma who are more likely to progress during treatment.

In a fairly recent study [58], MS imaging was used to generate spatial peptide signatures, which could be used to discriminate NB high from low and intermediate risk. As well as MALDI imaging, the authors also used a bottom-up nano-liquid chromatography electrospray ionization tandem mass spectrometry approach for protein identification. In these analyses, the authors used formalin-fixed, paraffin-embedded (FFPE) tissue sections, in which diagnostic biopsies from primary neuroblastoma categorized them as high (five samples) or other risk groups (low or intermediate risk, four samples). The acquired spatial peptide signatures allowed the identification of 11 proteins, most of which are associated with the extracellular matrix and cytoskeleton, which enabled the authors to distinguish high risk neuroblastomas from the tissue sections independently of conventional histology. Differential expression of the identified discriminative proteins, AHNAK and CRMP1, was immunohistochemically confirmed. These data showed a lower intensity distribution of CRMP1 in high-risk neuroblastomas and inversely higher intensity distribution in low- and intermediate-risk neuroblastomas. The authors claimed that such result is well in line with the reported role of CRMP1 in neuronal differentiation and its previous use as a marker gene in neuroblastoma gene expression panels as well as its usefulness as a prognostic and diagnostic marker in other cancers. The acquired data also identified AHNAK as a marker protein highly expressed in high-risk neuroblastoma, from which tryptic peptides have high intensity distributions in tumor cell-rich regions of sections analyzed by MALDI-MSI. The authors reported that AHNAK has not been previously associated with neuroblastoma but has been implicated in several cellular functions associated with cancer. Furthermore, discriminative spatial intensities of m/z peaks were validated in microarrayed tissue cores from tumor cell-rich regions in neuroblastomas. The imaging data generated by MALDI-MS allowed the detection of molecular heterogeneity in the investigated regions. In our opinion, the reported detection of molecular heterogeneity in NB by MS imaging needs further investigations, possibly involving much higher number of samples compared to those used in this study. Having said that, these initial data on a limited number of samples are a highly welcomed result. Currently, international risk classification of neuroblastoma is mainly based on clinical criteria plus MYCN oncogene amplification and more recently complemented by transcriptomic data, proving its central role for making therapy decisions and for disease management. Adding diagnostic information derived from proteomic analyses can only improve the precision of current risk classification approaches. The data presented by Wu et al. [58] provide a proof-of-concept for the technical feasibility of this approach. Furthermore, detection of tumor heterogeneity reported in the same study is likely to be a useful contribution to future efforts aimed at more reliable selection of prognostic or predicative biomarkers and signatures at the protein level in neuroblastoma.

Recent progress in epigenetic research has given hope for cancer patients, particularly those suffering from forms resistant to existing conventional therapies. Epigenetic therapies are generally designed to reverse the oncogenic alterations in chromatin components. These therapies are considered an emerging alternative to existing therapies against aggressive tumors that are or will become resistant to conventional treatments. In principle, these therapies target regulators, which are proteins that are involved in the creation, detection, and interpretation of epigenetic signals, such as methylation or histone post-translational modifications. MS-based proteomics is giving a substantial contribution to current efforts to investigate and understand these protein modifications. A recent article [59] described MS-based workflow that is capable of tracking all possible histone PTMs in an untargeted approach that makes use of human cells. In this workflow, histones were extracted from harvested cell culture, chemical derivatization by propionylation, and tryptic digestion followed by LC/MS, MS-MS. The derivatization step was necessary [60] because of the unusually high levels of lysines and arginines within the sequence of histone proteins; such high levels have the consequence that proteins digestion by trypsin would result in relatively short tryptic peptides and would vary based on the modification status of the histones. Derivatization by propionylation has two benefits: Firstly, it modifies all free primary amines, resulting in an Arg-C specificity instead of a tryptic specificity. Secondly, short tryptic peptides will show less retention on a C18 column during reversed-phase high-performance liquid chromatography. The presence of a propionyl group increases the hydrophobicity, thereby enhancing the retention and separation of the peptides in the LC analyses. That being said, the optimization of the derivatization step is not as straight forward as it sounds. In a careful examination of the various derivatization procedures [59], the authors investigated the pitfalls in histone propionylation during bottom-up mass spectrometry analysis.

5. Epigenetic-Based Therapies

Epigenetic therapies are an emerging alternative for overcoming drug resistance. This approach proposes targeting of epigenetic regulators, which are proteins involved in the creation, detection, and interpretation of epigenetic signals. The reversible nature of the epigenetic changes that occur in cancer has led to the possibility of 'epigenetic therapy' as an alternative to conventional therapies. The aim of epigenetic therapy is to reverse the epigenetic aberrations that occur in cancer, leading to the restoration of a 'normal epigenome'. A number of epigenetic drugs have been discovered in the last ten years that can effectively reverse DNA methylation and histone modification aberrations that occur in cancer. DNA methylation inhibitors were among the first epigenetic drugs proposed for use as cancer therapeutics. The potential of these drugs was realized over 50 years ago with the publication by Constantinides [61], showing that treatment with cytotoxic agents, 5-azacytidine (5-aza-CR) and 5-aza-2'-deoxycytidine (5-aza-CdR), leads to the inhibition of DNA methylation that induced gene expression and caused differentiation in cultured cells. The authors are not in a position to list and discuss the epigenetic mechanisms, which led to the discovery and development of various drugs, which gave hope to cancer patients, in particular those in pediatric age. That being said, the following general observations are in order: The recent literature has amply demonstrated that these epigenetic modifications are central in the initiation and progression of various forms of cancer. Furthermore, the information on the type and on the position of these modifications provided by MS-based proteomics are highly relevant to current and future efforts to discover new epigenetic therapies. However, further analytical data are needed before considering such technology a source for diagnostic and prognostic biomarkers to suggest therapeutic path for various forms of cancer. Despite the great potential of DNA methylation inhibitors as therapeutic option, their reaction with the DNA is known to be non-specific, causing genome-wide hypermethylation, which results in undesirable effects regarding the activation and/or silencing of various genes. It has been argued that such side effect could be mitigated by chemically synthesized small molecules, which are more effective than cytidine analogues. The attractive characteristic of these small molecules is that they do not require incorporation into DNA and bind directly to the catalytic site of the DNA methyl transferases [62].

In recent years, it has been established that aberrant gene silencing is linked to histone acetylation, bringing histone acetylation pattern to its normal state through treatment with histone deacetylase inhibitors (HDAC). These agents have been shown to have antitumor effects, including growth arrest, apoptosis, and the induction of differentiation. These effects by HDAC inhibitors are due to their ability to reactivate silenced suppressor genes [63]. A representative member of this class of inhibitors is suberoylanilide hydroxamic acid (SAHA), which has been approved for use in clinic over fifteen years ago for the treatment of T cell cutaneous lymphoma [64]. The well-studied interaction between the different components of the epigenetic machinery renders the use of combinatorial cancer strategies a highly attractive therapeutic option. A representative example of this combinatorial cancer treatment is the use of both DNA methylation in combination with HDCA inhibitors. Synergistic activities of DNA methylation and HDAC inhibitors were also demonstrated in a study showing greater reduction of lung tumor formation in mice when treated with phenylbutyrate and 5-Aza-CdR together [65].

6. Mass Spectrometry Monitoring of Therapeutic Drugs

Chemotherapeutic drugs are still a principal player in the treatment of various forms of cancer, particularly those in advanced stages. The determination of appropriate dosing regimens for the treatment of infants and very young children with cancer represents a major challenge in pediatric oncology. Dose reductions are commonly employed for many chemotherapeutic regimes; however, the suitability of dose reductions for various anticancer drugs remains unclear due to the lack of deep knowledge of the pharmacokinetics of these drugs in the infant patient population. In any disease, the efficacy of a given drug is measured by considering both its therapeutic effect and its toxicity. It is also well established that most anticancer drugs are cytotoxic in nature and have low specificity, which means that the optimal range of a therapeutic dose for a given patient is likely to be narrow. Recent works on this argument have shown that for most anticancer drugs, the concentration at which serious toxicity tends to manifest is many times higher than the concentration at which the therapeutic efficacy is achieved. This observation underlines the central role of therapeutic drug monitoring (TDM). Numerous works have demonstrated that failure of systemic cancer treatment can be, at least in part, due to the drug not being delivered to the tumor at sufficiently high concentration and/or sufficiently homogeneous distribution. The last decade has witnessed an increased use of mass spectrometry for TDM analyses. Aghai et al. [66] used LC/MS-MS for the simultaneous determination of ten kinase inhibitors in human serum and plasma. This method was designed for application in daily clinical routine. The authors reported that the development and validation of the method was according to the US Food and Drug Administration (FDA) and European Medicines Agency (EMA) validation guidelines for bioanalytical methods. The main steps in this method included proteins precipitation of the plasma samples and room temperature LC separation; eluted components were injected into positive electrospray ion source and the resulting ions were analyzed and detected using multiple reaction monitoring mode. Stable isotopically labeled compounds of each kinase inhibitor were used as internal standards. This method has a number of interesting elements, which should be underlined: (i) The method has a relatively short analysis time (7 min), which renders it highly suitable for high throughput analyses, particularly in clinical environment. (ii) A number of therapeutic regimes use multiple anticancer drugs simultaneously, which renders the simultaneous monitoring of multiple compounds highly informative regarding the response of the patients and the therapeutic usefulness of the combination of these drugs.

The relatively recent introduction of oral anticancer drugs resulted in significant improvement in the treatment of various forms of cancer. Patients undergoing this type of therapy tend to have variable concentrations of plasma, resulting in reduced therapeutic efficacy of the drug, and in some cases, unforeseen side effects One approach to mitigate these effects is regular TDM analyses of the patients receiving such treatment. Kehl et al. [67] described a method to simultaneously quantify the plasma concentrations of 57 oral antitumor agents. The authors used liquid chromatography coupled to high-resolution mass spectrometry and the method was fully validated according to the FDA guidelines. The application of this method to clinical routine was tested by the analysis of 71 plasma samples taken from 39 patients.

Mass spectrometry imaging (MSI) is a label-free molecular imaging technique that provides spatial as well as temporal information on the spatial distribution of drugs and their metabolites in a wide range of biological samples, a capability which lacks in the more diffused LC/MS methods. In recent years, (MSI) started to give relevant contribution to the emerging field of precision pharmacology. In this approach, various analytical techniques, including MSI, are used to understand whether an administered anticancer drug is being adequately delivered to the tumor region. Such information is central to both the assessment of the adequacy of the therapy and the resistance to the drug. In a relatively recent study [68], the authors reviewed the role of MSI in pre-clinical studies to characterize anticancer drug distribution within the body and the tumor, and the application of MSI in pre-clinical studies to define optimal drug dose or schedule, combinations, or new drug delivery systems. In their review, the authors underlined the following observations: the characterization of drug concentrations, and in particular drug distribution, within tumors or normal tissues is a challenge that the rapidly developing technique of MALDI-MSI has started to address and may have an important role in drug development. MALDI-MSI already has the potential to support pre-clinical studies by comparing the penetration of candidate molecules into different regions of spheroids in vitro and xenografts in vivo.

Published works in the last few years clearly show that LC coupled to tandem mass spectrometry is the preferred method for TDM analyses. It is also interesting to note that these works indicate a limited use of high-resolution mass spectrometry. This limited use can be justified by the following considerations: First, TDM analyses detect and quantify chemical entities with known molecular structure(s) and predetermined molecular weights; therefore, instruments with mass resolution of one atomic mass unit (amu) are sufficient for this type of analyses. This explains the extensive use of triple quadrupole instruments hyphenated with liquid chromatography. That being said, certain analyses conditions do necessitate the use of high-resolution mass spectrometry. For example, simultaneous monitoring of multiple anticancer drugs, some of which happen to have the same nominal molecular mass but different elemental composition. Identification of some untargeted metabolites of the monitored compounds is another analyses condition in which high resolution can be the only route for an unambiguous identification of the detected metabolites. Second, the relatively limited use of high-resolution instruments for TDM analyses can be partially attributed to higher costs and more demanding operational skills compared to their low-resolution counterparts.

7. Conclusions and Perspectives

Works discussed in this review underline the central role of MS-based proteomics in cancer research. The cited examples show how such approach is providing a wealth of information relevant to various aspects of cancer research, including biomarkers discovery, in particular those which could be used to discriminate tumor subgroups which happen to have similar or even overlapping histopathological features. The same approach furnishes much needed information on metabolic profiles, therapeutic drug monitoring, protein post-translational modifications, and molecular mechanisms in cancer, and signaling pathways associated with various forms of cancer. In recent years, such contribution has been enhanced by more frequent use of high-resolution mass spectrometry in combination with more efficient separation, fractionation, and metabolic labelling methods. MS-based proteomics has been given a fresh momentum by recent epigenetic findings, showing the central role of protein modifications in the landscape of epigenetic events. The involvement of epigenetic abnormalities in the initiation and progression of cancer is now widely accepted. Consequently, targeting the enzymatic machinery that controls the epigenetic regulation of the genome has emerged as a highly promising strategy for therapeutic intervention, in particular for forms of cancer showing drug resistance. It is also becoming more evident that the development of epigenetic drugs requires a detailed knowledge of the processes that govern chromatin regulation. Mass spectrometry-based proteomics is becoming a major source for such knowledge. There are various scientific opinions predicting that in the next few years more cancer therapies will be approved, as many are currently in advanced clinical trials. The authors are convinced that MS-based proteomics will greatly contribute to such anticipated developments.

Author Contributions: Conceptualization, M.A., P.T. and M.H.; writing—original draft preparation, P.T. and M.H.; writing—review and editing, P.T. and M.H.; supervision, M.A., P.T. and M.H. All authors have read and agreed to the published version of the manuscript.

Funding: This research received no external funding.

Acknowledgments: The authors wish to thank Andrea Biccari for his valid and fruitful collaboration.

Conflicts of Interest: The authors declare no conflict of interest.

References

1. Kirana, C.; Peng, L.; Miller, R.; Keating, J.P.; Glenn, C.; Shi, H.; Jordan, T.W.; Maddern, G.J.; Stubbs, R.S. Combination of laser microdissection, 2D-DIGE and MALDI-TOF MS to identify protein biomarkers to predict colorectal cancer spread. *Clin. Proteom.* **2019**, *16*, 3–13. [CrossRef]
2. Pusztaszeri, M.; Matter, M.; Kuonen, A.; Bouzourene, H. Nodal staging in colorectal cancer: Should distant lymph nodes be recovered in surgical specimens? *Hum. Pathol.* **2009**, *40*, 552–557. [CrossRef] [PubMed]
3. Guo, L.; Ren, H.; Zeng, H.; Gong, Y.; Ma, X. Proteomic analysis of cerebrospinal fluid in pediatric acute lymphoblastic leukemia patients: A pilot study. *OncoTargets Ther.* **2019**, *12*, 3859–3868. [CrossRef]
4. Xu, Y.; Zhuo, J.; Duan, Y.; Shi, B.; Chen, X.; Zhang, X.; Xiao, L.; Lou, J.; Huang, R.; Zhang, Q.; et al. Construction of protein profile classification model and screening of proteomic signature of acute leukemia. *Int. J. Clin. Exp. Pathol.* **2014**, *7*, 5569–5581. [PubMed]
5. Drake, R.R.; Elschenbroich, S.; Lopez-Perez, O.; Kim, Y.; Ignatchenko, V.; Ignatchenko, A.; Nyalwidhe, J.O.; Basu, G.; Wilkins, C.E.; Gjurich, B.; et al. In-depth proteomic analyses of direct expressed prostatic secretions. *J. Proteome Res.* **2010**, *9*, 2109–2116. [CrossRef]
6. Wu, C.C.; Chu, H.W.; Hsu, C.W.; Chang, K.P.; Liu, H.P. Saliva proteome profiling reveals potential salivary biomarkers for detection of oral cavity squamous cell carcinoma. *Proteomics* **2015**, *15*, 3394–3404. [CrossRef]
7. de Godoy, L.M.; Olsen, J.V.; de Souza, G.A.; Li, G.; Mortensen, P.; Mann, M. Status of complete proteome analysis by mass spectrometry: SILAC labeled yeast as a model system. *Genome Biol.* **2006**, *7*, R50. [CrossRef] [PubMed]
8. Priola, G.M.; Foster, M.W.; Deal, A.M.; Richardson, B.M.; Thompson, J.W.; Blatt, J. Cerebrospinal fluid proteomics in children during induction for acute lymphoblastic leukemia: A pilot study. *Pediatr. Blood Cancer* **2015**, *62*, 1190–1194. [CrossRef] [PubMed]
9. McEachron, T.A.; Helman, L.J. Recent Advances in Pediatric Cancer Research. *Cancer Res.* **2021**, *81*, 5783–5799. [CrossRef]
10. Mertins, P.; Mani, D.R.; Ruggles, K.V.; Gillette, M.A.; Clauser, K.R.; Wang, P.; Wang, X.; Qiao, J.W.; Cao, S.; Petralia, F.; et al. NCI CPTAC. Proteogenomics connects somatic mutations to signalling in breast cancer. *Nature* **2016**, *534*, 55–62. [CrossRef]
11. Sinha, A.; Huang, V.; Livingstone, J.; Wang, J.; Fox, N.S.; Kurganovs, N.; Ignatchenko, V.; Fritsch, K.; Donmez, N.; Heisler, L.E.; et al. The Proteogenomic Landscape of Curable Prostate Cancer. *Cancer Cell* **2019**, *35*, 414–427. [CrossRef]
12. Aebersold, R.; Agar, J.N.; Amster, I.J.; Baker, M.S.; Bertozzi, C.R.; Boja, E.S.; Costello, C.E.; Cravatt, B.F.; Fenselau, C.; Garcia, B.A.; et al. How many human proteoforms are there? *Nat. Chem. Biol.* **2018**, *14*, 206–214. [CrossRef]
13. Smith, L.M.; Kelleher, N.L. Consortium for Top Down Proteomics. Proteoform: A single term describing protein complexity. *Nat. Methods* **2013**, *10*, 186–187. [CrossRef]

14. Luger, K.; Mader, A.W.; Richmond, R.K.; Sargent, F.; Richmond, T.J. Crystal structure of the nucleosome core particle at 2.8 Å resolution. *Nature* **1997**, *389*, 251–260. [CrossRef]
15. Kouzarides, T. Chromatin modifications and their function. *Cell* **2007**, *128*, 693–705. [CrossRef]
16. Soldi, M.; Cuomo, A.; Bremang, M.; Bonaldi, T. Mass spectrometry-based proteomics for the analysis of chromatin structure and dynamics. *Int. J. Mol. Sci.* **2013**, *14*, 5402–5431. [CrossRef]
17. Bonaldi, T.; Imhoff, A.; Regula, J.T. A combination of different mass spectroscopic techniques for the analysis of dynamic changes of histone modifications. *Proteomics* **2004**, *4*, 1382–1396. [CrossRef]
18. Thomas, C.E.; Kelleher, N.L.; Mizzen, C.A. Mass spectrometric characterization of human histone H3: A bird's eye view. *J. Proteome Res.* **2006**, *5*, 240–247. [CrossRef]
19. Young, N.L.; DiMaggio, P.A.; Plazas-Mayorca, M.D.; Baliban, R.C.; Floudas, C.A.; Garcia, B.A. High throughput characterization of combinatorial histone codes. *Mol. Cell Proteom.* **2009**, *8*, 2266–2284. [CrossRef]
20. Yates, J.R.; McCormack, A.L.; Schieltz, D.; Carmack, E.; Link, A. Direct analysis of protein mixtures by tandem mass spectrometry. *J. Protein Chem.* **1997**, *16*, 495–497. [CrossRef]
21. Marcus, K.; Lelong, C.; Thierry Rabilloud, T. What Room for Two-Dimensional Gel-Based Proteomics in a Shotgun Proteomics World? *Proteomes* **2020**, *8*, 17. [CrossRef]
22. O'Farrell, P.H. High resolution two-dimensional electrophoresis of proteins. *J. Biol. Chem.* **1975**, *250*, 4007–4021. [CrossRef]
23. Ünlü, M.; Morgan, M.E.; Minden, J.S. Difference gel electrophoresis. A single gel method for detecting changes in protein extracts. *Electrophoresis* **1997**, *18*, 2071–2077. [CrossRef]
24. Braoudaki, M.; Lambrou, G.I.; Vougas, K.; Karamolegou, K.; George, T.; Tsangaris, G.T.; Tzortzatou-Stathopoulou, F. Protein biomarkers distinguish between high- and low-risk pediatric acute lymphoblastic leukemia in a tissue specific manner. *J. Hematol. Oncol.* **2013**, *6*, 52. [CrossRef]
25. Sinha, P.; Poland, J.; Kohl, S.; Schnölzer, M.; Helmbach, H.; Hütter, G.; Lage, H.; Schadendorf, D. Study of the development of chemoresistance in melanoma cell lines using proteome analysis. *Electrophoresis* **2003**, *23*, 2386–2404. [CrossRef]
26. Sarto, C.; Binz, P.A.; Mocarelli, P. Heat shock proteins in human cancer. *Electrophoresis* **2000**, *21*, 1218–1226. [CrossRef]
27. Crul, M.; van Waardenburg, R.C.; Beijnen, J.H.; Schellens, J.H. DNA-based drug interactions of cisplatin. *Cancer Treat. Rev.* **2002**, *28*, 291–303. [CrossRef]
28. Dai, Z.; Yin, J.; He, H.; Li, W.; Hou, C.; Qian, X.; Mao, N.; Pan, L. Mitochondrial comparative proteomics of human ovarian cancer cells and their platinum-resistant sublines. *Proteomics* **2010**, *10*, 3789–3799. [CrossRef]
29. Dzobo, K. Taking a Full Snapshot of Cancer Biology: Deciphering the Tumor Microenvironment for Effective Cancer Therapy in the Oncology Clinic. *OMICS* **2020**, *24*, 175–179. [CrossRef]
30. Gygi, S.P.; Corthals, G.L.; Zhang, Y.; Rochon, Y.; Aebersold, R. Evaluation of two-dimensional gel electrophoresis-based proteome analysis technology. *Proc. Natl. Acad. Sci. USA* **2000**, *97*, 9390–9395. [CrossRef]
31. Rabilloud, T. Two-dimensional gel electrophoresis in proteomics: Old, old fashioned, but it still climbs up the mountains. *Proteomics* **2002**, *2*, 3–10. [CrossRef]
32. Liu, X.; Hummon, A.B. Mass spectrometry imaging of therapeutics from animal models to three-dimensional cell cultures. *Anal. Chem.* **2015**, *87*, 9508–9519. [CrossRef]
33. Hayashi, A.; Konishi, I. Correlation of anti-tumor drug resistance with epigenetic regulation. *Br. J. Cancer* **2021**, *124*, 681–682. [CrossRef]
34. Aziz, M.H.; Ahmad, A. Epigenetic basis of cancer drug resistance. *Cancer Drug Resist.* **2020**, *3*, 113–116. [CrossRef]
35. Meyer, L.K.; Hermiston, M.L. The epigenome in pediatric acute lymphoblastic leukemia: Drug resistance and therapeutic opportunities. *Cancer Drug Resist.* **2019**, *2*, 313–325. [CrossRef]
36. Andersson, D.; Fagman, H.; Dalin, M.G.; Ståhlberg, A. Circulating cell-free tumor DNA analysis in pediatric cancers. *Mol. Asp. Med.* **2020**, *72*, 100819. [CrossRef]
37. Di Minno, A.; Gelzo, M.; Caterino, M.; Costanzo, M.; Ruoppolo, M.; Castaldo, G. Challenges in Metabolomics-Based Tests, Biomarkers Revealed by Metabolomic Analysis, and the Promise of the Application of Metabolomics in Precision Medicine. *Int. J. Mol. Sci.* **2022**, *23*, 5213. [CrossRef]
38. Veenstra, T.D.; Conrads, T.P.; Hood, B.L.; Avellino, A.M.; Ellenbogen, R.G.; Morrison, R.S. Biomarkers: Mining the biofluid proteome. *Mol. Cell Proteom.* **2005**, *4*, 409–418. [CrossRef]
39. Pinu, F.R.; Beale, D.J.; Paten, A.M.; Kouremenos, K.; Swarup, S.; Schirra, H.J.; Wishart, D. Systems Biology and Multi-Omics Integration: Viewpoints from the Metabolomics Research Community. *Metabolites* **2019**, *9*, 76. [CrossRef]
40. Petrick, L.; Imani, P.; Perttula, K.; Yano, Y.; Whitehead, T.; Metayer, C.; Schiffman, C.; Dolios, G.; Dudoit, S.; Rappaport, S. Untargeted metabolomics of newborn dried blood spots reveals sex-specific associations with pediatric acute myeloid leukemia. *Leuk. Res.* **2021**, *106*, 106585. [CrossRef]
41. Liu, X.; Li, J.; Hao, X.; Sun, H.; Zhang, Y.; Zhang, L.; Jia, L.; Tian, Y.; Sun, W. LC-MS-Based Urine Metabolomics Analysis for the Diagnosis and Monitoring of Medulloblastoma. *Front. Oncol.* **2022**, *12*, 949513. [CrossRef]
42. Metayer, C.; Zhang, L.; Wiemels, J.L.; Bartley, K.; Schiffman, J.; Ma, X.; Aldrich, M.C.; Chang, J.S.; Selvin, S.; Fu, C.H.; et al. Tobacco smoke exposure and the risk of childhood acute lymphoblastic and myeloid leukemias by cytogenetic subtype. *Cancer Epidemiol. Biomark. Prev.* **2013**, *22*, 1600–1611. [CrossRef]

43. Bennett, J.M.; Catovsky, D.; Daniel, M.T.; Flandrin, G.; Galton, D.A.; Gralnick, H.R.; Sultan, C. Proposals for the classification of the acute leukaemia. French-American-British (FAB) co-operative group. *Br. J. Heamatol.* **1976**, *33*, 451–458. [CrossRef]
44. Bennett, J.M. World Health Organization classification of the acute leukemias and myelodysplastic syndrome. *Int. J. Hematol.* **2000**, *72*, 131–133.
45. Roboz, J.; Roboz, G.J. Mass spectrometry in leukemia research and treatment. *Expert Rev. Hematol.* **2015**, *8*, 225–235. [CrossRef]
46. Geiger, T.; Cox, J.; Ostasiewicz, P.; Wisniewski, J.; Mann, M. Super-SILAC mix for quantitative proteomics of human tumor tissue. *Nat. Methods* **2010**, *7*, 383–385. [CrossRef]
47. Simpson, K.L.; Whetton, A.D.; Dive, C. Quantitative mass spectrometry-based techniques for clinical use: Biomarker identification and quantification. *J. Chromatogr. B Analyt. Technol. Biomed. Life Sci.* **2009**, *877*, 1240–1249. [CrossRef]
48. Nicolas, E.; Ramus, C.; Berthier, S.; Arlotto, M.; Bouamrani, A.; Lefebvre, C.; Morel, F.; Garin, J.; Ifrah, N.; Berger, F.; et al. Expression of S100A8 in leukemic cells predicts poor survival in *de novo* AML patients. *Leukemia* **2011**, *25*, 57–65. [CrossRef]
49. Bai, J.; He, A.; Huang, C.; Yang, J.; Zhang, W.; Yang, Y.; Yang, J.; Zhang, P.; Zhang, Y.; Zhou, F. Serum peptidome based biomarkers searching for monitoring minimal residual disease in adult acute lymphocytic leukemia. *Proteome Sci.* **2014**, *12*, 49. [CrossRef]
50. Alcolea, M.P.; Casado, P.; Rodríguez-Prados, J.C.; Vanhaesebroeck, B.; Cutillas, P.R. Phosphoproteomic analysis of leukemia cells under basal and drug-treated conditions identifies markers of kinase pathway activation and mechanisms of resistance. *Mol. Cell Proteom.* **2012**, *11*, 453–466. [CrossRef]
51. Kline, N.E.; Sevier, N. Solid tumors in children. *J. Pediatr. Nurs.* **2003**, *18*, 96–102. [CrossRef]
52. Paine, M.R.L.; Liu, J.; Huang, D.; Ellis, S.R.; Trede, D.; Kobarg, J.H.; Heeren, R.M.A.; Fernández, F.M.; MacDonald, T.J. Three-Dimensional Mass Spectrometry Imaging Identifies Lipid Markers of Medulloblastoma Metastasis. *Sci. Rep.* **2019**, *9*, 2205. [CrossRef]
53. Clark, A.R.; Calligaris, D.; Regan, M.S.; Pomeranz Krummel, D.; Agar, J.N.; Kallay, L.; MacDonald, T.; Schniederjan, M.; Santagata, S.; Pomeroy, S.L.; et al. Rapid discrimination of pediatric brain tumors by mass spectrometry imaging. *J. Neurooncol.* **2018**, *140*, 269–279. [CrossRef]
54. Woolman, M.; Kuzan-Fischer, C.M.; Ferry, I.; Kiyota, T.; Luu, B.; Wu, M.; Munoz, D.G.; Das, S.; Aman, A.; Taylor, M.D.; et al. Picosecond Infrared Laser Desorption Mass Spectrometry Identifies Medulloblastoma Subgroups on Intrasurgical Timescales. *Cancer Res.* **2019**, *79*, 2426–2434. [CrossRef]
55. Maris, J.M. Recent advances in neuroblastoma. *N. Engl. J. Med.* **2010**, *362*, 2202–2211. [CrossRef]
56. Cohn, S.L.; Pearson, A.D.; London, W.B.; Monclair, T.; Ambros, P.F.; Brodeur, G.M.; Faldum, A.; Hero, B.; Iehara, T.; Machin, D.; et al. The International Neuroblastoma Risk Group (INRG) classification system: An INRG Task Force report. *J. Clin. Oncol.* **2009**, *27*, 289–297. [CrossRef]
57. Quintás, G.; Yáñez, Y.; Gargallo, P.; Juan Ribelles, A.; Cañete, A.; Castel, V.; Segura, V. Metabolomic profiling in neuroblastoma. *Pediatr. Blood Cancer* **2020**, *67*, e28113. [CrossRef]
58. Wu, Z.; Hundsdoerfer, P.; Schulte, J.H.; Astrahantseff, K.; Boral, S.; Schmelz, K.; Eggert, A.; Klein, O. Discovery of Spatial Peptide Signatures for Neuroblastoma Risk Assessment by MALDI Mass Spectrometry Imaging. *Cancers* **2021**, *13*, 3184. [CrossRef]
59. Meert, P.; Govaert, E.; Scheerlinck, E.; Dhaenens, M.; Deforce, D. Pitfalls in histone propionylation during bottom-up mass spectrometry analysis. *Proteomics* **2015**, *15*, 2966–2971. [CrossRef]
60. De Clerck, L.; Willems, S.; Noberini, R.; Restellini, C.; Van Puyvelde, B.; Daled, S.; Bonaldi, D.; Deforce, D.; Dhaenens, M. hSWATH: Unlocking SWATH's full potential for an untargeted histone perspective. *J. Proteome Res.* **2019**, *18*, 3840–3849. [CrossRef]
61. Constantinides, P.G. Functional striated muscle cells from non-myoblast precursors following 5-azacytidine treatment. *Nature* **1977**, *267*, 364–366. [CrossRef]
62. Yoo, C.B.; Jones, P.A. Epigenetic therapy of cancer: Past, present and future. *Nat. Rev. Drug Discov.* **2006**, *5*, 37–50. [CrossRef]
63. Carew, J.S. Histone deacetylase inhibitors: Mechanisms of cell death and promise in combination cancer therapy. *Cancer Lett.* **2008**, *269*, 7–17. [CrossRef]
64. Cortez, C.C.; Jones, P.A. Chromatin, cancer and drug therapies. *Mutat. Res.* **2008**, *647*, 44–51.
65. Belinsky, S.; Donna, M.; Klinge, D.M.; Stidley, C.A.; Issa, J.-P.; Herman, J.G.; March, T.H.; Baylin, S.B. Inhibition of DNA methylation and histone deacetylation prevents murine lung cancer. *Cancer Res.* **2003**, *63*, 7089–7093.
66. Aghai, F.; Zimmermann, S.; Kurlbaum, M.; Jung, P.; Pelzer, T.; Klinker, H.; Isberner, N.; Scherf-Clavel, O. Development and validation of a sensitive liquid chromatography tandem mass spectrometry assay for the simultaneous determination of ten kinase inhibitors in human serum and plasma. *Anal. Bioanal. Chem.* **2021**, *413*, 599–612. [CrossRef]
67. Kehl, N.; Schlichtig, K.; Dürr, P.; Bellut, L.; Dörje, F.; Fietkau, R.; Pavel, M.; Mackensen, A.; Wullich, B.; Maas, R.; et al. An Easily Expandable Multi-Drug LC-MS Assay for the Simultaneous Quantification of 57 Oral Antitumor Drugs in Human Plasma. *Cancers* **2021**, *13*, 6329. [CrossRef]
68. Jove, M.; Spencer, J.; Clench, M.; Loadman, P.M.; Twelves, C. Precision pharmacology: Mass spectrometry imaging and pharmacokinetic drug resistance. *Crit. Rev. Oncol. Hematol.* **2019**, *141*, 153–162. [CrossRef]

Disclaimer/Publisher's Note: The statements, opinions and data contained in all publications are solely those of the individual author(s) and contributor(s) and not of MDPI and/or the editor(s). MDPI and/or the editor(s) disclaim responsibility for any injury to people or property resulting from any ideas, methods, instructions or products referred to in the content.

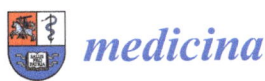

Review

Interstitial Cells of Cajal—Origin, Distribution and Relationship with Gastrointestinal Tumors

Petru Radu [1], Mihai Zurzu [1,*], Vlad Paic [1], Mircea Bratucu [1], Dragos Garofil [1], Anca Tigora [1], Valentin Georgescu [1], Virgiliu Prunoiu [2], Florian Popa [1], Valeriu Surlin [3] and Victor Strambu [1]

[1] General Surgery Department, Carol Davila Nephrology Hospital Bucharest, 020021 Bucharest, Romania
[2] Oncological Institute "Prof. Dr. Alexandru Trestioreanu", 022328 Bucharest, Romania
[3] Sixth Department of Surgery, University of Medicine and Pharmacy of Craiova, Craiova Emergency Clinical Hospital, 200642 Craiova, Romania
* Correspondence: zurzu_mihai@yahoo.com

Abstract: The interstitial cells of Cajal (ICC) represent a particular network formed by some peculiar cells that were first described by the great neuroanatomist, S. Ramon y Cajal. Nowadays, the ICC have become a fascinating topic for scientists, arousing their curiosity; as a result, there is a vast number of published articles related to the ICC. Today, everybody widely accepts that the ICC represent the pacemaker of the gastrointestinal tract and are highly probable to be the origin cells for gastrointestinal tumors (GISTs). Recently, Cajal-like cells (ICLC) were described, which are found in different organs but with an as yet unknown physiological role that needs further study. New information regarding intestinal development indicates that the ICC (fibroblast-like and muscle-like) and intestinal muscle cells have the same common embryonic cells, thereby presenting the same cellular ultrastructure. Nowadays, there is a vast quantity of information that proves the connection of the ICC and GISTs. Both of them are known to present c-kit expression and the same ultrastructural cell features, which includes minimal myoid differentiation that is noticed in GISTs, therefore, supporting the hypothesis that GISTs are ICC-related tumors. In this review, we have tried to highlight the origin and distribution of Cajal interstitial cells based on their ultrastructural features as well as their relationship with gastrointestinal stromal tumors.

Keywords: interstitial cells of Cajal; cancer; gastrointestinal tumors; c-kit

Citation: Radu, P.; Zurzu, M.; Paic, V.; Bratucu, M.; Garofil, D.; Tigora, A.; Georgescu, V.; Prunoiu, V.; Popa, F.; Surlin, V.; et al. Interstitial Cells of Cajal—Origin, Distribution and Relationship with Gastrointestinal Tumors. *Medicina* **2023**, *59*, 63. https://doi.org/10.3390/medicina59010063

Academic Editors: Valentin Titus Grigorean and Daniel Alin Cristian

Received: 29 November 2022
Revised: 23 December 2022
Accepted: 25 December 2022
Published: 28 December 2022

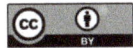

Copyright: © 2022 by the authors. Licensee MDPI, Basel, Switzerland. This article is an open access article distributed under the terms and conditions of the Creative Commons Attribution (CC BY) license (https://creativecommons.org/licenses/by/4.0/).

1. Introduction

The story of the ICC is a fascinating story of ever-changing medical concepts that emerged as a result of the interplay between researchers' limitless scientific intuition and its formal constraints through the continuous development of medical methodology but always limited [1]. It is this interplay that lies behind the evolution of fundamentally correct concepts many decades before the methods moved to the stage of providing sound theories if not providing the evidence itself [1].

Thus, the great Spanish neuroanatomist, Santiago Ramon y Cajal, conducting studies on these cells, arrived at the hypothesis (1893, 1911) that networks of interstitial cells anastomosed to each other are influenced "primarily" by components of the nervous system, while interstitial cells (seen as primitive "accessory" neurons) exert direct regulatory effects on the contraction of smooth muscle in the gastrointestinal tract [1].

Despite the fact that more than a century has passed since Ramon y Cajal described the staining characteristics of the "interstitial nerve cell" located between the external longitudinal muscle and the circular muscle of the intestine at the level of the Auerbach's plexus (1893, 1911), the function and developmental origin of these cells have remained unclear [2]. Although Ramon y Cajal and other contemporary researchers believed that these interstitial cells of Cajal were primitive neurons, it has been suggested that these cells are specialized smooth muscle cells [3], while other researchers have characterized them as fibroblasts [4].

Independent of Cajal's research, Sir Arthur Keith (1914, 1915), the scientist who described the sino-atrial cardiac pacemaker and was apparently unaware of Cajal's research, considered these cells to be a real pacemaker of the intestinal muscle layers [5]. The methods needed to prove or disprove these theories were not developed until 7–8 decades later, subsequently proving both to be essentially correct [1].

Between 1925 and 1965, several controversial papers were recorded with scientists presenting different opinions regarding the origin, function and distribution of the ICC. In 1970, after the development of electron microscopy, many mysteries were elucidated. The ICC presents similar properties to smooth muscle cells but also specific characteristics to perform the function of intestinal pacemaker. In the early 1980s, these cells were again brought back to the attention of gastroenterologists by Thunenberg and Faussone-Pellegrini [4,6].

Nowadays, the ICC are the object of study in many medical fields in order to understand the motility of the gut, their involvement in the development of GIST pathology, as well as to elucidate the pathogenesis of various motility disorders [7].

The main function of the digestive system is considered to be the digestion and absorption of nutrients. However, the digestive tract possesses a number of other important functions, namely motor, evacuatory, secretory and incretory immune functions [8]. The motility of the digestive tract is constantly under the control of several regulatory factors, among which are the intrinsic and extrinsic nervous system as well as the humoral system. The main cell types involved in regulating gastrointestinal motor function are enteric neurons, the ICC and effector cells (smooth muscle cells) [9].

The activity of the ICC has been shown to be fundamental, generating and propagating slow electrical waves that regulate the contractile activity of intestinal smooth muscle as well as mediating neurotransmission from intestinal motor neurons towards the intestinal muscle cells. Slow-wave amplitude is under the control of local factors, such as distention and intraluminal chemical stimulation [10,11].

Cajal cell damage leads to hypokinesis and hypotonia of the intestine, which causes severe constipation. In turn, impaired motor function of the digestive tract triggers pathological conditions in the whole body, such as autointoxication due to the absorption of toxic products and deregulation of the absorption of microelements and vitamins, which accelerate the aging process of the body [10].

For this review, we discuss the origin and distribution in the human gastrointestinal tract of the ICC as well as the relationship between these cells and GISTs based on their common ultrastructural features and biomarkers.

2. Origin of the Interstitial Cells of Cajal

The gastrointestinal system consists of cells that arise from all embryonic layers [12]. The endoderm gives rise to the epithelial cells of the intestinal lumen and the epithelial cells of the intestinal glands [13]. From the mesoderm, all muscle cells, connective tissue and lymphatic and blood structures are born [12]. Neural crest cells are derived from the ectoderm. Neural crest cells migrate in the digestive system and, after that, they give birth to all enteric neurons [12–14].

Despite the fact that the ICC was described more than 100 hundred years ago, their origin has long been an enigma, which is due to the fact that the ICC share structural features with neural crest-derived cells (neurons, glial cells) but also share features with mesoderm-derived cells (muscle cells, fibroblasts) [13]. Despite this debate over the years, some research conducted on chickens, quails [15] and rats [16] demonstrated that the origin of the ICC is in the mesoderm. This fact, demonstrated by the previous research teams, is reinforced by other subsequent studies on rats [2,17].

In the past years, Faussone-Pellegrini [3,6] analyzed the ultrastructural evolution of the ICC in the Auerbach's plexus and deep muscle plexus. They identified the ICC progenitor cells in newborn rats that are closely related to the nerve fibers of the myenteric plexus, but they could not establish the embryological origin of these cells [12]. Several studies from the past suggested that the ICC is derived from the mesoderm and share the same progenitor cells with cells from the smooth muscle [2,17].

Furthermore, Torihashi studied the evolution of c-kit reactivity markers for smooth muscles and neural crest-derived cell markers on embryonic small intestine specimens from rats [17], thus finding the existence of c-kit+ cells in the outer layers of the intestine in day 12 embryos. However, the cells at this level were not differentiated, and they did not present structural characteristics of an adult muscle cell or the ICC [17].

At embryonic day 15, cells at the level of the circular muscle layer, which are located inside the myenteric plexus, present immunoreactivity for actin and muscle myosin; in contrast, cells that develop at the place where the future longitudinal muscle tissue will be located are c-kit+ cells, but they lack the expression for actin and smooth muscle myosin [17]. In the late stages of embryonic development, a c-kit+ cell subpopulation was found to differentiate into smooth muscle cells showing positive expression for myofilament proteins; consequently, these cells lose the ability to show c-kit+ expression [17]. It is thus assumed that the ICC and smooth muscle cells have a common origin from c-kit+ progenitor cells in the primitive intestine, and all c-kit+ cells will differentiate into the ICC [17].

Another study from the literature carried out in 1998 by Kluppel [2] confirmed the previous results that the ICC and smooth muscle cells have the same embryonic progenitor cell. Kluppel studied the mRNA expression of smooth muscle myosin heavy chain (SMMHC) and c-kit immunoreactivity [2]. He found that all intestinal muscle cells initially show c-kit+ expression and expression for SMMHC; later in the developmental stages, they lose the ability to show c-kit+ expression, while all cells that will further become the ICC will keep c-kit expression but will lose expression for SMMHC [2]. The main conclusion of all this data is that the ICC and smooth muscle cells present the same progenitor cell [12,18].

In conclusion, the origin of the ICC is from the progenitor cells that arise from the mesoderm of the primitive intestine and possess the tyrosine kinase receptor c-kit [19]. However, there are a number of mesenchymal cells with c-kit+ expression that are destined to differentiate into smooth muscle cells, which lose expression for c-kit in the process of development but retain expression for myofilament proteins [18]. Furthermore, information is required to fully understand the entire process [12].

3. ICC Distribution in the Human Gastrointestinal Tract

The presence of the ICC in the human gastrointestinal tract has been demonstrated over the years from the esophagus [20] to the anal canal [21]; however, these cells present different morphological features and different tissue distribution.

The ICC exhibit a specific cell position, arrangement and shape based on the localization in different anatomical locations and different layers of the gastrointestinal tract (Figure 1). Therefore, these cells present several cellular subpopulations [22]. In the gastric region, there are reported different subtypes of the ICC and, in the small intestine and colon, the ICC present the same pattern of the subtype of the ICC in each segment [22]. All the subtypes of the ICC have the same ultrastructural characteristics, presence of numerous mitochondria, abundant intermediate filaments and gap junctions with the same cell and smooth muscle cells [22]. The structure of the ICC helps us understand the physiology of the gastrointestinal tract [22].

The ICC include a vast array of specialized cell types within the musculature of the gastrointestinal system. A number of these cell types play a pacemaker role within the gastrointestinal musculature, while others are heavily involved in the modulation of enteric neurotransmission. The most important cell types with a role in intestinal tract motility are the ICC of the myenteric plexus (MP), ICC intramuscular (IM) and ICC of the deep muscle plexus (DMP) (Table 1) [23].

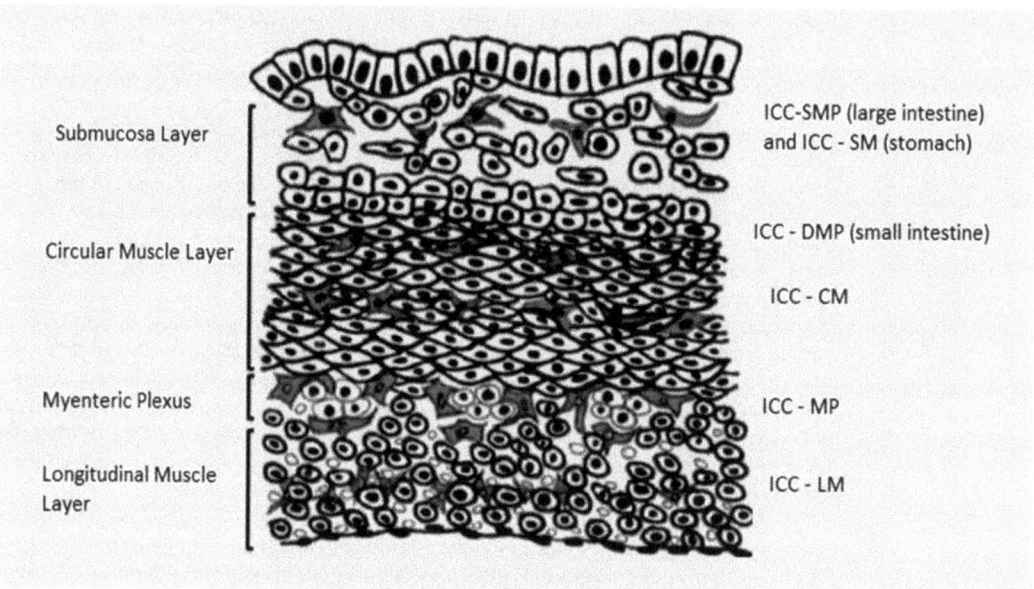

Figure 1. Distribution of the ICC.

Table 1. Features of the ICC subtypes.

Subtypes	Distribution	Morphology	Function
ICC progenitor	Stomach Intestine	Groups of round or oval cells	Possess the ability to repair or replenish damaged ICC. [24]
ICC of the myenteric plexus (Auerbach): MY	Stomach Ileon and jejunum Colon	Multipolar cells, possessing multiple interconnected branches	Generate and propagate slow electrical waves. [24]
ICC of longitudinal muscle tissue: LM	Distal oesophagus Stomach Ileon and jejunum Colon	Bipolar cells, oriented along the long axis of the surrounding smoth muscle cells	Important role in neurotransmission between the intestinal nervous system and smooth muscle cells. [25]
ICC of circular muscle tissue: CM	Distal oesophagus Stomach Ileon and jejunum Colon	Bipolar cells, oriented along the long axis of the surrounding smoth muscle cells	Important role in neurotransmission between the intestinal nervous system and smooth muscle cells. [26]
ICC-IM: mixed form, combining ICC-CM and ICC-LM	Distal oesophagus Stomach Ileon and jejunum Colon	Bipolar cells, oriented along the long axis of the surrounding smoth muscle cells	Important role in neurotransmission between the intestinal nervous system and smooth muscle cells. [24]
ICC of deep muscular plexus: DMP	Ileon and jejunum	Multipolar cells, located in the deep muscular plexus; in close association with the nerve fascicles of the deep muscular plexus	Neural transmission. [27]
ICC of submucosa and submucosal plexus: SM and SMP	Pylorus–SM Colon–SMP	Bipolar or Multipolar cells	Pacemakers and neurotransmission roles. [24]

4. ICC and GISTs

The concept of "gastrointestinal stromal tumor" was first expressed by Mazur and Clark [28], whom mentioned that all spindle cell tumors from the gastrointestinal system do not present the characteristics of smooth muscle cells. GISTs present diverse structural features, and therefore, a range of tumor subtypes are described, such as plexosarcomas [29] and myenteric plexomas [30]. All of these different features were given only based on the structural features of the progenitor cells. Data from the literature state that tumors with a diameter of less than 3 cm are generally considered benign; however, all GISTs can degenerate malignantly [31]. According to data from the literature, most gastrointestinal tumors are present in the entire gastrointestinal tract with predominant involvement of the stomach (60–70%) but with lesser involvement of the small intestine (20–30%) and large intestine (10%), generally occurring in middle-aged patients [32]. A number of similar tumors have been described with structural features similar to GISTs but with some particular differences and are referred to as extra-gastrointestinal stromal tumors [31].

GISTs often have minimum myoid differentiation and a big number of cytoplasmic filaments [33]. GISTs show ultrastructural features similar to the ICC, namely an elongated cell body and a series of cytoplasmic processes. In order to distinguish ICC from fibroblasts, it should be taken into account that the cytoplasmic processes of fibroblasts are usually thin, very broad, fascia-like structures, whereas the cytoplasmic processes of the ICC are narrow, round in shape and present as slightly flattened. The nucleus is ovoid with one or more nucleoli and has limited content located at the periphery. The cytoplasm of the cell body is in the form of a thin frame around the nucleus often enlarged at the origin of the primary cytoplasmic processes. These extensions are two to five in number, giving rise to numerous secondary and tertiary extensions, and the basal lamina is present but often incomplete [7]. The ultrastructural features between Cajal interstitial cells, smooth muscle cells, fibroblasts and gastrointestinal tumor cells are shown in Table 2.

Table 2. Cytological characteristics of ICC, Fibroblasts, Smooth muscle cells and GIST.

Cell Type	C-Kit	CV	BL	MIT	NC	IF	RER	GJ
ICC	+	+	-	++	++	++	+	++
Fibroblats	-	-	-	+	+	+	++	+
Smooth muscle cells	+	++	++	++	++	++	+	++
GIST	+	+	-	++	+	+	++	-

Abbreviations: CV = caveolae, BL = basal lamina, MIT = mitochondria, NC = nerve contact, IF = intermediate filaments, RER=Rough endoplasmic reticulum, GJ = gap junction, C = kit reactivity [7,34,35].

Diffuse hyperplasia of the ICC is observed in these patients, which is considered a pre-neoplastic lesion [31]. Also in the literature data, it is stated that almost 80% of all GISTs express CD 34 [36]. Germline c-kit mutations have also been detected in patients with GISTs at exons 11 and 13 [37].

GISTs express multiple biomarkers in common with the ICC; some of them, as for example Anoctamin1 and Kit, have been identified as key markers in the diagnosis of GISTs [37].

Additional common biomarkers between the ICC and GISTs have revealed important biological mechanisms in the genesis of GISTs; one of these is ETV1 that is a part of the ETS domain of transcription factors, which holds a key role in the regulation of transcription of ICC and GIST, thereby stimulating tumorigenesis and GIST development [37].

5. Discussions

It is assumed that the ICC showing myoid features are not the ICC originally depicted by Raymon y Cajal almost a century ago. The cells around the enteric lymph nodes with immunohistochemical expression of CD117 more likely represent the initially described ICC [7].

The physiological role of these interstitial cells has not yet been fully elucidated. Also, from multiple studies, we can see encouraging information to fully understand the intercellular relationships of the ICC and their role in gastrointestinal tract pathology [38].

The ICC and GISTs show the same precursor cells, most likely stem cells present in the muscle wall of the intestine. These cells retain a certain feature of the evolving germ stem cell and can associate RNA expression of both c-kit and SMMHC protein. Furthermore, the ICC and GISTs share other common biomarkers, such as Anoctamin1 ETV1, which is an important factor in the genesis of GISTs [37] and, in addition, can present muscle cells [7].

New information and data from future studies will be able to clarify all questions regarding this topic.

Author Contributions: Conceptualization, P.R. and M.Z.; methodology, P.R. and V.P. (Vlad Paic); software, M.B.; validation, P.R., F.P. and V.S. (Victor Strambu); formal analysis, D.G.; investigation, A.T.; resources, V.S. (Valeriu Surlin); data curation, V.P. (Virgiliu Prunoiu) and V.G.; writing—original draft preparation, M.Z. and V.S. (Victor Strambu); writing—review and editing, all authors. All authors have read and agreed to the published version of the manuscript.

Funding: This research received no external funding.

Institutional Review Board Statement: Not applicable.

Informed Consent Statement: Not applicable.

Data Availability Statement: Data sharing is not applicable to this article.

Conflicts of Interest: The authors declare no conflict of interest.

References

1. Thuneberg, L. One hundred years of interstitial cells of Cajal. *Microsc. Res. Tech.* **1999**, *47*, 223–238. [CrossRef]
2. Kluppel, M.; Huizinga, J.D.; Malysz, J.; Bernstein, A. Developmental origin and Kit-dependent development of the interstitial cells of cajal in the mammalian small intestine. *Dev. Dyn.* **1998**, *211*, 60–71. [CrossRef]
3. Faussone Pellegrini, M.S. Ultrastructural peculiarities of the inner portion of the circular layer of the colon. II. Research on the mouse. *Acta Anat.* **1985**, *122*, 187–192. [CrossRef]
4. Thuneberg, L. Interstitial cells of Cajal: Intestinal pacemaker cells? *Adv. Anat. Embryol. Cell Biol.* **1982**, *71*, 1–130.
5. Hanani, M. Introduction to interstitial cells of Cajal. *Microsc. Res. Tech.* **1999**, *47*, 221–222. [CrossRef]
6. Faussone Pellegrini, M.S.; Cortesini, C. Some ultrastructural features of the muscular coat of human small intestine. *Acta Anat.* **1983**, *115*, 47–68. [CrossRef]
7. Min, K.W.; Leabu, M. Interstitial cells of Cajal (ICC) and gastrointestinal stromal tumor (GIST): Facts, speculations, and myths. *J. Cell Mol. Med.* **2006**, *10*, 995–1013. [CrossRef]
8. Faussone-Pellegrini, M.S. Interstitial cells of Cajal: Once negligible players, now blazing protagonists. *Ital. J. Anat. Embryol.* **2005**, *110*, 11–31.
9. Gfroerer, S.; Rolle, U. Interstitial cells of Cajal in the normal human gut and in Hirschsprung disease. *Pediatr. Surg. Int.* **2013**, *29*, 889–897. [CrossRef]
10. Lee, J.C.; Thuneberg, L.; Berezin, I.; Huizinga, J.D. Generation of slow waves in membrane potential is an intrinsic property of interstitial cells of Cajal. *Am. J. Physiol.* **1999**, *277*, G409–G423. [CrossRef]
11. Iino, S.; Horiguchi, K. Interstitial cells of cajal are involved in neurotransmission in the gastrointestinal tract. *Acta Histochem. Cytochem.* **2006**, *39*, 145–153. [CrossRef]
12. Young, H.M. Embryological origin of interstitial cells of Cajal. *Microsc. Res. Tech.* **1999**, *47*, 303–308. [CrossRef]
13. Roberts, D.J. Molecular mechanisms of development of the gastrointestinal tract. *Dev. Dyn.* **2000**, *219*, 109–120. [CrossRef]
14. Burns, A.J.; Le Douarin, N.M. Enteric nervous system development: Analysis of the selective developmental potentialities of vagal and sacral neural crest cells using quail-chick chimeras. *Anat. Rec.* **2001**, *262*, 16–28. [CrossRef]
15. Lecoin, L.; Gabella, G.; Le Douarin, N. Origin of the c-kit-positive interstitial cells in the avian bowel. *Development* **1996**, *122*, 725–733. [CrossRef]
16. Young, H.M.; Ciampoli, D.; Southwell, B.R.; Newgreen, D.F. Origin of interstitial cells of Cajal in the mouse intestine. *Dev. Biol.* **1996**, *180*, 97–107. [CrossRef]
17. Torihashi, S.; Ward, S.M.; Sanders, K.M. Development of c-Kit-positive cells and the onset of electrical rhythmicity in murine small intestine. *Gastroenterology* **1997**, *112*, 144–155. [CrossRef]
18. Faussone-Pellegrini, M.S.; Thuneberg, L. Guide to the identification of interstitial cells of Cajal. *Microsc. Res. Tech.* **1999**, *47*, 248–266. [CrossRef]

19. Torihashi, S.; Horisawa, M.; Watanabe, Y. c-Kit immunoreactive interstitial cells in the human gastrointestinal tract. *J. Auton. Nerv. Syst.* **1999**, *75*, 38–50. [CrossRef]
20. Faussone-Pellegrini, M.S.; Cortesini, C. Ultrastructural features and localization of the interstitial cells of Cajal in the smooth muscle coat of human esophagus. *J. Submicrosc. Cytol.* **1985**, *17*, 187–197.
21. Hagger, R.; Gharaie, S.; Finlayson, C.; Kumar, D. Distribution of the interstitial cells of Cajal in the human anorectum. *J. Auton. Nerv. Syst.* **1998**, *73*, 75–79. [CrossRef]
22. Komuro, T. Structure and organization of interstitial cells of Cajal in the gastrointestinal tract. *J. Physiol.* **2006**, *576*, 653–658. [CrossRef]
23. Alaburda, P.; Lukosiene, J.I.; Pauza, A.G.; Kyguoliene, K.R. Ultrastructural changes of the human enteric nervous system and interstitial cells of Cajal in diverticular disease. *Histol. Histopathol.* **2020**, *35*, 18136.
24. Zhou, J.; O'Connor, M.D.; Ho, V. The Potential for Gut Organoid Derived Interstitial Cells of Cajal in Replacement Therapy. *Int. J. Mol. Sci.* **2017**, *18*, 2059. [CrossRef]
25. Kwon, J.G.; Hwang, S.J.; Hennig, G.W.; Bayguinov, Y.; McCann, C.; Chen, H.; Rossi, F.; Besmer, P.; Sanders, K.M.; Ward, S.M. Changes in the structure and function of ICC networks in ICC hyperplasia and gastrointestinal stromal tumors. *Gastroenterology* **2009**, *136*, 630–639. [CrossRef]
26. Christensen, J.; Rick, G.A.; Lowe, L.S. Distributions of interstitial cells of Cajal in stomach and colon of cat, dog, ferret, opossum, rat, guinea pig and rabbit. *J. Auton. Nerv. Syst.* **1992**, *37*, 47–56. [CrossRef]
27. Vannucchi, M.G.; Zardo, C.; Corsani, L.; Faussone-Pellegrini, M.S. Interstitial cells of Cajal, enteric neurons, and smooth muscle and myoid cells of the murine gastrointestinal tract express full-length dystrophin. *Histochem. Cell Biol.* **2002**, *118*, 449–457. [CrossRef]
28. Mazur, M.T.; Clark, H.B. Gastric stromal tumors. Reappraisal of histogenesis. *Am. J. Surg. Pathol.* **1983**, *7*, 507–519. [CrossRef]
29. Herrera, G.A.; De Moraes, H.P.; Grizzle, W.E.; Han, S.G. Malignant small bowel neoplasm of enteric plexus derivation (plexosarcoma). Light and electron microscopic study confirming the origin of the neoplasm. *Dig. Dis. Sci.* **1984**, *29*, 275–284. [CrossRef]
30. Min, K.W. Small intestinal stromal tumors with skeinoid fibers. Clinicopathological, immunohistochemical, and ultrastructural investigations. *Am. J. Surg. Pathol.* **1992**, *16*, 145–155. [CrossRef]
31. da Silva Meirelles, L.; Chagastelles, P.C.; Nardi, N.B. Mesenchymal stem cells reside in virtually all post-natal organs and tissues. *J. Cell Sci.* **2006**, *119*, 2204–2213. [CrossRef]
32. Negreanu, L.M.; Assor, P.; Mateescu, B.; Cirstoiu, C. Interstitial cells of Cajal in the gut–a gastroenterologist's point of view. *World J. Gastroenterol.* **2008**, *14*, 6285–6288. [CrossRef]
33. Park, S.H.; Kim, M.K.; Kim, H.; Song, B.J.; Chi, J.G. Ultrastructural studies of gastrointestinal stromal tumors. *J. Korean Med. Sci.* **2004**, *19*, 234–244. [CrossRef]
34. Komuro, T. Comparative morphology of interstitial cells of Cajal: Ultrastructural characterization. *Microsc. Res. Tech.* **1999**, *47*, 267–285. [CrossRef]
35. Vij, M.; Agrawal, V.; Kumar, A.; Pandey, R. Cytomorphology of gastrointestinal stromal tumors and extra-gastrointestinal stromal tumors: A comprehensive morphologic study. *J. Cytol.* **2013**, *30*, 8–12. [CrossRef]
36. Nakayama, H.; Enzan, H.; Miyazaki, E.; Kuroda, N.; Naruse, K.; Hiroi, M. Differential expression of CD34 in normal colorectal tissue, peritumoral inflammatory tissue, and tumour stroma. *J. Clin. Pathol.* **2000**, *53*, 626–629. [CrossRef]
37. Schaefer, I.M.; Marino-Enriquez, A.; Fletcher, J.A. What is New in Gastrointestinal Stromal Tumor? *Adv. Anat. Pathol.* **2017**, *24*, 259–267. [CrossRef]
38. Streutker, C.J.; Huizinga, J.D.; Driman, D.K.; Riddell, R.H. Interstitial cells of Cajal in health and disease. Part I: Normal ICC structure and function with associated motility disorders. *Histopathology* **2007**, *50*, 176–189. [CrossRef]

Disclaimer/Publisher's Note: The statements, opinions and data contained in all publications are solely those of the individual author(s) and contributor(s) and not of MDPI and/or the editor(s). MDPI and/or the editor(s) disclaim responsibility for any injury to people or property resulting from any ideas, methods, instructions or products referred to in the content.

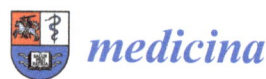
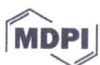

Systematic Review

Assessing the Predictive Power of the Hemoglobin/Red Cell Distribution Width Ratio in Cancer: A Systematic Review and Future Directions

Donatella Coradduzza [1], Serenella Medici [2], Carla Chessa [3], Angelo Zinellu [1], Massimo Madonia [3], Andrea Angius [4], Ciriaco Carru [1,5,*] and Maria Rosaria De Miglio [3,*]

1. Department of Biomedical Sciences, University of Sassari, 07100 Sassari, Italy; dcoradduzza@uniss.it (D.C.); azinellu@uniss.it (A.Z.)
2. Department of Chemical, Physical, Mathematical and Natural Sciences, University of Sassari, 07100 Sassari, Italy; sere@uniss.it
3. Department of Medicine, Surgery and Pharmacy, University of Sassari, 07100 Sassari, Italy; c.chessa17@studenti.uniss.it (C.C.); madonia@uniss.it (M.M.)
4. Istituto di Ricerca Genetica e Biomedica (IRGB), Consiglio Nazionale delle Ricerche (CNR), Cittadella Universitaria di Cagliari, 09042 Cagliari, Italy; andrea.angius@irgb.cnr.it
5. Control Quality Unit, Azienda-Ospedaliera Universitaria (AOU), 07100 Sassari, Italy
* Correspondence: carru@uniss.it (C.C.); demiglio@uniss.it (M.R.D.M.)

Abstract: *Background and Objectives*: The hemoglobin (Hb)/red cell distribution width (RDW) ratio has emerged as an accessible, repeatable, and inexpensive prognostic factor that may predict survival in cancer patients. The focus of this systematic review is to investigate the prognostic role of the Hb/RDW ratio in cancer and the implications for clinical practice. *Materials and Methods*: A literature search of PubMed, Scopus, and Web of Science databases was performed by an independent author between 18 March and 30 March 2023 to collect relevant literature that assessed the prognostic value of the Hb/RDW ratio in cancer. Overall survival (OS), progression-free survival (PFS), and the association of these with the Hb/RDW ratio were considered to be the main endpoints. *Results*: Thirteen retrospective studies, including 3818 cancer patients, were identified and involved in this review. It was observed that, when patients with a high vs. low Hb/RDW ratio were compared, those with a lower Hb/RDW ratio had significantly poorer outcomes ($p < 0.05$). In lung cancer patients, a one-unit increase in the Hb/RDW ratio reduces mortality by 1.6 times, whilst in esophageal squamous-cell carcinoma patients, a lower Hb/RDW ratio results in a 1.416-times greater risk of mortality. *Conclusions*: A low Hb/RDW ratio was associated with poor OS and disease progression in patients with cancer. This blood parameter should be considered a standard biomarker in clinical practice for predicting OS and PFS in cancer patients. Future searches will be necessary to determine and standardize the Hb/RDW cut-off value and to assess whether the Hb/RDW ratio is optimal as an independent prognostic factor or if it requires incorporation into risk assessment models for predicting outcomes in cancer patients.

Keywords: hemoglobin to red cell distribution width; Hb/RDW ratio; cancer; risk assessment

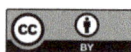

1. Introduction

Cancer poses a significant global health challenge, accounting for substantial morbidity and mortality, with 19.3 million new cases and 10 million deaths reported worldwide in 2020 [1]. There is a high prevalence of cancers such as female breast cancer, lung cancer, and colorectal cancer, influenced by factors like lifestyle, environment, and screening practices. Notably, breast cancer has become the most-diagnosed cancer globally, and thyroid cancer rates have surged due to overdiagnosis [2,3]. While developed countries exhibit higher cancer incidence rates, mortality rates vary less. Globally, prostate cancer is frequently diagnosed, with the highest rates in specific regions, but mortality rates for breast and cervical cancers are notably higher in developing countries due to lifestyle, environmental, and healthcare disparities [4–9]. The global cancer burden is projected to increase by 47% from 2020 to 2040, with a more substantial increase in developing countries [10]. This growth is fueled by demographic changes and increasing risk factors associated with globalization and economic growth [11]. Addressing this challenge necessitates the establishment of sustainable infrastructure for cancer prevention and care in developing countries [12]. Tailored interventions can reduce the future cancer burden and bridge disparities between developing and developed nations [13]. Public health policies should prioritize building such infrastructure to mitigate the growing cancer challenge [12].

In this context, the development of novel tools is critical and must emphasize clinical applications and translational research [14–16].

An augmented red cell distribution width (RDW) serves as a crucial measure, indicating the variability in red blood cell (RBC) size. The RDW, expressed as a percentage in the complete blood count, aids in the diagnosis and monitoring of various medical conditions [17].

An elevated RDW often indicates a mix of large and small red blood cells, signifying diverse potential causes for anemia. Scientific interest in the clinical utility of the RDW has been observed in specific disease states, such as obstructive sleep apnea syndrome (OSAS), chronic obstructive pulmonary disease (COPD), immune disorders, surgical procedures, retinal artery occlusion, and even COVID-19 [18–20].

The clinical relevance of the RDW extends beyond anemia, demonstrating significance for various disease states, including OSAS, COPD, immune disorders, surgical procedures, retinal artery occlusion, and even COVID-19 [21]. Conditions such as iron, vitamin B12, and folate deficiencies contribute to alterations in the RDW by impacting the production and size of RBCs [22]. Additionally, hemoglobinopathies like thalassemia and chronic inflammatory conditions such as rheumatoid arthritis and lupus are associated with an elevated RDW [21,23]. Diseases affecting the bone marrow, including myelodysplastic syndromes and leukemia, further influence the production of RBCs, which is reflected in the RDW. Moreover, the RDW emerges as a potential biomarker in cardiovascular diseases, linking an increased RDW to a higher risk of adverse cardiovascular events [24]. It is crucial to emphasize that while the RDW is valuable, its interpretation is most effective when considered in conjunction with other clinical and laboratory parameters [9,25–31]. This comprehensive evaluation is vital for informed clinical decision making. Its proposed role as a biomarker extends to certain cancers, potentially indicating larger tumors and advanced cancer stages.

Similarly, hemoglobin (Hb) levels have historically been indicators of a patient's tolerance to treatment. Changes in Hb levels can influence decisions about the intensity and duration of therapy. Low Hb levels may indicate malnutrition, such as anemia, which potentially indicates a low tolerance to treatment [24,25]. Substantial evidence suggests that anemia before treatment may predict poor outcomes in cancer patients, including nasopharyngeal carcinoma, head and neck cancer, cervical cancer [26–30], and colorectal cancer [32]. Hb levels play a crucial role in diagnosing and monitoring various medical conditions. In anemia diagnosis, Hb levels are a primary indicator, suggesting the reduced blood oxygen-carrying capacity that is characteristic of various types of anemia [29,30]. Hb levels can reflect nutritional deficiencies, especially iron-deficiency anemia. Insufficient iron intake can lead to decreased Hb production, affecting overall health [28].

Hb levels are monitored to assess blood loss, either due to acute events like trauma or due to chronic conditions such as gastrointestinal bleeding. Certain chronic diseases, such as chronic kidney disease, can impact Hb levels, necessitating monitoring for effective management [29]. Hb is essential for transporting oxygen throughout the body, and abnormal Hb levels may indicate issues with oxygen delivery, affecting overall tissue and organ function. Various blood disorders, including sickle cell anemia and thalassemia, which are characterized by an abnormal Hb structure or production, can be diagnosed and managed through monitoring Hb levels [30]. Hb is linked to cardiovascular health, and abnormal levels may be associated with conditions such as heart failure and COPD [33]. In pregnant women, monitoring Hb levels is essential to detect and manage conditions like iron-deficiency anemia, which impacts both maternal and fetal health [34]. Hb levels are monitored postoperatively to assess blood loss during surgery and to guide transfusion decisions if necessary [35]. In summary, Hb levels are a versatile marker used in the diagnosis and the monitoring of various medical conditions, providing valuable insights into overall health, nutritional status, blood disorders, and treatment tolerance [36].

The relationship between the RDW and Hb levels in the context of cancer is intricately influenced by various non-neoplastic factors. These include deficiencies in essential nutrients, such as iron, vitamin B12, and folate [37]. Additionally, chronic inflammatory conditions, such as rheumatoid arthritis, systemic lupus erythematosus, and inflammatory bowel diseases, can exert an impact on both the RDW and Hb levels [38]. Certain chronic diseases, including chronic kidney disease and COPD, contribute to alterations in the RDW and Hb. Conditions leading to the increased destruction of red blood cells (hemolysis) can significantly influence both the RDW and Hb levels. Moreover, impaired kidney function has repercussions on erythropoiesis, manifesting as changes in the RDW and Hb. Diseases affecting the bone marrow, such as myelodysplastic syndromes and leukemia, play a role in shaping the production and maturation of red blood cells, thereby affecting the RDW and Hb [39]. Furthermore, specific drugs and medications may impact the production and survival of RBCs, exerting an influence on the RDW and Hb [40]. Inherited conditions, like thalassemia and sickle cell anemia, contribute to variations in both the RDW and Hb [41]. Disorders influencing the structure or synthesis of hemoglobin, such as thalassemia, can similarly impact both the RDW and Hb.

In the realm of cancer research, the Hb/RDW ratio emerges as a pivotal biomarker that was initially proposed as a prognostic indicator in esophageal squamous-cell carcinoma (ESCC) [23] and subsequently applied across diverse cancer types [34,42,43]. Demonstrating its utility as an independent prognostic factor, the Hb/RDW ratio significantly influences both overall survival (OS) and disease-free survival.

This ratio provides valuable insights into RBCs' size distribution and oxygen-carrying capacity, which are essential aspects influenced by cancer-related factors. As cancer often induces alterations in blood parameters, the Hb/RDW ratio gains particular significance [43,44]. Changes in the RDW and Hb levels, influenced by factors like inflammation, nutritional deficiencies, or bone marrow disorders, directly impact the Hb/RDW ratio. Monitoring this ratio over time becomes crucial for gaining valuable information on cancer progression and prognosis, establishing itself as a promising tool in cancer prognosis research. The Hb/RDW ratio acts as a composite measure, offering a comprehensive perspective on RBCs' distribution and oxygen-carrying capacity, which are both critical elements that are affected by various cancer-related factors.

The Hb/RDW ratio has been investigated in various cancer types, demonstrating its correlation with tumor characteristics and progression. In hepatocellular carcinoma (HCC), the Hb/RDW ratio was identified as a significant factor influencing progression-free survival (PFS) and OS [45]. Studies in hematologic cancers revealed a significantly higher Hb/RDW ratio in patients with endometrial carcinoma and primary HCC, which was associated with poor survival outcomes [46,47].

Cancer-related physiological changes play a substantial role in influencing the Hb/RDW ratio [48]. The systemic nature of cancer induces physiological stress, triggering changes in blood parameters such as the RDW and Hb, subsequently affecting the Hb/RDW ratio [49]. Chronic inflammation, a common response to cancer, impacts both the RDW and Hb levels, contributing to alterations in the Hb/RDW ratio [50]. Conditions often associated with cancer, such as deficiencies in iron, vitamin B12, and folate, can impact the production and size of RBCs, further affecting the Hb/RDW ratio [17]. Tumors affecting the bone marrow, as seen in myelodysplastic syndromes and leukemia, can disrupt the normal production of RBCs, manifesting as changes in the RDW and Hb levels, ultimately influencing the Hb/RDW ratio [51].

Furthermore, advanced tumor stages and larger tumor sizes have been linked to changes in the RDW, offering insights into tumor characteristics and progression [52]. Therapies like chemotherapy and radiation, which directly affect bone marrow and the production of RBCs, contribute to the composite nature of the Hb/RDW ratio, making it a valuable indicator of a patient's overall condition [53,54].

This systematic review aims to comprehensively explore the prognostic value of the Hb/RDW ratio in cancer, shedding light on its implications for clinical practice. Figure 1 provides a visual representation of the key components and relationships discussed in this review.

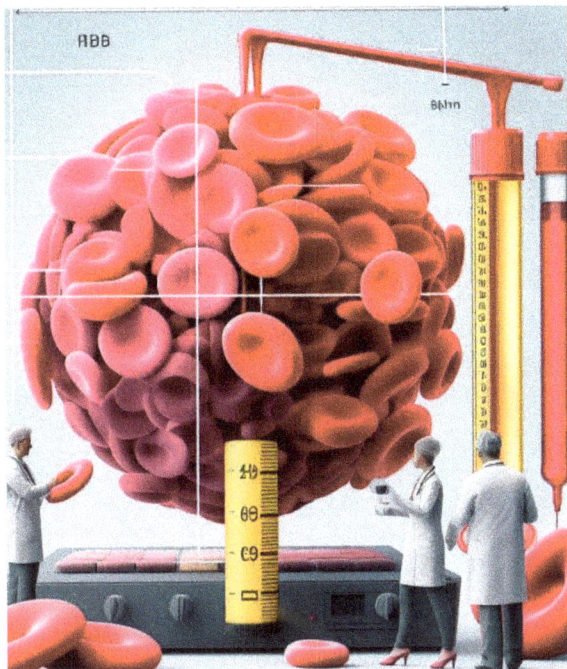

Figure 1. Critical role of hemoglobin (Hb)/Red Cell Distribution Width (RDW) ratios in utilizing blood cell data for diagnostic and prognostic purposes. Hb levels and RDW are fundamental parameters analyzed from blood samples, and their ratio (Hb/RDW) serves as a valuable metric in clinical assessment.

2. Materials and Methods

2.1. Search Strategy and Selection Criteria

This systematic review adheres to the PRISMA guidelines and aligns with the Grades of Recommendation, Assessment, Development, and Evaluation (GRADE) criteria [45,47,55]. From 18 March to 30 March 2023, the authors conducted a comprehensive search on the PubMed, Scopus, and Web of Science databases. Utilizing keywords such as "Hb/RDW", "hemoglobin to red cell distribution width", "HRR", "hemoglobin", "red cell distribution width", "cancer", "prognosis", "prognostic value", "overall survival", "progression-free survival", and "event-free survival", the search aimed to refine the scope of the literature.

Inclusion criteria involved the exploration and reporting of the Hb/RDW ratio's value in cancer patients. Literature was excluded if it fell into categories such as review articles, pre-2013 publications, or non-English language articles. Additional relevant material was sought by screening the reference lists of the identified literature and previous review articles.

The exclusion criteria were carefully applied, encompassing materials like abstracts, letters, reviews, case reports, etc. Studies with insufficient data for comprehensive analysis were omitted. Research lacking specific data regarding hematologic malignancies or the RDW was excluded. In cases where multiple publications originated from the same cohort, only the most recent report was included for our meta-analysis.

2.2. Data Collection and Quality Assessment

The literature satisfying our eligibility criteria and incorporated into this review underwent data extraction by the authors. The key data points comprised details of the study (author and date), the study design, the total number of patients, their cancer diagnoses, the specific outcomes measured, and the study results. The assessment of the literature incorporated in this review aligned with the GRADE criteria, which assesses the quality of evidence and provides recommendations for use [45]. These criteria encompass the quality of the methodology, the directness of evidence, heterogeneity, the precision of effect estimates, and the potential for publication bias. This resulted in assigning a level of evidence and recommendation for use, categorized as high, moderate, or low.

3. Results

3.1. Literature Search and Study Characteristics

The search revealed 421 papers, with 213 duplicates among them. Following the assessment of titles and abstracts from the remaining 208 papers, 72 full texts underwent review. In total, 13 studies met the specified criteria, and no further literature was identified in the references of the incorporated studies or by the reviewer team (Figure 2). All studies integrated in this systematic review and meta-analysis followed a retrospective design, in alignment with the inclusion criteria depicted in the methodology. The number of patients investigated ranged from 80 to 840, with a total of 3818 patients included across all 13 studies. The value of the Hb/RDW ratio as a prognostic measure was evaluated in lung cancer, upper tract urothelial carcinoma, esophageal carcinoma, renal cell cancer, bladder cancer, gastric carcinoma, lymphoma, head and neck cancer, breast cancer, and nasopharyngeal cancer. The comprehensive data extraction is described in Table 1.

Table 1. Data extraction and baseline characteristics of the identified literature.

Reference	Author (Year)	Study Design	Patient Population	Outcome Measures	Results
[56]	Su et al. (2021)	Retrospective	730 patients with upper tract urothelial carcinoma	Clinicopathological measures compared with Hb/RDW ratio	Patients with an Hb/RDW ratio below 1.05 showed a poorer renal function, tumor with high pathological stage, and high grade.
[57]	Figen et al. (2023)	Retrospective	840 patients with small-cell lung cancer	OS PFS RDW and Hb and associated ratios	A one-unit increase in Hb/RDW ratio reduced mortality and increased survival by 1.6 times.
[58]	Petrella et al. (2021)	Retrospective	342 patients with lung adenocarcinoma operated in the last two years	Preoperative Hb/RDW, Pathological stage Disease characteristics	DFS had an increased HR of relapse for preoperative Hb/RDW ratio lower than 1.01 ($p < 0.004$).
[59]	Sun et al. (2016)	Retrospective	362 patients ESCC patients	Hb/RDW ratio, OS, 5-year OS	Patients with a lower Hb/RDW ratio showed a 1.416 times greater risk of dying through the follow-up compared to healthy patients.

Table 1. Cont.

Reference	Author (Year)	Study Design	Patient Population	Outcome Measures	Results
[60]	Yilmaz et al. (2021)	Retrospective	198 patients with RCC	Hb/RDW ratio, systemic immune-inflammation index, LMR, NLR, OS, PFS	Hb/RDW ratio is an independent prognostic factor for predicting PFS and OS in RCC patients.
[61]	Zhao et al. (2022)	Retrospective	80 patients with pulmonary large-cell neuroendocrine carcinoma	Hb/RDW ratio, characteristics, risk factors for OS	Patients with low Hb/RDW ratio exhibited a poorer OS than those with a high ratio ($p < 0.001$).
[62]	Yilmaz et al. (2020)	Retrospective	152 patients with muscle-invasive bladder cancer	Hb/RDW ratio, systemic immune-inflammation index, LMR, NLR, OS, PFS	Hb/RDW ratio is an independent prognostic factor for PFS and OS in patients with muscle-invasive bladder cancer
[63]	Yilmaz et al. (2020)	Retrospective	85 patients with gastric cancer who were treated with neoadjuvant FLOT	Hb/RDW ratio, DFS, PFS, NLR, systemic immune-inflammation index	Hb/RDW ratio was an independent prognostic factor for DFS and OS ($p = 0.001$ and $p = 0.037$, respectively); higher Hb/RDW was associated with better DFS and OS in gastric cancer.
[64]	Dong et al. (2022)	Retrospective	265 patients with DLBCL	Hb/RDW ratio, OS, PFS	Hb/RDW ratio is an independent prognostic factor for OS ($p < 0.001$) and PFS ($p < 0.001$) in DLBCL patients.
[65]	Tham et al. (2018)	Retrospective	205 patients with head and neck cancer	Hb/RDW ratio, EFS, OS	Multivariate analysis identified as independent prognostic factors associated with EFS: BMI ($p = 0.0364$), advanced T stage ($p = 0.001$), and low Hb/RDW ratio ($p = 0.017$). Hb/RDW was not associated with OS.
[66]	Bozkaya et al. (2019)	Retrospective	153 patients with NSCLC	Hb/RDW ratio, Glasgow prognostic scores, NLR, OS, PFS	Low Hb/RDW was an independent prognostic factor for OS ($p = 0.03$) and PFS ($p < 0.001$) in advanced NSCLC.
[67]	Zhang et al. (2022)	Retrospective	226 patients with breast cancer	Hb/RDW ratio, PLR, monocyte to high-density lipoprotein ratio, risk of breast cancer	Hb/RDW and monocyte to high-density lipoprotein ratio were independent prognostic factors for breast cancer ($p < 0.001$). Low Hb/RDW was linked with prolonged hospitalization, higher RDW, and lower Hb levels ($p < 0.05$).
[68]	Lin et al. (2021)	Retrospective	180 patients with NPC	Hb/RDW ratio, NLR and PLR for the diagnosis of nasopharyngeal cancer	NLR and PLR were notably higher in NPC patients than in healthy subjects ($p < 0.001$). Hb/RDW ratio was extensively lower in NPC patients than in healthy subjects ($p < 0.001$).

Hb: hemoglobin; RDW: red cell distribution width; OS: overall survival; PFS: progression-free survival; DFS: disease-free survival; HR: hazard ratio; ESCC: esophageal squamous-cell carcinoma; RCC: renal cell cancer; LMR: lymphocyte-to-monocyte ratio; NLR: neutrophil-to-lymphocyte ratio; FLOT: fluorouracil, leucovorin, oxaliplatin, docetaxel; DLBCL: diffuse large b-cell lymphoma; EFS: event-free survival; BMI: body mass index; NSCLC: non-small-cell lung cancer; PLR: platelet-to-lymphocyte ratio; NPC: nasopharyngeal cancer.

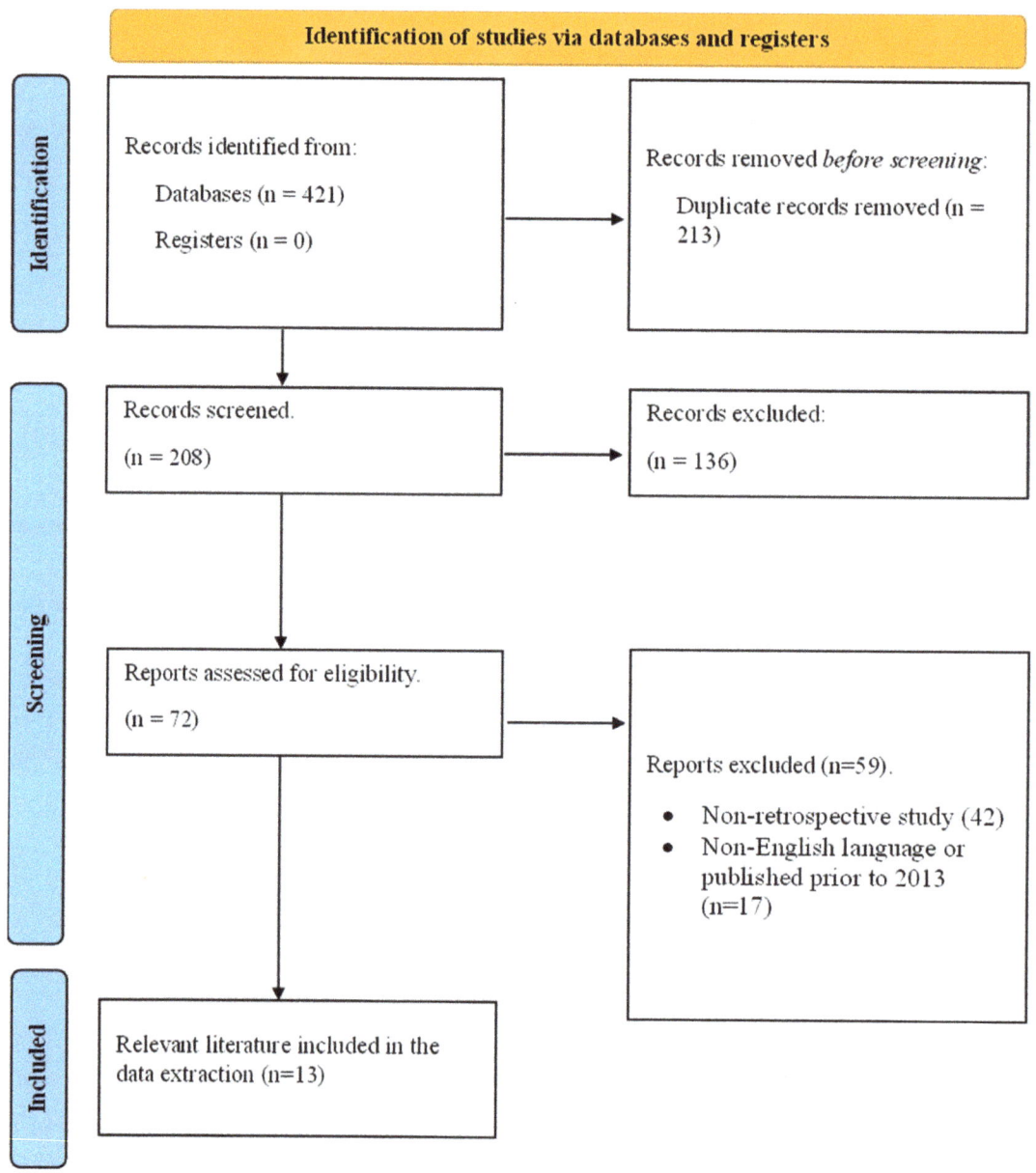

Figure 2. PRISMA flow diagram representing the literature search and study selection process.

3.2. Prognostic Value of Hb/RDW

All included literature reported a significant association between the Hb/RDW and prognostic outcomes of patients with cancer, including OS, PFS, and EFS ($p < 0.05$ to $p < 0.001$). In patients with small-cell lung cancer, a one-unit increase in the Hb/RDW ratio reduced death and increased survival by 1.6 times and had a statistically significant effect on OS and PFS [69,70]. Similarly, in patients with esophageal cancer, a lower Hb/RDW ratio was associated with a 1.416-times greater risk of mortality through the follow-up [71]. These associations were observed across all included cancer types aside from head and neck carcinoma. However, Tham et al. reported that the Hb/RDW ratio was independently related to event-free survival (EFS, $p = 0.017$) [42,43,72–75].

3.3. Other Outcomes

Beyond the association of the Hb/RDW ratio with primary parameters of survival, the identified literature also reported the prognostic value of the Hb/RDW ratio for predicting renal function and pathological staging in upper tract urothelial carcinoma patients. In these patients, a Hb/RDW ratio below 1.05 was related to a poorer renal function, and a tumor with a high pathological stage and grade [76]. It was observed in one study that a low Hb/RDW was linked with prolonged hospitalization, a higher RDW, and lower Hb levels ($p < 0.05$) [53,77–79].

3.4. Risk of Bias and Quality of Evidence

The assessment of the included studies' risk of bias and the quality of evidence has been crucial for interpreting the findings and making informed conclusions. In this systematic review, the retrospective nature of the included literature presents inherent limitations in the study design, primarily in terms of selection and recall biases, as described by Talari et al. [80], Table 2.

Table 2. GRADE criteria for risk-of-bias evaluation. Green: No Risk of Bias; Yellow: Low or Maybe Risk of Bias; Red: High Risk of Bias.

Reference	Author (Year)	Methodological Quality	Directness of Evidence	Heterogeneity	Precision of Effect Estimates	Publication Bias	Overall Quality of Evidence
[56]	Su et al. (2021)	Yellow	Yellow	Yellow	Green	Yellow	Yellow
[57]	Figen et al. (2023)	Green	Yellow	Yellow	Yellow	Red	Yellow
[58]	Petrella et al. (2021)	Green	Yellow	Yellow	Yellow	Yellow	Yellow
[59]	Sun et al. (2016)	Yellow	Green	Red	Yellow	Red	Yellow
[60]	Yilmaz et al. (2021)	Yellow	Green	Yellow	Yellow	Red	Yellow
[61]	Zhao et al. (2022)	Yellow	Yellow	Yellow	Yellow	Yellow	Yellow
[62]	Yilmaz et al. (2020)	Yellow	Yellow	Yellow	Yellow	Yellow	Yellow
[63]	Yilmaz et al. (2020)	Yellow	Green	Yellow	Yellow	Yellow	Yellow
[64]	Dong et al. (2022)	Yellow	Yellow	Yellow	Yellow	Yellow	Yellow
[65]	Tham et al. (2018)	Yellow	Green	Yellow	Yellow	Yellow	Yellow
[66]	Bozkaya et al. (2019)	Yellow	Yellow	Yellow	Green	Yellow	Yellow
[67]	Zhang et al. (2022)	Yellow	Yellow	Yellow	Yellow	Yellow	Yellow
[68]	Lin et al. (2021)	Yellow	Yellow	Yellow	Yellow	Yellow	Yellow

Risk of Bias:

All the studies included in this systematic review followed a retrospective design, aligning with the predefined inclusion criteria. However, retrospective studies inherently carry risks of bias, particularly in terms of patient selection, data collection, and potential recall biases. The absence of a prospective approach limits the ability to control for confounding variables and may impact the robustness of the findings. Moreover, the inclusion of only retrospective studies may introduce a selection bias, as certain relevant data from prospective studies might have been excluded.

Quality of Evidence:

The GRADE evaluation encompasses considerations such as the methodological quality, the directness of the evidence, heterogeneity, the precision of effect estimates, and the risk of publication bias. All studies included in the review followed a retrospective design, but, as per the GRADE criteria, retrospective studies are considered lower in methodological quality compared to prospective ones. This limitation is acknowledged in the risk-of-bias assessment. The evidence directly addresses the prognostic value of the Hb/RDW ratio in various cancers, aligning with the research question. However, the retrospective nature of the studies may have impacted the directness of the evidence due to potential biases and confounding factors. Moreover, the included studies cover a diverse range of cancer types, which may contribute to heterogeneity in the findings. Heterogeneity can affect the generalizability of the results and should be considered in the interpretation.

The precision of effect estimates relies on the consistency and accuracy of the data. The retrospective design and potential biases may have impacted the precision of the effect estimates, and this limitation is reflected in the risk-of-bias assessment.

4. Discussion

This systematic review delves into the prognostic significance of the Hb/RDW ratio in cancer, aiming to shed light on its potential implications for clinical practice. The Hb/RDW ratio emerges from the literature and our findings as an accessible, repeatable, and cost-effective prognostic factor that is capable of predicting survival across various cancer types [23,29,81].

Our results consolidate evidence demonstrating the substantial prognostic value of the Hb/RDW ratio in lung, breast, gastric, esophageal, and lymphoma cancers [82]. The overarching trend establishes a correlation between a low Hb/RDW ratio and poorer OS, PFS, and EFS compared to cases with a higher ratio. This association is not only consistent but also notably significant in specific cancer subtypes, such as ESCC and pulmonary large-cell neuroendocrine carcinoma [16,30].

Moreover, the Hb/RDW ratio demonstrates its predictive capabilities post-treatment, as observed in gastric cancer patients treated with neo-adjuvant fluorouracil, leucovorin, oxaliplatin, and docetaxel (FLOT) [32]. These findings advocate for the broad clinical applications of the Hb/RDW ratio in cancer, warranting further exploration of its potential as a reliable prognostic marker.

In the era of advanced technologies like genomics, proteomics, and imaging, the financial implications of biomarker screening programs are well-documented [83]. Our study underscores the cost-effectiveness of the Hb/RDW ratio, positioning it as a practical and valuable screening tool for cancer. The observations of Toumazis et al. on the limited cost-effectiveness of biomarkers costing USD 750 or more highlight the pragmatic appeal of the Hb/RDW ratio, easily obtained from routine complete blood cell counts [41,42].

While the primary focus of this systematic review is the prognostic value of the Hb/RDW ratio, its diagnostic potential in cancer patients is noteworthy. The findings of Lin et al. on its utility in the auxiliary diagnosis of nasopharyngeal cancer, especially when combined with other ratios like the neutrophil-to-lymphocyte ratio or the platelet-to-lymphocyte ratio (PLR), extend its clinical relevance beyond prognosis [37]. Zhai et al.'s proposed combination of the Hb/RDW ratio with platelet/lymphocyte ratios (HP + PLR) further validates its efficacy as a simple and reliable prognostic marker, surpassing alternative indicators [43,44].

However, it is imperative to consider certain exclusions for the Hb/RDW ratio to maintain its prognostic value. Chronic inflammatory and autoimmune diseases must be ruled out, as emphasized by Su et al. [27]. Additional factors, including white blood cell count and platelet count, should be factored into the assessment, particularly in upper tract urothelial cancer patients.

Transitioning to the physiological underpinnings, the Hb/RDW ratio becomes a dynamic parameter reflecting changes during cancer development. The increased production of red blood cells, stimulated by tumor-induced metabolic demands and cytokines/growth factors, offers mechanistic insights. The nuanced relationship between cancer cells' higher rate of cell division, the cytokine-induced production of RBCs, and the body's response to cancer-induced anemia contributes to the variability in the Hb/RDW ratio.

The co-analysis of Hb and the RDW underscores their roles as crucial physiological markers during cancer progression and treatment. Hemoglobin's susceptibility to decreasing due to chemotherapy-induced anemia and due to direct effects on the bone marrow positions it as a prognostic marker, especially in head and neck cancer. The association of the RDW with adverse prognostic factors in hematological lymphoma signifies its potential inclusion in prognostic scores for HL, given its simplicity, affordability, and easy availability [84].

In conclusion, the Hb/RDW ratio emerges as a promising, cost-effective, and easily accessible prognostic and diagnostic tool in cancer. Its versatility across cancer types, coupled with its mechanistic insights into physiological changes, warrants further exploration and validation in prospective studies. The limitations, particularly the retrospective nature of the included literature, advocate for future large-scale, multicenter prospective studies to standardize the Hb/RDW cut-off values and solidify its prognostic value.

5. Conclusions

In conclusion, this systematic review explores the prognostic significance of the Hb/RDW ratio in various cancers, shedding light on its potential implications for clinical practice. The global cancer burden is on the rise, necessitating innovative approaches to diagnosis, monitoring, and prognosis. As established in the introduction, cancer is a complex and multifaceted challenge influenced by various factors, including lifestyle, environment, and screening practices.

The review emphasizes the critical role of Hb and the RDW in cancer prognosis, with a focus on their dynamic interplay in the Hb/RDW ratio. An elevated RDW and altered Hb levels can serve as indicators of diverse medical conditions, ranging from nutritional deficiencies to chronic diseases and cancers. The systematic literature search and the meta-analysis, conducted in accordance with established guidelines, reveal a significant association between the Hb/RDW ratio and prognostic outcomes in various cancer types.

The findings underscore the versatility of the Hb/RDW ratio as a prognostic marker, demonstrating its value in predicting OS, PFS, and EFS. Notably, the association holds across different cancer subtypes, indicating the potential broad clinical applicability of this ratio.

Moreover, this review addresses the cost-effectiveness of the Hb/RDW ratio as a screening tool, contrasting it with more expensive biomarkers. The simplicity and the accessibility of the Hb/RDW ratio, derived from routine complete blood cell counts, position it as a practical and valuable option for cancer prognosis.

While focusing primarily on prognosis, this review also acknowledges the diagnostic potential of the Hb/RDW ratio, especially when combined with other ratios or parameters. The physiological underpinnings of the ratio are explored, highlighting its dynamic nature reflecting changes during cancer development.

Despite the compelling findings, this review acknowledges the limitations inherent in the retrospective nature of the included studies. To address this, we call for future large-scale, multicenter prospective studies, aiming to standardize the Hb/RDW cut-off values and to solidify its prognostic value across different cancer contexts.

In summary, the Hb/RDW ratio emerges from this review as a promising, cost-effective, and easily accessible prognostic and diagnostic tool in cancer. Its versatility, coupled with mechanistic insights into physiological changes, warrants further exploration and validation in prospective studies, offering a potential breakthrough in the landscape of cancer prognosis and patient management.

Author Contributions: Conceptualization, D.C. and S.M.; methodology, D.C. and S.M.; software, D.C., A.Z. and C.C. (Carla Chessa); formal analysis, D.C., A.Z. and C.C. (Carla Chessa); investigation, D.C. and S.M.; resources, M.R.D.M. and C.C. (Ciriaco Carru); writing—original draft preparation, D.C. and S.M.; writing—review and editing, M.R.D.M., S.M. and C.C. (Ciriaco Carru); supervision, C.C. (Ciriaco Carru) and A.A.; funding acquisition, M.R.D.M., S.M. and M.M. All authors have read and agreed to the published version of the manuscript.

Funding: This work was supported by grants from Fondazione Banco di Sardegna, Italy-2022.

Institutional Review Board Statement: Not applicable.

Informed Consent Statement: Not applicable.

Data Availability Statement: Not applicable.

Conflicts of Interest: The authors declare no conflict of interest.

References

1. Bray, F.; Ferlay, J.; Soerjomataram, I.; Siegel, R.L.; Torre, L.A.; Jemal, A. Global cancer statistics 2018: Globocan estimates of incidence and mortality worldwide for 36 cancers in 185 countries. *CA Cancer J. Clin.* **2018**, *68*, 394–424. [CrossRef] [PubMed]
2. Sung, H.; Ferlay, J.; Siegel, R.L.; Laversanne, M.; Soerjomataram, I.; Jemal, A.; Bray, F. Global cancer statistics 2020: Globocan estimates of incidence and mortality worldwide for 36 cancers in 185 countries. *CA Cancer J. Clin.* **2021**, *71*, 209–249. [CrossRef]
3. Siegel, R.L.; Miller, K.D.; Fuchs, H.E.; Jemal, A. Cancer statistics, 2021. *CA Cancer J. Clin.* **2021**, *71*, 7–33. [CrossRef] [PubMed]
4. Schottenfeld, D.; Beebe-Dimmer, J.L.; Buffler, P.A.; Omenn, G.S. Current perspective on the global and united states cancer burden attributable to lifestyle and environmental risk factors. *Annu. Rev. Public Health* **2013**, *34*, 97–117. [CrossRef] [PubMed]
5. Dunn, B.K.; Woloshin, S.; Xie, H.; Kramer, B.S. Cancer overdiagnosis: A challenge in the era of screening. *J. Natl. Cancer Cent.* **2022**, *2*, 235–242. [CrossRef] [PubMed]
6. Torre, L.A.; Siegel, R.L.; Ward, E.M.; Jemal, A. Global cancer incidence and mortality rates and trends—An update. *Cancer Epidemiol. Biomark. Prev.* **2016**, *25*, 16–27. [CrossRef] [PubMed]
7. Sitki Copur, M. State of cancer research around the globe. *Oncology* **2019**, *33*, 181–185.
8. Singh, D.; Vignat, J.; Lorenzoni, V.; Eslahi, M.; Ginsburg, O.; Lauby-Secretan, B.; Arbyn, M.; Basu, P.; Bray, F.; Vaccarella, S. Global estimates of incidence and mortality of cervical cancer in 2020: A baseline analysis of the who global cervical cancer elimination initiative. *Lancet Glob. Health* **2023**, *11*, e197–e206. [CrossRef]
9. Iyengar, S.; Hall, I.J.; Sabatino, S.A. Racial/ethnic disparities in prostate cancer incidence, distant stage diagnosis, and mortality by US census region and age group, 2012–2015. *Cancer Epidemiol. Biomark. Prev.* **2020**, *29*, 1357–1364. [CrossRef]
10. Morgan, E.; Arnold, M.; Gini, A.; Lorenzoni, V.; Cabasag, C.J.; Laversanne, M.; Vignat, J.; Ferlay, J.; Murphy, N.; Bray, F. Global burden of colorectal cancer in 2020 and 2040: Incidence and mortality estimates from globocan. *Gut* **2023**, *72*, 338–344. [CrossRef]
11. Jakovljevic, M.; Timofeyev, Y.; Ranabhat, C.L.; Fernandes, P.O.; Teixeira, J.P.; Rancic, N.; Reshetnikov, V. Real gdp growth rates and healthcare spending–comparison between the g7 and the em7 countries. *Glob. Health* **2020**, *16*, 64. [CrossRef]
12. World Health Organization. *Who Report on Cancer: Setting Priorities, Investing Wisely and Providing Care for All*; WHO: Geneva, Switzerland, 2020.
13. Dickerson, J.C.; Ragavan, M.V.; Parikh, D.A.; Patel, M.I. Healthcare delivery interventions to reduce cancer disparities worldwide. *World J. Clin. Oncol.* **2020**, *11*, 705. [CrossRef]
14. Coradduzza, D.; Bellu, E.; Congiargiu, A.; Pashchenko, A.; Amler, E.; Necas, A.; Carru, C.; Medici, S.; Maioli, M. Role of nano-mirnas in diagnostics and therapeutics. *Int. J. Mol. Sci.* **2022**, *23*, 6836. [CrossRef]
15. Medici, S.; Peana, M.; Coradduzza, D.; Zoroddu, M.A. Gold nanoparticles and cancer: Detection, diagnosis and therapy. *Semin. Cancer Biol.* **2021**, *76*, 27–37. [CrossRef]
16. Coradduzza, D.; Solinas, T.; Azara, E.; Culeddu, N.; Cruciani, S.; Zinellu, A.; Medici, S.; Maioli, M.; Madonia, M.; Carru, C. Plasma polyamine biomarker panels: Agmatine in support of prostate cancer diagnosis. *Biomolecules* **2022**, *12*, 514. [CrossRef] [PubMed]
17. Li, N.; Zhou, H.; Tang, Q. Red blood cell distribution width: A novel predictive indicator for cardiovascular and cerebrovascular diseases. *Dis. Markers* **2017**, *2017*, 7089493. [CrossRef]
18. Akceoglu, G.A.; Saylan, Y.; Inci, F. A snapshot of microfluidics in point-of-care diagnostics: Multifaceted integrity with materials and sensors. *Adv. Mater. Technol.* **2021**, *6*, 2100049. [CrossRef]
19. Marks, P.W. Anemia: Clinical approach. In *Concise Guide to Hematology*; Springer International Publishing: Berlin/Heidelberg, Germany, 2019; pp. 21–27.
20. Lee, J.J.; Montazerin, S.M.; Jamil, A.; Jamil, U.; Marszalek, J.; Chuang, M.L.; Chi, G. Association between red blood cell distribution width and mortality and severity among patients with covid-19: A systematic review and meta-analysis. *J. Med. Virol.* **2021**, *93*, 2513–2522. [CrossRef]
21. Ye, X.; Liu, J.; Chen, Y.; Wang, N.; Lu, R. The impact of hemoglobin level and transfusion on the outcomes of chemotherapy in gastric cancer patients. *Int. J. Clin. Exp. Med.* **2015**, *8*, 4228–4235.
22. Durie, B.G.; Salmon, S.E. A clinical staging system for multiple myeloma correlation of measured myeloma cell mass with presenting clinical features, response to treatment, and survival. *Cancer* **1975**, *36*, 842–854. [CrossRef] [PubMed]
23. Coradduzza, D.; Bo, M.; Congiargiu, A.; Azara, E.; De Miglio, M.R.; Erre, G.L.; Carru, C. Decoding the Microbiome's influence on rheumatoid arthritis. *Microorganisms* **2023**, *11*, 2170. [CrossRef]
24. Zhang, F.; Han, H.; Wang, C.; Wang, J.; Zhang, G.; Cao, F.; Cheng, Y. A retrospective study: The prognostic value of anemia, smoking and drinking in esophageal squamous cell carcinoma with primary radiotherapy. *World J. Surg. Oncol.* **2013**, *11*, 249. [CrossRef] [PubMed]
25. Zhang, F.; Cheng, F.; Cao, L.; Wang, S.; Zhou, W.; Ma, W. A retrospective study: The prevalence and prognostic value of anemia in patients undergoing radiotherapy for esophageal squamous cell carcinoma. *World J. Surg. Oncol.* **2014**, *12*, 244. [CrossRef] [PubMed]
26. Coradduzza, D.; Congiargiu, A.; Chen, Z.; Zinellu, A.; Carru, C.; Medici, S. Ferroptosis and senescence: A systematic review. *Int. J. Mol. Sci.* **2023**, *24*, 3658. [CrossRef] [PubMed]

27. Qu, J.; Zhou, T.; Xue, M.; Sun, H.; Shen, Y.; Chen, Y.; Tang, L.; Qian, L.; You, J.; Yang, R.; et al. Correlation analysis of hemoglobin-to-red blood cell distribution width ratio and frailty in elderly patients with coronary heart disease. *Front. Cardiovasc. Med.* **2021**, *8*, 728800. [CrossRef] [PubMed]
28. Williams, A.M.; Brown, K.H.; Allen, L.H.; Dary, O.; Moorthy, D.; Suchdev, P.S. Improving anemia assessment in clinical and public health settings. *J. Nutr.* **2023**. [CrossRef] [PubMed]
29. Pasricha, S.-R.; Tye-Din, J.; Muckenthaler, M.U.; Swinkels, D.W. Iron deficiency. *Lancet* **2021**, *397*, 233–248. [CrossRef]
30. An, R.; Huang, Y.; Man, Y.; Valentine, R.W.; Kucukal, E.; Goreke, U.; Sekyonda, Z.; Piccone, C.; Owusu-Ansah, A.; Ahuja, S.; et al. Emerging point-of-care technologies for anemia detection. *Lab Chip* **2021**, *21*, 1843–1865. [CrossRef]
31. Arishi, W.A.; Alhadrami, H.A.; Zourob, M. Techniques for the detection of sickle cell disease: A review. *Micromachines* **2021**, *12*, 519. [CrossRef]
32. Coradduzza, D.; Arru, C.; Culeddu, N.; Congiargiu, A.; Azara, E.G.; Scanu, A.M.; Zinellu, A.; Muroni, M.R.; Rallo, V.; Medici, S.; et al. Quantitative metabolomics to explore the role of plasma polyamines in colorectal cancer. *Int. J. Mol. Sci.* **2022**, *24*, 101. [CrossRef]
33. Cordeiro dos Santos, N.; Fernández, M.M.; Camelier, A.; de Almeida, V.D.C.; Maciel, R.R.B.T.; Camelier, F.W.R. Prevalence and impact of comorbidities in individuals with chronic obstructive pulmonary disease: A systematic review. *Tuberc. Respir. Dis.* **2022**, *85*, 205–220. [CrossRef] [PubMed]
34. Shi, H.; Chen, L.; Wang, Y.; Sun, M.; Guo, Y.; Ma, S.; Wang, X.; Jiang, H.; Wang, X.; Lu, J.; et al. Severity of anemia during pregnancy and adverse maternal and fetal outcomes. *JAMA Netw. Open* **2022**, *5*, e2147046. [CrossRef] [PubMed]
35. Awada, W.N.; Mohmoued, M.F.; Radwan, T.M.; Hussien, G.Z.; Elkady, H.W. Continuous and noninvasive hemoglobin monitoring reduces red blood cell transfusion during neurosurgery: A prospective cohort study. *J. Clin. Monit. Comput.* **2015**, *29*, 733–740. [CrossRef] [PubMed]
36. Hasan, M.N.; Fraiwan, A.; An, R.; Alapan, Y.; Ung, R.; Akkus, A.; Xu, J.Z.; Rezac, A.J.; Kocmich, N.J.; Creary, M.S.; et al. Based microchip electrophoresis for point-of-care hemoglobin testing. *Analyst* **2020**, *145*, 2525–2542. [CrossRef] [PubMed]
37. Azimi, S.; Faramarzi, E.; Sarbakhsh, P.; Ostadrahimi, A.; Somi, M.H.; Ghayour, M. Folate and vitamin b12 status and their relation to hematological indices in healthy adults of iranians: Azar cohort study. *Nutr. Health* **2019**, *25*, 29–36. [CrossRef]
38. Lin, F.; Wang, X.; Liang, Y.; Liu, D.; Zhang, Y.; Zhong, R.; Yang, Z. Red blood cell distribution width in rheumatoid arthritis, ankylosing spondylitis and osteoarthritis: True inflammatory index or effect of anemia? *Ann. Clin. Lab. Sci.* **2018**, *48*, 301–307.
39. Sankar, V.; Villa, A. Hematologic diseases. In *Burket's Oral Medicine*; Wiley: Hoboken, NJ, USA, 2021; pp. 627–664.
40. Poz, D.; De Falco, E.; Pisano, C.; Madonna, R.; Ferdinandy, P.; Balistreri, C.R. Diagnostic and prognostic relevance of red blood cell distribution width for vascular aging and cardiovascular diseases. *Rejuvenation Res.* **2019**, *22*, 146–162. [CrossRef]
41. Nandi, A.; Talukdar, M.; Bhattacharya, S.; Sen, S.; Biswas, S.; Roy, K. Red blood cell indices in different hemoglobinopathies: A cross-sectional study in eastern india. *Indian J. Pathol. Microbiol.* **2022**, *65*, 1–6.
42. Angius, A.; Pira, G.; Cossu-Rocca, P.; Sotgiu, G.; Saderi, L.; Muroni, M.R.; Virdis, P.; Piras, D.; Vincenzo, R.; Carru, C.; et al. Deciphering clinical significance of bcl11a isoforms and protein expression roles in triple-negative breast cancer subtype. *J. Cancer Res. Clin. Oncol.* **2023**, *149*, 3951–3963. [CrossRef]
43. Karakochuk, C.D.; Hess, S.Y.; Moorthy, D.; Namaste, S.; Parker, M.E.; Rappaport, A.I.; Wegmüller, R.; Dary, O.; HEmoglobin MEasurement (HEME) Working Group. Measurement and interpretation of hemoglobin concentration in clinical and field settings: A narrative review. *Ann. N. Y. Acad. Sci.* **2019**, *1450*, 126–146. [CrossRef]
44. Das, R.; Saleh, S.; Nielsen, I.; Kaviraj, A.; Sharma, P.; Dey, K.; Saha, S. Performance analysis of machine learning algorithms and screening formulae for β–thalassemia trait screening of Indian antenatal women. *Int. J. Med. Inform.* **2022**, *167*, 104866. [CrossRef] [PubMed]
45. Brożek, J.; Akl, E.A.; Alonso-Coello, P.; Lang, D.; Jaeschke, R.; Williams, J.W.; Phillips, B.; Lelgemann, M.; Lethaby, A.; Bousquet, J. Grading quality of evidence and strength of recommendations in clinical practice guidelines: Part 1 of 3. An overview of the grade approach and grading quality of evidence about interventions. *Allergy* **2009**, *64*, 669–677. [CrossRef] [PubMed]
46. Wiciński, M.; Liczner, G.; Cadelski, K.; Kołnierzak, T.; Nowaczewska, M.; Malinowski, B. Anemia of chronic diseases: Wider diagnostics—Better treatment? *Nutrients* **2020**, *12*, 1784. [CrossRef] [PubMed]
47. Coradduzza, D.; Congiargiu, A.; Chen, Z.; Cruciani, S.; Zinellu, A.; Carru, C.; Medici, S. Humanin and its pathophysiological roles in aging: A systematic review. *Biology* **2023**, *12*, 558. [CrossRef] [PubMed]
48. Zhai, Z.; Gao, J.; Zhu, Z.; Cong, X.; Lou, S.; Han, B.; Yin, X.; Zhang, Y.; Xue, Y. The ratio of the hemoglobin to red cell distribution width combined with the ratio of platelets to lymphocytes can predict the survival of patients with gastric cancer liver metastasis. *BioMed Res. Int.* **2021**, *2021*, 8729869. [CrossRef]
49. Fang, Y.; Sun, X.; Zhang, L.; Xu, Y.; Zhu, W. Hemoglobin/red blood cell distribution width ratio in peripheral blood is positively associated with prognosis of patients with primary hepatocellular carcinoma. *Med. Sci. Monit. Int. Med. J. Exp. Clin. Res.* **2022**, *28*, e937146. [CrossRef]
50. Koma, Y.; Onishi, A.; Matsuoka, H.; Oda, N.; Yokota, N.; Matsumoto, Y.; Koyama, M.; Okada, N.; Nakashima, N.; Masuya, D.; et al. Increased red blood cell distribution width associates with cancer stage and prognosis in patients with lung cancer. *PLoS ONE* **2013**, *8*, e80240. [CrossRef]
51. Turgutkaya, A.; Akın, N.; Sargın, G.; Bolaman, Z.; Yavaşoğlu, İ. The relationship between red cell distribution width and prognostic scores in myelodysplastic syndrome. *Hematol. Transfus. Cell Ther.* **2022**, *44*, 332–335. [CrossRef]

52. Eoh, K.-J.; Lee, T.-K.; Nam, E.-J.; Kim, S.-W.; Kim, Y.-T. Clinical relevance of red blood cell distribution width (rdw) in endometrial cancer: A retrospective single-center experience from Korea. *Cancers* **2023**, *15*, 3984. [CrossRef]
53. Baker, L.; Park, L.; Gilbert, R.; Ahn, H.; Martel, A.; Lenet, T.; Davis, A.; McIsaac, D.I.; Tinmouth, A.; Fergusson, D.A. Intraoperative red blood cell transfusion decision-making: A systematic review of guidelines. *Ann. Surg.* **2021**, *274*, 86–96. [CrossRef]
54. Jayasudha, D. Assessment of Red Cell Distribution Width in Portal Hypertension and Its Correlation with Child Turcotte Pugh Score among Patients with Chronic Liver Disease. Ph.D. Thesis, Madras Medical College, Chennai, India, 2017.
55. Jameus, A.; Kennedy, A.E.; Thome, C. Hematological changes following low dose radiation therapy and comparison to current standard of care cancer treatments. *Dose-Response* **2021**, *19*, 15593258211056196. [CrossRef] [PubMed]
56. Moher, D.; Liberati, A.; Tetzlaff, J.; Altman, D.G.; The PRISMA Group. Preferred reporting items for systematic reviews and meta-analyses: The prisma statement. *Ann. Intern. Med.* **2009**, *151*, 264–269. [CrossRef] [PubMed]
57. Aslan, M.; Bekmez, E.T. The Ratio of Hemoglobin to Red Cell Distribution Width Predicts Pathological Complete Response with Rectal Cancer Treated by Neoadjuvant Chemoradiotherapy. *EJMI* **2023**, *7*, 283–289.
58. Wen, X.; Coradduzza, D.; Shen, J.; Scanu, A.M.; Muroni, M.R.; Massidda, M.; Rallo, V.; Carru, C.; Angius, A.; De Miglio, M.R. Harnessing Minimal Residual Disease as a Predictor for Colorectal Cancer: Promising Horizons Amidst Challenges. *Medicina* **2023**, *59*, 1886. [CrossRef] [PubMed]
59. Sun, P.; Zhang, F.; Chen, C.; Bi, X.; Yang, H.; An, X.; Wang, F.; Jiang, W. The ratio of hemoglobin to red cell distribution width as a novel prognostic parameter in esophageal squamous cell carcinoma: A retrospective study from southern China. *Oncotarget* **2016**, *7*, 42650–42660. [CrossRef]
60. Yılmaz, A.; Yılmaz, H.; Tekin, S.B.; Bilici, M. The prognostic significance of hemoglobin-to-red cell distribution width ratio in muscle-invasive bladder cancer. *Biomark. Med.* **2020**, *14*, 727–738. [CrossRef] [PubMed]
61. Yılmaz, A.; Mirili, C.; Tekin, S.B.; Bilici, M. The ratio of hemoglobin to red cell distribution width predicts survival in patients with gastric cancer treated by neoadjuvant flot: A retrospective study. *Ir. J. Med. Sci.* **2020**, *189*, 91–102. [CrossRef] [PubMed]
62. Lin, Z.; Zhang, X.; Luo, Y.; Chen, Y.; Yuan, Y. The value of hemoglobin-to-red blood cell distribution width ratio (hb/rdw), neutrophil-to-lymphocyte ratio (nlr), and platelet-to-lymphocyte ratio (plr) for the diagnosis of nasopharyngeal cancer. *Medicine* **2021**, *100*, e26537. [CrossRef]
63. Su, Y.-C.; Wen, S.-C.; Li, C.-C.; Su, H.-C.; Ke, H.-L.; Li, W.-M.; Lee, H.-Y.; Li, C.-Y.; Yang, S.-F.; Tu, H.-P. Low hemoglobin-to-red cell distribution width ratio is associated with disease progression and poor prognosis in upper tract urothelial carcinoma. *Biomedicines* **2021**, *9*, 672. [CrossRef]
64. Ergür, F.Ö.; Öztürk, A. A new prognostic marker in small cell lung cancer: Red cell distribution ratio of hemoglobin. *Anatol. Curr. Med. J.* **2023**, *5*, 148–152. [CrossRef]
65. Xiu, W.-J.; Zheng, Y.-Y.; Wu, T.-T.; Hou, X.-G.; Yang, Y.; Ma, Y.-T.; Xie, X. Hemoglobin-to-red-cell distribution width ratio is a novel predictor of long-term patient outcomes after percutaneous coronary intervention: A retrospective cohort study. *Front. Cardiovasc. Med.* **2022**, *9*, 726025. [CrossRef]
66. Yılmaz, H.; Yılmaz, A.; Demirağ, G. Prognostic significance of hemoglobin-to-red cell distribution width ratio in patients with metastatic renal cancer. *Future Oncol.* **2021**, *17*, 3853–3864. [CrossRef]
67. Zhao, W.; Shi, M.; Zhang, J. Preoperative hemoglobin-to-red cell distribution width ratio as a prognostic factor in pulmonary large cell neuroendocrine carcinoma: A retrospective cohort study. *Ann. Transl. Med.* **2022**, *10*, 42. [CrossRef]
68. Dong, X.-Y.; Tang, G.-F.; Chen, W.; Cao, J.; Cheng, H.; Li, Z.-Y.; Xu, K.-L. Influence of the ratio of peripheral hemoglobin-to-red cell distribution width on the prognosis of patients with diffuse large b-cell lymphoma. *Zhongguo Shi Yan Xue Ye Xue Za Zhi* **2022**, *30*, 765–770.
69. Tham, T.; Olson, C.; Wotman, M.; Teegala, S.; Khaymovich, J.; Coury, J.; Costantino, P. Evaluation of the prognostic utility of the hemoglobin-to-red cell distribution width ratio in head and neck cancer. *Eur. Arch. Oto-Rhino-Laryngol.* **2018**, *275*, 2869–2878. [CrossRef]
70. Zhao, W.; Shen, X.; Hua, Q.; Yang, L.; Zhou, R.; Zhou, C.; Xu, P. Red cell distribution width—A potential prognostic indicator for colorectal cancer patients after radical resection in China. *J. Gastrointest. Oncol.* **2023**, *14*, 1746–1758. [CrossRef] [PubMed]
71. Bozkaya, Y.; Kurt, B.; Gürler, F. A prognostic parameter in advanced non-small cell lung cancer: The ratio of hemoglobin-to-red cell distribution width. *Int. J. Clin. Oncol.* **2019**, *24*, 798–806. [CrossRef] [PubMed]
72. Zhang, X.; Tan, X.; Li, J.; Wei, Z. Relationship between certain hematological parameters and risk of breast cancer. *Future Oncol.* **2022**, *18*, 3409–3417. [CrossRef] [PubMed]
73. Coradduzza, D.; Azara, E.; Medici, S.; Arru, C.; Solinas, T.; Madonia, M.; Zinellu, A.; Carru, C. A preliminary study procedure for detection of polyamines in plasma samples as a potential diagnostic tool in prostate cancer. *J. Chromatogr. B* **2021**, *1162*, 122468. [CrossRef]
74. Wu, F.; Yang, S.; Tang, X.; Liu, W.; Chen, H.; Gao, H. Prognostic value of baseline hemoglobin-to-red blood cell distribution width ratio in small cell lung cancer: A retrospective analysis. *Thorac. Cancer* **2020**, *11*, 888–897. [CrossRef]
75. Petrella, F.; Casiraghi, M.; Radice, D.; Cara, A.; Maffeis, G.; Prisciandaro, E.; Rizzo, S.; Spaggiari, L. Prognostic value of the hemoglobin/red cell distribution width ratio in resected lung adenocarcinoma. *Cancers* **2021**, *13*, 710. [CrossRef] [PubMed]
76. Coradduzza, D.; Ghironi, A.; Azara, E.; Culeddu, N.; Cruciani, S.; Zinellu, A.; Maioli, M.; De Miglio, M.R.; Medici, S.; Fozza, C.; et al. Role of polyamines as biomarkers in lymphoma patients: A pilot study. *Diagnostics* **2022**, *12*, 2151. [CrossRef]

77. Herraez, I.; Bento, L.; Del Campo, R.; Sas, A.; Ramos, R.; Ibarra, J.; Mestre, F.; Alemany, R.; Bargay, J.; Sampol, A.; et al. Prognostic role of the red blood cell distribution width (rdw) in hodgkin lymphoma. *Cancers* **2020**, *12*, 3262. [CrossRef]
78. Rahamim, E.; Zwas, D.R.; Keren, A.; Elbaz-Greener, G.; Ibrahimli, M.; Amir, O.; Gotsman, I. The ratio of hemoglobin to red cell distribution width: A strong predictor of clinical outcome in patients with heart failure. *J. Clin. Med.* **2022**, *11*, 886. [CrossRef]
79. Song, J.; Yu, T.; Yan, Q.; Zhang, Q.; Wang, L. Association of Hemoglobin to Red Blood Cell Distribution Width-Standard Deviation (RDW-SD) Ratio and 3-Month Readmission in Elderly Chinese Patients with Heart Failure: A Retrospective Cohort Study. *Int. J. Gen. Med.* **2023**, *16*, 303–315. [CrossRef] [PubMed]
80. Talari, K.; Goyal, M. Retrospective studies–utility and caveats. *J. R. Coll. Physicians Edinb.* **2020**, *50*, 398–402. [CrossRef] [PubMed]
81. Chen, H.; Zhen, Z.; Dong, Y.; Liu, C.; Dong, B.; Xue, R. Hemoglobin to red cell distribution width ratio: A predictor of clinical outcome and diuretic response in patients with acute heart failure. *Int. J. Cardiol.* **2023**, *394*, 131368. [CrossRef]
82. Jang, T.K.; Kim, H.; Eo, W.; Kim, K.H.; Lee, C.M.; Kim, M. Clinical Significance of the Combination of Serum HE4 Levels, Hemoglobin-to-Red Cell Distribution Width Ratio, and CT Imaging for the Pretreatment Assessment of Adnexal Masses. *J. Cancer* **2023**, *14*, 600. [CrossRef]
83. Li, J.; Wuethrich, A.; Dey, S.; Lane, R.E.; Sina, A.A.; Wang, J.; Wang, Y.; Puttick, S.; Koo, K.M.; Trau, M. The growing impact of micro/nanomaterial-based systems in precision oncology: Translating "multiomics" technologies. *Adv. Funct. Mater.* **2020**, *30*, 1909306. [CrossRef]
84. Ai, L.; Mu, S.; Hu, Y. Prognostic role of RDW in hematological malignancies: A systematic review and meta-analysis. *Cancer Cell Int.* **2018**, *18*, 61. [CrossRef]

Disclaimer/Publisher's Note: The statements, opinions and data contained in all publications are solely those of the individual author(s) and contributor(s) and not of MDPI and/or the editor(s). MDPI and/or the editor(s) disclaim responsibility for any injury to people or property resulting from any ideas, methods, instructions or products referred to in the content.

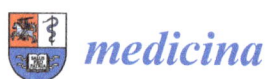 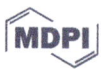

Case Report

Spindle Cell Rhabdomyosarcoma of the Inguinal Region Mimicking a Complicated Hernia in the Adult—An Unexpected Finding

Valentin Titus Grigorean [1,2], Radu Serescu [3], Andrei Anica [3,4], Violeta Elena Coman [1,2], Ştefan Iulian Bedereag [5], Roxana Corina Sfetea [6], Mircea Liţescu [7,8,*], Iancu Emil Pleşea [5], Costin George Florea [2,4], Cosmin Burleanu [2,4], Anwar Erchid [2,4] and Ionuţ Simion Coman [1,2]

1. Discipline of General Surgery, "Bagdasar-Arseni" Clinical Emergency Hospital, 10th Clinical Department—General Surgery, Faculty of Medicine, "Carol Davila" University of Medicine and Pharmacy, 37 Dionisie Lupu Street, 020021 Bucharest, Romania; valentin.grigorean@umfcd.ro (V.T.G.); elena.coman@umfcd.ro (V.E.C.); ionut.coman@umfcd.ro (I.S.C.)
2. General Surgery Department, "Bagdasar-Arseni" Clinical Emergency Hospital, 12 Berceni Road, 041915 Bucharest, Romania; costinflorea1990@gmail.com (C.G.F.); burleanucosmin@gmail.com (C.B.); erchid.anwar@yahoo.com (A.E.)
3. Amethyst Medical Center, 42 Odăii Street, 075100 Otopeni, Romania; raduserescu@gmail.com (R.S.); dr.andrei.anica@gmail.com (A.A.)
4. Ph.D. School, "Carol Davila" University of Medicine and Pharmacy, 37 Dionisie Lupu Street, 020021 Bucharest, Romania
5. Pathology Department, "Bagdasar-Arseni" Clinical Emergency Hospital, 12 Berceni Road, 041915 Bucharest, Romania; stefanbedereag@gmail.com (Ş.I.B.); pie1956@yahoo.com (I.E.P.)
6. Discipline of Modern Languages, 3rd Preclinical Department—Complementary Sciences, Faculty of Medicine, "Carol Davila" University of Medicine and Pharmacy, 37 Dionisie Lupu Street, 020021 Bucharest, Romania; roxana.sfetea@umfcd.ro
7. Discipline of Surgery and General Anesthesia, "Sf. Ioan" Clinical Emergency Hospital, 2nd Department, Faculty of Dental Medicine, "Carol Davila" University of Medicine and Pharmacy, 37 Dionisie Lupu Street, 020021 Bucharest, Romania
8. General Surgery Department, "Sf. Ioan" Clinical Emergency Hospital, 13 Vitan-Bârzeşti Road, 042122 Bucharest, Romania
* Correspondence: mircea.litescu@umfcd.ro

Citation: Grigorean, V.T.; Serescu, R.; Anica, A.; Coman, V.E.; Bedereag, Ş.I.; Sfetea, R.C.; Liţescu, M.; Pleşea, I.E.; Florea, C.G.; Burleanu, C.; et al. Spindle Cell Rhabdomyosarcoma of the Inguinal Region Mimicking a Complicated Hernia in the Adult—An Unexpected Finding. *Medicina* 2023, *59*, 1515. https://doi.org/10.3390/medicina59091515

Academic Editor: Vishal G. Shelat

Received: 29 July 2023
Revised: 15 August 2023
Accepted: 16 August 2023
Published: 23 August 2023

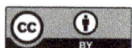

Copyright: © 2023 by the authors. Licensee MDPI, Basel, Switzerland. This article is an open access article distributed under the terms and conditions of the Creative Commons Attribution (CC BY) license (https://creativecommons.org/licenses/by/4.0/).

Abstract: Rhabdomyosarcoma is a rare tumor that is diagnosed mostly in children and adolescents, rarely in adults, representing 2–5% of all soft tissue sarcomas. It has four subtypes that are recognized: embryonal (50%), alveolar (20%), pleomorphic (20%), and spindle cell/sclerosing (10%). The diagnosis of rhabdomyosarcoma is based on the histological detection of rhabdomyoblasts and the expression of muscle-related biomarkers. Spindle cell/sclerosing rhabdomyosarcoma consists morphologically of fusiform cells with vesicular chromatin arranged in a storiform pattern or long fascicles, with occasional rhabdomyoblasts. Also, dense, collagenous, sclerotic stroma may be seen more commonly in adults. We present a rare case of an adult who presented to the hospital with a tumor in the left inguinal area, was first diagnosed with a left strangulated inguinal hernia and was operated on as an emergency, although the diagnosis was ultimately a spindle cell rhabdomyosarcoma of the inguinal region.

Keywords: rhabdomyosarcoma; spindle cell; inguinal; hernia; adult

1. Introduction

Rhabdomyosarcoma is defined as a malignant mesenchymal tumor that has skeletal muscle differentiation, with four subtypes that are recognized: embryonal (50%), alveolar (20%), pleomorphic (20%), and spindle cell/sclerosing (10%) [1]. A more detailed classification includes the botryoid rhabdomyosarcoma, which is a subtype of the embryonal rhabdomyosarcoma, characteristic of the mucosal surfaces on the walls of hollow organs, such as the vagina, the uterine cervix, the bladder, the biliary tract, or the nasopharynx of infants [2,3].

Rhabdomyosarcoma is a rare tumor that is diagnosed mostly in children and adolescents, but rarely in adults, representing 2–5% of all soft tissue sarcomas [4]. Around two-thirds of the cases occur in children younger than 6 years of age [5]. Rhabdomyosarcomas account for 3% of childhood cancers and 2% of adolescent cancers and its incidence makes information regarding its characteristics very limited [6–8].

The diagnosis of rhabdomyosarcoma is based on the histological detection of rhabdomyoblasts and the expression of muscle-related biomarkers. Despite showing elements of skeletal muscle differentiation, rhabdomyosarcomas can develop in areas where skeletal muscle is absent [9].

Following the efforts of the Intergroup Rhabdomyosarcoma Study, Newton and al. proposed a classification for the prediction of the outcome of patients with various types of rhabdomyosarcomas (Table 1) [10,11]:

Table 1. Prognosis of various types of rhabdomyosarcoma.

Prognosis	Type
Superior prognosis	Botryoid rhabdomyosarcoma Spindle cell rhabdomyosarcoma
Intermediate prognosis	Embryonal rhabdomyosarcoma
Poor prognosis	Alveolar rhabdomyosarcoma Undifferentiated rhabdomyosarcoma

Cavazzana et al. first described spindle cell rhabdomyosarcomas in children [12], while Rubin et al. published the first occurrence of spindle cell rhabdomyosarcomas in adults [13]. Furthermore, Mentzel et al. reported sclerosing pseudovascular rhabdomyosarcoma, an additional morphological variant of spindle cell rhabdomyosarcoma, in adults [14]. Although initial classifications included the spindle cell/sclerosing rhabdomyosarcoma as a subtype of embryonal rhabdomyosarcoma [15], it was classified as a separate entity by the World Health Organization in 2013 [16]. Morphologically, it consists of fusiform cells with vesicular chromatin arranged in a storiform pattern or long fascicles, with occasional rhabdomyoblasts. Also, dense, collagenous, sclerotic stroma may be seen more commonly in adults [1].

We present a rare case of an adult who presented to the hospital with a tumor in the left inguinal area, was first diagnosed with a left strangulated inguinal hernia and was operated on as an emergency before diagnosis with a spindle cell rhabdomyosarcoma of the inguinal region.

2. Detailed Case Description

A 69-year-old male patient, known to have type I obesity, arterial hypertension, and type II diabetes, for which he takes oral medication, presents to the Emergency Department of our hospital with a tumor in the left inguinal region. The patient reports that he observed the tumor several months ago, during which it grew and was accompanied by local pain.

The local clinical exam reveals, in the left inguinal region, a mass of approximately 8/5 cm (cm), that has an increased consistency, adherent to the superficial and profound planes. Given its location, the pain reported by the patient, and our inability to mobilize the tumor, we establish an initial diagnosis of a strangulated left inguinal hernia.

A chest X-ray exam reveals right lateral-basal right pleurisy in small quantity, while the abdominal X-ray exam does not reveal pneumoperitoneum or air-fluid levels. Biologically, we find hyperglycemia, with a value of 170 milligrams (mg)/deciliter (dL).

We perform an emergency surgical procedure using a left inguinal approach. We identify a tumoral mass in the inguinal canal, which encompasses the spermatic cord up to the profound inguinal orifice and modifies the local anatomy, making it difficult to identify the normal structures of this area. We are not able to identify a hernia sac, but the certain exclusion of a strangulated hernia is only made after we perform an additional midline incision in the lower abdomen, with the endo-abdominal inspection of the inguinofemoral region. The dissection in the inguinal area is difficult due to the infiltrative characteristic of the tumor, which also invades the inguinal ligament and is in close vicinity to the external iliac vessels and the left pubic ramus. Due to the lack of an extemporaneous histopathological analysis and the impossibility of performing a complete resection of the tumor without the sacrifice of the left testicle, we limit our procedure to a biopsy from the tumor.

Subsequently, the patient has a favorable surgical evolution, being discharged on the fifth postoperative day.

The histopathological examination of the biopsy specimen reveals adipose and muscle tissue that includes a diffuse infiltrative mesenchymal tumoral proliferation, with a fasciculated pattern made by elongated cells, with obvious pleomorphism. Associated with these elements, a component of multinucleated cells with eosinophilic cytoplasm, of the rhabdoid type (3 mitoses/high-power-field (HPF)) is observed.

Given the histopathologic result, suggesting a rhabdomyosarcoma, the patient receives an oncologic evaluation, including one from an expert based in an European Society for Medical Oncology (ESMO) Sarcoma reference center. The recommendation, taking into account the age and the associated diseases of the patient, is for a surgical procedure with microscopic complete resection (R_0) if possible, followed by adjuvant radiotherapy and adjuvant chemotherapy with Doxorubicin.

The patient returns to our department 10 days after the first discharge. A thoracic, abdominal, and pelvic computer tomography (CT) is performed, revealing a nodular tumor with left inguinal topography, imprecisely delimited outline, iodophil, dimensions of 51/33/73 mm (transverse/anteroposterior/craniocaudal diameters). The lesion is not distinguishable from the content of the inguinal canal and presents relations posteriorly and laterally with the external iliac vessels, with a fatty cleavage plane to them, superiorly and medially with the inferior epigastric vessels, without cleavage plane, invasive medially in the rectus abdominis muscle, superior and laterally invasive in the transversus abdominis muscle, and posteriorly and inferiorly in contact with the pectineus muscle. In addition to these relations the CT reveals a small lymph node of 15/10 mm between the portal vein and inferior cava vein. It also reveals multiple thyroid nodules and a pseudo-nodular pulmonary consolidation, with subpleural topography in the posterobasal segment of the right inferior pulmonary lobe, most probably of atelectatic origin (Figure 1A,B).

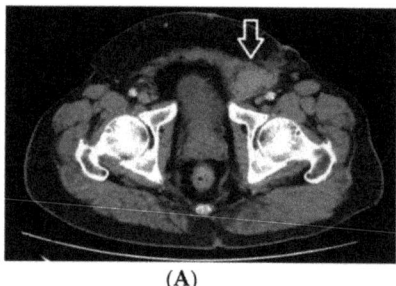 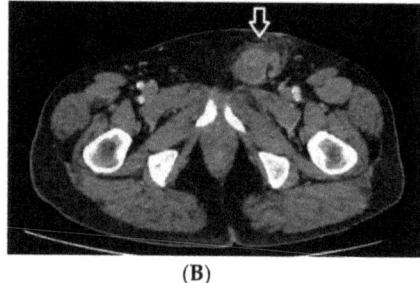

(A)   (B)

Figure 1. Abdominal CT image of the tumor (marked with white arrow) at different levels (**A**,**B**).

We perform the surgical procedure, in which we manage to resect the entire tumor en bloc with the spermatic cord and left testicle, including its invasion in the muscles, the invasion of the pubic ramus with resection of the periosteum and the dissection from the left external iliac vessels (Figure 2). Subsequently, the patient has a favorable surgical evolution, being discharged on the ninth postoperative day.

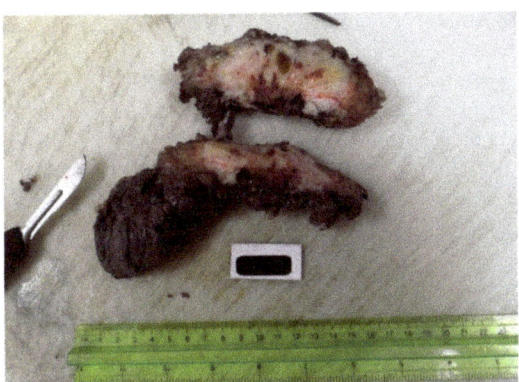

Figure 2. The resected tumor en bloc with the left testicle.

The histopathological examination of the resected tumor reveals a spermatic cord, with the architecture disrupted by malignant mesenchymal tumor proliferation. This has a nodular, fascicular pattern, in the form of intersecting, confluent bundles, forming extensive groups of spindle-shaped tumor cells and frequent tumor cells with abundant cytoplasm, intensely eosinophilic, with nuclei dislocated at the periphery of the cell having a rhabdoid appearance. In addition, some multinucleated giants can be seen, with marked cytonuclear atypia, relatively rare mitotic figures, and the presence of atypical mitoses (approximately 5 mitoses/10 HPF), narrow foci of tumor necrosis (<50% of the examined tumor mass), areas of hemorrhage, siderophagia and polymorphic inflammatory infiltrate with a diffuse intratumoral and peritumoral disposition. In addition, perineural invasion (PNI+) and lymphovascular invasion (LVI+) are present (Figure 3A–C). The proximal limit of resection is free, and the left testicle and epididymis are not invaded by the tumor.

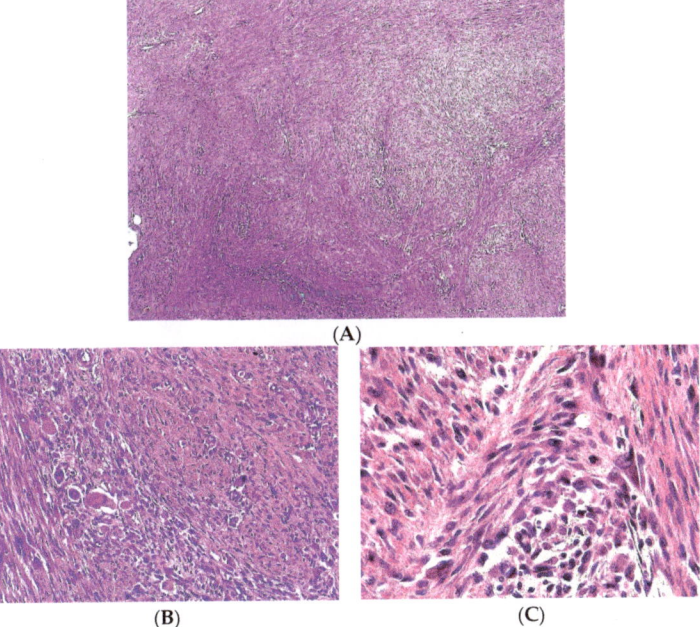

Figure 3. The histopathologic aspect of the specimen—optic microscopy, hematoxylin-eosin staining, magnifying of 4× (**A**), 20× (**B**), and 40× (**C**), respectively.

The histopathological analysis and the immunohistochemistry tests (Table 2) reveal a malignant paratesticular mesenchymal proliferation, compatible with a spindle cell rhabdomyosarcoma.

Table 2. Results of the immunohistochemistry exam.

Immunohistochemistry Marker	Result
Vimentin	Diffuse and intense positive in the tumoral proliferation
Myogenic determination gene (MyoD1)	Diffuse positive in the tumoral proliferation
Myogenin (Myf-4)	Focal positive in the tumoral proliferation
Desmin	Focal positive in the tumoral proliferation
Actin	Positive in the tumoral proliferation
Epithelial membrane antigen (EMA)	Negative in the tumoral proliferation
CD34	Negative in the tumoral proliferation; the presence of internal control
Ki67	Positive in approximately 25% of the tumoral cells

The patient is evaluated again by the oncologist who recommends a cardiology evaluation before starting the adjuvant therapy. The patient receives a transthoracic echocardiogram, revealing a normal global ejection fraction, normal aspect of both ventricles with preserved systolic function, and only mild diastolic dysfunction, but with normal filling pressures.

About one and a half months after the second surgical procedure, pelvic Magnetic Resonance Imaging (MRI) is performed (Figure 4A,B), revealing a recent postoperative aspect in the left inguinal and femoral area, with associated inflammatory modifications. In addition, it reveals external iliac lymph nodes of a maximum 21/7 mm size on the right side and 19/6 mm on the left side, and inguinofemoral lymph nodes of a maximum of 13/8 mm in size on the right side and 13/9 mm on the left side. In addition, the pectineal muscle presents in its 1/3 anterior region a few muscle bundles with modified signal (short tau inversion recovery (STIR) hypersignal), gadolinium enhancement—inflammatory modifications or tumor invasion, as well as a few satellite lymph nodes of maximum 7/6 mm in size.

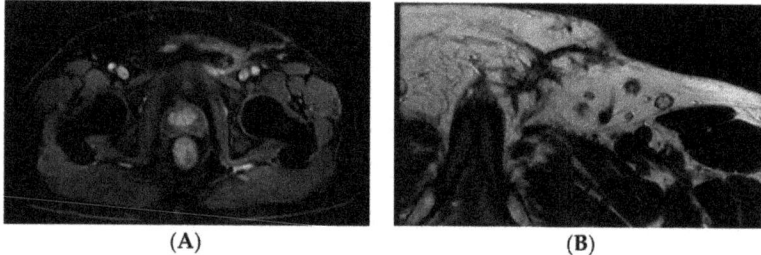

(A) (B)

Figure 4. Postoperative MRI aspect of the left inguinal area—axial sections at different levels showing inflammatory modifications (A) and several lymph nodes (B).

Shortly after the MRI exam, the patient undergoes radiotherapy for a month and a half, with external radiation in two areas at a planned target volume (PTV): left inguinal region (PTV1) and tumor bed (PTV2). The total dose for PTV1 was 50 Grays (Gy) (25 fractions of 2 Gy, 5 days a week, conventional fractionation), using arc therapy with volume modulation of intensity (IMRT-VMAT technique). The total dose for PTV2 was

66 Gy (33 fractions of 2 Gy, 5 days a week, conventional technique), using the IMRT-VMAT technique (Figure 5A–C).

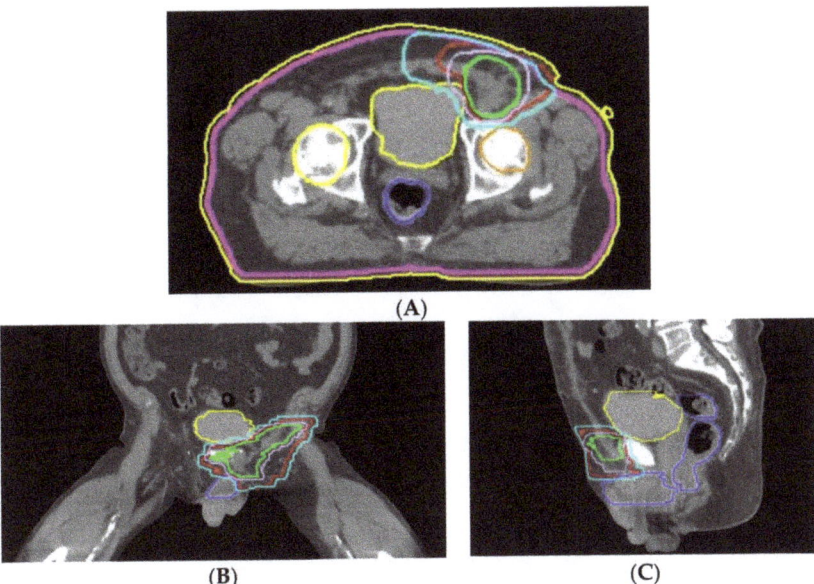

Figure 5. Sections of external radiation areas: clinical target volume (CTV) 1—red (50 Gy); PTV1—dark blue (50 Gy); CTV2—green (66 Gy); PTV2—purple (66 Gy); axial (**A**), coronal (**B**) and sagittal (**C**) sections. Sky blue, pink, yellow and orange have no clinical significance in this case.

A week after the completion of the radiotherapy, a CT scan of the thorax, abdomen and pelvis is performed, showing no suggestive CT signs for local left inguinal tumoral recurrence and no lumbar-aortic or pelvic suspect lymph nodes (Figure 6A,B).

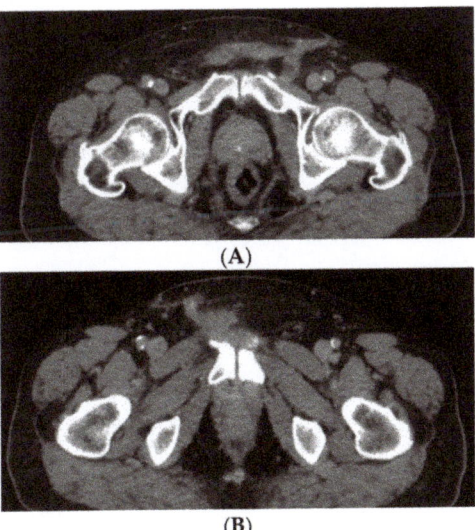

Figure 6. CT scan aspect, over three months after the tumor resection, at various levels, axial sections (**A**,**B**).

After the insertion of a port-a-cath, 5 months after the resection of the tumor, the patient undergoes six sessions of chemotherapy with Doxorubicin 60 mg/m^2, one dose every 3 weeks.

Interspersed with the chemotherapy sessions, 6 months after the surgical procedure, the patient undergoes a positronic emission tomography (PET-CT). This reveals: a few lymph nodes with low uptake for fluorodeoxyglucose (F18-FDG) located on the right side of the trachea (not suggesting oncological lesions), encapsulated pleural fluid with pachypleuritis and atelectasis, diffuse enhanced uptake of the mentioned substance in the colon in the context of the oral antidiabetic treatment, and left inguinal modifications, diffuse and with minimal uptake. The conclusion of the PET-CT is that there are no active metabolic lesions with oncologic interest (Figure 7A,B).

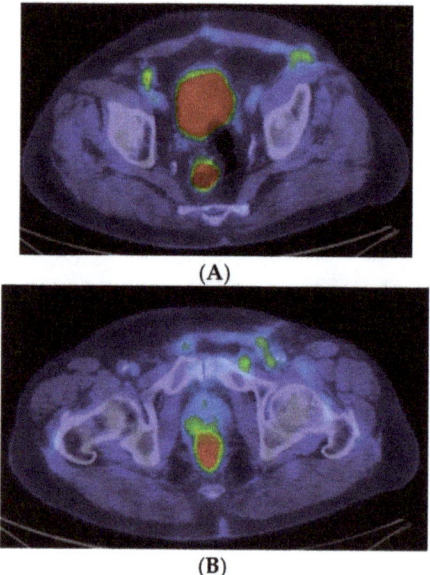

Figure 7. Postoperative PET-CT aspect, at different levels—axial sections (**A**,**B**).

After the chemotherapy, two more thoracic, abdominal, and pelvic CT scans are performed, as well as a head CT scan, with no evidence of tumor relapse or metastases, with the most recent being made just a few days before the submission of this research.

At present, 15 and a half months after the resection of the rhabdomyosarcoma, the patient is in good condition, monitored closely, and presenting with an incisional hernia at the site of the abdominal midline incision, which we will repair after the oncological assessment.

3. Discussion

Spindle cell/sclerosing rhabdomyosarcoma represents 3–10% of rhabdomyosarcomas, affecting infants, children, and adults (ICD-O coding—8912/3) [17]. Studies show a strong predilection for young patients, with a mean age of around 7 years [15,18]. It affects both sexes, but some studies report a male preponderance with a ratio of 6:1 [19,20], while the presence of the MYOD1-mutant genetic subtype reveals a decreased male-to-female ratio [21].

In contrast to the spindle cell rhabdomyosarcoma in children and adolescents, where the most commonly affected region is the genitourinary tract and the orbital area, the main location of the spindle cell rhabdomyosarcoma in adults is in the head and neck region (except the orbital area) and the deep soft tissue of the extremities [22–25]. In addition, although they have a better prognosis compared to other subtypes of rhabdomyosarcoma, spindle cell rhabdomyosarcoma tumors are very aggressive and associated with a poor prognosis in adults, compared to this subtype of tumors in children [14,26].

The particularity of our patient was the unusual age of discovery for this subtype of rhabdomyosarcoma and the location of the tumor, mimicking a strangulated inguinal hernia that forced us to perform an emergency surgical procedure at that moment.

Regarding the pathogenesis of spindle cell rhabdomyosarcoma, several groups have been described:

- Spindle cell/sclerosing rhabdomyosarcoma with a somatic activating mutation of the MYOD1 gene at position Lys122 that can be homo- or heterozygous. The mutated gene interacts with the MYC oncogene. This subtype can be encountered both in children in adults, being characterized by a poor prognosis, especially in children and adolescents, with the latter group age presenting a characteristic mutation of MyoD1 p.Leu122Arg [21,27,28];
- Variants with a rearrangement in the VGLL2/NCOA2 genes, that occur in children under the age of five or as congenital neoplasms. The prognosis is good, but with a high risk of local recurrence [16,29];
- Patients with spindle cell rhabdomyosarcoma developing in their bones, with EWSR1/FUS-TFCP2 or MEIS1-NCOA2 translocations. The presence of these mutations in adults has a very poor prognosis [30–35];
- Cases that do not have the alterations described above, encountered most commonly around the area of the testis or within the abdominal cavity [36];
- Patients with spindle cell rhabdomyosarcoma without molecular alterations [27].

Spindle cell/sclerosing rhabdomyosarcoma appears as a variably circumscribed tumor, with a size ranging between 1.5 and 35 cm. It shows a white-to-tan surface with a whorled appearance. Necrosis and cystic degeneration can also be present [17].

Histopathologically, spindle cell rhabdomyosarcoma is identified by cellular fascicles in spindle cells, with an intersecting or herringbone growth pattern, similar to fibrosarcoma or leiomyosarcoma. The spindled cells have pale eosinophilic cytoplasm and blunted, fusiform or ovoid, centrally located nuclei with small undistinguished nucleoli. Hyperchromatic nuclei, mitotic figures, and nuclear atypia are often present. In addition, primitive undifferentiated areas with round cells and hyperchromatic nuclei can also be present focally. Tadpole or strap cells, rhabdomyoblasts with elongated eosinophilic tails with cross-striations, can sometimes be identified [17]. Sclerosing rhabdomyosarcomas have prominent sclerosis/hyalinization, with tumor cells in various arrangements:cords, nests, microalveoli, or trabeculae in pseudovascular growth pattern. Areas with sclerosis may mimic osteosarcoma due to the extensive formation of the matrix [12,14,21,23,36]. Intraosseous spindle cell rhabdomyosarcoma, described recently, presents, apart from the typical spindle cell morphology, as areas of distinctly epithelioid cells arranged in fascicles and sheets [29,30,33].

Immunohistochemically, spindle cell/sclerosing rhabdomyosarcoma is characterized by the diffuse expression of desmin in all cases, with only the focal expression of myogenin (Myf-4) in most cases. MyoD1 staining can be diffuse or focal in the spindle cell tumors, but it is usually present in a diffuse pattern in sclerosing cases. Staining for smooth muscle actin (SMA) and muscle-specific actin (MSA) is usually absent. In addition, a positive result in cytokeratin and anaplastic lymphoma kinase (ALK) can be seen in the intraosseous spindle cell rhabdomyosarcoma [17].

According to the acknowledged histopathological description of spindle cell rhabdomyosarcoma, histopathological examination of the resected specimen in our patient revealed extensive groups of spindle-shaped tumor cells and frequent tumor cells with eosinophilic cytoplasm, with nuclei of rhabdoid appearance. At the immunohistochemical exam: desmin was focally positive, MyoD1 was diffuse positive, myogenin was focally positive, and, atypically, actin was positive in the tumoral proliferation. Furthermore, vimentin was diffuse and intensely positive, while Ki67 was positive in approximately 25% of the tumoral cells in our patient. Various published cases in the literature have shown variable values of Ki67 expression. Kacar et al. presented a case of spindle cell rhabdomyosarcoma with a Ki67 proliferation index < 2% [37], Jakkampudi et al. published a case with positivity of 40–50% for Ki67 [19] and Zhao et al. described a series of cases diagnosed with spindle cell/sclerosing rhabdomyosarcoma in which the proliferative index Ki67 varied from 15% to 80% [38]. The markers EMA and CD34 were negative in tumoral proliferation. Also, characteristically, spindle cell rhabdomyosarcoma has a negative expression for caldesmon, S-100 protein or glial fibrillary acidic protein (GFAP) [39], but the immunohistochemical examination for our patient did not include these markers.

Rhabdomyosarcoma should be treated by a multidisciplinary team. Surgery is the basic therapeutic option for these patients, regardless of the risk group to which they belong. It should first be considered after diagnosis with the intent of complete resection of the tumor and obtaining microscopically radical surgical margins—R_0 [27,40]. If metastases to lymph nodes are present, radical radiotherapy is used, but given the complications of radiotherapy, a histopathological examination of the lymph nodes should be made to exclude a reactive, non-neoplastic lymphadenopathy. Sparring treatment is usually preferred in case of the involvement of extremities.

In the case of our patient, we resected the recommended 5 cm of normal tissue cranially to the tumor and the histopathological result revealed a tumor-free limit of resection. Distally, we were forced to perform a left orchiectomy, with the histopathological analysis revealing no invasion of the left testicle and epididymis. Circumferentially, the limit of 5 cm could not be achieved because of the particular area involved, the inguinal canal, but we managed to perform a complete resection of the tumor after dissecting it from the external iliac vessels and a resection of the pubic ramus periosteum.

Radical radiotherapy should be considered in the case of extensive local tumoral invasion without the possibility of radical surgery, or in the case of other contraindications for surgical treatment [4,27,41]. Depending on the localization and clinical group (radical radiotherapy or supplementary radiotherapy after the surgical procedure), the total doses for radiotherapy vary between 50 and 65 Gy, with individual, personalized regiments for each patient, also taking into account the age of the patient [42,43].

Regarding chemotherapy, adding neoadjuvant and adjuvant therapy to the patients with metastases obtained a from 60% to 90% 5-year survival. In patients over 16 years of age and adults, the results were determined to be worse, with a 5-year survival of only 30–40% [27]. Various chemotherapy drugs are used, either in monotherapy or in association with two or three drugs: Vincristine, Doxorubicin, Ifosfamide, Dactinomycin, Cyclophosphamide, Actinomycin, and Etoposide. The subject of adjuvant and neoadjuvant radiotherapy and chemotherapy is one of actuality and several research studies are trying to determine the optimal protocols for the treatment of these tumors [36,44–48].

After finishing the oncological treatment, the patient should be observed carefully. The recommended procedure involves a physical examination and imaging studies such as CT and MRI of the primary localization, and CT of the chest, abdomen, and pelvis. Medical evaluation should take place every three months for the first two years, then every six months for the next three years, and subsequently once a year [27].

The most important factors for predicting the overall survival in patients with spindle cell rhabdomyosarcoma are the presence of metastatic disease at the first evaluation, tumor size, obtaining a negative margin status after primary surgical resection, and the response to chemotherapy [22,24,44].

In our case, after the complete surgical resection of the tumor, the patient responded well to radiotherapy and chemotherapy, whilst being closely monitored clinically and imagistically by multiple CT scans of the chest, abdomen, and pelvis, a pelvic MRI, and a PET-CT scan. These images showed no tumor relapse up until this moment, 15 months after the surgery.

4. Conclusions

Spindle cell rhabdomyosarcoma is a rare form of malignant mesenchymal tumor that occurs especially often in children and adolescents. In adults, especially the elderly, the presence of this type of tumor in the inguinal area is very uncommon and may come as a surprise, due to its resemblance to a complicated inguinal hernia.

The management of these cases is complex and involves the complete surgical resection of the tumor when possible, and associated radiotherapy and chemotherapy, as well as a strict follow-up, with frequent clinical and imagistic evaluations.

Author Contributions: Conceptualization, I.S.C. and V.T.G.; methodology, V.E.C. and I.E.P.; software, C.B. and C.G.F.; validation, V.T.G., M.L. and I.S.C.; formal analysis, A.E.; investigation, R.S. and A.A.; resources, Ș.I.B.; writing—original draft preparation, I.S.C.; writing—review and editing, R.C.S. and V.T.G.; supervision, V.T.G.; project administration, I.S.C.; funding acquisition, V.T.G. All authors have read and agreed to the published version of the manuscript.

Funding: The publication of this paper was supported by the University of Medicine and Pharmacy "Carol Davila", through the institutional program "Publish not Perish".

Informed Consent Statement: Informed consent was obtained from the patient involved in the study.

Data Availability Statement: Data is unavailable due to privacy or ethical restrictions.

Conflicts of Interest: The authors declare no conflict of interest.

References

1. Horvai, A. Bones, Joints and Soft Tissue Tumors. In *Pathologic Basis of Disease*, 10th ed.; Kumar, V., Abbas, A., Aster, J., Turner, J., Eds.; Elsevier Inc.: Philadelphia, PA, USA, 2021; pp. 1171–1218.
2. Villella, J.A.; Bogner, P.N.; Jani-Sait, S.N.; Block, A.M.W.; Lele, S. Rhabdomyosarcoma of the cervix in sisters with review of the literature. *Gynecol. Oncol.* **2005**, *99*, 742–748. [CrossRef] [PubMed]
3. Margioula-Siarkou, C.; Petousis, S.; Almperis, A.; Margioula-Siarkou, G.; Laganà, A.S.; Kourti, M.; Papanikolaou, A.; Dinas, K. Sarcoma Botryoides: Optimal Therapeutic Management and Prognosis of an Unfavorable Malignant Neoplasm of Female Children. *Diagnostics* **2023**, *13*, 924. [CrossRef] [PubMed]
4. Ferrari, A.; Dileo, P.; Casanova, M.; Bertulli, R.; Meazza, C.; Gandola, L.; Navarria, P.; Collini, P.; Gronchi, A.; Olmi, P.; et al. Rhabdomyosarcoma in adults. A retrospective analysis of 171 patients treated at a single institution. *Cancer* **2003**, *98*, 571–580. [CrossRef] [PubMed]
5. Yuan, G.; Yao, H.; Li, X.; Li, H.; Wu, L. Stage 1 embryonal rhabdomyosarcoma of the female genital tract: A retrospective clinical study of nine cases. *World J. Surg. Oncol.* **2017**, *15*, 42. [CrossRef] [PubMed]
6. Wang, X.; Feng, J.; Li, Z.; Zhang, X.; Chen, J.; Feng, G. Characteristics and prognosis of embryonal rhabdomyosarcoma in children and adolescents: An analysis of 464 cases from the SEER database. *Chin. Med. Assoc. Pediatr. Investig.* **2020**, *4*, 242–249. [CrossRef] [PubMed]
7. Ward, E.; DeSantis, C.; Robbins, A.; Kohler, B.; Jemal, A. Childhood and adolescent cancer statistics, 2014. *CA Cancer J. Clin.* **2014**, *64*, 83–103. [CrossRef] [PubMed]
8. Koscielniak, E.; Morgan, M.; Treuner, J. Soft tissue sarcoma in children: Prognosis and management. *Paediatr. Drugs* **2002**, *4*, 21–28. [CrossRef]
9. Kabir, W.; Choong, P. The Epidemiology and Pathogenesis of Sarcoma. In *Sarcoma, A Practical Guide to Multidisciplinary Management*; Choong, P., Ed.; Springer: Singapore, 2021; pp. 11–28.
10. Newton, W.A.J.; Gehan, E.A.; Webber, B.L.; Marsden, H.B.; van Unnik, A.J.; Hamoudi, A.B.; Tsokos, M.C.; Shimada, H.; Harms, D.; Schmidt, D.; et al. Classification of rhabdomyosarcomas and related sarcomas. Pathologic aspects and proposal for a new classification--an Intergroup Rhabdomyosarcoma Study. *Cancer* **1995**, *76*, 1073–1085.
11. Parham, D.M.; Ellison, D.A. Rhabdomyosarcomas in Adults and Children: An Update. *Arch. Pathol. Lab. Med.* **2006**, *130*, 1454–1465. [CrossRef]
12. Cavazzana, A.O.; Schmidt, D.; Ninfo, V.; Harms, D.; Tollot, M.; Carli, M.; Treuner, J.; Betto, R.; Salviati, G. Spindle cell rhabdomyosarcoma. A prognostically favorable variant of rhabdomyosarcoma. *Am. J. Surg. Pathol.* **1992**, *16*, 229–235. [CrossRef]
13. Rubin, B.P.; Hasserjian, R.P.; Singer, S.; Janecka, I.; Fletcher, J.A.; Fletcher, C.D.M. Spindle cell rhabdomyosarcoma (so-called) in adults: Report of two cases with emphasis on differential diagnosis. *Am. J. Surg. Pathol.* **1998**, *22*, 459–464. [CrossRef] [PubMed]
14. Mentzel, T.; Katenkamp, D. Sclerosing, pseudovascular rhabdomyosarcoma in adults. Clinicopathological and immunohistochemical analysis of three cases. *Virchows Arch.* **2000**, *436*, 305–311. [CrossRef] [PubMed]
15. Carroll, S.J.; Nodit, L. Spindle cell rhabdomyosarcoma: A brief diagnostic review and differential diagnosis. *Arch. Pathol. Lab. Med.* **2013**, *137*, 1155–1158. [CrossRef] [PubMed]

16. Alaggio, R.; Zhang, L.; Sung, Y.S.; Huang, S.C.; Chen, C.L.; Bisogno, G.; Zin, A.; Agaram, N.P.; LaQuaglia, M.P.; Wexler, L.H.; et al. A Molecular Study of Pediatric Spindle and Sclerosing Rhabdomyosarcoma: Identification of Novel and Recurrent VGLL2-related Fusions in Infantile Cases. *Am. J. Surg. Pathol.* **2016**, *40*, 224–235. [CrossRef] [PubMed]
17. Agaram, N.; Szuhai, K. Spindle cell/sclerosing rhabdomyosarcoma. In *WHO Classification of Tumours Editorial Board—Soft Tissue and Bone Tumours*, 5th ed.; WHO Press: Geneve, Switzerland; International Agency for Research on Cancer: Lyon, France, 2020; pp. 211–213.
18. Weiss, S.; Goldblum, J. *Soft Tissue Tumors*, 5th ed.; Applied Pathology; Elsevier-Saunders: Philadelphia, PA, USA, 1988; Volume 6, pp. 153–240.
19. Jakkampudi, A.; Kaliyath, S.; Hegde, P.; Mathias, M.; Shetty, V. Spindle cell rhabdomyosarcoma in the adult: A rare case report. *J. Oral Maxillofac. Pathol.* **2022**, *26* (Suppl. S1), S103.
20. Parham, D.M.B.F. Embryonal rhabdomyosarcoma. In *WHO Classification of Tumours. Pathology and Genetics of Tumours of Soft Tissue and Bone*; Fletcher, C.D., Bridge, J.A., Hogendoorn, P.C.M.F., Eds.; IARC Press: Lyon, France, 2013; pp. 127–129.
21. Agaram, N.P.; LaQuaglia, M.P.; Alaggio, R.; Zhang, L.; Fujisawa, Y.; Ladanyi, M.; Wexler, L.H.; Antonescu, C.R. MYOD1-mutant spindle cell and sclerosing rhabdomyosarcoma: An aggressive subtype irrespective of age. A reappraisal for molecular classification and risk stratification. *Mod. Pathol.* **2019**, *32*, 27–36. [CrossRef] [PubMed]
22. Little, D.J.; Ballo, M.T.; Zagars, G.K.; Pisters, P.W.T.; Patel, S.R.; El-Naggar, A.K.; Garden, A.S.; Benjamin, R.S. Adult rhabdomyosarcoma: Outcome following multimodality treatment. *Cancer* **2002**, *95*, 377–388. [CrossRef]
23. Nascimento, A.F.; Fletcher, C.D.M. Spindle cell rhabdomyosarcoma in adults. *Am. J. Surg. Pathol.* **2005**, *29*, 1106–1113. [CrossRef]
24. Hawkins, W.G.; Hoos, A.; Antonescu, C.R.; Urist, M.J.; Leung, D.H.; Gold, J.S.; Woodruff, J.M.; Lewis, J.J.; Brennan, M.F. Clinicopathologic analysis of patients with adult rhabdomyosarcoma. *Cancer* **2001**, *91*, 794–803. [CrossRef]
25. Stock, N.; Chibon, F.; Nguyen Binh, M.B.; Terrier, P.; Michels, J.J.; Valo, I.; Robin, Y.M.; Guillou, L.; Ranchère-Vince, D.; Decouvelaere, A.V.; et al. Adult-type rhabdomyosarcoma: Analysis of 57 cases with clinicopathologic description, identification of 3 morphologic patterns and prognosis. *Am. J. Surg. Pathol.* **2009**, *33*, 1850–1859. [CrossRef]
26. Hartmann, S.; Lessner, G.; Mentzel, T.; Kübler, A.C.; Müller-Richter, U.D.A. An adult spindle cell rhabdomyosarcoma in the head and neck region with long-term survival: A case report. *J. Med. Case Rep.* **2014**, *8*, 208. [CrossRef] [PubMed]
27. Łomiak, M.; Świtaj, T.; Spałek, M.; Radzikowska, J.; Chojnacka, M.; Falkowski, S.; Wągrodzki, M.; Kukwa, W.; Szumera-Ciećkiewicz, A.; Rutkowski, P.; et al. Diagnosis and treatment of rhabdomyosarcomas. *Oncol. Clin. Pract.* **2023**. [CrossRef]
28. Kohsaka, S.; Shukla, N.; Ameur, N.; Ito, T.; Ng, C.K.Y.; Wang, L.; Lim, D.; Marchetti, A.; Viale, A.; Pirun, M.; et al. A recurrent neomorphic mutation in MYOD1 defines a clinically aggressive subset of embryonal rhabdomyosarcoma associated with PI3K-AKT pathway mutations. *Nat. Genet.* **2014**, *46*, 595–600. [CrossRef] [PubMed]
29. Watson, S.; Perrin, V.; Guillemot, D.; Reynaud, S.; Coindre, J.M.; Karanian, M.; Guinebretière, J.M.; Freneaux, P.; Le Loarer, F.; Bouvet, M.; et al. Transcriptomic definition of molecular subgroups of small round cell sarcomas. *J. Pathol.* **2018**, *245*, 29–40. [CrossRef] [PubMed]
30. Agaram, N.P.; Zhang, L.; Sung, Y.S.; Cavalcanti, M.S.; Torrence, D.; Wexler, L.; Francis, G.; Sommerville, S.; Swanson, D.; Dickson, B.C.; et al. Expanding the Spectrum of Intraosseous Rhabdomyosarcoma: Correlation between Two Distinct Gene Fusions and Phenotype. *Am. J. Surg. Pathol.* **2019**, *43*, 695. [CrossRef]
31. Chrisinger, J.S.A.; Wehrli, B.; Dickson, B.C.; Fasih, S.; Hirbe, A.C.; Shultz, D.B.; Zadeh, G.; Gupta, A.A.; Demicco, E.G. Epithelioid and spindle cell rhabdomyosarcoma with FUS-TFCP2 or EWSR1-TFCP2 fusion: Report of two cases. *Virchows Arch.* **2020**, *477*, 725–732. [CrossRef]
32. Wong, D.D.; van Vliet, C.; Gaman, A.; Giardina, T.; Amanuel, B. Rhabdomyosarcoma with FUS re-arrangement: Additional case in support of a novel subtype. *Pathology* **2019**, *51*, 116–120. [CrossRef] [PubMed]
33. Dashti, N.K.; Wehrs, R.N.; Thomas, B.C.; Nair, A.; Davila, J.; Buckner, J.C.; Martinez, A.P.; Sukov, W.R.; Halling, K.C.; Howe, B.M.; et al. Spindle cell rhabdomyosarcoma of bone with FUS–TFCP2 fusion: Confirmation of a very recently described rhabdomyosarcoma subtype. *Histopathology* **2018**, *73*, 514–520. [CrossRef]
34. Tagami, Y.; Sugita, S.; Kubo, T.; Iesato, N.; Emori, M.; Takada, K.; Tsujiwaki, M.; Segawa, K.; Sugawara, T.; Kikuchi, T.; et al. Spindle cell rhabdomyosarcoma in a lumbar vertebra with FUS-TFCP2 fusion. *Pathol. Res. Pract.* **2019**, *215*, 152399. [CrossRef]
35. Le Loarer, F.; Cleven, A.H.G.; Bouvier, C.; Castex, M.P.; Romagosa, C.; Moreau, A.; Salas, S.; Bonhomme, B.; Gomez-Brouchet, A.; Laurent, C.; et al. A subset of epithelioid and spindle cell rhabdomyosarcomas is associated with TFCP2 fusions and common ALK upregulation. *Mod. Pathol.* **2020**, *33*, 404–419. [CrossRef]
36. Leuschner, I.; Newton, W.; Schmidt, D.; Sachs, N.; Asmar, L.; Hamoudi, A.; Harms, D.; Maurer, H.M. Spindle Cell Variants of Embryonal Rhabdomyosarcoma in the Paratesticular Region A Report of the Intergroup Rhabdomyosarcoma Study. *Am. J. Surg. Pathol.* **1993**, *17*, 858. [CrossRef] [PubMed]
37. Kaçar, A.; Demir, H.A.; Durak, H.; Dervişoğlu, S. Spindle cell rhabdomyosarcoma displaying CD34 positivity: A potential diagnostic pitfall; report of two pediatric cases. *Turk. Patoloji Derg.* **2013**, *29*, 221–226. [PubMed]
38. Zhao, Z.; Yin, Y.; Zhang, J.; Qi, J.; Zhang, D.; Ma, Y.; Wang, Y.; Li, S.; Zhou, J. Spindle cell/sclerosing rhabdomyosarcoma: Case series from a single institution emphasizing morphology, immunohistochemistry and follow-up. *Int. J. Clin. Exp. Pathol.* **2015**, *8*, 13814. [PubMed]

39. Smith, M.H.; Atherton, D.; Reith, J.D.; Islam, N.M.; Bhattacharyya, I.; Cohen, D.M. Rhabdomyosarcoma, Spindle Cell/Sclerosing Variant: A Clinical and Histopathological Examination of this Rare Variant with Three New Cases from the Oral Cavity. *Head. Neck Pathol.* **2017**, *11*, 494. [CrossRef]
40. Meza, J.L.; Anderson, J.; Pappo, A.S.; Meyer, W.H. Analysis of prognostic factors in patients with nonmetastatic rhabdomyosarcoma treated on intergroup rhabdomyosarcoma studies III and IV: The children's oncology group. *J. Clin. Oncol.* **2006**, *24*, 3844–3851. [CrossRef] [PubMed]
41. Borinstein, S.C.; Steppan, D.; Hayashi, M.; Loeb, D.M.; Isakoff, M.S.; Binitie, O.; Brohl, A.S.; Bridge, J.A.; Stavas, M.; Shinohara, E.T.; et al. Consensus and controversies regarding the treatment of rhabdomyosarcoma. *Pediatr. Blood Cancer* **2018**, *65*, e26809. [CrossRef] [PubMed]
42. Ladra, M.M.; Szymonifka, J.D.; Mahajan, A.; Friedmann, A.M.; Yeap, B.Y.; Goebel, C.P.; MacDonald, S.M.; Grosshans, D.R.; Rodriguez-Galindo, C.; Marcus, K.J.; et al. Preliminary results of a phase II trial of proton radiotherapy for pediatric rhabdomyosarcoma. *J. Clin. Oncol.* **2014**, *32*, 3762–3770. [CrossRef]
43. Benkhaled, S.; Mané, M.; Jungels, C.; Shumelinsky, F.; Aubain, N.D.; Saint Van Gestel, D. Successful treatment of synchronous chemoresistant pulmonary metastasis from pleomorphic rhabdomyosarcoma with stereotaxic body radiation therapy: A case report and a review of the literature. *Cancer Treat. Res. Commun.* **2021**, *26*, 100282. [CrossRef]
44. Esnaola, N.F.; Rubin, B.P.; Baldini, E.H.; Vasudevan, N.; Demetri, G.D.; Fletcher, C.D.M.; Singer, S. Response to Chemotherapy and Predictors of Survival in Adult Rhabdomyosarcoma. *Ann. Surg.* **2001**, *234*, 215. [CrossRef]
45. Kojima, Y.; Hashimoto, K.; Ando, M.; Yonemori, K.; Yamamoto, H.; Kodaira, M.; Yunokawa, M.; Shimizu, C.; Tamura, K.; Hosono, A.; et al. Comparison of dose intensity of vincristine, dactinomycin, and cyclophosphamide chemotherapy for child and adult rhabdomyosarcoma: A retrospective analysis. *Cancer Chemother. Pharmacol.* **2012**, *70*, 391–397. [CrossRef]
46. Raney, R.B.; Maurer, H.M.; Anderson, J.R.; Andrassy, R.J.; Donaldson, S.S.; Qualman, S.J.; Wharam, M.D.; Wiener, E.S.; Crist, W.M. The Intergroup Rhabdomyosarcoma Study Group (IRSG): Major Lessons From the IRS-I Through IRS-IV Studies as Background for the Current IRS-V Treatment Protocols. *Sarcoma* **2001**, *5*, 925281. [CrossRef]
47. Simon, J.H.; Paulino, A.C.; Ritchie, J.M.; Mayr, N.A.; Buatti, J.M. Presentation, Prognostic Factors and Patterns of Failure in Adult Rhabdomyosarcoma. *Sarcoma* **2003**, *7*, 147. [CrossRef]
48. Keskin, S.; Ekenel, M.; Basaran, M.; Kilicaslan, I.; Tunc, M.; Bavbek, S. Clinicopathological characteristics and treatment outcomes of adult patients with paratesticular rhabdomyosarcoma (PRMS): A 10-year single-centre experience. *Can. Urol. Assoc. J.* **2012**, *6*, 42. [CrossRef]

Disclaimer/Publisher's Note: The statements, opinions and data contained in all publications are solely those of the individual author(s) and contributor(s) and not of MDPI and/or the editor(s). MDPI and/or the editor(s) disclaim responsibility for any injury to people or property resulting from any ideas, methods, instructions or products referred to in the content.

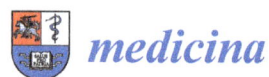 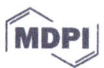

Case Report

The Philadelphia Chromosome, from Negative to Positive: A Case Report of Relapsed Acute Lymphoblastic Leukemia Following Allogeneic Stem Cell Transplantation

Elena-Cristina Marinescu [1,2,*], Horia Bumbea [1,2], Iuliana Iordan [1,2,3], Ion Dumitru [2], Dan Soare [1,2], Cristina Ciufu [1,2] and Mihaela Gaman [2,4]

1. Department of Methodology and Scientific Research, "Carol Davila" University of Medicine and Pharmacy, Eroilor Sanitari Boulevard, No. 8, 050474 Bucharest, Romania
2. Department of Hematology, Emergency University Hospital of Bucharest, Splaiul Independentei, No. 169, 050098 Bucharest, Romania
3. Department of Medical Semiology and Nephrology, "Carol Davila" University of Medicine and Pharmacy, 050474 Bucharest, Romania
4. Department of Hematology, "Carol Davila" University of Medicine and Pharmacy, Eroilor Sanitari Boulevard, No. 8, 050474 Bucharest, Romania
* Correspondence: mecrystyna13@yahoo.com; Tel.: +40-213180522

Abstract: Relapsed acute lymphoblastic leukemia (ALL) represents a continuous challenge for the clinician. Despite recent advances in treatment, the risk of relapse remains significant. The clinical, biological, cytogenetic, and molecular characteristics may be different at the time of relapse. Current comprehensive genome sequencing studies suggest that most relapsed patients, especially those with late relapses, acquire new genetic abnormalities, usually within a minor clone that emerges after ALL diagnosis. We report the case of a 23-year-old young woman diagnosed with Philadelphia chromosome-negative B cell acute lymphoblastic leukemia. The patient underwent allogeneic stem cell transplantation (allo-HSCT) after complete remission. Despite having favorable prognostic factors at diagnosis, the disease relapsed early after allo-HSCT. The cytogenetic and molecular exams at relapse were positive for the Philadelphia chromosome, respectively for the Bcr-Abl transcript. What exactly led to the recurrence of this disease in a more aggressive cytogenetic and molecular form, although there were no predictive elements at diagnosis?

Keywords: acute lymphoblastic leukemia; Philadelphia chromosome; relapse; allogeneic stem cell transplantation

Citation: Marinescu, E.-C.; Bumbea, H.; Iordan, I.; Dumitru, I.; Soare, D.; Ciufu, C.; Gaman, M. The Philadelphia Chromosome, from Negative to Positive: A Case Report of Relapsed Acute Lymphoblastic Leukemia Following Allogeneic Stem Cell Transplantation. *Medicina* **2023**, *59*, 671. https://doi.org/10.3390/medicina59040671

Academic Editors: Valentin Titus Grigorean and Daniel Alin Cristian

Received: 9 February 2023
Revised: 14 March 2023
Accepted: 22 March 2023
Published: 28 March 2023

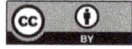

Copyright: © 2023 by the authors. Licensee MDPI, Basel, Switzerland. This article is an open access article distributed under the terms and conditions of the Creative Commons Attribution (CC BY) license (https://creativecommons.org/licenses/by/4.0/).

1. Introduction

Acute lymphoblastic leukemia (ALL) is the most common childhood cancer, but is less common in adolescents and young adults (AYA) and is rare in older adults. AYA is an age between 15 and 49 years, depending on the study. Patients with B precursor ALL-AYA are known to have worse outcomes and more treatment-related toxicities compared with children. The 5-year survival rate of ALL is higher than 90% in children [1], but falls significantly to 60–85% in adolescents and young adults ([2], pp. 3660–3668) and to less than 30% in older adults [3].

In terms of clinical and biological characteristics and response to treatment, AYA-ALL differs from the pediatric ALL population. Lower event-free and survival rates in AYA patients are due in part to unfavorable tumor biology. Although survival of adolescents and young adults with acute lymphoblastic leukemia has improved with the use of pediatric-inspired protocols [4], the results of those who relapse remain poor.

The Philadelphia chromosome (Ph) is the most common cytogenetic abnormality in adult patients with acute lymphoblastic leukemia, occurring in about 20% to 30% of all cases [5]. The incidence increases with age and represents the most common form of ALL in the elderly population and is therefore a relatively rare event in AYA (less than 20%) [6]. Patients with Ph-positive ALL are at increased risk for central nervous system (CNS) involvement and an aggressive clinical course. Historically, they have had worse outcome compared to their Ph-negative counterparts [7]. However, the outcomes of patients with Ph-ALL have changed dramatically with the addition of tyrosine kinase inhibitors (TKI) to cytotoxic chemotherapy, increasing the rate of complete response to as high as 90% [8].

Risk stratification by cytogenetics and molecular genetics reflects the prognostic heterogeneity of ALL that determines which patients are at a high risk of relapse and should be considered for more intensive treatment strategies, including allogeneic stem cell transplantation.

Also, minimal residual disease (MRD) assessment plays a central role in risk stratification and treatment guidance in patients with ALL. MRD assessment is of extreme prognostic importance, as MRD is one of the most important risk factors for relapse, as confirmed by multivariate prognostic analyses in many studies [9]. Measurable residual disease is the amount of cancer cells that remain after therapy. MRD is not a classic biomarker, but a measure of actual disease burden. Patients with morphologic complete remission (CR) may also have MRD. Laboratory techniques for MRD testing in ALL provide a higher degree of sensitivity and specificity than morphology. Current MRD testing includes flow cytometry (FC), polymerase chain reaction (PCR), and more recently, next-generation sequencing (NGS). MRD assessment by FC has a sensitivity of 10^{-4} (standard) to 10^{-5}, by PCR a sensitivity of 10^{-4} to 10^{-5}, while the NGS method has the highest sensitivity, at 10^{-6}.

Various studies show that the lower the level of MRD before HSCT and the better the results, the lower the risk of relapse [10]. However, it is still unclear what is the best treatment approach in case of MRD positivity. Early systemic relapses, occurring within the first 12 months after allogeneic hematopoietic stem cell transplantation, have a poor prognosis with a median survival of 7.4 months and a long-term survival rate of only 20–30% [11].

Although therapy for ALL has made great strides in recent years, relapses are still present in a high percentage of cases and present a challenge to the clinician. Identification of predictive risk factors for relapse is necessary at diagnosis and it is also necessary to evaluate them during the development and treatment of the disease.

The case of ALL, presented below, represents a rarer situation of early relapse after bone marrow transplantation, involving the occurrence of a cytogenetic change with an unfavorable prognosis that was not present at diagnosis. It was a challenge to identify the possible factors that could have caused this rather atypical relapse (Figure 1).

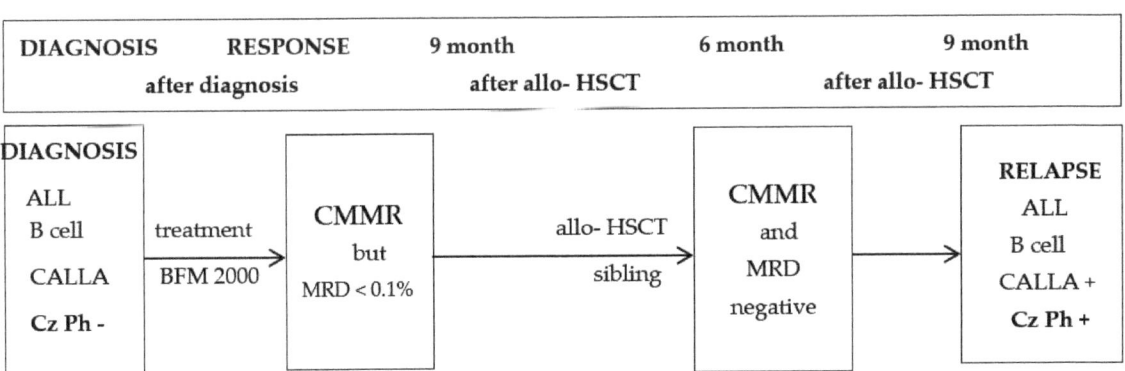

Figure 1. Evolution of disease. CMMR = complete medullary morphological remission; MRD = minimum residual disease; Allo-HSCT = allogeneic hematopoietic stem cell transplantation; Cz Ph = Philadelphia Chromosome.

2. Presentation

We discuss the case of a 21-year-old woman who came to the emergency department with altered general condition, fatigue, loss of appetite, cough, fever, and purpura. Her medical history was irrelevant. Laboratory findings on admission revealed life-threatening anemia (a hemoglobin of 2.3 g/dL), severe thrombocytopenia (a platelet count of 24×10^9/L), and a normal leukocyte count of 6.8×10^9/L. In the peripheral blood smear (PBS), we found 6% medium-sized blasts with a morphological aspect suggestive of lymphoblasts (ALL-1, according to the FAB classification). Bone marrow examination revealed involvement of 38% blasts similar to those described in PBS.

Immunophenotyping by flow cytometry from bone marrow aspirate identified 33% cells with the following aspect: SSC low, CD34+, cMPO-, cCD79a+, cCD3-, CD3-, CD7-, CD117-, CD13-, CD33-, CD10+ (CALLA), CD19+, CD20-, sIgM kappa, lambda-, CD66c- (KOR-SA), NG.2-, CD123-, cTdT-, CD58-. The described are based on the diagnosis of acute B-cell lymphoblastic leukemia, positive for CALLA, not otherwise specified, according to the 2016 World Health Organization (WHO) criteria.

Cytogenetic examination carried out on 10 metaphases revealed that there were no numerical or structural alterations in chromosomes at this level of resolution (it should be noted that the cellularity of the bone marrow aspirate was low). In addition, a molecular study was performed that did not detect the Bcr-Abl transcript or the MLL fusion gene.

At the time of diagnosis, the patient had no neurologic signs or symptoms. Cerebrospinal fluid (CSF) studies and imaging also did not describe central nervous system (CNS) involvement.

Taking into account the available data—young age, normal white blood cells, precursor of the B lineage, positive for CALLA (CD10+), no evidence of CNS involvement, and no Philadelphia chromosome—we classified the patient in a standard risk group.

Based on the preponderance of the data presented in the review, the best therapeutic approach for this patient would be intensive pediatric treatment. We decided to treat according to the Berlin-Frankfurt-Münster (BFM) protocol because we knew the following data from the literature. The BFM 2000 protocol consisted of the following stages: induction (prednisone, vincristine, daunorubicin, PEG -asparaginase, intrathecal methotrexate), early intensification (cyclophosphamide, cytarabine, 6-mercaptopurine, intrathecal methotrexate), consolidation (combination of dexamethasone, vincristine, vindensine HD-cytarabine, HD-methotrexate, cyclophosphamide, ifosfamide, PEG–asparaginase, etoposide, intrathecal therapy), and re-induction therapy (dexamethasone, vincristine, doxorubicin, PEG–asparaginase, cyclophosphamide, cytarabine, 6-thioguanine), followed by maintenance (6-mercaptopurine, methotrexate).

The patient achieved complete morphological marrow remission immediately after the induction phase. After the reinduction phase, i.e., 9 months after the start of treatment, the patient was still in complete morphologic remission, without CNS damage, but with the presence of minimal residual disease of less than 0.1% as determined by flow cytometry. It should be noted that no major infectious or hemorrhagic complications or other severe toxicities occurred during chemotherapy according to the BFM protocol, except for grade 2–3 hepatic cytolysis, which was controlled by hepatoprotective treatment.

At this time, the patient underwent allo-HSCT from a matched related donor, knowing that MRD is the most important prognostic information and decision support for allocation to allogeneic hematopoietic stem cell transplantation. The procedure was successful, with no major complications and no graft-versus-host disease (GVHD). Chemotherapy-based myeloablative transplant conditioning regimens were applied without total body irradiation (TBI) for technical reasons. Six months after allo-HSCT, the patient was in complete remission, with negative MRD and 100% chimerism.

After another three months, the patient came to the scheduled follow-up in good general condition. However, PBS revealed a recurrence of blast cells, which raised suspicion of relapse of the disease. We performed a reexamination to determine the current state of the disease. Morphologically, the blasts had a similar appearance to that at diagnosis (ALL-1). The bone marrow aspirate showed the presence of 85% lymphoblasts.

The immunophenotypic aspect of the bone marrow blast cells showed some changes from the time of diagnosis, namely the positivity of the CD66c marker (KOR-SA), indicating the likelihood of the presence of the Philadelphia chromosome (Figure 2). This suspicion was confirmed by the result of the cytogenetic and molecular examinations. The Philadelphia chromosome was detected in 34% of the analyzed 10 metaphases. In 45.1% of malignant cells, molecular analysis identified the Bcr-Abl e1a2 transcript (m-Bcr) corresponding to protein p190. An examination of the central nervous system was also performed, and no relapse was found at this level.

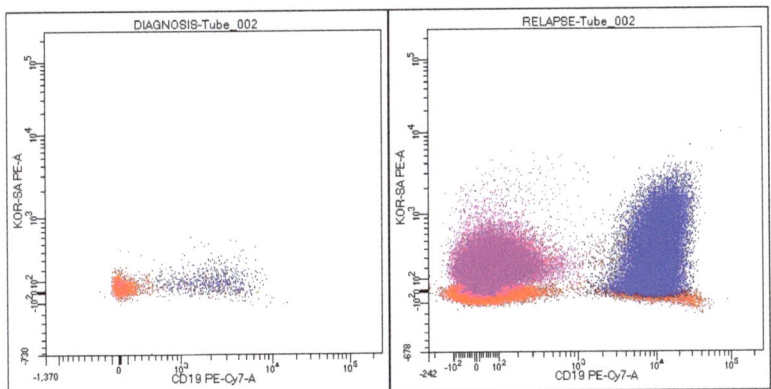

Figure 2. Immunophenotypic expression of KOR-SA at diagnosis versus relapse. In blue: CD19+ blasts (and CD34+). In violet: granulocytes as internal control (almost absent at diagnosis due to the hypocellular marrow sample and consequently few events).

At this point, in the face of a relapse with the presence of the Philadelphia chromosome, we decided to initiate treatment with dasatinib, knowing that this TKI has the advantage of preventing CNS involvement. The selected dose of dasatinib was 70 mg/day. Given the corticosteroid sensitivity the disease exhibited at the time of diagnosis, dexamethasone therapy was also administered.

After only 3 days of TKI treatment, we observed the disappearance of blast precursors from peripheral blood. The occurrence of grade 2–3 liver toxicity was noted, which required the interruption of TKI treatment. Complete remission of liver toxicity occurred after 7 days of dasatinib treatment. Subsequently, TKI was administered again, but at a dose reduced to 50 mg/day. It should be mentioned that there were no other toxicities, either hematologic or nonhematologic of higher magnitude, that would require interruption of treatment.

Very quickly, after another week of treatment with dasatinib, bone marrow evaluation already showed morphologic remission and Bcr-Abl transcript was no longer detected. It should be noted that the sample studied was from peripheral blood and the number of copies was reduced.

At this time, the patient is on treatment with dasatinib 3 months after relapse after bone marrow transplantation, with maintenance of morphologic and molecular remission, and is awaiting CAR-T therapy as a bridge to a second bone marrow transplantation.

3. Discussion

AYA with ALL represent a special subset of patients compared with the pediatric or adult population.

Although the survival rate for most children with ALL is now 90%, older adolescents and young adults historically have a much worse prognosis, with an event-free survival rate (EFS) of only 30% to 45% [12].

Over the past decade, treatment outcomes for AYA patients have improved with a disease-free survival rate of 60% to 70% when treated with pediatric approaches [13].

The superiority of pediatric approaches for the AYA population has now been demonstrated in several retrospective analyses, with higher complete remission rates, higher event-free survival, lower risk of relapse, and with comparable rates of nonrelapse mortality.

However, the number of cases of AYA-ALL that relapse remains high and is a challenge.

This case of acute lymphoblastic leukemia with a precursor of the B lineage, Ph-negative, with early relapse less than one year after HSCT (although the initial features of the disease placed the patient in a low-risk group) raises several questions. There are certain biological characteristics that influence treatment response and survival.

In our case, the biological, morphological, immunophenotypic, cytogenetic, and molecular characteristics at the time of diagnosis were not predictive of relapse. Certain characteristics of blast cells might allow predictions of the presence of certain genetic or molecular alterations and of the prognosis. It is well known that the expression of the markers CD66c [14], CD33 [15] or CD13 [16] can be correlated with the presence of the Philadelphia chromosome. NG2 (neuronal glial antigen 2) also has predictive value for MLL rearrangements [17]. In our case, the absence of the Philadelphia chromosome, the BCR-ABL1 fusion gene, and the absence of the MLL gene was later confirmed by cytogenetic and molecular studies. The presence of CALLA provides a good prognosis for the disease.

On the other hand, the pattern of ALL cytogenetics at AYA differ from that of the pediatric population. For example, a newly recognized unfavorable risk entity, BCR-ABL1-like (Ph-like) ALL, describes a category of B cells in ALL characterized by gene expression profiles similar to those of BCR-ABL1 ALL but lacking BCR-ABL1 translocation [18]. The incidence of Ph-like ALL appears to peak in adolescents, with a prevalence of nearly 30% (compared with 10% in children and 20–25% in older adults), and Ph-like ALL is associated with a poor prognosis across the age spectrum [19].

Overall, the lower incidence of cytogenetic abnormalities associated with favorable outcome, combined with the higher proportion of patients with low-risk genetic features, such as Ph+ and Ph-like ALL, in AYA patients contributes to their poorer survival compared with children. In our case, this evaluation of the presence or absence of this genetic abnormality could not be performed.

The choice of treatment was made with knowledge of the data from the literature, which states that the patients with AYA-ALL treated with the BFM protocol had high overall survival (OS) and complete remission (CRD) rates and tolerated this pediatric regimen with acceptable toxicity. The OS and CRD rates were comparable to those achieved with hyper-CVAD, an adult leukemia therapy ([2], pp. 3589–3754)

The persistence of minimal residual disease at the end of chemotherapy led to the indication of bone marrow allotransplantation. When feasible, allogeneic HSCT is preferable to standard intensive pediatric chemotherapy in MRD-positive patients to reduce the risk of relapse and increase survival from ≤25% without HSCT to approximately 45–55% (GMALL, NILG, GRAALL studies, reviewed by Bassan et al.) [9].

However, 9 months after bone marrow transplantation, the patient relapsed with a new chromosomal change (Philadelphia chromosome) compared to the time of diagnosis, although 9 months after transplantation, minimal residual disease was negative and chimerism was 100%.

Measurement of donor chimerism using peripheral blood and/or bone marrow samples is an alternative method for detecting residual or impending disease recurrence. Assessment of donor chimerism may be particularly valuable in patients for early detection of impending relapse when a reliable MRD marker has been lost and/or cannot be determined after transplantation [20]. Data suggest that the relevance of low MRD positivity after allo-HCT depends on the time elapsed since transplantation. In a study of pediatric patients, the longer the time has elapsed from the time of transplantation, the higher the risk of treatment failure in the presence of low-level MRD [10].

Several hypotheses can be considered that underlie the relapse of the disease: Was there a dormant clone that could not be identified at diagnosis that escaped immune system control? Is this mutation acquired during the development of the disease or is it secondary to treatment? Could possible contamination by the donor also be considered? Did the use of a myeloablative conditioning regimen in TBI potentially favor relapse?

In view of all this, the question arises of whether it would not be more effective to include TKIs in treatment in prophylactic doses and after certain clinical trials, starting from the diagnosis of ALL.

Relapse after allo-HSCT in patients with ALL has a poor prognosis. However, in modern times, outcomes and management of this group of patients have improved. The advent of immunotherapy, deep insights into the molecular mechanisms leading to resistance, and the discovery of new targeted therapies have led to numerous clinical trials and provide new hope for this patient group.

4. Conclusions

The Philadelphia chromosome is the most common cytogenetic alteration associated with acute lymphoblastic leukemia. It leads to an unfavorable prognosis for the disease. However, the introduction and development of TKIs have improved response rate and survival in this disease. The Philadelphia chromosome may be present at diagnosis or may occur later in the course of the disease and contribute to relapse of the disease.

It is extremely important that, in the case of acute leukemia relapse but also throughout the evolution of the disease, a complete and thorough reevaluation, both morphological and immunophenotypic, as well as cytogenetic and molecular, is carried out, because there may be acquisitions of new changes compared to the time of diagnosis, which require other targeted lines of treatment.

Author Contributions: Conceptualization, E.-C.M. and H.B.; methodology, E.-C.M.; software, E.-C.M., I.I. and I.D.; validation, H.B. and I.D.; formal analysis, E.-C.M.; investigation, E.-C.M.; resources, I.I.; data curation, I.D.; writing—original draft preparation, E.-C.M.; writing—review and editing, D.S.; visualization, M.G.; spuervision, C.C.; project administration, E.-C.M.; funding acquisition, E.-C.M. All authors have read and agreed to the published version of the manuscript.

Funding: This research received no external funding.

Institutional Review Board Statement: Not applicable.

Informed Consent Statement: Not applicable.

Data Availability Statement: Not applicable.

Conflicts of Interest: The authors declare no conflict of interest.

References

1. Inaba, H.; Mullighan, C.G. Pediatric acute lymphoblastic leukemia. *Haematologica* **2020**, *105*, 2524–2539. [CrossRef] [PubMed]
2. Rytting, M.E.; Thomas, D.A.; O'Brien, S.M.; Ravandi-Kashani, F.; Jabbour, E.J.; Franklin, A.R.; Kadia, T.M.; Pemmaraju, N.; Daver, N.G.; Ferrajoli, A.; et al. Augmented Berlin-Frankfurt-Münster therapy in adolescents and young adults (AYAs) with acute lymphoblastic leukemia (ALL). *Cancer* **2014**, *120*, 3660–3668. [CrossRef] [PubMed]
3. Sive, J.I.; Buck, G.; Fielding, A.; Lazarus, H.M.; Litzow, M.R.; Luger, S.; Marks, D.I.; McMillan, A.; Moorman, A.V.; Richards, S.M.; et al. Outcomes in older adults with acute lymphoblastic leukaemia (ALL): Results from the international MRC UKALL XII/ECOG2993 trial. *Br. J. Haematol.* **2012**, *157*, 463–471. [CrossRef] [PubMed]
4. Stock, W.; Luger, S.M.; Advani, A.S.; Yin, J.; Harvey, R.C.; Mullighan, C.G.; Willman, C.L.; Fulton, N.; Laumann, K.M.; Malnassy, G.; et al. A pediatric regimen for older adolescents and young adults with acute lymphoblastic leukemia: Results of CALGB 10403. *Blood J. Am. Soc. Hematol.* **2019**, *133*, 1548–1559. [CrossRef] [PubMed]
5. Burmeister, T.; Schwartz, S.; Bartram, C.R.; Gokbuget, N.; Hoelzer, D.; Thiel, E. Patients' age and BCR-ABL frequency in adult B-precursor ALL: A retrospective analysis from the GMALL study group. *Blood J. Am. Soc. Hematol.* **2008**, *112*, 918–919. [CrossRef] [PubMed]
6. Moorman, A.V. New and emerging prognostic and predictive genetic biomarkers in B-cell precursor acute lymphoblastic leukemia. *Haematologica* **2016**, *101*, 407–416. [CrossRef] [PubMed]

7. Gleibetaner, B.; Gleißner, B.; Gökbuget, N.; Bartram, C.R.; Janssen, B.; Rieder, H.; Janssen, J.W.G.; Fonatsch, C.; Heyll, A.; Voliotis, D.; et al. Leading prognostic relevance of the BCR-ABL translocation in adult acute B-lineage lymphoblastic leukemia: A prospective study of the German Multicenter Trial Group and confirmed polymerase chain reaction analysis. *Blood* **2002**, *99*, 1536–1543. [CrossRef] [PubMed]
8. Sasaki, K.; Kantarjian, H.M.; Short, N.J.; Samra, B.; Khoury, J.D.; Shamanna, R.K.; Konopleva, M.; Jain, N.; DiNardo, C.D.; Khouri, R.; et al. Prognostic factors for progression in patients with Philadelphia chromosome-positive acute lymphoblastic leukemia in complete molecular response within 3 months of therapy with tyrosine kinase inhibitors. *Cancer* **2021**, *127*, 2648–2656. [CrossRef] [PubMed]
9. Bassan, R.; Intermesoli, T.; Scattolin, A.; Viero, P.; Maino, E.; Sancetta, R.; Carobolante, F.; Gianni, F.; Stefanoni, P.; Tosi, M.; et al. Minimal residual disease assessment and risk-based therapy in acute lymphoblastic leukemia. *Clin. Lymphoma Myeloma Leuk.* **2017**, *17S*, S2–S9. [CrossRef] [PubMed]
10. Balduzzi, A.; Di Maio, L.; Silvestri, D.; Songia, S.; Bonanomi, S.; Rovelli, A.; Conter, V.; Biondi, A.; Cazzaniga, G.; Valsecchi, M.G. Minimal residual disease before and after transplantation for childhood acute lymphoblastic leukaemia: Is there any room for intervention? *Br. J. Haematol.* **2014**, *164*, 396–408. [CrossRef] [PubMed]
11. Kuhlen, M.; Willasch, A.M.; Dalle, J.H.; Wachowiak, J.; Yaniv, I.; Ifversen, M.; Sedlacek, P.; Guengoer, T.; Lang, P.; Bader, P.; et al. Outcome of relapse after allogeneic HSCT in children with ALL enrolled in the ALL-SCT 2003/2007 trial. *Br. J. Haematol.* **2018**, *180*, 82–89. [CrossRef] [PubMed]
12. Pulte, D.; Gondos, A.; Brenner, H. Trends in survival after diagnosis with hematologic malignancy in adolescence or young adulthood in the United States, 1981–2005. *Cancer* **2009**, *115*, 4973–4979. [CrossRef] [PubMed]
13. Boissel, N.; Auclerc, M.F.; Lhéritier, V.; Perel, Y.; Thomas, X.; Leblanc, T.; Rousselot, P.; Cayuela, J.M.; Gabert, J.; Fegueux, N.; et al. Should adolescents with acute lymphoblastic leukemia be treated as old children or young adults? Comparison of the French FRALLE-93 and LALA-94 trials. *J. Clin. Oncol.* **2003**, *21*, 774–780. [CrossRef] [PubMed]
14. Owaidah, T.M.; Rawas, F.I.; Al khayatt, M.F.; Elkum, N.B. Expression of CD66c and CD25 in Acute Lymphoblastic Leukemia as a Predictor of the Presence of BCR/ABL Rearrangement. *Hematol. Oncol. Stem Cell Ther.* **2008**, *1*, 34–37. [CrossRef] [PubMed]
15. Corrente, F.; Bellesi, S.; Metafuni, E.; Puggioni, P.L.; Marietti, S.; Ciminello, A.M.; Za, T.; Sorà, F.; Fianchi, L.; Sica, S.; et al. Role of Flow-Cytometric Immunophenotyping in Prediction of BCR/ABL1 Gene Rearrangement in Adult B-Cell Acute Lymphoblastic Leukemia: FLOW-CYTOMETRY IN BCR/ABL1 ADULT B-ALL. *Cytom. Clin. Cytom.* **2018**, *94*, 468–476. [CrossRef] [PubMed]
16. Hrušák, O.; Porwit-MacDonald, A. Antigen Expression Patterns Reflecting Genotype of Acute Leukemias. *Leukemia* **2002**, *16*, 1233–1258. [CrossRef] [PubMed]
17. Lopez-Millan, B.; Sanchéz-Martínez, D.; Roca-Ho, H.; Gutiérrez-Agüera, F.; Molina, O.; Diaz de la Guardia, R.; Torres-Ruiz, R.; Fuster, J.L.; Ballerini, P.; Suessbier, U.; et al. NG2 antigen is a therapeutic target for MLL-rearranged B-cell acute lymphoblastic leukemia. *Leukemia* **2019**, *33*, 1557–1569. [CrossRef] [PubMed]
18. Arber, D.A.; Orazi, A.; Hasserjian, R.; Thiele, J.; Borowitz, M.J.; Le Beau, M.M.; Bloomfield, C.D.; Cazzola, M.; Vardiman, J.W. The 2016 revision to the World Health Organization classification of myeloid neoplasms and acute leukemia. *Blood* **2016**, *127*, 2391–2405. [CrossRef] [PubMed]
19. Roberts, K.G.; Gu, Z.; Payne-Turner, D.; McCastlain, K.; Harvey, R.C.; Chen, I.-M.; Pei, D.; Iacobucci, I.; Valentine, M.; Pounds, S.B.; et al. High Frequency and Poor Outcome of Philadelphia Chromosome–Like Acute Lymphoblastic Leukemia in Adults. *J. Clin. Oncol.* **2017**, *35*, 394–401. [CrossRef] [PubMed]
20. Terwey, T.H.; Hemmati, P.G.; Nagy, M.; Pfeifer, H.; Gökbuget, N.; Brüggemann, M.; Le Duc, T.M.; le Coutre, P.; Dörken, B.; Arnold, R. Comparison of Chimerism and Minimal Residual Disease Monitoring for Relapse Prediction after Allogeneic Stem Cell Transplantation for Adult Acute Lymphoblastic Leukemia. *Biol. Blood Marrow Transplant.* **2014**, *20*, 1522–1529. [CrossRef] [PubMed]

Disclaimer/Publisher's Note: The statements, opinions and data contained in all publications are solely those of the individual author(s) and contributor(s) and not of MDPI and/or the editor(s). MDPI and/or the editor(s) disclaim responsibility for any injury to people or property resulting from any ideas, methods, instructions or products referred to in the content.

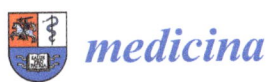

Case Report

The Use of Liquid Biopsy in the Molecular Analysis of Plasma Compared to the Tumour Tissue from a Patient with Brain Metastasis: A Case Report

Veronica Aran [1,*], Vinicius Mansur Zogbi [2], Renan Lyra Miranda [3], Felipe Andreiuolo [3], Nathalie Henriques Silva Canedo [3], Carolina Victor Nazaré [2], Paulo Niemeyer Filho [2] and Vivaldo Moura Neto [1]

1. Laboratório de Biomedicina do Cérebro, Instituto Estadual do Cérebro Paulo Niemeyer, Rua do Rezende156-Centro, Rio de Janeiro 20231-092, Brazil
2. Neurosurgery Division, Instituto Estadual do Cérebro Paulo Niemeyer, Rua do Rezende156-Centro, Rio de Janeiro 20231-092, Brazil
3. Neuropathology and Molecular Genetics Laboratory, Instituto Estadual Do Cérebro Paulo Niemeyer, Rua do Rezende156-Centro, Rio de Janeiro 20231-092, Brazil
* Correspondence: varanponte@gmail.com; Tel.: +55-2-19-7208-8811

Abstract: Different cancers have multiple genetic mutations, which vary depending on the affected tumour tissue. Small biopsies may not always represent all the genetic landscape of the tumour. To improve the chances of identifying mutations at different disease stages (early, during the disease course, and refractory stage), liquid biopsies offer an advantage to traditional tissue biopsy. In addition, it is possible to detect mutations related to metastatic events depending on the cancer types analysed as will be discussed in this case report, which describes a patient with brain metastasis and lung cancer that harboured *K-RAS* mutations both in the brain tumour and in the ctDNA present in the bloodstream.

Keywords: brain metastases; lung hepatoid adenocarcinoma; *K-RAS*; liquid biopsy; ddPCR

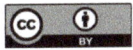

1. Introduction

The minimally invasive technique known as liquid biopsy can detect tumour-derived biomarkers in body fluids such as in blood. Circulating tumour DNA (ctDNA) refers to DNA of tumour origin, and being cell-free [1]. In fact, there are two sources of DNA that can be noninvasively assessed in blood circulation: cell-free circulating DNA (cfDNA) and the tumour-derived DNA fraction (ctDNA). They consist of small fragments of nucleic acid that are not associated with cells or cell fragments, and several studies have shown that ctDNA is present in advanced neoplasia [2]. This probably occurs because of apoptosis, cell necrosis, and active tumour secretion since tumour cell division occurs faster than normal cell division [3]. Thus, analysis of ctDNA is considered helpful in the prognosis, identification of alterations in different genes, selection of targeted therapies, and disease monitoring in cancer [4]. In addition, apart from blood (serum or plasma), sources of cfDNA/ctDNA include urine, saliva, cerebrospinal fluid, seminal fluid, and pleural fluid samples [3,5].

Plasma offers the possibility to give crucial molecular information via the analysis of ctDNA to detect cancer-related mutations in distinct tumour types, such as already described in the profiling of lung, colorectal, brain, and breast tumours, showing a promising perspective for clinical monitoring [6–9]. The first Food and Drug Administration (FDA) approval of a ctDNA liquid biopsy test occurred in 2016, being developed to detect epidermal growth factor receptor (*EGFR*) gene mutations in patients with non-small-cell lung cancer (NSCLC) as a companion diagnostic test. In recent years, multigene panel assays of liquid biopsy have been approved as companion diagnostics taking advantage of NGS methods for sequencing analyses [10]. The European Society for Medical Oncology

(ESMO) guidelines recommend validated liquid biopsies for genotyping of patients with advanced cancer even when tissue-based testing remains the gold standard procedure, due to limitations of ctDNA assays in detecting certain molecular alterations [11]. Nevertheless, ctDNA analysis is an important choice when tissue biopsies are not possible [11].

The anatomical site of tumours was shown to correlate with variable amounts of ctDNA levels in plasma, with brain tumours showing the lowest levels probably due to the presence of the blood−brain barrier (BBB) [2,12]. The brain is composed of unique cells that perform tissue-specific functions (e.g., neurons, astrocytes, oligodendrocytes, etc). Brain tumours are heterogeneous, and depending on the tumour type, are considered among the most lethal, such as glioblastoma [13]. Brain metastases are one of the most frequent intracranial lesions, which develop via tumour cells passing from the bloodstream to the central nervous system through the breakdown of the BBB, resulting in distribution throughout the central nervous system, especially in areas of blood flow [14].

The colonisation of tumour cells from the primary tumour site into distant organs results in the formation of metastatic tumours. With regards to frequent metastatic sites in the body, usually the most common are the lung, liver, and brain, which were shown to present organ-specific patterns, brain metastases being one of the most lethal among them [15]. When comparing the genetic landscape of primary versus metastatic tumours, some studies have reported genetic heterogeneity in paired primary tumours and brain metastases [16], while others revealed high similarity among them [17]. In that sense, through the search for ctDNA mutations in different brain cancer patients that undergo surgery in our Institute, we detected *K-RAS* mutations in one patient's plasma sample. This was unusual since *K-RAS* mutations are not frequently found in primary brain tumours but are, for example, commonly present in lung tumours, being also considered a therapeutic target in lung cancer. A recent study showed that in 242 gliomas analyzed for RAS gene alterations, only 3 showed *K-RAS* mutations confirming its infrequency [18]. Therefore, we gathered both molecular and clinical information to report this case.

The patient arrived at our Institute, transferred from an emergency care unit with an image of an expansive lesion on her occipital and parietal lobe and an infiltrative lesion on the occipital bone. After careful evaluation of the patient's clinical and molecular data, the case described in this report was considered to represent an interesting example of the importance of liquid biopsy being performed alongside conventional biopsy. This case study was approved by the Human Ethics Committee of the *Instituto Estadual do Cérebro Paulo Niemeyer* (protocol N° CAAE 90680218.6.0000.8110). The patient's case will be discussed in this article as follows.

2. Case Report

A female, sixty-year-old patient presented with syncope, a history of headache, paresis in the right side of the body, and an occipital bulge with progressive growth in the past nine months. After being admitted to the first hospital, she underwent a chest x-ray that showed a pulmonary mass on the left side (Figure 1). Regarding clinical history, the patient was an ex-smoker with a smoking load of 1 pack/year for 40 years, with systemic arterial hypertension, dyslipidaemia, and a history of an acute heart infarct treated with stent placement 2 years before. No further investigation was performed at that time. She was then transferred to the *Instituto Estadual do Cérebro Paulo Niemeyer* (Rio de Janeiro, Brazil) for further evaluation and surgical programming.

A brain CT scan revealed a parietal-temporal-occipital (PTO) lesion and a transcranial tumour (Figure 2). She underwent the surgical procedure to remove both lesions resulting in deficit improvement.

The histopathological analysis was also performed and revealed an epithelial neoplasia composed of cells with rounded, vesicular nuclei and eosinophilic cytoplasm, forming glands. There were extensive areas of necrosis. Immunostains (Figure 3) showed positivity for cytokeratin 7 (CK7), with cytoplasmic and nuclear positivity for thyroid transcription factor 1 (TTF1), cytoplasmic positivity for both napsin A, and hepatocyte antigen (Hep-

Par). Cytokeratin 20 was not expressed by tumour cells. The immunoprofile favoured a metastatic adenocarcinoma with hepatoid features.

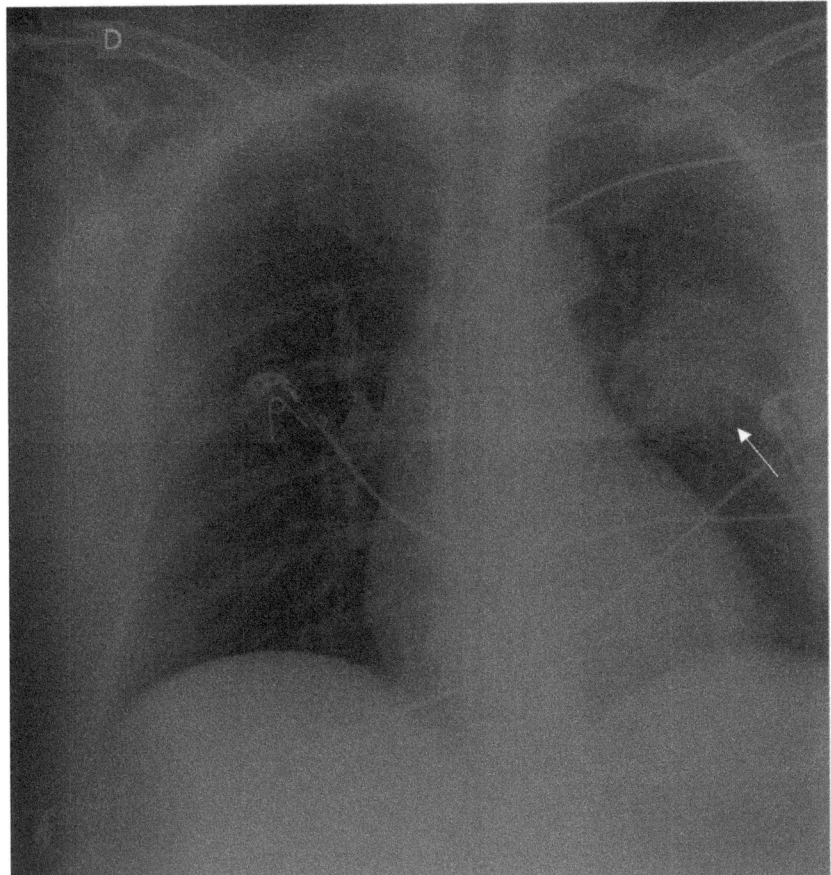

Figure 1. Chest X-ray showing a round mass in the upper lobe of the left lung (indicated with an arrow) suggestive of lung cancer (D in the image means right side).

We next investigated whether the ctDNA in the patient's plasma could be detected and analysed using Droplet Digital PCR (ddPCR) following the methodology described in our previously published study [19]. Briefly, presurgical plasma samples were obtained and analysed for the presence of ctDNA via ddPCR using Bio-Rad's mutation-specific assays (i.e., Bio-Rad's ddPCR G12/13 screening kit able to detect seven KRAS mutations: G12A, G12C, G12D, G12R, G12S, G12V, G13D). The liquid biopsy revealed the presence of K-RAS mutations in the samples analysed, which could be any of the G12/13 mutations detected in the assay. The two-dimensional scatter plot shows blue and orange dots representing, respectively, mutant-only and wild-type plus mutant K-RAS ctDNA in the patient's plasma (Figure 4A), with a mutation frequency of 1.2%. In addition, we performed the same analysis on the patient's tumour sample that was removed during surgery followed by formalin fixation and paraffin embedding. Interestingly, we found the same K-RAS mutations tested in the plasma sample, but at a much higher rate, 68.8% (Figure 4B).

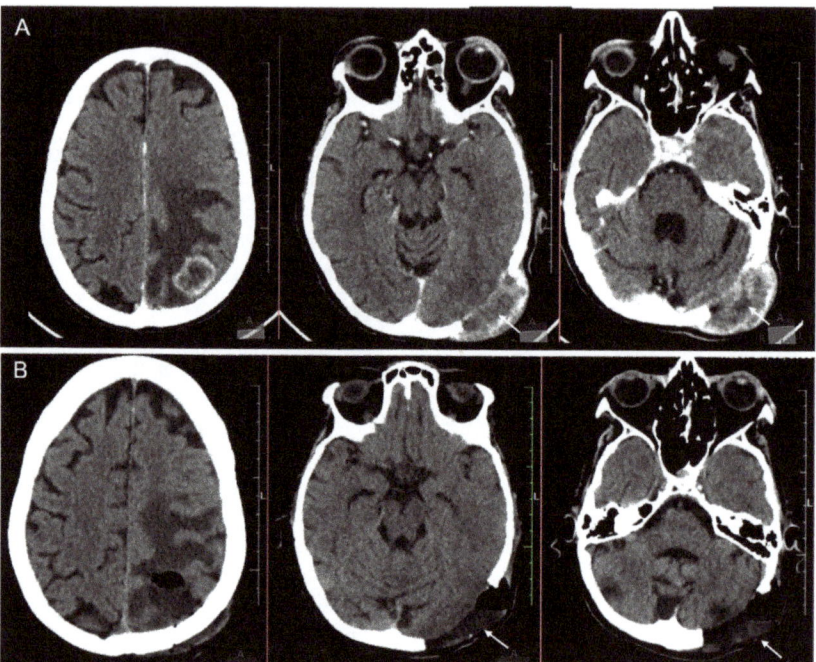

Figure 2. Computer tomography (CT scan) of the brain showing pre- (**A**) and postoperative images (**B**). (**A**) CT scan with venous contrast showing an intra-axial lesion on the occipital/parietal lobes and an infiltrative transcranial lesion in the occipital bone. (**B**) Postoperative image of both intracranial and transcranial lesions.

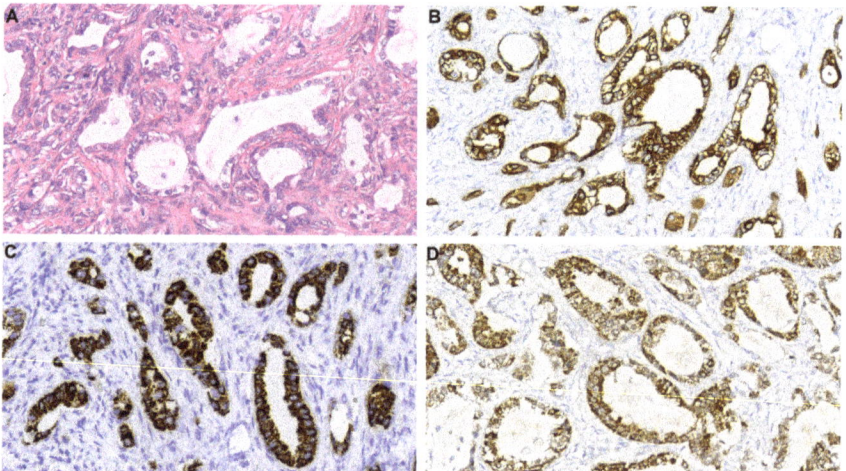

Figure 3. Histopathologic analysis of the brain metastasis tumour sample. Hematoxylin and eosin-stained histological sections show adenocarcinoma, comprised cells with increased nuclear/cytoplasmic ratio and prominent nucleoli forming glands (**A**). Neoplastic cells display strong cytoplasmic positivity for cytokeratin 7 (**B**), strong cytoplasmic positivity for HEP-PAR (**C**), and both nuclear and cytoplasmic staining for TTF1 (**D**). Magnification: 300×.

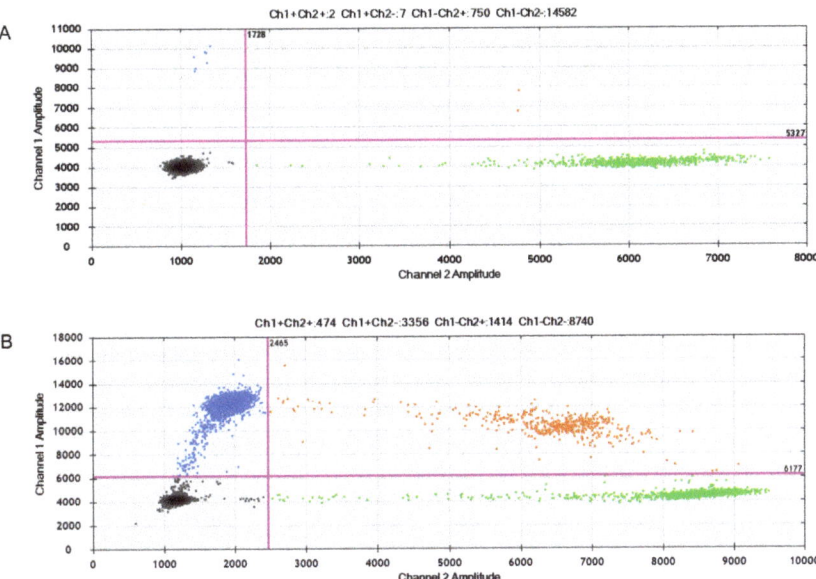

Figure 4. Two-dimensional scatter plot presenting four clusters obtained with mutant *K-RAS* and its wild-type allele. (**A**) Analysis of ctDNA extracted from patient's plasma. (**B**) Analysis of ctDNA extracted from patient's brain tumour mass. In both graphs (**A**,**B**), the fluorescence of channel 1 (FAM) is plotted against the fluorescence of channel 2 (HEX) for each drop (colour: blue, black, orange, or green). Drops are grouped into the following groups: FAM negative, negative HEX (doubly negative drops—black marking); FAM positive, HEX negative (positive drops for the sample with mutation—blue marking); FAM negative, HEX positive (positive drops for wild-type sample—green marking); FAM positive, HEX positive (doubly positive drops, containing both wild-type and mutated DNA—orange labelling). The ddPCR™ *KRAS G12/G13* Screening Kit (Bio-Rad's catalogue number 1863506) detects seven *K-RAS* mutations: G12A, G12C, G12D, G12R, G12S, G12V, G13D (blue labelling), without discriminating each one of them.

3. Discussion

There is not enough knowledge regarding pathways that control blood–brain barrier (BBB) permeability in the normal brain versus brain tumours; however there is consensus that an important step during the metastatic cancer cell journey to the brain is the invasion through the BBB [20]. The most frequent primary tumours that metastasize to the brain are lung, breast, and melanoma, being magnetic resonance imaging (MRI) and CT scan, commonly used in the initial diagnosis of brain tumours [21]. Regarding the molecular profile of brain metastasis, it was previously observed that *K-RAS* mutations were significantly increased in primary lung tumours metastasized to the brain via next-generation sequencing (NGS) analysis [22]. Interestingly, the ddPCR performance has demonstrated more accuracy when compared to NGS in distinct tumour analysis [23]. The main difference between NGS versus ddPCR techniques is that the latter is mainly restricted to the detection of known mutations, with limited capability of detecting several mutations per assay, whereas NGS more broadly detects multiple specific genetic changes at once but cannot efficiently detect mutation frequencies below 1% as the ddPCR does [24].

There are insufficient studies evaluating the precision of the ddPCR analysis performed in plasma versus brain tumour tissues, probably due to the difficulty in obtaining enough levels of nucleic acids extracted from plasma for analysis. In addition, only a small portion of cfDNA contains ct-DNA. Thus, the present report contributes to the field since it indicates the high sensitivity of the ddPCR technology in identifying low-frequency mutations both in the plasma and in the tumour tissue of the same patient. Our analysis showed the presence of K-RAS mutations in both samples, which are not frequently found in brain tumours but have been reported in lung hepatoid adenocarcinoma [25], a tumour that was also found in the patient analysed. In addition, lung cancers frequently harbour K-RAS mutations, and it is also one of the most common origins of brain metastases [22], which could potentially explain the present finding in the tumour tissue analysed. Besides, it has been shown that K-RAS alterations found in plasma are significantly predictive of K-RAS tumour status with significant tumour and plasma status consensus [26,27].

Although one limitation of ctDNA detection relies on the low abundance of ctDNA fragments in plasma samples making its detection difficult, the ddPCR method can successfully detect low-frequency mutations, even below 1% [28]. In our study, we were able to detect a K-RAS mutation frequency of 1.2% compared to 68.8% in the tumour sample analysed. Thus, the ddPCR method could be potentially employed to detect metastatic events and serve as a monitoring tool for the evaluation of gene mutations, such as K-RAS, in both primary and metastatic brain tumours. The major limitation of our report is that we were unable to obtain plasma samples after the brain tumour's surgical resection, which could have been useful to check if the levels of circulating K-RAS ctDNA were affected after surgery.

Even though liquid biopsies have been established in various clinical settings, there are still important validations to be made in the brain tumours' scenario, including noninvasive diagnosis of different brain tumour types, prognosis, disease monitoring and prediction of minimal residual disease.

4. Conclusions

Although the evaluation of ctDNA alone cannot yet bypass the need for tissue biopsies, it may be complementary to other diagnostic and disease monitoring tools, such as in brain metastases. A study including large numbers of paired samples will be important to further confirm this finding and to support liquid biopsy as a noninvasive and reliable screening method that could potentially benefit patients with brain tumours.

Author Contributions: Conceptualization, V.A. and V.M.N.; methodology, V.A., V.M.Z., R.L.M., F.A. and N.H.S.C.; writing—V.A. and V.M.Z.; writing—review and editing, all authors. All authors have read and agreed to the published version of the manuscript.

Funding: For the development of this report, no specific grant from funding agencies in the public, commercial, or not-for-profit sectors was received.

Institutional Review Board Statement: The study was conducted in accordance with the Declaration of Helsinki and approved by the Ethics Committee of *Instituto Estadual do Cérebro Paulo Niemeyer* (protocol N° CAAE 90680218.6.0000.8110, 28 June 2018).

Informed Consent Statement: Informed consent was obtained from the patient involved in the study.

Data Availability Statement: Not applicable.

Acknowledgments: The authors thank the IDEAS association for all the support at the IECPN, and the Brazilian agencies: *Conselho Nacional de Desenvolvimento Científico e Tecnológico (CNPq) and Fundação de Amparo à Pesquisa do Rio de Janeiro (FAPERJ)*.

Conflicts of Interest: The authors declare no conflict of interest.

References

1. Husain, H.; Velculescu, V.E. Cancer DNA in the Circulation: The Liquid Biopsy. *JAMA* **2017**, *318*, 1272–1274. [CrossRef]
2. Bettegowda, C.; Sausen, M.; Leary, R.J.; Kinde, I.; Wang, Y.; Agrawal, N.; Bartlett, B.R.; Wang, H.; Luber, B.; Alani, R.M.; et al. Detection of circulating tumor DNA in early- and late-stage human malignancies. *Sci. Transl. Med.* **2014**, *6*, 224ra24. [CrossRef] [PubMed]
3. Yan, Y.-Y.; Guo, Q.-R.; Wang, F.-H.; Adhikari, R.; Zhu, Z.-Y.; Zhang, H.-Y.; Zhou, W.-M.; Yu, H.; Li, J.-Q.; Zhang, J.-Y. Cell-Free DNA: Hope and Potential Application in Cancer. *Front. Cell Dev. Biol.* **2021**, *9*, 639233. [CrossRef] [PubMed]
4. Poulet, G.; Massias, J.; Taly, V. Liquid Biopsy: General Concepts. *Acta Cytol.* **2019**, *63*, 449–455. [CrossRef] [PubMed]

5. Ponti, G.; Maccaferri, M.; Mandrioli, M.; Manfredini, M.; Micali, S.; Cotugno, M.; Bianchi, G.; Ozben, T.; Pellacani, G.; Del Prete, C.; et al. Seminal Cell-Free DNA Assessment as a Novel Prostate Cancer Biomarker. *Pathol. Oncol. Res.* **2018**, *24*, 941–945. [CrossRef] [PubMed]
6. Yao, Y.; Liu, J.; Li, L.; Yuan, Y.; Nan, K.; Wu, X.; Zhang, Z.; Wu, Y.; Li, X.; Zhu, J.; et al. Detection of circulating tumor DNA in patients with advanced non-small cell lung cancer. *Oncotarget* **2017**, *8*, 2130–2140. [CrossRef] [PubMed]
7. Sant, M.; Bernat-Peguera, A.; Felip, E.; Margelí, M. Role of ctDNA in Breast Cancer. *Cancers* **2022**, *14*, 310. [CrossRef]
8. Malla, M.; Loree, J.M.; Kasi, P.M.; Parikh, A.R. Using Circulating Tumor DNA in Colorectal Cancer: Current and Evolving Practices. *J. Clin. Oncol.* **2022**, *40*, 2846–2857. [CrossRef]
9. Piccioni, D.E.; Achrol, A.S.; Kiedrowski, L.A.; Banks, K.C.; Boucher, N.; Barkhoudarian, G.; Kelly, D.F.; Juarez, T.; Lanman, R.B.; Raymond, V.M.; et al. Analysis of cell-free circulating tumor DNA in 419 patients with glioblastoma and other primary brain tumors. *CNS Oncol.* **2019**, *8*, CNS34. [CrossRef]
10. Sato, Y. Clinical utility of liquid biopsy-based companion diagnostics in the non-small-cell lung cancer treatment. *Explor. Target. Anti-Tumor Ther.* **2022**, *3*, 630–642. [CrossRef]
11. Pascual, J.; Attard, G.; Bidard, F.-C.; Curigliano, G.; De Mattos-Arruda, L.; Diehn, M.; Italiano, A.; Lindberg, J.; Merker, J.; Montagut, C.; et al. ESMO recommendations on the use of circulating tumour DNA assays for patients with cancer: A report from the ESMO Precision Medicine Working Group. *Ann. Oncol.* **2022**, *33*, 750–768. [CrossRef] [PubMed]
12. De Mattos-Arruda, L.; Mayor, R.; Ng, C.K.Y.; Weigelt, B.; Martínez-Ricarte, F.; Torrejon, D.; Oliveira, M.; Arias, A.; Raventos, C.; Tang, J.; et al. Cerebrospinal fluid-derived circulating tumour DNA better represents the genomic alterations of brain tumours than plasma. *Nat. Commun.* **2015**, *6*, 8839. [CrossRef]
13. Perus, L.J.M.; Walsh, L.A. Microenvironmental Heterogeneity in Brain Malignancies. *Front. Immunol.* **2019**, *10*, 2294. [CrossRef] [PubMed]
14. Quattrocchi, C.C.; Errante, Y.; Gaudino, C.; Mallio, C.A.; Giona, A.; Santini, D.; Tonini, G.; Zobel, B.B. Spatial brain distribution of intra-axial metastatic lesions in breast and lung cancer patients. *J. Neurooncol.* **2012**, *110*, 79–87. [CrossRef] [PubMed]
15. Rehman, A.U.; Khan, P.; Maurya, S.K.; Siddiqui, J.A.; Santamaria-Barria, J.A.; Batra, S.K.; Nasser, M.W. Liquid biopsies to occult brain metastasis. *Mol. Cancer* **2022**, *21*, 113. [CrossRef]
16. Mansfield, A.; Aubry, M.; Moser, J.; Harrington, S.; Dronca, R.; Park, S.; Dong, H. Temporal and spatial discordance of programmed cell death-ligand 1 expression and lymphocyte tumor infiltration between paired primary lesions and brain metastases in lung cancer. *Ann. Oncol.* **2016**, *27*, 1953–1958. [CrossRef] [PubMed]
17. Matsumoto, S.; Takahashi, K.; Iwakawa, R.; Matsuno, Y.; Nakanishi, Y.; Kohno, T.; Shimizu, E.; Yokota, J. Frequent EGFR mutations in brain metastases of lung adenocarcinoma. *Int. J. Cancer* **2006**, *119*, 1491–1494. [CrossRef]
18. Makino, Y.; Arakawa, Y.; Yoshioka, E.; Shofuda, T.; Minamiguchi, S.; Kawauchi, T.; Tanji, M.; Kanematsu, D.; Nonaka, M.; Okita, Y.; et al. Infrequent RAS mutation is not associated with specific histological phenotype in gliomas. *BMC Cancer* **2021**, *21*, 1025. [CrossRef]
19. Aran, V.; Heringer, M.; da Mata, P.J.; Kasuki, L.; Miranda, R.L.; Andreiuolo, F.; Chimelli, L.; Filho, P.N.; Gadelha, M.R.; Neto, V.M. Identification of mutant K-RAS in pituitary macroadenoma. *Pituitary* **2021**, *24*, 746–753. [CrossRef]
20. Fares, J.; Kanojia, D.; Rashidi, A.; Ulasov, I.; Lesniak, M.S. Genes that Mediate Metastasis across the Blood-Brain Barrier. *Trends Cancer* **2020**, *6*, 660–676. [CrossRef]
21. Bertolini, F.; Spallanzani, A.; Fontana, A.; Depenni, R.; Luppi, G. Brain metastases: An overview. *CNS Oncol.* **2015**, *4*, 37–46. [CrossRef] [PubMed]
22. Vassella, E.; Kashani, E.; Zens, P.; Kündig, A.; Fung, C.; Scherz, A.; Herrmann, E.; Ermis, E.; Schmid, R.A.; Berezowska, S. Mutational profiles of primary pulmonary adenocarcinoma and paired brain metastases disclose the importance of KRAS mutations. *Eur. J. Cancer* **2021**, *159*, 227–236. [CrossRef] [PubMed]
23. Garcia, J.; Forestier, J.; Dusserre, E.; Wozny, A.-S.; Geiguer, F.; Merle, P.; Tissot, C.; Ferraro-Peyret, C.; Jones, F.S.; Edelstein, D.L.; et al. Cross-platform comparison for the detection of RAS mutations in cfDNA (ddPCR Biorad detection assay, BEAMing assay, and NGS strategy). *Oncotarget* **2018**, *9*, 21122–21131. [CrossRef]
24. Singh, R.R. Next-Generation Sequencing in High-Sensitive Detection of Mutations in Tumors: Challenges, Advances, and Applications. *J. Mol. Diagn.* **2020**, *22*, 994–1007. [CrossRef] [PubMed]
25. Chen, L.; Han, X.; Gao, Y.; Zhao, Q.; Wang, Y.; Jiang, Y.; Liu, S.; Wu, X.; Miao, L. Anti-PD-1 Therapy Achieved Disease Control After Multiline Chemotherapy in Unresectable KRAS-Positive Hepatoid Lung Adenocarcinoma: A Case Report and Literature Review. *Onco Targets Ther.* **2020**, *13*, 4359–4364. [CrossRef]
26. Xu, J.M.; Liu, X.J.; Ge, F.J.; Lin, L.; Wang, Y.; Sharma, M.R.; Liu, Z.-Y.; Tommasi, S.; Paradiso, A. KRAS mutations in tumor tissue and plasma by different assays predict survival of patients with metastatic colorectal cancer. *J. Exp. Clin. Cancer Res.* **2014**, *33*, 104. [CrossRef]
27. Zhang, M.; Wu, J.; Zhong, W.; Zhao, Z.; Guo, W. Comparative study on the mutation spectrum of tissue DNA and blood ctDNA in patients with non-small cell lung cancer. *Transl. Cancer Res.* **2022**, *11*, 1245–1254. [CrossRef]
28. Dong, L.; Wang, S.; Fu, B.; Wang, J. Evaluation of droplet digital PCR and next generation sequencing for characterizing DNA reference material for KRAS mutation detection. *Sci. Rep.* **2018**, *8*, 9650. [CrossRef]

Disclaimer/Publisher's Note: The statements, opinions and data contained in all publications are solely those of the individual author(s) and contributor(s) and not of MDPI and/or the editor(s). MDPI and/or the editor(s) disclaim responsibility for any injury to people or property resulting from any ideas, methods, instructions or products referred to in the content.

MDPI AG
Grosspeteranlage 5
4052 Basel
Switzerland
Tel.: +41 61 683 77 34
www.mdpi.com

Medicina Editorial Office
E-mail: medicina@mdpi.com
www.mdpi.com/journal/medicina

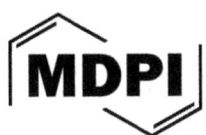

Disclaimer/Publisher's Note: The statements, opinions and data contained in all publications are solely those of the individual author(s) and contributor(s) and not of MDPI and/or the editor(s). MDPI and/or the editor(s) disclaim responsibility for any injury to people or property resulting from any ideas, methods, instructions or products referred to in the content.